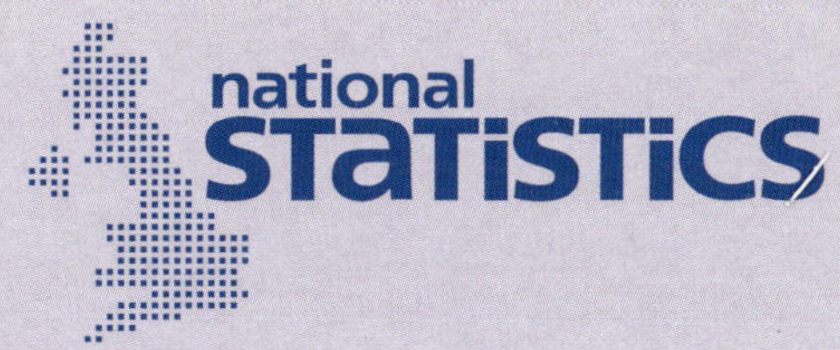

Geographic Variations in Health

Editors:

Clare Griffiths

Justine Fitzpatrick

London: The Stationery Office

Contact points

For enquiries about this publication, contact
Health Variations Team
Tel: 020 7533 5210
E-mail: healthgeog@ons.gov.uk

To order this publication, call The Stationery Office on
0870 600 5522. See also back cover.

For general enquiries, contact the National Statistics Public
Enquiry Service on 0845 601 3034 (minicom: 01633 812399)
E-mail: info@statistics.gov.uk
Fax: 01633 652747
Letters: Room DG/18, 1 Drummond Gate, London SW1V 2QQ

You can also find National Statistics on the internet at
www.statistics.gov.uk

About the Office for National Statistics

The Office for National Statistics (ONS) is the government
agency responsible for compiling, analysing and disseminating
many of the United Kingdom's economic, social and
demographic statistics, including the retail prices index, trade
figures and labour market data, as well as the periodic census of
the population and health statistics. The Director of ONS is
also the National Statistician and the Registrar General for
England and Wales, and the agency that administers the
registration of births, marriages and deaths there.

A National Statistics publication

National Statistics are produced to high professional standards
set out in the National Statistics Code of Practice. They
undergo regular quality assurance reviews to ensure that they
meet customer needs. They are produced free from any political
interference.

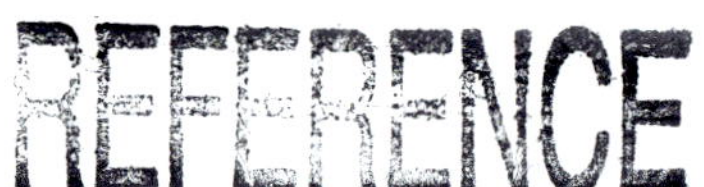

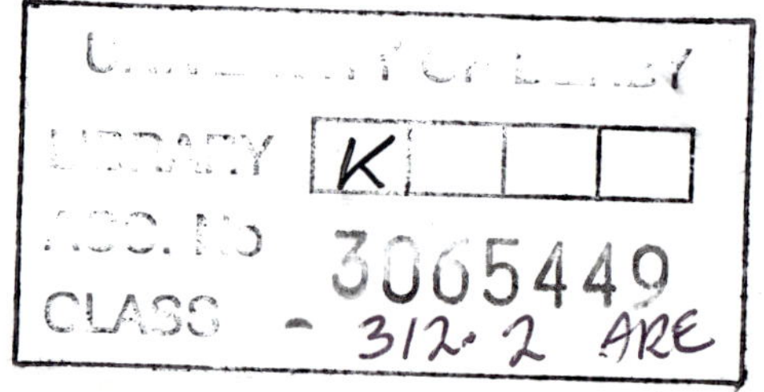

Contents

CHAPTER 1: INTRODUCTION TO THE VOLUME

Justine Fitzpatrick, Clare Griffiths and Peter Goldblatt

CHAPTER 2: DEMOGRAPHIC BACKGROUND

Clare Griffiths

CHAPTER 3: SOCIO-ECONOMIC CHARACTERISTICS OF THE PEOPLE

Clare Griffiths and Justine Fitzpatrick

CHAPTER 4: CLASSIFICATIONS USED IN THIS VOLUME

Justine Fitzpatrick

CHAPTER 5: PATTERNS AND TRENDS IN FERTILITY

Clare Griffiths and Liz Kirby

CHAPTER 6: PATTERNS AND TRENDS IN STILLBIRTHS AND INFANT MORTALITY

Justine Fitzpatrick and Nicola Cooper

CHAPTER 7: ANALYSIS OF INFANT MORTALITY BY RISK FACTORS AND BY CAUSE OF DEATH IN ENGLAND AND WALES

Nicola Cooper

CHAPTER 8: GEOGRAPHIC VARIATION IN CONGENITAL ANOMALY NOTIFICATIONS IN ENGLAND AND WALES

Ruth Yates and Lois Cook

CHAPTER 9: GEOGRAPHIC PATTERNS IN CANCER INCIDENCE

Penny Babb, Anita Brock, Jenny Jones and Mike Quinn

CHAPTER 10: DESCRIPTIVE ANALYSIS OF GEOGRAPHIC PATTERNS AND TRENDS IN ADULT MORTALITY BY CAUSE OF DEATH

Justine Fitzpatrick, Clare Griffiths, Mike Kelleher and Stan McEvoy

CHAPTER 11: ANALYSIS OF MORTALITY BY DEPRIVATION AND CAUSE OF DEATH

Zoe Uren and Justine Fitzpatrick

CHAPTER 12: GEOGRAPHIC VARIATION IN MORTALITY BY SOCIAL CLASS AND ALTERNATIVE SOCIAL CLASSIFICATIONS

Zoe Uren, Justine Fitzpatrick, Alison Reid and Peter Goldblatt

CHAPTER 13: GEOGRAPHIC VARIATIONS IN HEALTH: MAIN FINDINGS AND IMPLICATIONS FOR THE FUTURE

Clare Griffiths, Peter Goldblatt and Justine Fitzpatrick

LIST OF TABLES, FIGURES AND MAPS

Chapter 2
Figures

Maps

Chapter 3
Tables

Figures

Maps

Chapter 4
Tables

Figures

Chapter 5
Tables

Figures

Maps

Chapter 6
Tables

Figures

Contents

Chapter 10
Tables

Figures

Chapter 11

Figures

Chapter 12

Figures

Appendices
Tables

Maps

Foreword

This volume, on geographic variations in health, builds on the
tradition started in the nineteenth century of undertaking in-
depth analyses of mortality by area in decennial supplements to
the annual statistical publications.

The volume considerably extends the coverage and range of
analyses available in previous supplements. For the first time, it
takes a broader view of health outcomes than are reflected by
mortality alone, by including reviews of variations in congenital
anomalies, cancer incidence, infant mortality, births,
conceptions and abortions. It makes far more extensive use of
maps to illustrate statistically significant variations.

As in previous supplements, there is a strong emphasis on
identifying the factors associated with geographic variation in
the outcomes studied and to interpret these in terms of
demographic patterns and material inequality. To these ends,
there are separate chapters summarising demographic and
socio-economic influences and all analyses draw on the recently
revised ONS classification of local authorities.

Last, but by no means least, wherever possible the analyses of
local variation are, for the first time, presented on a comparable
basis for all parts of the United Kingdom. This comprehensive
view has made it possible to place the geographic patterns
observed in a wider context than was previously possible. The
support of the Scottish, Welsh and Northern Irish
administrations was essential in achieving this.

Len Cook
National Statistician

Acknowledgements

It would not have been possible to produce a book covering such a wide range of topics without the committed support of many people both within and outside ONS, for which we are very grateful. The overall plan and outline for this volume were originally prepared with Karen Dunnell and Gillian Dollamore. The main contributors to each chapter are of course listed as authors. Many others assisted in preparing data for analysis, including Angela Donkin, David Edwards, Mike Kelleher, Aysha Malik, Ian Thurman, Claire Dighton, Moira Mickleburgh and Kevin Davy.

Others in ONS and in the Department of Health have given professional advice on the many drafts of individual chapters including Patsy Bailey, Allan Baker, Bev Botting, Nirupa Dattani, Chris Denham, Tim Devis, Frances Drever, Peter Goldblatt, John Haskey, Lesz Lancucki, Hugh Markowe, David Pearce, Vera Ruddock and Judith Walton.

The contributions of the following staff in Wales, Scotland and Northern Ireland were essential in making this a comprehensive United Kingdom analysis:

> Graham Jackson and Ian Brown at the General Register Office for Scotland;

> Roger Black, Ross Elder, Scott Heald, Mark Hollinsworth, Mary Smalls and Brian Whiteman at the Information and Statistics Division of the National Health Service in Scotland;

> Clive Lewis and Cath Roberts at the National Assembly for Wales;

> John Steward at the Welsh Cancer Intelligence and Surveillance Unit;

> Mairé Rodgers at the Northern Ireland Statistics and Research Agency;

> John Gordon at the General Register Office for Northern Ireland and

> Anna Gavin at the Northern Ireland Cancer Registry.

We are also grateful to the regional cancer registries for England for their contribution and close co-operation with the national registry at ONS.

The preparation of the maps for publication was carried out by Alistair Dent, Alan Smith, Pam Owen and Nick Richardson from ONS Geography. Special mention should also go to the proof readers Stan McEvoy, Mike Kelleher, Nigel Physick, Claire Dighton, Glenn Meredith, Moira Mickleburgh and Anita Brock.

The advice of the independent referees listed in Appendix C was crucial in assuring the quality of the final product.

Introduction to the volume

Justine Fitzpatrick, Clare Griffiths and Peter Goldblatt

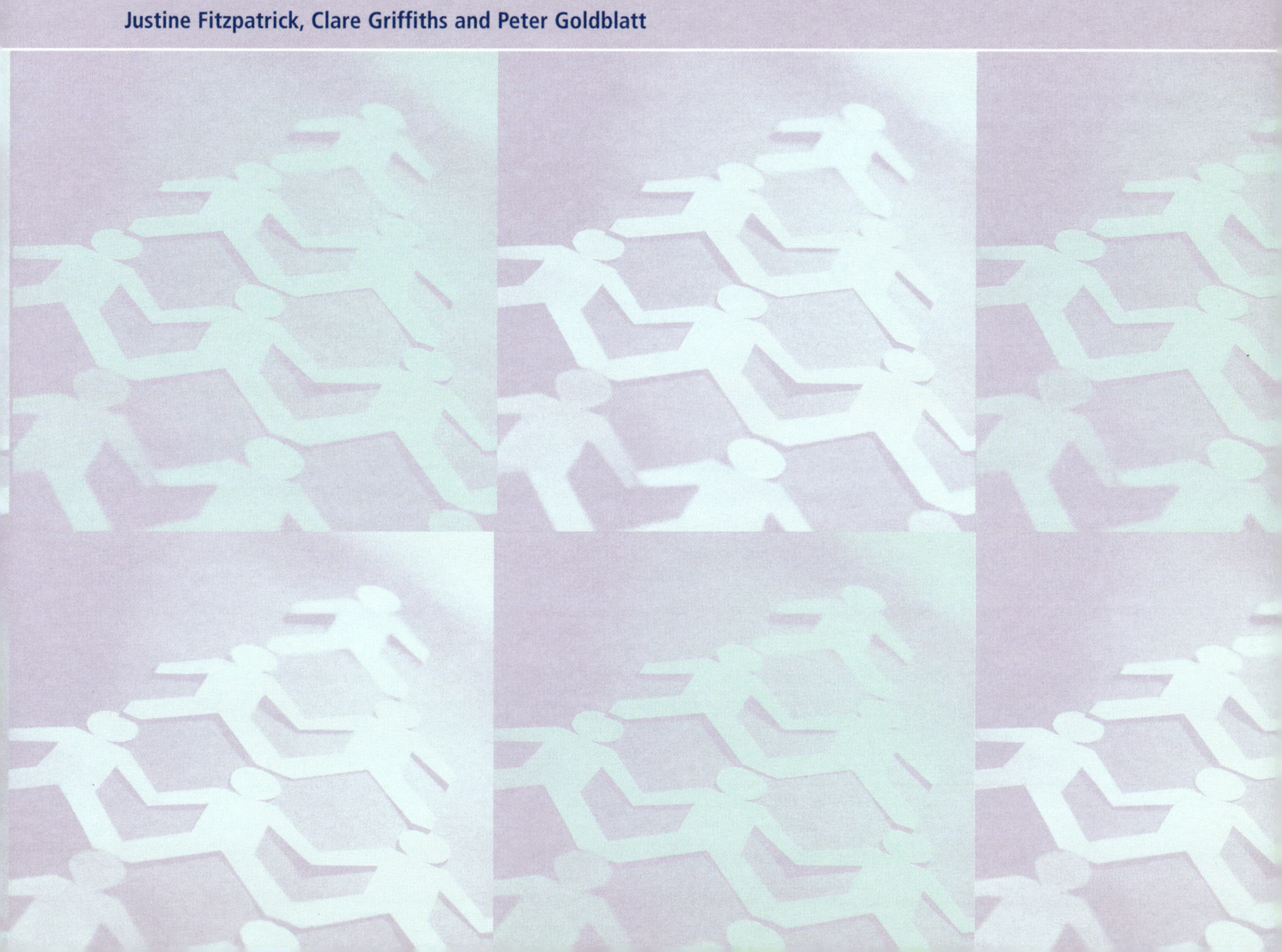

Chapter 1
Introduction to the volume

This report, *Geographic Variations in Health*, is the latest in a series of decennial supplements in which the Registrar General for England and Wales presents an in-depth review of the geography of health. Previous decennial supplements on geography were restricted to England and Wales and, for many years, largely concentrated on variations in mortality.[1,2,3,4] This report is broader in its focus, covering geographic variations in mortality (including infant mortality and stillbirths), fertility-related topics (including conceptions, abortions, live births and congenital anomalies) and cancer incidence. In addition these geographic analyses are extended to cover the whole of the United Kingdom wherever possible.

1.1 Why analyse geographic variations in health?

There is a long history to the measurement of health inequalities in this country. This tradition has always recognised the contribution made by the social circumstances of individuals and the places in which they live. The Poor Law Commissioners, set up to review the workings of the New Poor Law Act 1834, presented evidence from inspectors[5] and commented:

"Such is the filthy, close and crowded state of the houses, and the poisonous condition of the localities in which the greater part of the houses are situated from the total want of drainage, and the masses of putrefying matters of all sorts which are allowed to remain and accumulate indefinitely … Yet in these pestilential places the industrious poor are obliged to take their abode."

Analyses developed subsequently by the General Register Office, following its foundation in 1837, focused on representing inequalities in health in both geographic and occupational terms.[6] Recent analyses have identified individual circumstances as having the greatest impact on area differences.[7,8] Areas with poor levels of health are predominantly those with the largest proportion of poor people and area averages largely reflect this distribution. However, in many of these analyses the impact of area characteristics on the health of individuals in that area is also evident. Graham[9] summarises these as follows:

"How can places damage health? Both material and psychosocial pathways have been suggested. For example, the areas populated by poorer people score higher on material hazards like environmental pollution… These areas are also less well resourced in terms of shops, recreational facilities, …

With respect to psychosocial pathways, research has focused particularly on the ways in which communities operate to resource and support the well-being of residents…. The concept of social capital has gained particular currency in research concerned with these social dimensions of areas."

Geographic inequalities in health - differences in the health experiences of the population according to the area in which they live - must therefore continue to be viewed as an important dimension of inequality.

Socio-economic differentials in health were the focus of the previous decennial supplement, *Health Inequalities*.[10] This report confirmed that socio-economic differences in health persisted into the 1990s and had widened since previous analyses were undertaken. There is also evidence of a polarisation between areas, for example in levels of deprivation between local authorities in recent years[11] and between those authorities in the top and bottom deciles of mortality under age 65 since the 1970s.[7]

Concern that the quality of life in many poor neighbourhoods has become increasingly detached from the rest of society has prompted Government to launch a number of initiatives in deprived areas, as indicated in the Social Exclusion Unit Report, *A New Commitment to Neighbourhood Renewal*.[12] This strategy aims to ensure that *"within 10 to 20 years, no-one should be seriously disadvantaged by where they live."* Narrowing the health gap, as well as the gap in some of the determinants of health, between the most deprived neighbourhoods and the rest of the country is a central part of this vision.

Each of the administrations in the United Kingdom has already developed strategies for health in which the reduction of inequalities is an integral part. Emphasis on deprived neighbourhoods is likely to form an increasingly important element in implementing these. In July 1999 the White Paper *Saving Lives: Our Healthier Nation*[13] was published. It has a commitment to *"improve the health of everyone and the worst-off in particular."* More recently, the *NHS Plan*[14] for England aims to bring improvements in health across the board and to reduce health inequalities. The White Paper *Towards a Healthier Scotland*[15] calls for a *"coherent attack on health inequalities with a special focus on improving the health of children and young people."* The recent consultation paper produced by the Department of Health, Social Security and Public Safety in Northern Ireland, *Investing for Health*,[16] and the Health Strategy for Wales, *Better Health Better Wales*,[17] both have a commitment to targeting health inequalities.

The report of the *Independent Inquiry into Inequalities in Health*,[18] commissioned by the Secretary of State for Health, identified several elements in achieving equity in health care that underlies the NHS:

"ensuring that health care services serving disadvantaged populations are not of poorer quality or less accessible; that the allocation and application of resources are in relation to need; and ensuring that positive efforts are made to achieve greater uptake and use of effective services by making extra efforts to reach those whose health is worse."

All these policy aims require a clear understanding of health status in different areas and how this relates to disadvantage. In particular, there is considerable debate on the circumstances in which mainstream programmes that target deprived individuals are likely to be more effective than area-based targeting.[19] Better understanding of spatial patterning and its causes will assist in ensuring that resources can be appropriately targeted and that appropriate baselines can be set to monitor the impact of policies and initiatives on outcomes.

The geography of health variations also has a place in epidemiological analysis, to suggest possible causal pathways. Early examples of this type include the well-known study by Snow in 1855,[20] demonstrating the transmission of cholera through water supplied from different sources. More recently, small area analyses have been used to look at, for example, health in the vicinity of nuclear installations,[21, 22] waste disposal facilities[23, 24] and electricity power lines.[25, 26]

1.2 The approach taken in this volume

This volume aims to describe the spatial pattern of health across the United Kingdom during the 1990s, both in terms of variations between areas over the whole of the period studied and in terms of trends. It also sets out to identify factors associated with these variations, which might suggest possible causal links or common explanations. This comprehensive picture of geographic inequalities in health in the United Kingdom during the 1990s and how they relate to the characteristics of areas should help to provide a baseline for any future monitoring of health inequalities.

The analyses in this volume are presented using a common set of administrative boundaries - those at 1999. This is intended to make the findings more relevant to current health policy and research and to facilitate comparisons now and in the future (for example, by providing the best available baseline for trend analysis). Data are presented in 11 main chapters. Chapters 2 to 4 are scene-setting analyses. Chapter 2 presents an overview of the main demographic features of the United Kingdom population at national, regional and local authority level. Chapter 3 looks at the socio-economic characteristics of the population, drawing extensively on data from the 1991 Census. Chapter 4 describes the classifications used in this volume to describe patterns in health, namely the ONS classification of local authorities[27] and the Carstairs and Morris index of deprivation.[28] This type of analysis is useful as it groups areas with similar characteristics together and thus helps to put forward potential explanations for the differences in health presented for administrative areas. As these classifications are Great Britain-based and no comparable data are available for Northern Ireland, analyses that use these classifications are necessarily restricted to Great Britain. In some analyses, for which individual level data were not available for all constituent countries of the United Kingdom, coverage is restricted to England and Wales.

Chapter 5 examines geographic variations in fertility, including conceptions, abortions and live births, focusing on two age groups of particular current interest in relation to one or more of these outcomes - teenagers and women in their late thirties. The relationship between conceptions, abortions and live births and deprivation is also examined. Data on live births are presented for the whole of the United Kingdom, but in the case of conceptions and abortions data are presented for Great Britain only. The analysis of conceptions and abortions by deprivation is restricted to England and Wales.

Geographic variations in stillbirth and infant mortality rates within the United Kingdom are examined in chapter 6, based on country, region, local authority, ONS classification and deprivation. Chapter 7 then looks in more detail at some of the factors that might contribute to mortality variation in infancy across England and Wales. For this latter analysis the ONS linked infant mortality file is used. This file links infant death records to their birth registration, thus enabling mortality rates to be analysed using factors collected at birth registration, for example, birthweight, Social Class, registration type, mother's country of birth and mother's age at birth. The linked file is also used to examine geographic variation in infant mortality by cause of death.

Two chapters look at aspects of geographic variations in morbidity. Geographic variation in the notification of congenital anomalies for England and Wales is examined in chapter 8, based primarily on data for the regions of England and for Wales. This chapter uses both the Carstairs and Morris index of deprivation and the ONS classification of local authorities, where relevant. Chapter 9 concerns geographic variation in cancer incidence. This chapter reviews the incidence of the top three cancers in men (lung, prostate and colorectal) and in women (breast, colorectal and lung). These account for over 50 per cent of all registrations for each sex. The incidence for each of these cancers is then examined, for individual local authorities in Great Britain, for regions within England and for groups of authorities based on the ONS classification. Incidence data are also examined using the Carstairs and Morris deprivation index.

Chapter 10 provides a descriptive analysis of geographic variation in mortality at all ages in the United Kingdom. Variations in all-cause mortality and also the main causes of death at all geographic levels are studied in detail. As in other chapters, the relationship with the ONS classification of local authorities is also examined. Chapter 11 examines variations in mortality by cause of death and deprivation. Chapter 12 looks at Social Class variations in mortality within the countries and regions of the United Kingdom for a large number of causes of death. It also uses data from the ONS Longitudinal Study to investigate the relationship between alternative social classifications (such as housing tenure and car access) and variations in mortality at country and regional level within England and Wales.

1.3 Administrative geography used in this volume

Traditionally the geography used for the analysis of variations in health has been constrained by the administrative geography in use at the time. Any results obtained will therefore be strongly influenced by the boundaries in use and trends over time cannot be examined. In addition, it is not unusual to find very different types of areas geographically adjacent to each other within the United Kingdom. The larger the administrative area, the greater the variation in the types of areas and the population within that area. Health does not necessarily follow administrative boundaries. In this volume we have presented all data for areas as at April 1999; in order to achieve this it was necessary to recast all data to the boundaries as at that date.

Where possible data are presented for the constituent parts of the United Kingdom (England, Wales, Scotland and Northern Ireland) and for all local authorities within these. Data are also presented for the nine Government Office Regions within England: North East, North West, Yorkshire and the Humber, East Midlands, West Midlands, East of England, London, South East and South West.

Throughout this volume, 'local authority' is used as a generic term to refer to all local authority districts, London boroughs and metropolitan districts in England, unitary authorities in England and Wales, local council areas in Scotland and district councils in Northern Ireland. Similarly, the term 'country' is used generically to describe each of the four main parts of the United Kingdom.

1.4 Availability of data electronically

The data behind all the maps at local authority level will be made available through our website at www.statistics.gov.uk.

References

1 Office of Population Censuses and Surveys. *Area mortality: the Registrar General's Decennial Supplement for England and Wales 1969-1973*. HMSO (London: 1981).

2 Office of Population Censuses and Surveys. *The Registrar General's Decennial Supplement for England and Wales 1961, Area mortality tables*. HMSO (London: 1967).

3 Office of Population Censuses and Surveys. *The Registrar General's Decennial Supplement for England and Wales 1951, Area mortality tables*. HMSO (London: 1958).

4 Britton M. *Mortality and Geography: a review in the mid-1980s, England and Wales*. HMSO (London: 1990).

5 Smith S. Quoted in Simon J. *English sanitary institutions*. Cassell (London: 1890).

6 Registrar General. *Sixteenth annual report*. HMSO (London: 1856).

7 Shaw M, Dorling D, Gordon D and Davey Smith G. *The Widening Gap. Health inequalities and policy in Britain*. The Policy Press (Bristol: 1999).

8 Sloggett A and Joshi H. Higher mortality in deprived areas: community or personal disadvantage? *British Medical Journal* 309 (1994), 1470-1474.

9 Graham H. (ed.) *Understanding health inequalities*. Open University Press (Buckingham: 2001).

10 Drever F and Whitehead M. (eds.) *Health inequalities*. The Stationery Office (London: 1997).

11 Robson B, Bradford M and Tomlinson R. *Updating and revising the Index of Local Deprivation*. DETR Regeneration Research Series (London: 1998).

12 Social Exclusion Unit. *A New Commitment to Neighbourhood Renewal: National Strategy Action Plan*. Cabinet Office (London: 2001).

13 Department of Health. White Paper. *Saving Lives: Our Healthier Nation*. The Stationery Office (London: 1999).

14 Department of Health. White Paper. *The NHS Plan*. The Stationery Office (London: 2000).

15 Scottish Executive. White Paper. *Towards a Healthier Scotland*. The Stationery Office (Edinburgh: 1999).

16 Department of Health, Social Security and Personal Services. *Investing for Health*. Department of Health, Social Security and Personal Services (Belfast: 2000).

17 Welsh Office. *Better Health Better Wales*. The Stationery Office (Cardiff: 1998).

18 Acheson D. *Independent Inquiry into Inequalities in Health Report*. The Stationery Office (London: 1998).

19 Smith G. *Area-based initiatives: the rationale for and options for area targeting*. CASE paper 25. London School of Economics (London: 1999).

20 Snow J. *On the mode of communication of cholera*. (2nd edition) Churchill (London: 1855) reproduced in *Snow on cholera*. Hafner (New York: 1965).

21 Gardner MJ, Hall AJ, Downes S and Terrell JD. Follow-up study of children born to mothers resident in Seascale, West Cumbria (birth cohort). *British Journal of Industrial Medicine* 295 (1987), 822-827.

22 Craft AW, Parker L, Openshaw S, Charlton M, Newell J, Birch JM and Blair V. Cancer in young people in the north of England, 1968-85: analysis by Census wards. *Journal of Epidemiology and Community Health* 47 (1993), 109-115.

23 Elliott P, Hills M, Beresford J, Kleinschmidt I, Jolley D, Pattenden S, Rodrigues L, Westlake A and Rose G. Incidence of cancers of the larynx and lung near incinerators of waste solvents and oils in Great Britain. *Lancet* 339 (1992), 854-858.

24 Elliott P, Shaddick G, Kleinschmidt I, Jolley D, Walls P, Beresford J and Grundy C. Cancer incidence near municipal solid waste incinerators in Great Britain. *British Journal of Cancer* 73 (1996), 702-710.

25 Repacholi MH and Ahlbom A. Exposure to power-frequency magnetic fields and the risk of childhood cancer. *Lancet* 354 (1999), 1925-1931.

26 McDowall ML. Mortality of persons resident in the vicinity of electricity transmission facilities. *British Journal of Cancer* 53 (1986), 271-279.

27 Office for National Statistics. *The ONS classification of local and health authorities of Great Britain: revised in 1999*. Series SMPS no. 63. The Stationery Office (London: 1999).

28 Carstairs V and Morris R. *Deprivation and health in Scotland*. Aberdeen University Press (Aberdeen: 1991).

Chapter 2
Demographic background

Clare Griffiths

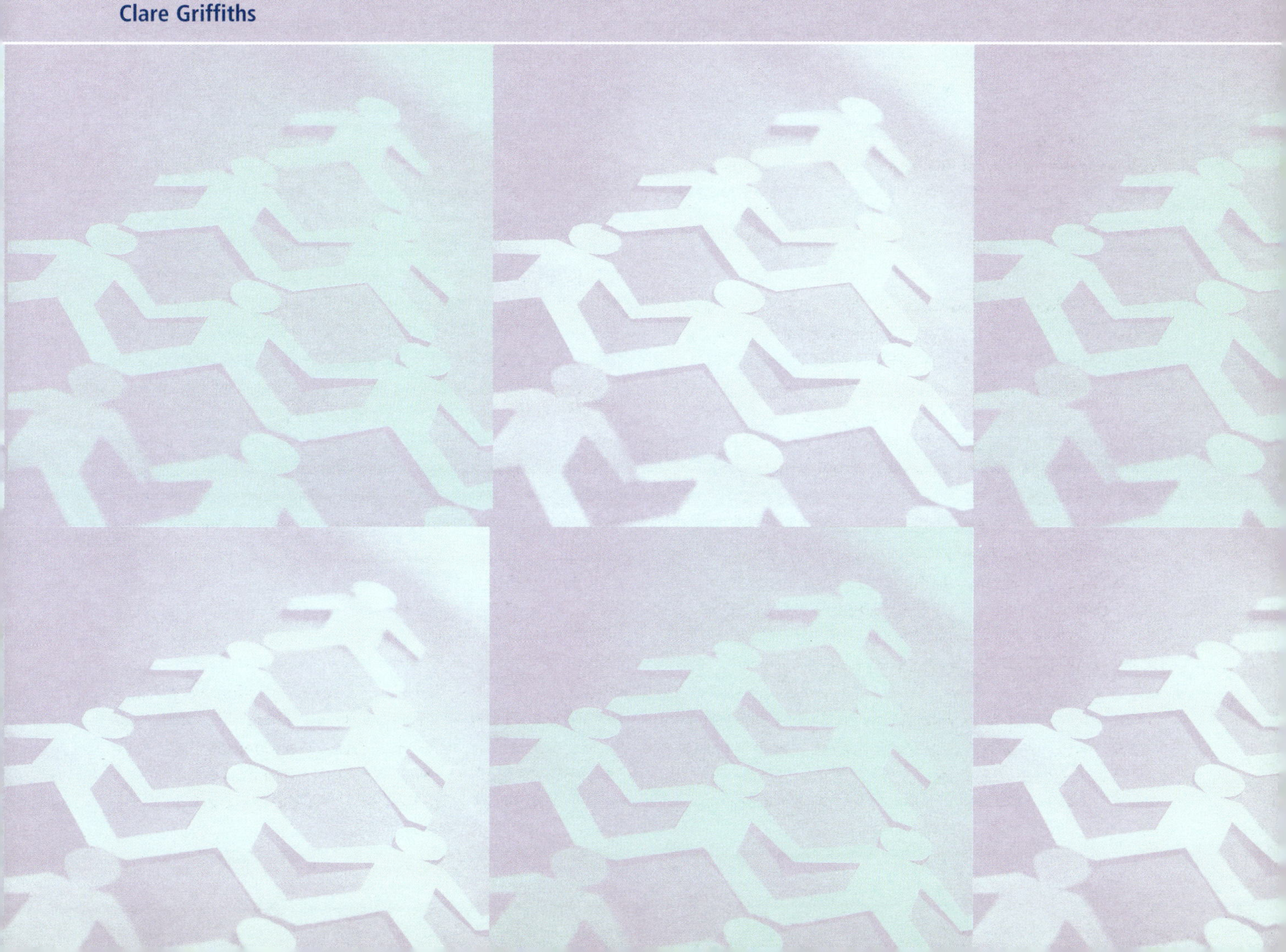

Chapter 2
Demographic background

2.1 Introduction

This chapter provides a brief introduction and overview of the main features of the United Kingdom population. It examines the number of people resident in the United Kingdom in 1997, their ages and how they are distributed throughout the United Kingdom. It then goes on to look at how the population has changed between 1991 and 1997 and looks at the factors underlying this - natural change and migration. This is followed by an examination of projected changes in the future.

The chapter analyses data for 1991 and 1997, as the analysis in following chapters looks at variations in health over this time period. Population estimates for 1991 and 1997 form the basis of the majority of the analysis in this chapter, but analysis of components of change between these two dates and population projections to 2011 have also been used.

Other authors have produced similar but far more detailed examinations of the British and United Kingdom populations;[1,2,3] this chapter does not attempt to duplicate this, but merely to provide a brief overview to put the rest of this book into context.

2.2 The number of people

Figures 2.1 and 2.2 show the number of people in particular age groups for countries and regions of the United Kingdom, for males and females separately, in 1997. The most populous region was the South East which had a population of around 8 million in 1997. London was the second largest region in terms of population with around 7 million people living there. Although the North East was the region of England with the smallest population, less people lived in Northern Ireland than in this region or any of the other countries of the United Kingdom (1.7 million). Scotland's population was around 5 million in 1997 and Wales' around 3 million.

Each country and region had a larger number of females than males (Figures 2.1, 2.2). This is largely because women outnumbered men significantly in the over 65 age group. There were also slightly more women than men aged 45 to 64, but men were in a majority under age 45.

The largest five local authorities were Bradford, Sheffield, Glasgow City, Leeds and Birmingham, with populations ranging from just under 500,000 to just over 1,000,000. These authorities comprised about 6 per cent of the total population of the United Kingdom and the largest 42 authorities (out of a total of 434) made up 25 per cent of the total population. The size of local authorities within London ranged from just under 150,000 in Kingston-upon-Thames to just over 300,000 in

Barnet, excluding the City of London which had a population of around 5,000. The smallest local authority in the United Kingdom was the Isles of Scilly, which had a population of about 2,000. Maps B to E in Appendix B show the distribution of local authorities within countries and regions.

Population pyramids give an overall picture of the population structure of an area by age and sex. They show the percentage of the total population in each age and sex grouping. The overall shape of the pyramid depends upon the age and sex structure of the population. This is influenced not only by births and deaths but also by migration, both internal and international. The age-distribution of a population is best regarded as being primarily determined by fertility and modified by mortality and migration.[4] The shape of the pyramids presented here (Figures 2.3 and 2.4) are typical of that seen in countries with low fertility, low mortality and relatively little migration.[5]

The four countries of the United Kingdom had very similar population pyramids in 1997 (Figure 2.3). There was a substantial peak in the population in the age groups between 25 and 40. This roughly corresponds to people born between the mid 50s and late 60s, when fertility was higher than in recent years.[6] There were more women than men in the older ages, as women have lower mortality than men.[7] Northern Ireland's pyramid differed more from the other three in that it had a larger proportion of population at younger ages and a smaller proportion in the older ages.

The age-sex structures of the regions of England, excluding London, were all broadly similar. London had a very different structure (Figure 2.4), with a high proportion of the population aged 0 to 4 reflecting high fertility, but low proportions aged 10 to 14, suggesting that people may migrate out of London once they have had children. It had a peak of population between the ages of 30 and 34, and much higher proportions in the working ages than the other regions. The South West, by contrast, had larger proportions aged over 60 and it is known that the South West tends to be a focus for migration of people once they have retired, although the strength of this has been debated.[8,9] Figures 3.20 and 3.21 in chapter 3 also show these trends.

2.3 Dependency ratios

The dependency ratio is a frequently used index that summarises the age distribution of a population. Though strictly the ratio of economically active to economically inactive persons in a population, the ratio of age groups - children and elderly to working ages - is often used. The most appropriate age cut-offs for the United Kingdom are the school leaving age (16) and retirement age (65 for men, 60 for

Figure 2.1

**Size of population by country, region and age group, males
United Kingdom 1997**

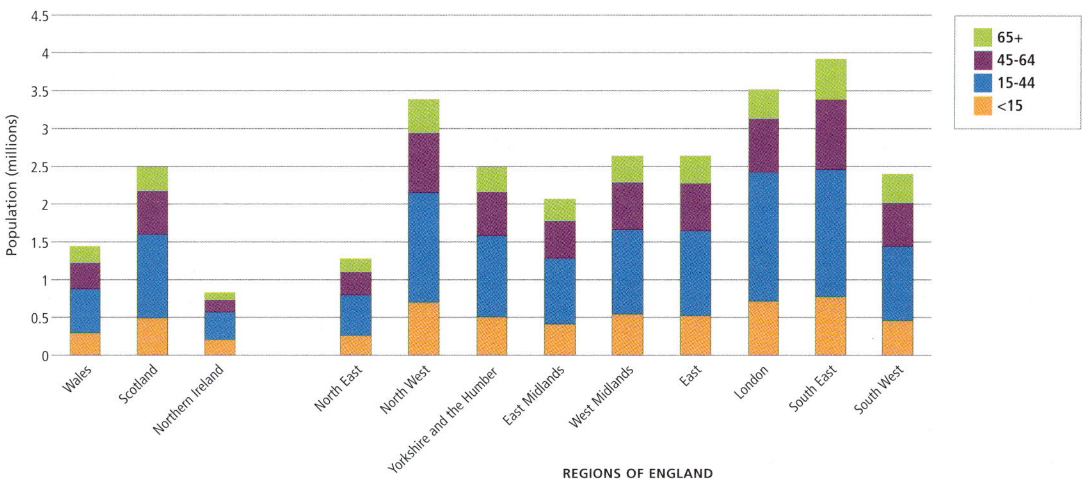

Figure 2.2

**Size of population by country, region and age group, females
United Kingdom 1997**

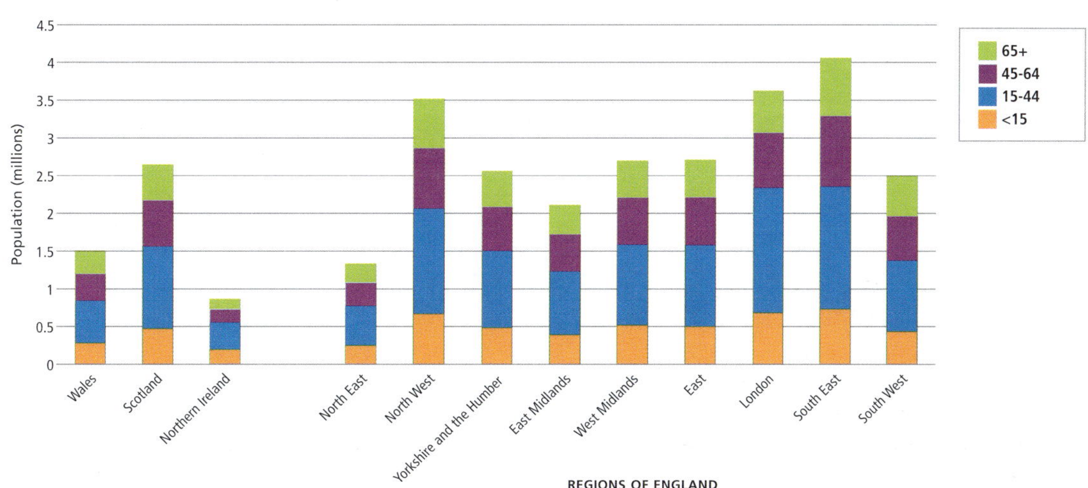

women),[4] although this may change as more 16 to 18 year olds remain in full-time education and changes in the retirement age begin to have an impact.

The dependency ratio for the United Kingdom as a whole in 1997 was 630 per 1,000, meaning that for every 1,000 people of working age there were 630 dependants. London (556 per 1,000) and Scotland (608 per 1,000) had substantially lower dependency ratios than the United Kingdom. The South West (677 per 1,000) and Wales (679 per 1,000) had markedly higher ratios.

Separate ratios can be presented to indicate childhood and elderly dependency. Most of the countries and regions had similar values for childhood dependency (Figure 2.5), the exception being Northern Ireland, which had a higher value,

determined by the relatively larger proportion of Northern Ireland's population that were aged under 16, as shown in the population pyramids discussed earlier. This is a result of previously higher levels in annual birth rates.[10]

There was more variation across countries and regions in the figures for elderly dependency (Figure 2.5). Elderly dependency ratios were low compared to the United Kingdom as a whole in London and Northern Ireland, determined by the large proportion of London's population in the working ages and low proportion of the population of pensionable age in Northern Ireland, as seen in the population pyramids described earlier. The high proportion of people of working age in London is due to inward migration in order to seek out a career. This pull of London for working age people is well documented.[8] The elderly dependency ratio was high compared to the United Kingdom in the South West and in Wales,

Figure 2.3

**Population pyramids by country
United Kingdom 1997**

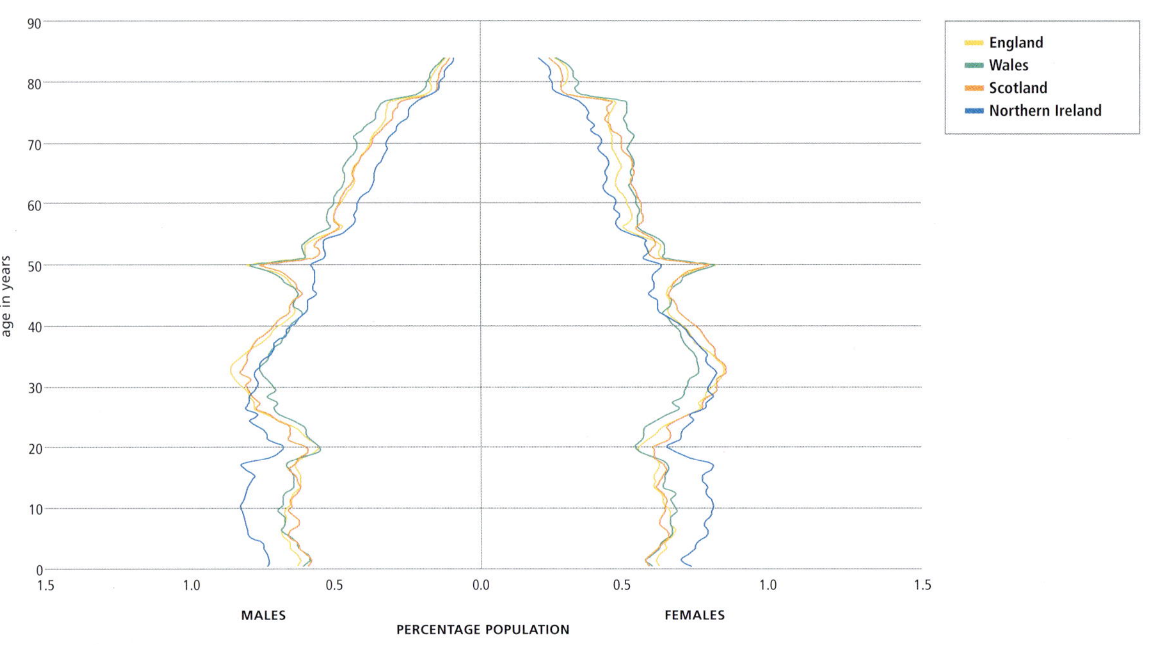

Figure 2.4

**Population pyramids by region
England 1997**

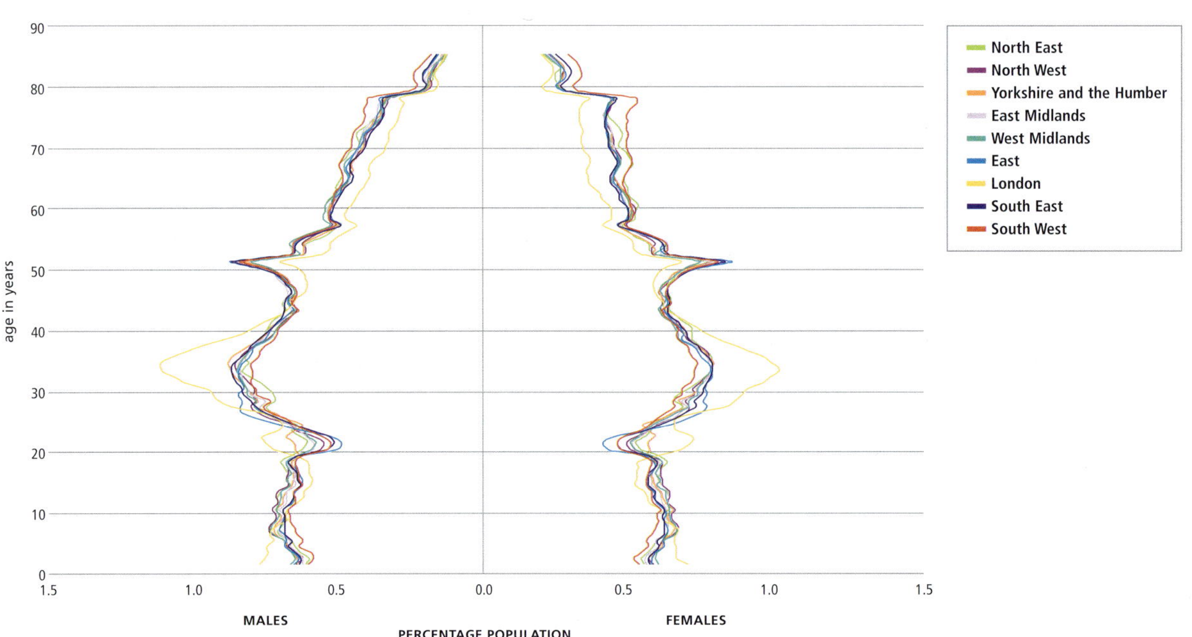

Figure 2.5

**Childhood and elderly dependency ratios by country and region
United Kingdom 1997**

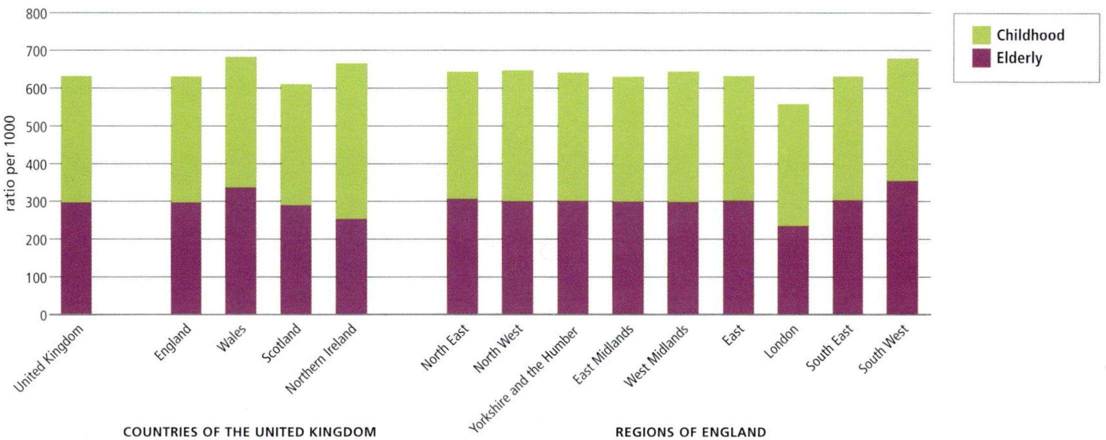

determined by the larger proportions of those of pensionable age in these two areas. This is likely to be the result of older people migrating to the South West and Wales after retirement, as suggested earlier.

Map 2.1 shows the overall picture of childhood dependency by local authority. There were clusters of local authorities with high levels of childhood dependency throughout the United Kingdom, mainly in Northern Ireland, east inner London, Liverpool and Manchester. The west of inner London, by contrast, had low childhood dependency; a pattern hidden in the overall figures for London described above. The majority of local authorities with the highest levels of childhood dependency were in Northern Ireland, which would be expected given the picture for Northern Ireland as a whole described above.

The overall picture of elderly dependency by local authority contrasts with the pattern of childhood dependency. Areas which had high elderly dependency were spread throughout the United Kingdom in coastal and rural areas, and areas with low elderly dependency were located around cities and in more central locations, an exception to this being the Shetland Islands (Map 2.2). Authorities in the west of London also had low elderly dependency.

2.4 Population density

The distribution of the population across the United Kingdom is very uneven, reflecting the highly urbanised nature of the population, with over 90% of people living in urban areas,[11] and the physical character of the country, with upland areas that are largely uninhabitable and the remainder containing relatively densely settled urban areas. Following the 1991 Census, ONS published a volume of key statistics for urban and rural areas, giving in detail the differences in the characteristics of those who live in these area types,[12] but further examination of this is outside the scope of this volume.

Overall, in 1997, England was the most densely populated country and Scotland the least. Within England, London was more densely populated than any of the other regions, and the South West was the least densely populated region (Figure 2.6). Analysis at country and regional level, however, masks the picture of population density across the United Kingdom and can give a false impression. Although Scotland is described as the least densely populated of the four countries, it had more people living at higher densities at local level than Northern Ireland or Wales, which had the least number of people living at higher population density (Figure 2.7).

Examining variation in the population densities of local authorities within countries and regions, Figure 2.8 shows clearly that London was a more homogeneous area in terms of population density than other parts of the United Kingdom, with all its local authorities having substantially higher population density than the United Kingdom as a whole. Each other region or country had a spread of variation in population density around the United Kingdom average.

Looking at the distribution of population across the United Kingdom (Map 2.3), the lowest densities were found in rural areas of Scotland, Cumbria, Northumberland and north Yorkshire, Wales, parts of Northern Ireland and more rural parts of the South West region of England. Areas of high population density stretched across England from the North West to South East and this broad distribution has not changed substantially over time.[11] There were a number of areas of high population density located away from this axis - parts of the North East of England, south Wales, the Forth/Clyde area of Scotland and the south coast of England including Portsmouth, Southampton and Brighton and Hove.

2.5 Population change

Between 1991 and 1997 there was an increase in the population of all the countries and regions, except for the North East,

Map 2.1

Childhood dependency ratios by local authority
United Kingdom 1997

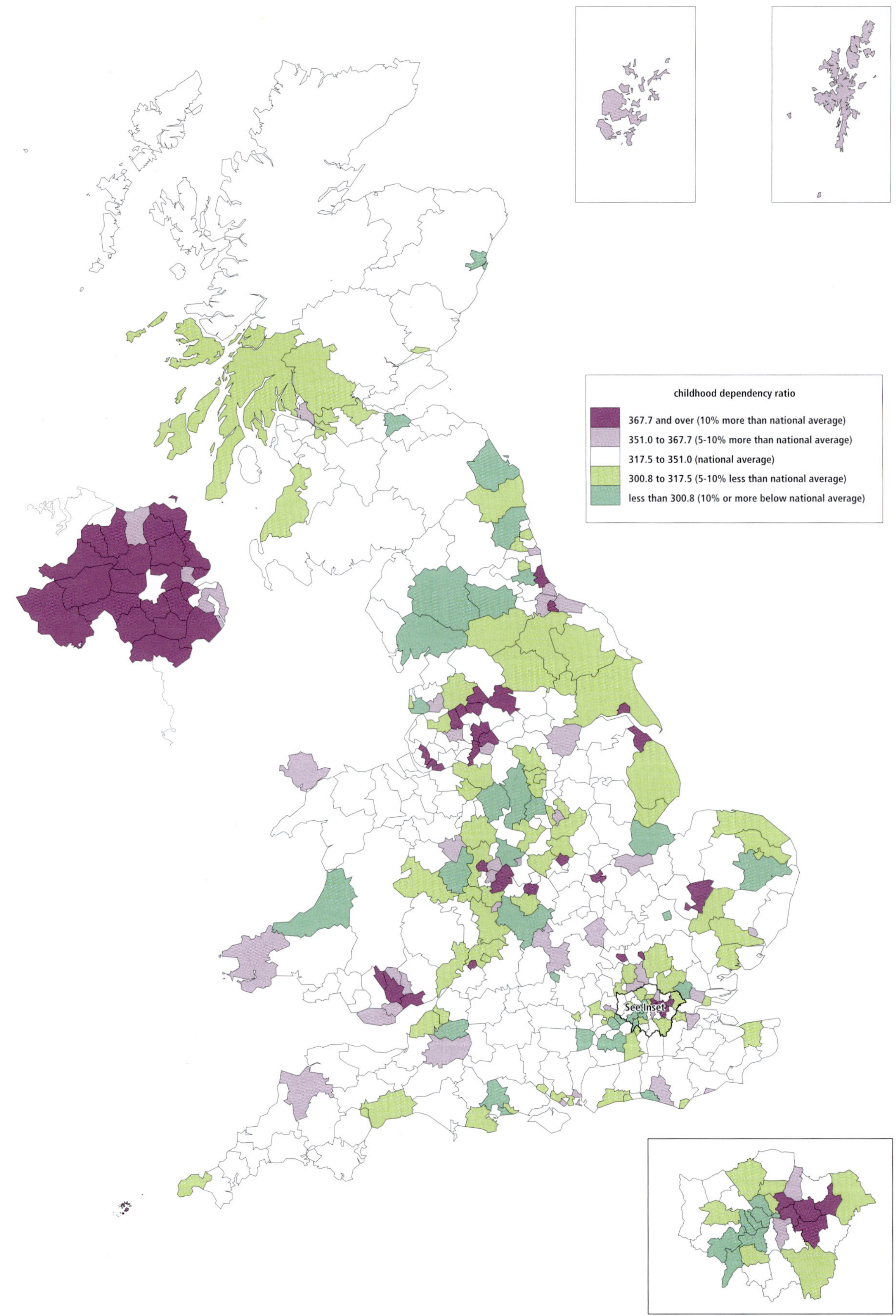

Map 2.2

**Elderly dependency ratios by local authority
United Kingdom 1997**

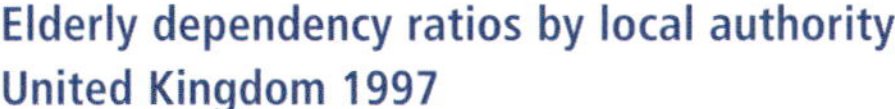

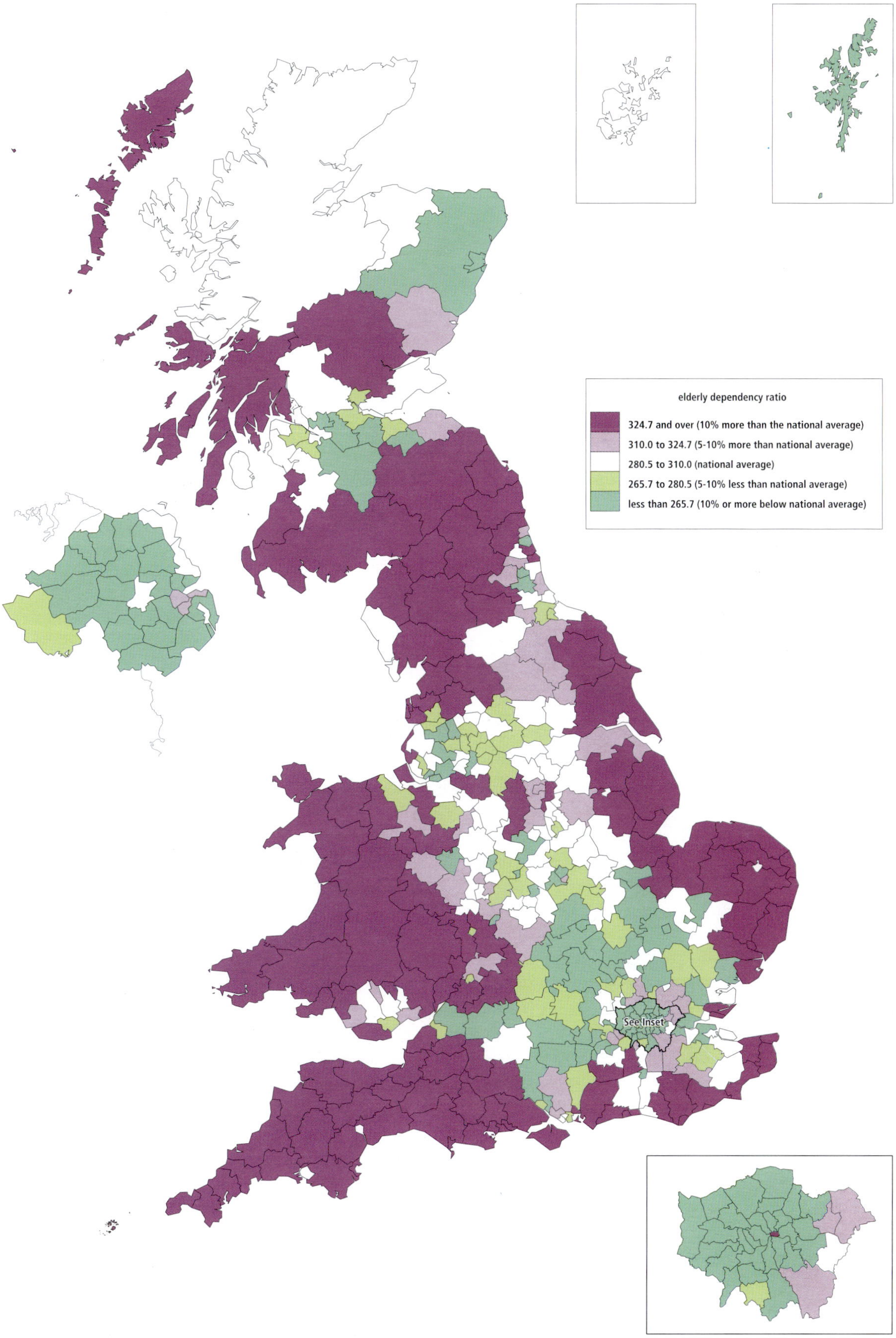

Figure 2.6

**Population density by country and region
United Kingdom 1997**

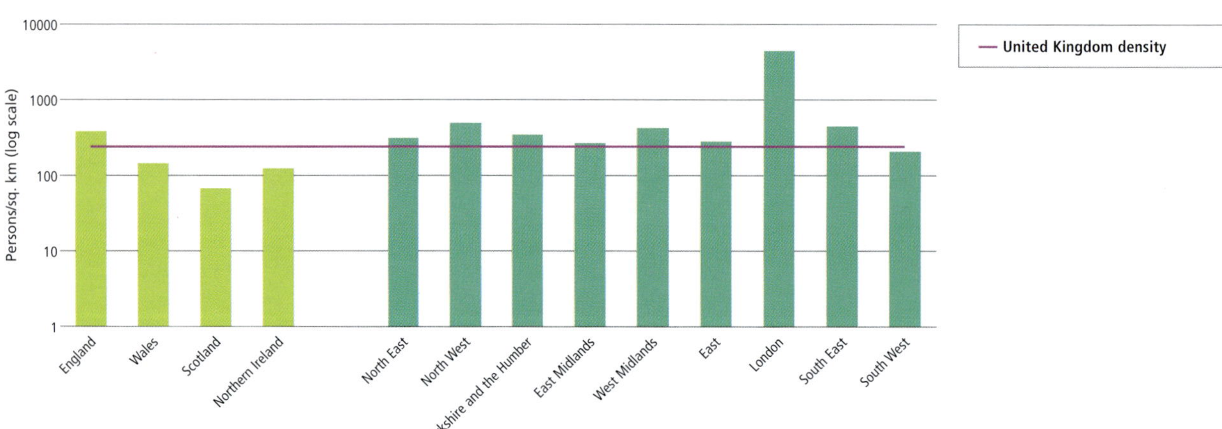

Figure 2.7

**Population-weighted* population density by country and region
United Kingdom 1997**

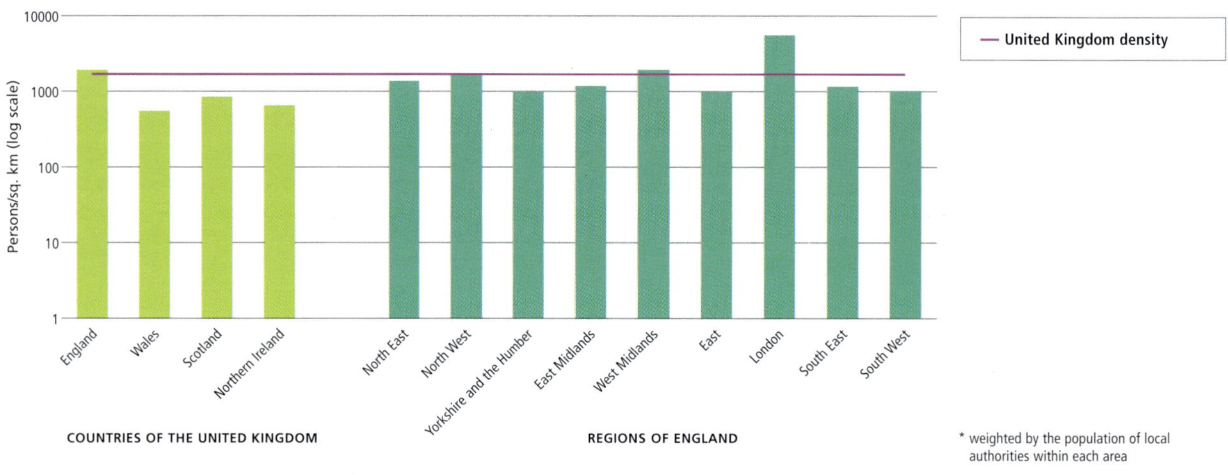

where the population declined, and North West, where there was no overall change in the size of the population (Figure 2.9). Reflecting this, many more local authorities had an increase in their population between 1991 and 1997 than had a decrease. Those with the most substantial increases were located in rural, suburban and coastal areas and Northern Ireland (outside Belfast). Authorities with the largest declines were in the major centres of population, including Belfast, Glasgow City, Manchester, Liverpool and other urban areas. A number of island authorities also had declines in population - Isles of Scilly, Isle of Anglesey, Isle of Wight and Eilean Siar (Map 2.4). These changes could be a result of changes in migration patterns or of natural change in population, that is the excess of births over deaths (or vice versa). The contribution of these two factors to overall population change is examined below.

2.6 Components of population change

Population change can be divided into two parts - that due to natural change (births less deaths) and that which is due to migration. Other small changes, such as changes to the resident population in the Armed Forces or boundary change, are included within the migration component. In presenting data for England, Wales and Scotland all boundary changes have been taken into account, therefore any 'other' changes are the result of movement in the Armed Forces population. In Northern Ireland they have not. One ward, Rathfriland, was reallocated to Banbridge from Newry and Mourne in 1993. The effect of this boundary change is included in the effects due to migration and other changes. The data on migration includes both internal and external migration.

Figure 2.8

Population density by local authority within countries and regions
United Kingdom 1997

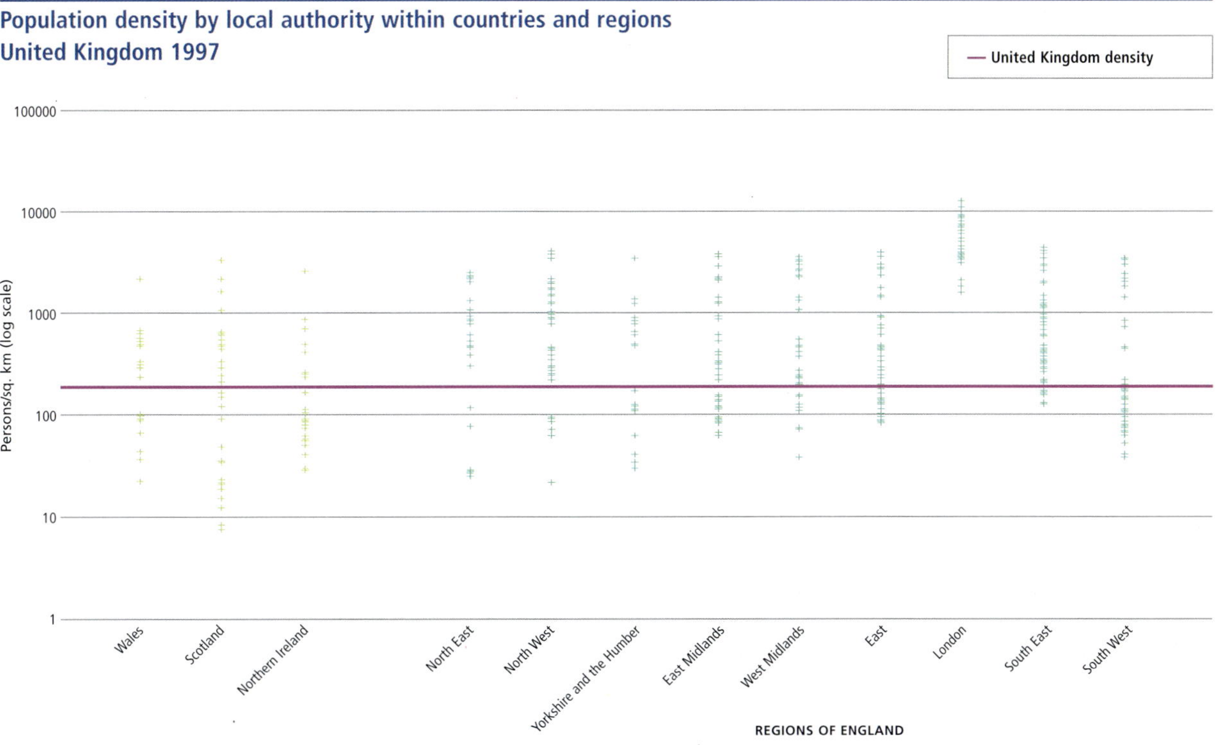

Figure 2.10 shows that between 1991 and 1997 declines in population due to migration occurred in the North East, North West and West Midlands. In the West Midlands this was counterbalanced by an increase in population due to natural change. In the North West the net effect was almost no overall change. In the North East however out-migration was greater than the increase in population from natural change, so the population of this region declined between 1991 and 1997.

The South West experienced a large increase in population due to in-migration, but deaths exceeded births in this region. In Yorkshire and the Humber, London and Northern Ireland the bulk of population increase was due to natural change, whereas in Wales, the South East, the East of England and East Midlands, the most substantial increases were due to migration.

Analysis at the country and regional level masks variation in population change by local authority. Map 2.5 shows that at a local authority level, deaths exceeded births in most of the rural and coastal areas of the United Kingdom between 1991 and 1997. All local authorities in London and Northern Ireland had births exceeding deaths by a substantial amount, contributing to the large increases for the region and the country as a whole respectively seen in Figure 2.10. In addition, central areas of England across Berkshire and Wiltshire had an excess of births over deaths (Map 2.5).

Map 2.6 shows that areas losing population as a result of out-migration in the 1990s were Liverpool, Birmingham and Manchester and their surrounding areas, urban areas of the

North East and parts of London, especially the east. Local authorities gaining population from migration were spread throughout the rest of the United Kingdom.

2.7 Population projections

Figure 2.11 shows the projected population in 2011 for countries of the United Kingdom and regions of England. Overall declines are projected in Scotland and the North East and North West of England. The largest increases are projected to occur in the East Midlands and southern regions of England. At local authority level, Map 2.7 shows the projected population change to 2011. Fewer authorities show a projected decline in population than an increase in population, particularly in the south of England. The only areas of substantial decline in the south of England are found to the east of London, in parts of Essex and Kent. Generally, local authorities that are expected to decline in population are found in more urban areas of the north of England, Scotland (as well as two island councils), parts of south Wales (as well as the Isle of Anglesey) and Belfast. Areas of expected substantial increase are found throughout the south of England and parts of the Midlands, as would be expected given the regional figures described above.

Figure 2.9

**Overall population change by country and region
United Kingdom 1991-1997**

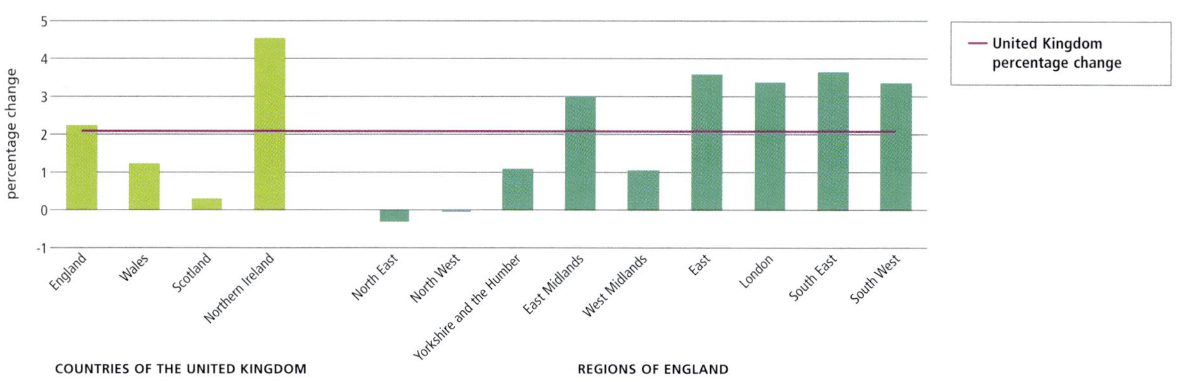

Figure 2.10

**Components of population change by country and region
United Kingdom 1991-1997**

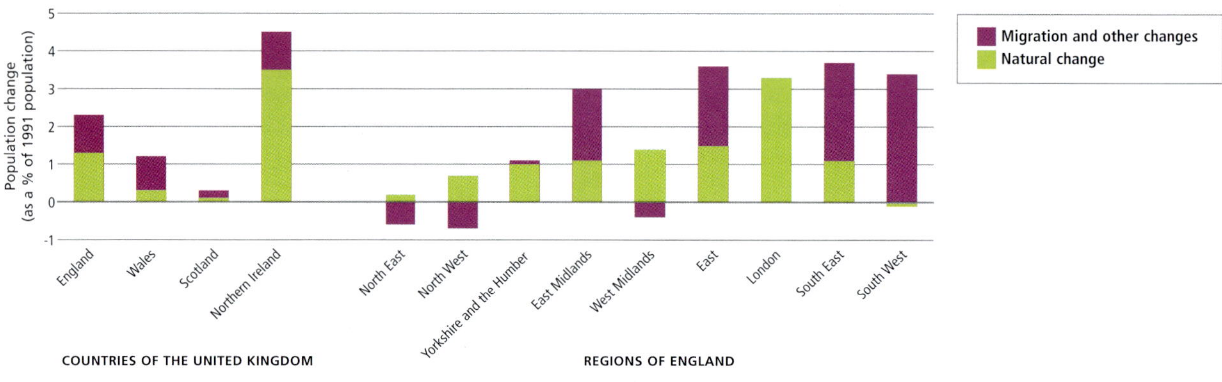

Figure 2.11

**Projected change in the population between 1997 and 2011 by country and region
United Kingdom 1996-based***

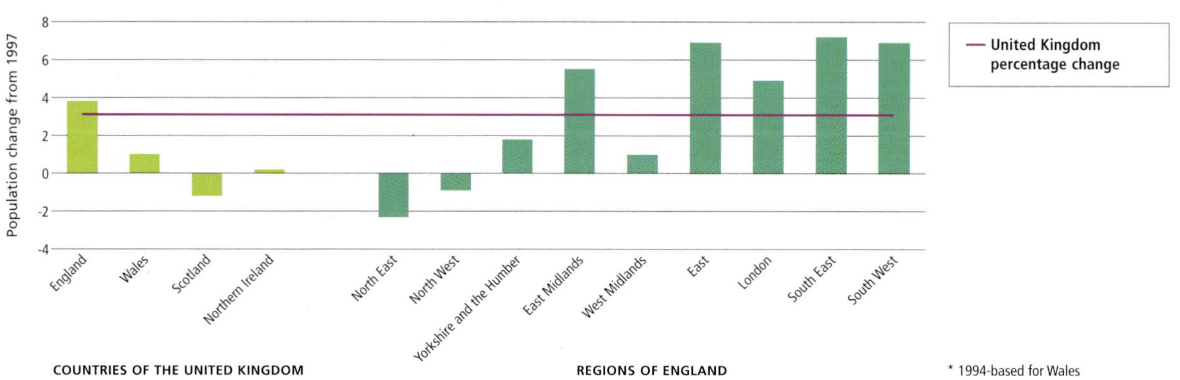

Map 2.3

**Population density by local authority
United Kingdom 1997**

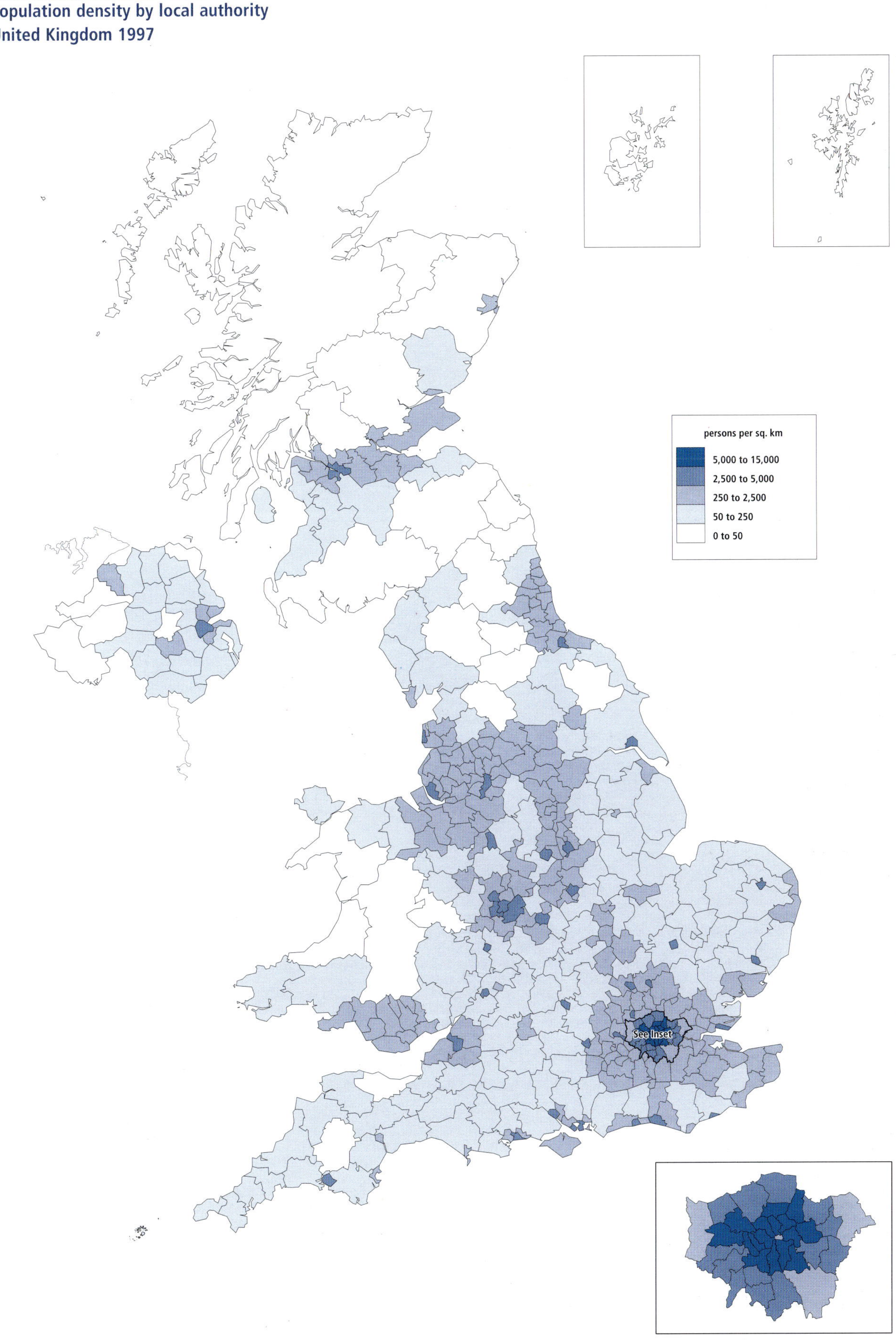

Map 2.4

**Overall percentage change in the population by local authority
United Kingdom 1991-1997**

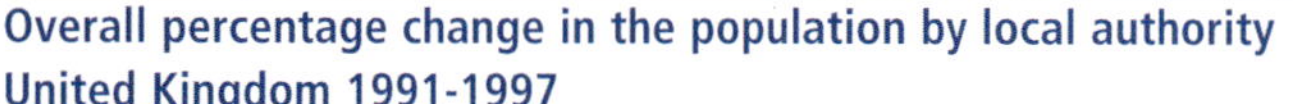

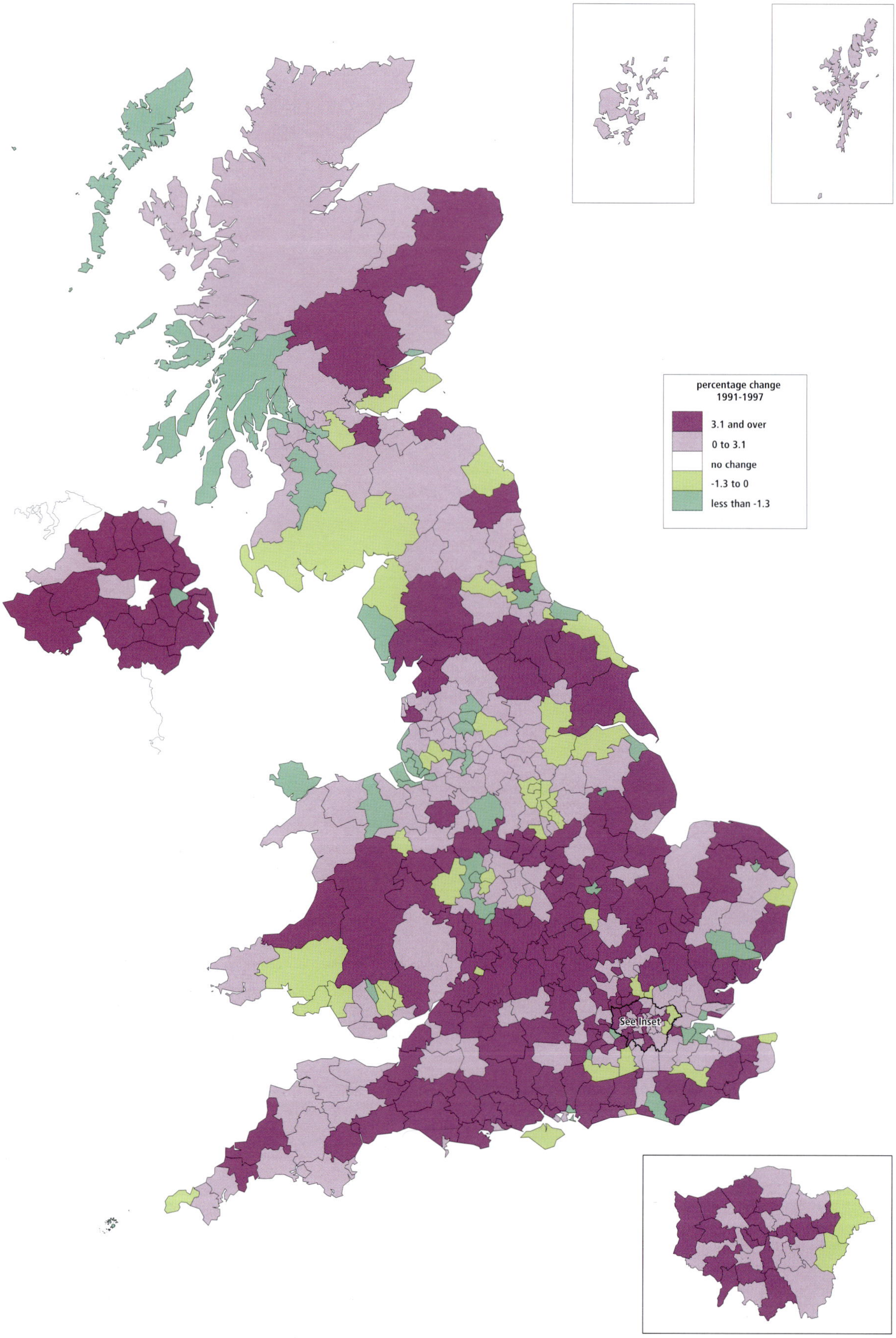

Map 2.5

Population change due to natural change by local authority
United Kingdom 1991-1997

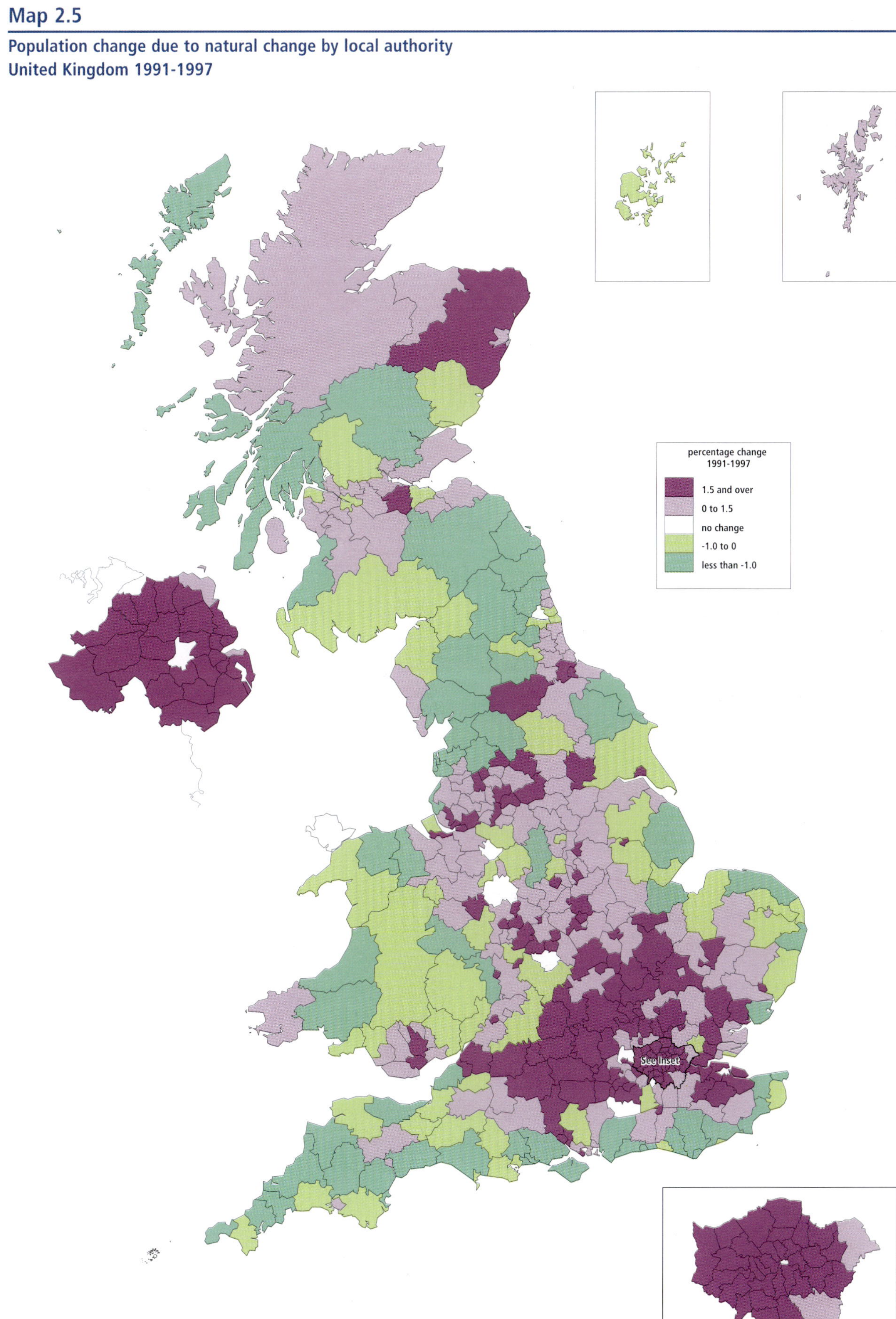

Map 2.6

**Population change due to migration* by local authority
United Kingdom 1991-1997**

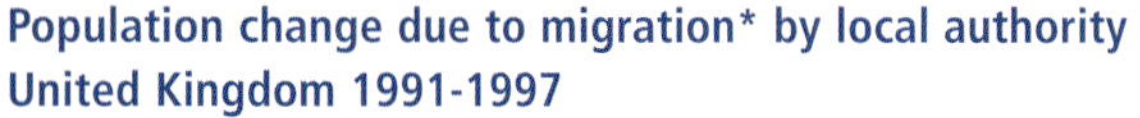

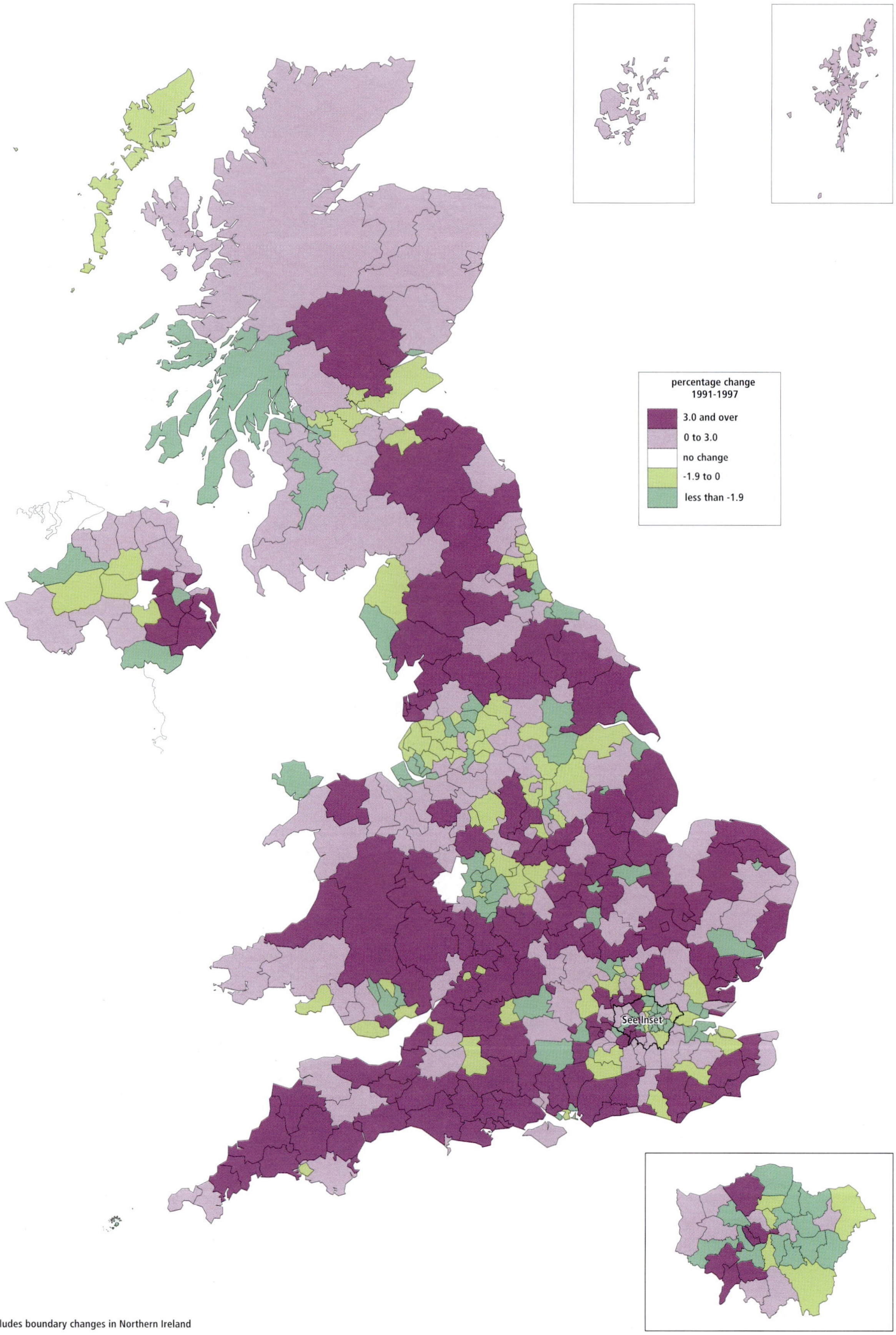

* Includes boundary changes in Northern Ireland

Map 2.7

Projected change in the population between 1997 and 2011 by local authority
United Kingdom 1996-based*

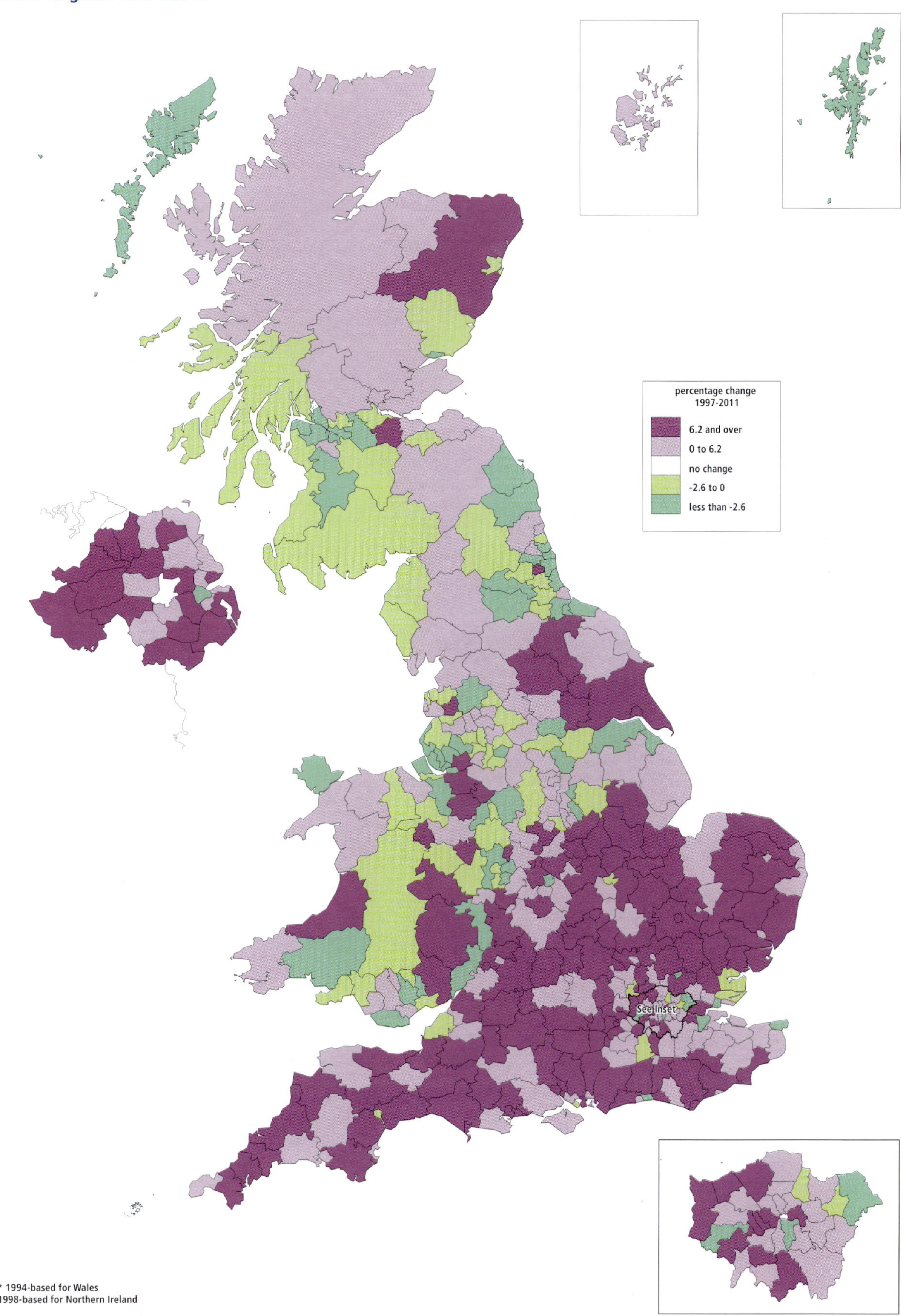

* 1994-based for Wales
1998-based for Northern Ireland

References

1 Coleman D and Salt J. *The British Population: Patterns, Trends, and Processes.* Oxford University Press (Oxford: 1992).

2 Champion T, Wong C, Rooke A, Dorling D, Coombes M and Brunsdon C. *The Population of Britain in the 1990s. A Social and Economic Atlas.* Clarendon Press (Oxford: 1996).

3 Dorling D. *A New Social Atlas of Britain.* Wiley (Chichester: 1995).

4 Newell C. *Methods and Models in Demography.* Wiley (Chichester: 1988).

5 Shyrock HS and Siegel J. *The Methods and Materials of Demography.* Academic Press (London: 1976).

6 Coleman D and Salt J. Fertility trends. In *The British Population: Patterns, Trends, and Processes.* Oxford University Press (Oxford: 1992), 113-174.

7 Office for National Statistics. Annual Update: 1998 mortality statistics general (England and Wales). *Health Statistics Quarterly* 8 (2000), 95-100.

8 Coleman D and Salt J. Internal migration. In *The British Population: Patterns, Trends, and Processes.* Oxford University Press (Oxford: 1992), 395-432.

9 Warnes AM and Law CM. The elderly population of Great Britain: locational trends and policy implications. *Institute of British Geographers: Transactions* 9 (1984), 37-59.

10 Armitage B and Babb P. Population review: (4) Trends in fertility. *Population Trends* 84 (1996), 7-13.

11 Coleman D and Salt J. The changing distribution of population in the United Kingdom. In *The British Population: Patterns, Trends, and Processes.* Oxford University Press (Oxford: 1992), 83-112.

12 Office for National Statistics, General Register Office for Scotland. *1991 Census. Key statistics for urban and rural areas. Great Britain.* The Stationery Office (London: 1997).

Socio-economic characteristics of the people

Clare Griffiths and Justine Fitzpatrick

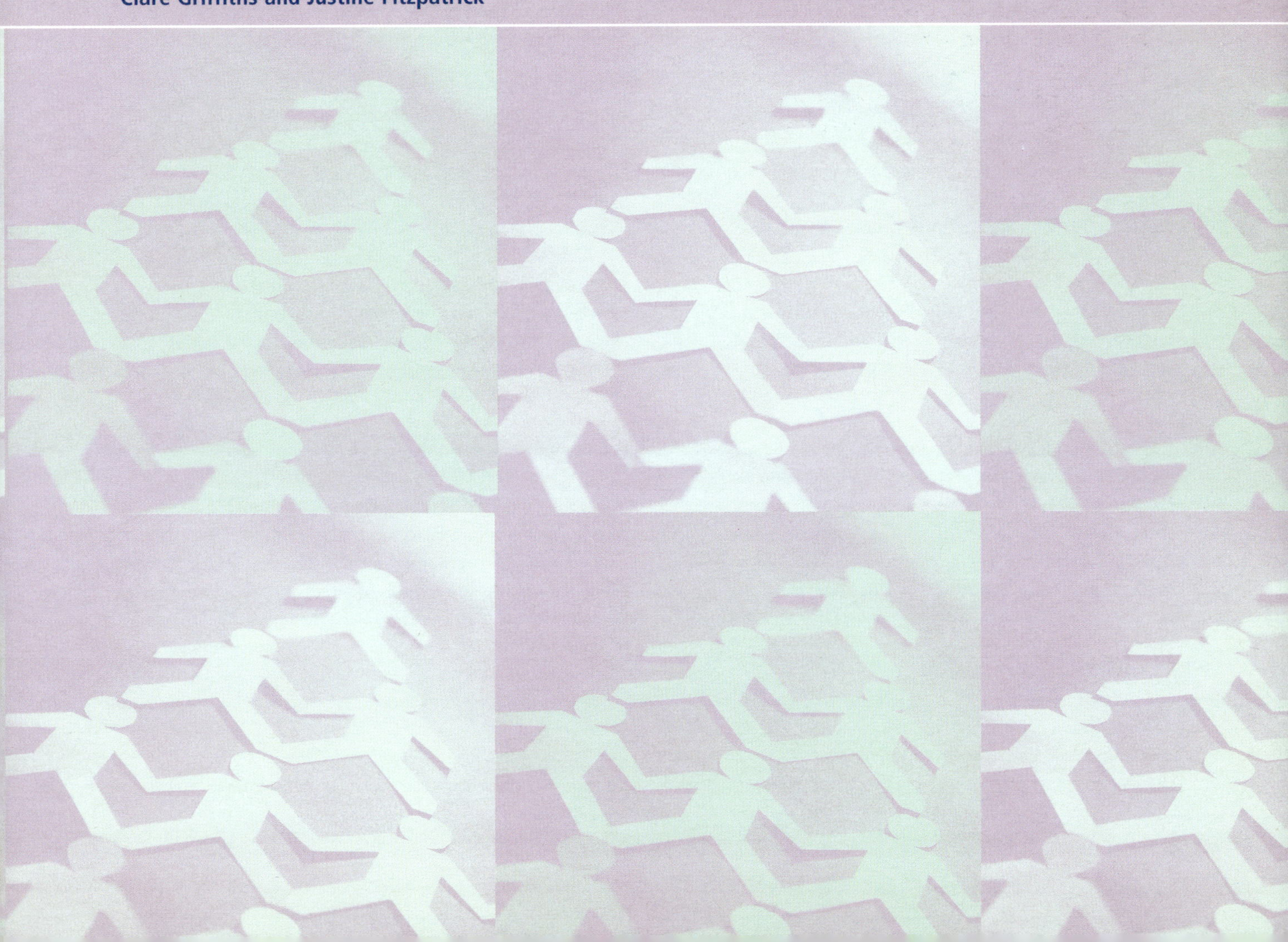

Chapter 3
Socio-economic characteristics of the people

3.1 Introduction

The health of individuals is influenced not simply by age, gender and genetic factors, but also by their environment, including their social and economic circumstances, as well as the circumstances in which they live. The relationships are complex and have been discussed in detail elsewhere.[1] This chapter examines geographic variation in just some of these social and economic factors, in order to provide background to the geographic patterns described in the later chapters of the volume. We have focused on marital status, Social Class, unemployment, ethnicity, country of birth, living arrangements, housing tenure, access to cars, migration and health-related behaviour. All these factors vary geographically, although some vary more than others, and so may also be associated with the geographic patterns of health described in later chapters. Factors such as housing tenure and access to cars are often used in the study of health variations as proxies for factors such as income. Social Class (based on occupation) is also used as a proxy, for income and also for factors which are not directly measurable such as social status. Occupation itself may also be a powerful determinant of health.

3.2 Sources of data

The sources used in this chapter are primarily the Labour Force Survey (LFS) and the 1991 Census. Data from the LFS and other social surveys are used to give more up-to-date figures for countries and regions. All local authority data relate to the 1991 Census, as this is the most up to date information available with this level of geographic detail. However, data for countries and regions will not be directly comparable to the local authority level data from the Census.

Data from the 1991 Census have been recast to current (1999) boundaries, in line with the rest of the volume. These local authority boundaries will be current in the 2001 Census so the information should be useful for comparison purposes. However this was not fully possible for the marital status and country of birth data for England and Wales. For these two groups of data it was not possible to take into account boundary changes that involved the reallocation of only one enumeration district (ED) from one authority to another. Account was taken of all other boundary changes and so this will have minimal effect on the patterns presented.

3.3 Marital status

The association between marital status and health, first noted by Farr in the 1850s[2] and Durkeim in the 1890s,[3] has also been the subject of more recent study. In 1967, an analysis of suicides by marital status was included in the Registrar General's Statistical Review and showed that the married had much lower mortality from suicide than the unmarried, with the divorced having the highest rates.[4] A number of more recent studies have also shown an association between marriage and health.[5] Analysis using the US National Longitudinal Mortality Study showed that the unmarried were found to be at increased risk of death compared to the married, for both men and women. This strong association was found to remain after adjustment for socio-economic factors.[6]

Work using the ONS Longitudinal Study for England and Wales has shown married men and women to have lower mortality rates than single, widowed or divorced men and women.[7] Migrants to England and Wales who were unmarried also had higher mortality than migrants who were married.[8]

Another study that followed men up during the 1980s found that single (never-married) men were at increased risk of cardiovascular mortality, and other causes of mortality excluding cancer, compared to married men. Divorced or separated men were not found to be at increased risk and widowed men were found to be at increased risk of non-cancer non-cardiovascular disease mortality. This was found after controlling for factors such as health and socio-economic status.[9]

A study using the United States National Longitudinal Mortality Study found that the divorced had a suicide rate twice as high as those who were married, after adjusting for factors such as age, race, education, income and region.[10] A further study of cause-specific mortality found unmarried men to be at increased risk of mortality from testicular cancer.[11]

It is not just risk of adult mortality that marital status is associated with. Young single women are less likely to attend antenatal classes than older married women, which has implications for the future health of their children[12] and variation in social support, including marital status, has been shown in one study to account for over 30 per cent of variation in foetal growth and subsequent birthweight.[13]

Infant mortality has also been shown to be strongly associated with the mother's marital status. A higher infant mortality rate has been found for those born outside marriage, with a 45 to 68 per cent higher rate for those babies that are solely registered by the mother or that are jointly registered by both parents, but whose parents are not living together.[14] The association between infant mortality and marital status across Wales and the regions of England is discussed in chapter 7.

The marital status profiles of men and women in the United Kingdom are different. In all countries and regions, a larger

Figure 3.1

**Percentage of the population aged 16 and over who are unmarried by country and region, males
United Kingdom 1997**

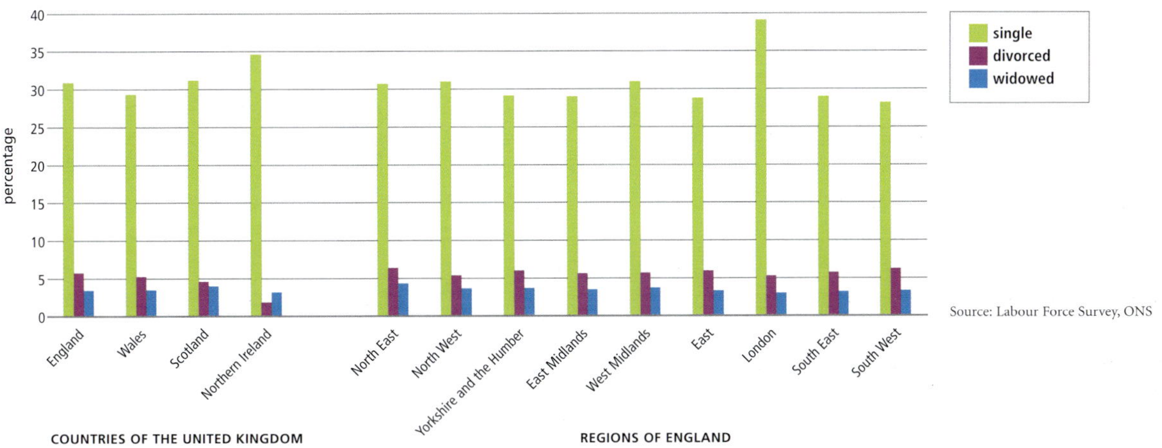

Figure 3.2

**Percentage of the population aged 16 and over who are unmarried by country and region, females
United Kingdom 1997**

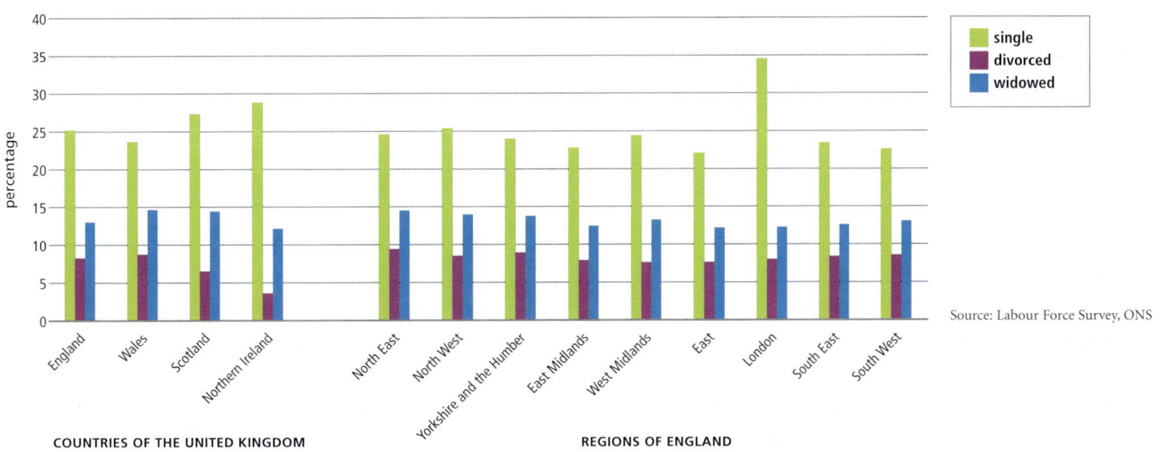

proportion of men than women were single in 1997, but a larger proportion of women were widowed. The proportion of widowed women was generally more than three times that of widowed men. Northern Ireland was the country with the largest proportion of single men and women in the United Kingdom and only 2 per cent of men and 4 per cent of women in Northern Ireland were divorced compared with 5 per cent or more in each of England, Scotland and Wales (Figures 3.1, 3.2). Of the regions of England, London had the highest proportion of single men, just under 40 per cent, and women, just under 35 per cent, compared with around 30 per cent or less of men and 25 per cent or less of women in the other regions.

When we examine variations at local authority level for 1991, the regional pattern is reflected in the maps for single people. High percentages of single men and women were found in authorities in Northern Ireland, London and major towns and cities and low proportions in the Humber area and south Wales for women and the Wash area and authorities along the south coast for men. The majority of authorities had 25 to 30 per cent of men and 20 to 25 per cent of women being single at the time of the 1991 Census (Maps 3.1, 3.2). The highest proportions of widowers were found in coastal areas, the far north of England and Scotland. Low proportions were found in Northern Ireland and central parts of England, close to London (Map 3.3). High proportions of divorced men were found in London, major towns and cities and Pennine areas. Low proportions were found in authorities in Northern Ireland and Scotland and parts of northern England (Map 3.4).

Map 3.1

**Percentage of men who were single at the 1991 Census by local authority
United Kingdom 1991**

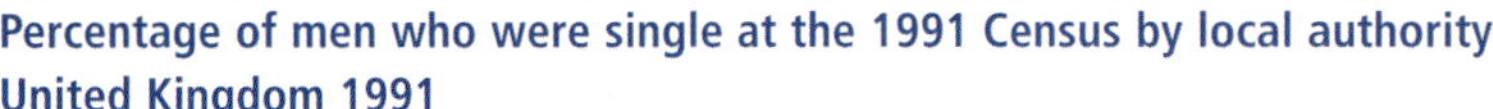

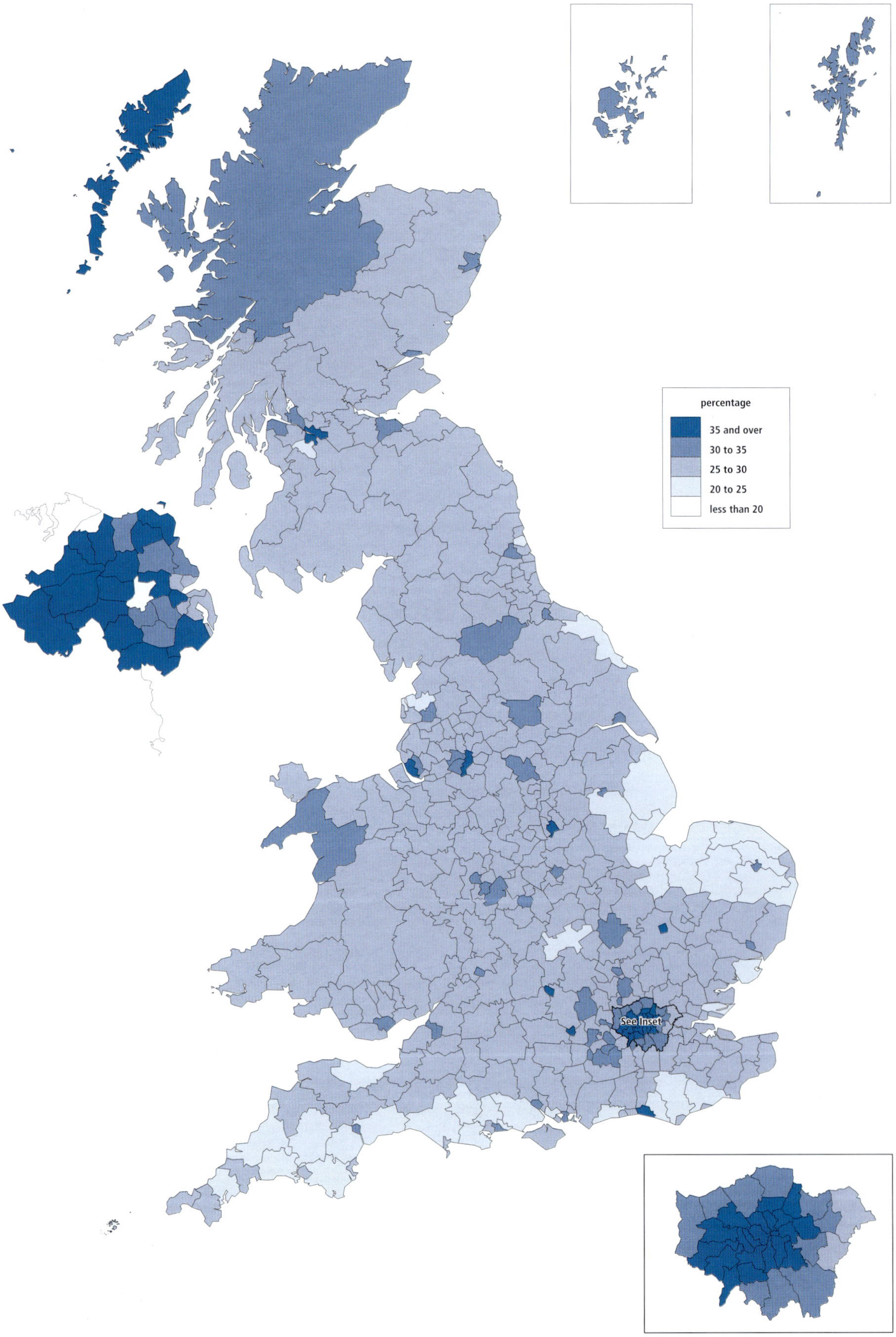

source: 1991 Census

Map 3.2

Percentage of women who were single at the 1991 Census by local authority
United Kingdom 1991

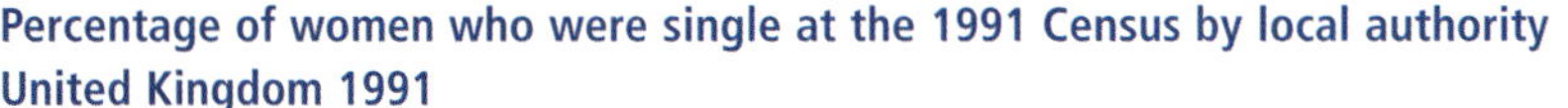

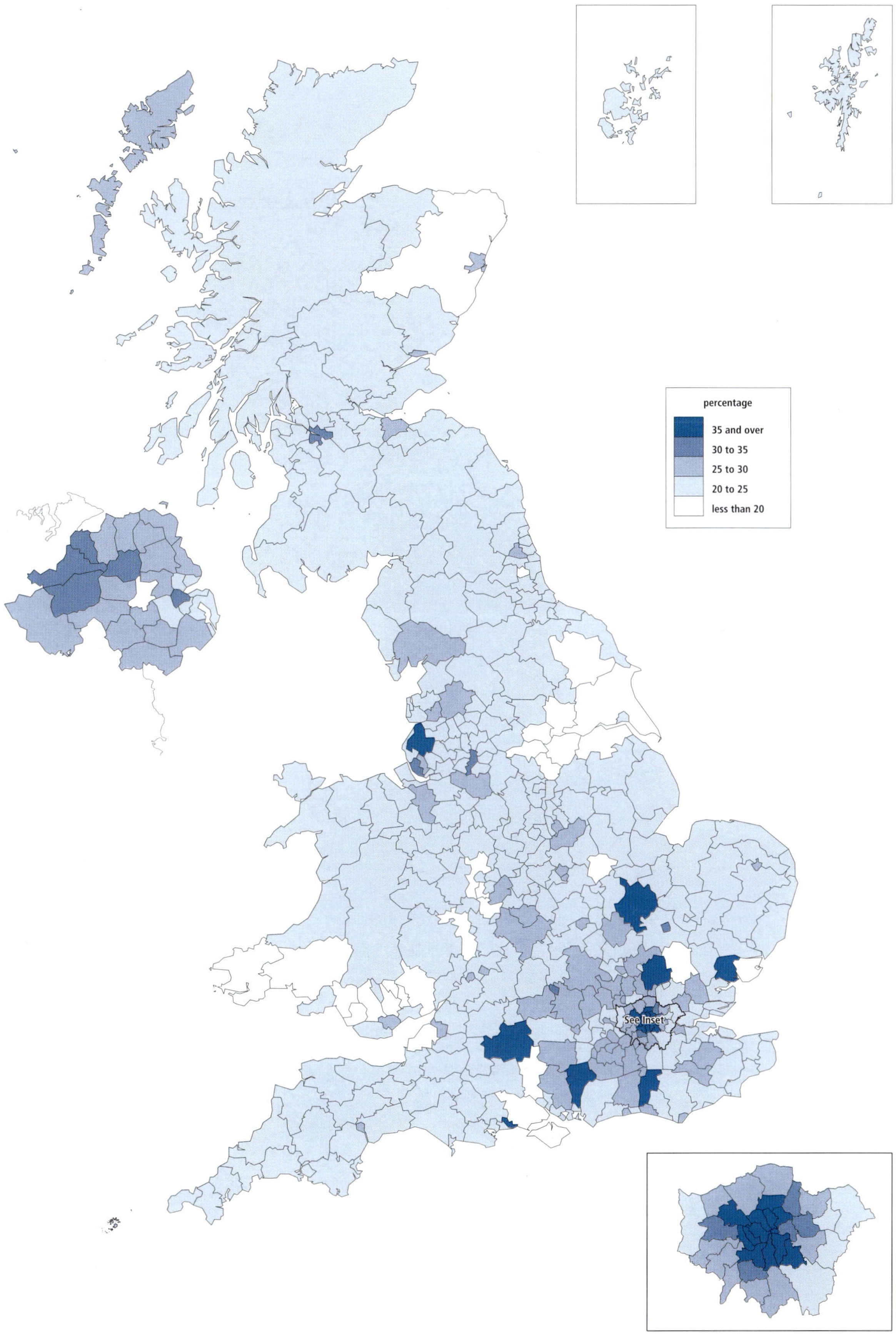

source: 1991 Census

Map 3.3

**Percentage of men who were widowered at the 1991 Census by local authority
United Kingdom 1991**

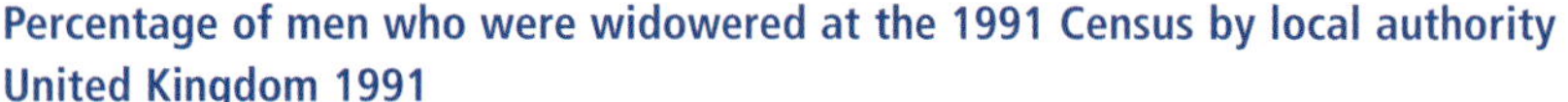

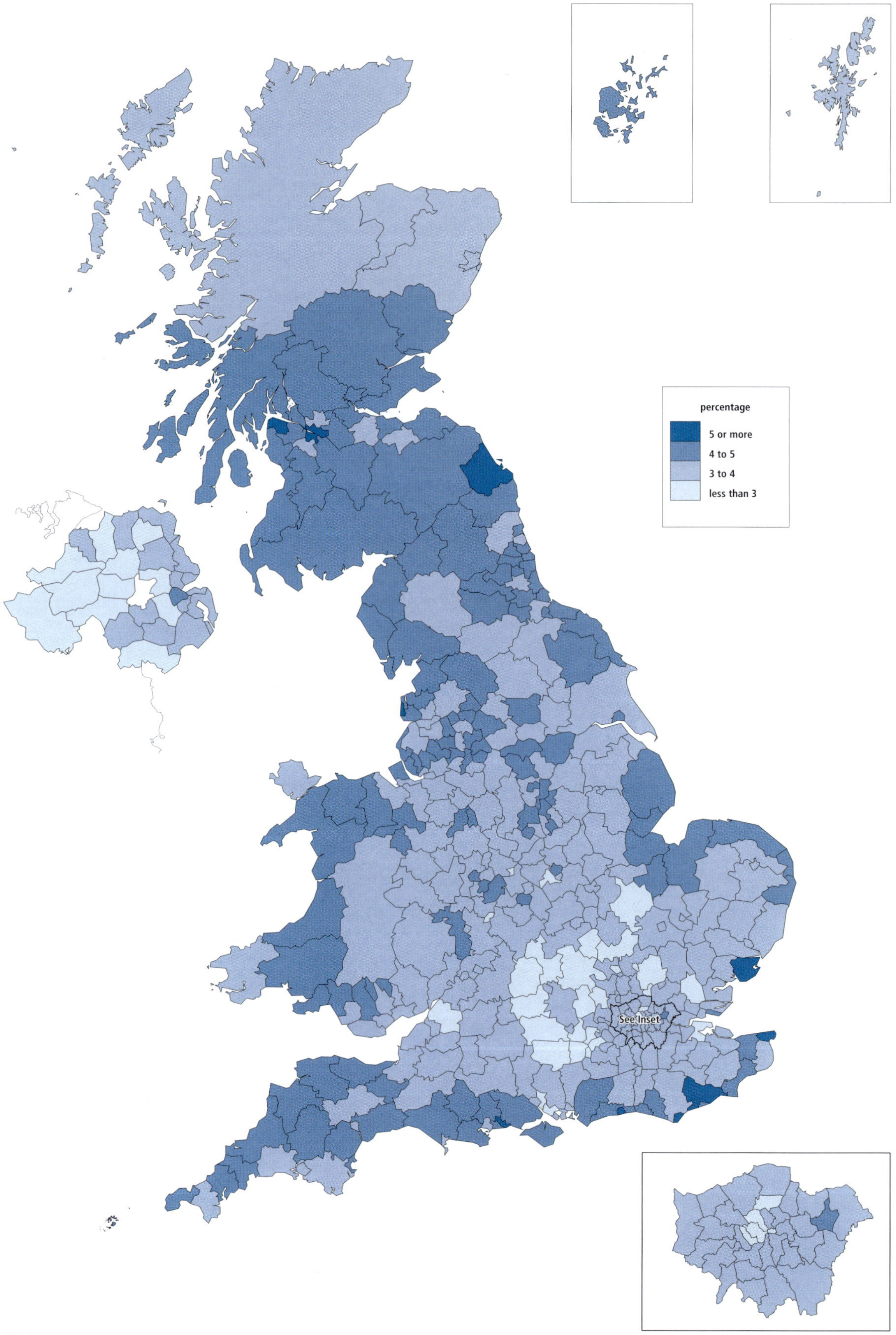

source: 1991 Census

Map 3.4

**Percentage of men who were divorced at the 1991 Census by local authority
United Kingdom 1991**

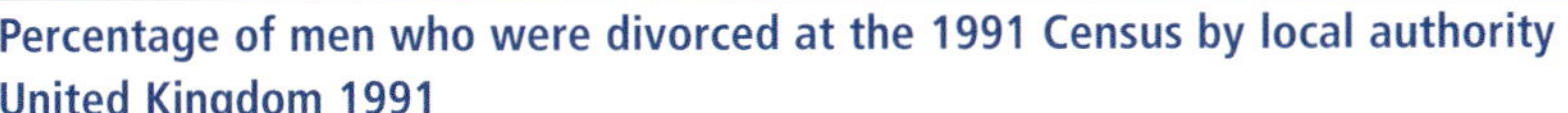

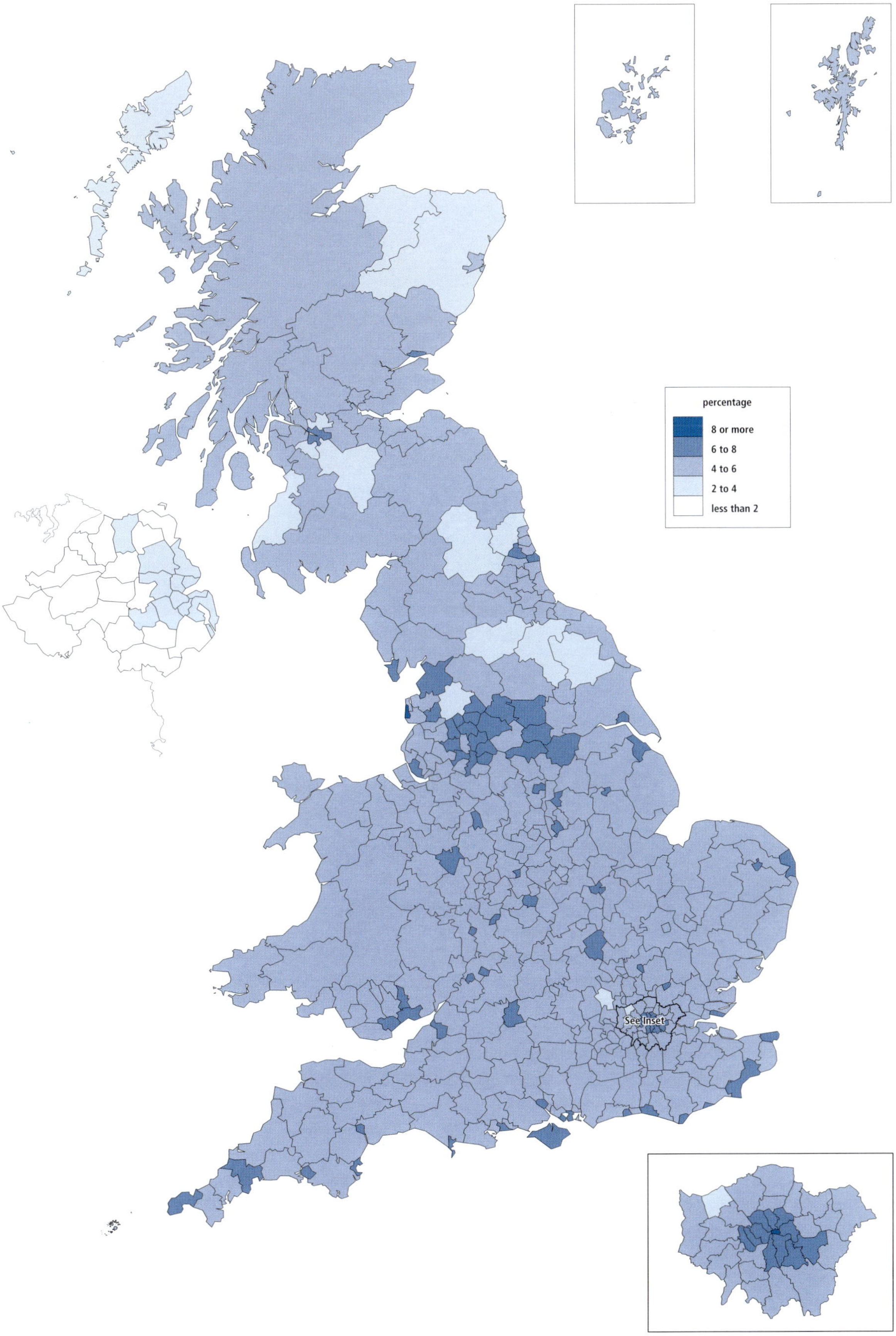

source: 1991 Census

3.4 Social Class

Box 3.1 Social Class

The Registrar General for England and Wales introduced the Social Class classification (based on occupation) to analyse the 1911 Census. The classification aimed to group together people of similar socio-economic status based on occupational skill. The classification is derived from two items of information, occupation and status in employment, that is employee, manager, foreman/supervisor or self-employed, with or without employees. The classification system used in the 1990s is shown below:

Social Class (based on occupation)

I   Professional (e.g. accountants, electronic engineers)

II   Managerial and technical/intermediate (e.g. proprietors and managers – sales, production, works and maintenance managers)

IIIN   Skilled non-manual (e.g. clerks and cashiers – not retail)

IIIM   Skilled manual (e.g. drivers of road goods vehicles, metal working and production fitters)

IV   Partly skilled (e.g. storekeepers and warehousemen, machine tool operators)

V   Unskilled (e.g. building and civil engineering labourers, cleaners)

Source: reproduced from Bunting (1997)[15]

In 1994 the Office for National Statistics commissioned the Economic and Social Research Council (ESRC) to carry out a review of the two social classifications widely used in official statistics – Social Class based on occupation (SC, formerly Registrar General's Social Class) and Socio-economic Group (SEG). This review was completed in June 1998 and the main recommendation, that both SC and SEG should be replaced by a new single-purpose classification scheme, was accepted. The new classification, implemented in 2001, is called the National Statistics - Socio-economic Classification (NS-SEC).

The development of the NS-SEC was described in *Population Trends*[16] and in more detail in two reports published as part of the ESRC review.[17, 18] Like both SC and SEG, the NS-SEC is based on occupation, although it differs fundamentally from these previous classifications in that classes within the scheme are based not on skill levels or concepts of manual/non-manual work, but on employment relations and conditions, such as job security, forms of wage payment and career prospects. Details of the classification can be found on the National Statistics website (www.statistics.gov.uk).

The ONS, and predecessors, have traditionally used occupationally based classifications - principally Social Class (based on occupation) - to measure and report on health differences between sub-groups within the population. Box 3.1 gives more detail on the Social Class classification. Since 1911 the Registrar General has included data on mortality by Social Class in England and Wales in decennial supplements.[19] Data from 1991-1993 showed that men aged 20-64 in Social Class V had almost three times the mortality of those in Social Class I.[20] Early analysis of the relationship between mortality and the National Statistics Socio-economic Classification (NS-SEC) showed similar results.[21]

Analysis of life expectancy by Social Class has shown that men in Social Classes IV or V had lower life expectancy than men in Social Classes I or II in 1987-1991[22] and in 1992-1996[23] and that between these two dates those in Social Classes I or II experienced greater gains in life expectancy than those in Social Classes IV or V. Similar results have also been found when comparing the 1970s with the 1990s.[24]

Infant mortality rates are higher for babies born to fathers in unskilled and partly skilled jobs compared with those whose fathers are in professional occupations.[25] The average birthweight for babies whose fathers are in unskilled occupations is lower than those born to fathers in professional occupations.[26] Children aged under 4 whose fathers were in Social Class V have also been found to have about twice the mortality rate of children under 4 whose fathers were in Social Class I, although a clear gradient across all Social Classes could only be seen for those aged under 1.[14]

Cause of childhood death in the 1960s, 70s and 80s has been found to vary by father's Social Class. An increased proportion of deaths in childhood due to respiratory diseases, accidents, poisoning and violence is found in manual Social Classes, compared to an increased proportion of deaths due to cancer in non-manual Social Classes.[27, 28, 29, 30]

More discussion of the influence of Social Class on the mortality of men of working ages by region is found in chapter 12 and on infant mortality by region in chapter 7.

In this chapter, data on Social Class for countries and regions are taken from the LFS and include all those people aged 16 to retirement if they were economically active and include the inactive and unemployed if they had a job within the last 8 years, taking their Social Class from this job. The data for local authorities come from the 1991 Census and include all those aged 16 and over if they were economically active. The unemployed are included if they had a job in the last 10 years, taking their Social Class from this job. The inactive, including the retired, are not included. However, people who were above retirement age but still working will be included. These differences in the data will lead to slight differences between the actual figures for countries and regions compared to local authorities. Only the overall geographic differences between countries and regions and between local authorities should be compared.

Figures 3.3 and 3.4 show the proportions of men and women of working ages in Social Classes I or II and IV or V in 1997. Of the countries of the United Kingdom, England had the highest

Figure 3.3

**Percentage of men and women of working ages in Social Classes I or II by country and region
United Kingdom 1997**

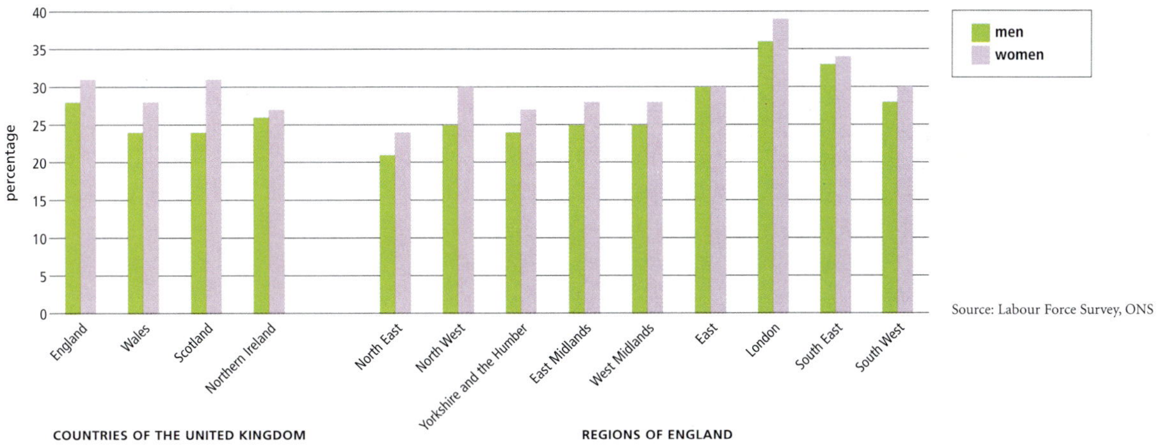

Figure 3.4

**Percentage of men and women of working ages in Social Classes IV or V by country and region
United Kingdom 1997**

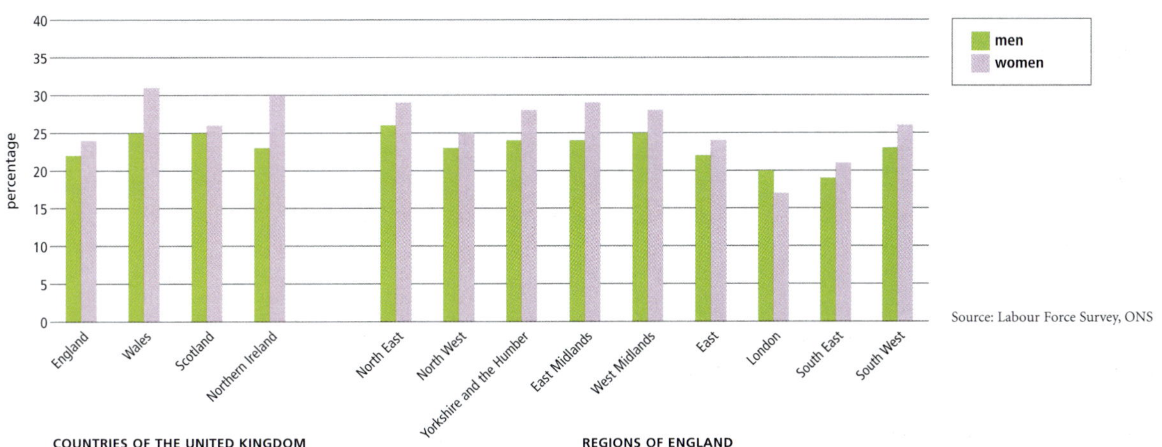

proportion of men in Social Classes I or II and Scotland and England the highest proportion of women. Wales and Scotland had the highest proportions of men in Social Classes IV or V and Wales and Northern Ireland the highest proportion of women.

Within England, London and the South East stood out as having the highest proportions of both men and women in Social Classes I or II and the North East the lowest. High proportions in Social Classes IV or V were found in the northern regions and the Midlands, although the North West region had a slightly lower proportion, similar to that in the East of England and South West. London and the South East had the lowest proportions in Social Classes IV or V.

The pattern by country and region presented above masks large variations in the Social Class distribution of the population by local authority. Map 3.5 shows that local authorities with high percentages in Social Classes I or II were found around London

and throughout the Home Counties, south Manchester and north Cheshire and parts of the East and West Midlands away from the urban centres. Authorities which had the lowest proportions in Social Classes I or II were found in a cluster in the North East region, parts of south Yorkshire and the Humber, a cluster on the east coast of England, mid to south Wales, parts of Devon and Cornwall and the majority of authorities in Northern Ireland. The pattern shown in the map is for men, but the pattern for women was very similar.

Map 3.6 shows that authorities with high percentages in Social Classes IV or V were found in south Wales, Lincolnshire and the Wash areas, Pennine areas and authorities around Tyne and Wear. Low percentages in Social Classes IV or V were generally found in authorities in London and the Home Counties, as would be expected from the regional figures described above. Although the map presented shows data for men, the patterns for women were broadly similar.

Map 3.5

Percentage of economically active men aged 16 and over in Social Classes I or II at the 1991 Census by local authority United Kingdom 1991

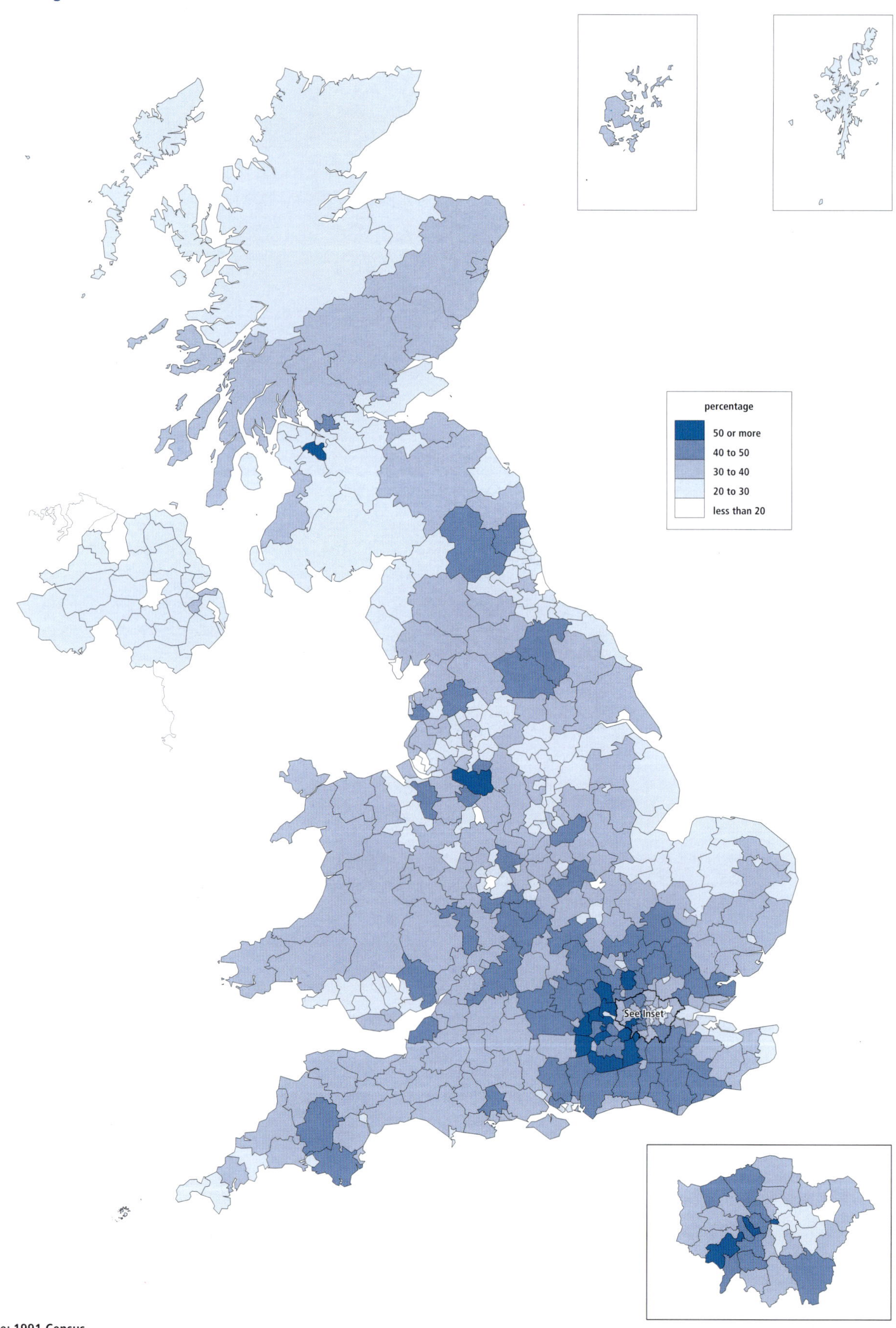

source: 1991 Census

Map 3.6

**Percentage of economically active men aged 16 and over in Social Classes IV or V at the 1991 Census by local authority
United Kingdom 1991**

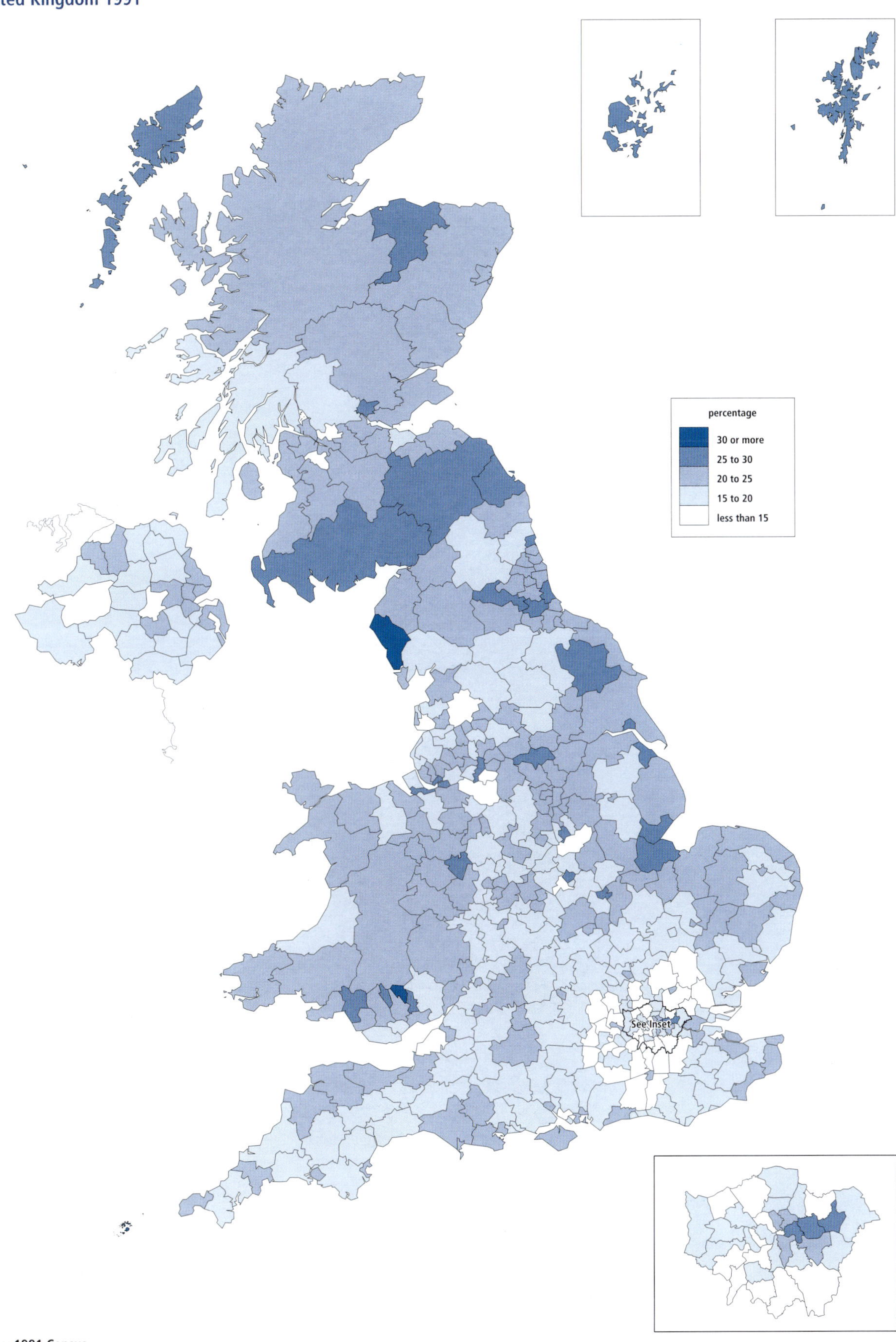

source: 1991 Census

Map 3.7

**Percentage of men aged 16-24 who were unemployed at the 1991 Census by local authority
United Kingdom 1991**

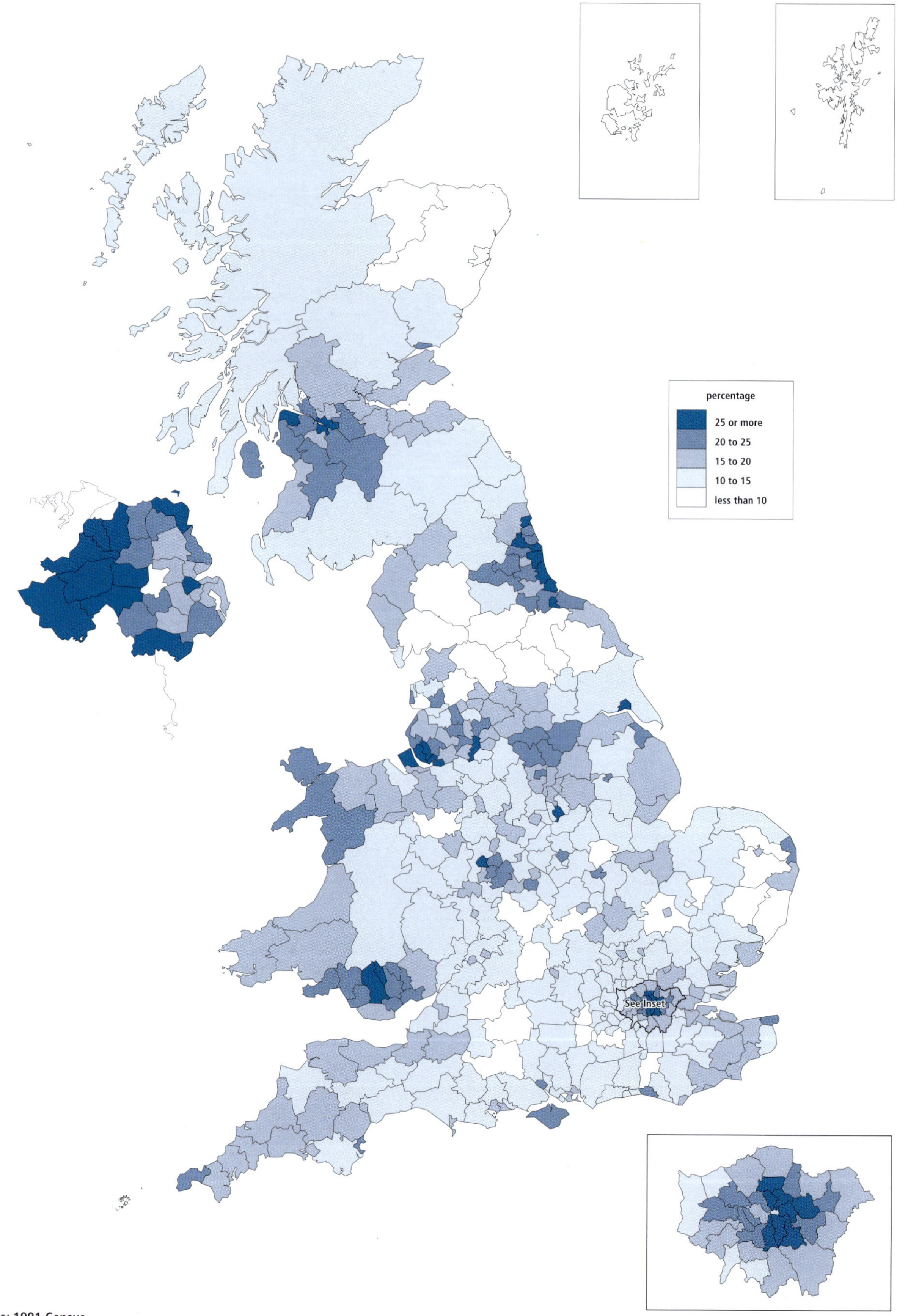

source: 1991 Census

3.5 Unemployment

The relationship between ill health and unemployment[31] and increased mortality risk and unemployment[32, 33] is well documented. Analysis of the 1981 Census cohort from the ONS Longitudinal Study showed that men and women of working ages who were unemployed at the time of the 1981 Census had an excess mortality risk of about 33 per cent between 1981 and 1992.[34]

Later work confirmed earlier findings and showed that between 1986 to 1995 women and men who were unemployed had higher mortality than those who were employed, 45 per cent higher in women.[24] It appears that it is in the regions of England where unemployment is at its highest and duration of unemployment is longest that the unemployed are at the highest risk of premature mortality compared with the general population.[35] Additionally unemployment has been shown to be associated with increased childhood mortality[36] and increased risk of Sudden Infant Death Syndrome (SIDS).[37]

Box 3.2 Differences in Definitions of Unemployment Between the 1991 Census and the 1997 Labour Force Survey

Labour Force Survey

The LFS uses an internationally agreed standard definition of unemployment, based on guidelines issued by the International Labour Office (ILO). This counts people as *unemployed* if they were:

- without a job, and
- available to start work in the 2 weeks following the survey, and
- had either been looking for a job in the 4 weeks before the survey; or
- were waiting to start a job they had obtained.

1991 Census

The Census form asked which of the following each person aged 16 or over was doing in the last week. If more than one box was ticked, the main activity was taken as the first one, in the following order of precedence:

a   On a government employment or training scheme;
b   full-time employee (more than 30 hours a week);
c   part-time employee (one hour or more a week);
d   self-employed, employing other people;
e   self-employed, not employing other people;
f   waiting to start a job;
g   unemployed and looking for a job;
h   at school or in other full-time education;
i   unable to work because of long-term sickness or disability;
j   retired;
k   looking after home or family;
l   other

The Census classification should approximate to that which would have been obtained by interviewers in the LFS, subject to differences resulting from self-classification. The Census included as *unemployed* anyone who ticked boxes f or g listed above.

Source: reproduced from Sly (1994)[38]

This section presents data from both the LFS and the 1991 Census. The LFS is used to present data on unemployment for countries of the United Kingdom and regions of England in 1997. The 1991 Census is used to present unemployment data for local authorities. Although there are differences in the way data are obtained in these two sources (see Box 3.2), results from the 1991 LFS and the 1991 Census have been found to be reassuringly similar.[38]

Figures 3.5 and 3.6 show unemployment rates in 1997 by age, using the International Labour Office (ILO) definition. Of the countries of the United Kingdom, Northern Ireland had the highest rate among men of working ages, but it had an average rate for women of working ages. For women aged 16-59 and men aged 16-24 Wales and Scotland had the highest unemployment. For women age 16-24 Wales had the highest levels. At regional level within England, the highest levels of unemployment for both men and women, aged 16-retirement and 16-24 were found in the North East and London. The lowest regional unemployment rates were in the South East and South West for both men and women.

The pattern of unemployment across the United Kingdom by local authority at the time of the 1991 Census was very similar for men and women and across age groups. Map 3.7 shows that local authorities with high unemployment among males aged 16-24 were located in inner London, Northern Ireland, South Wales, South Yorkshire, Merseyside, Birmingham, Glasgow and the surrounding area, the North East of England and also Cornwall. The highest proportions were found in Knowsley (38 per cent), Liverpool and Hackney (36 per cent). Hackney and Knowsley both also had 26 per cent of 16-24 year old women unemployed.

3.6 Ethnicity

Surveys are the main source of information on the health status of people from minority ethnic groups. Analysis from the General Household Survey showed that Pakistanis and Bangladeshis aged under 65 were more likely to report a limiting long term illness than those in the white ethnic group. However, those in the Indian and Black minority ethnic groups did not have differential rates of limiting long term illness to those in the white ethnic group.[39] Another survey found that those aged 16-74 in all minority ethnic groups were more likely to report their health status as poor than those in the white ethnic group, with Bangladeshis the most likely.[39]

We have used the LFS to update information on the proportion of the population in minority ethnic groups to 1997 for countries and regions. Therefore, for countries other than England and at regional level within England, the percentage of the population in particular minority ethnic groups cannot always be estimated with accuracy, as the sample is not sufficiently large. Data are therefore only included here if their standard errors are less than 20 per cent, as recommended by Schuman.[40] This means that no figures for individual minority ethnic groups are available for Wales, Scotland or Northern Ireland.

Figure 3.7 shows that of the countries of the United Kingdom, England had the largest proportion of its people in minority ethnic groups, 7 per cent compared to 1 per cent or less in the

Figure 3.5

**ILO unemployment rate by country and region, men aged 16-64 and women aged 16-59
United Kingdom 1997**

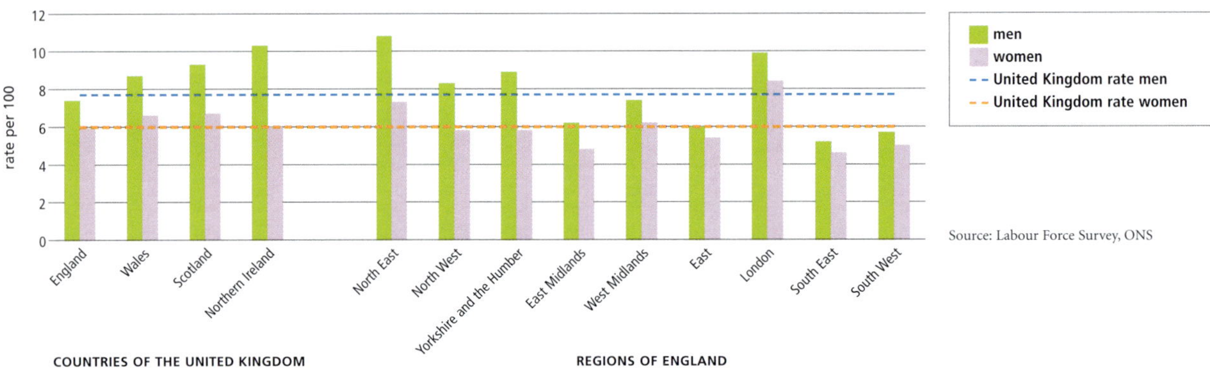

Source: Labour Force Survey, ONS

Figure 3.6

**ILO unemployment rate by country and region, men and women aged 16-24
United Kingdom 1997**

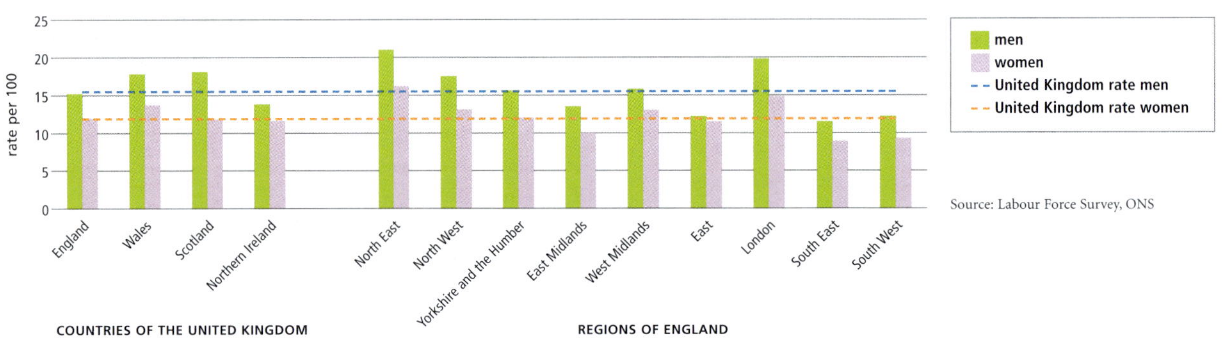

Source: Labour Force Survey, ONS

other three countries. Within the regions of England, London had the largest minority ethnic population - 1.8 million people in 1997. This amounted to a quarter of the total population of London and nearly half the entire minority ethnic population in England. The West Midlands was the region with the second largest minority ethnic population, nearly 10 per cent of the population, half of whom were of Indian and Pakistani origin. The North East and the South West regions had the smallest minority ethnic populations, and it was not possible to estimate numbers in individual groups for these two regions.

London was the only region with a substantial proportion of its population in the Black-African and Bangladeshi groups and London had the largest proportion of the population in the Indian and Black-Caribbean groups, followed by the West and East Midlands. Yorkshire and the Humber had the largest proportion of the population in the Pakistani group, followed by the West Midlands, North West and London. London and the South East were the only regions with large enough Chinese populations to be accurately measured (Figure 3.8).

Data from the 1991 Census allowed a full analysis of the patterns of ethnicity by local authority to be carried out, using detailed categories. This resulted in the publication of a detailed volume on the geography of minority ethnic groups.[41] For this volume, we have not attempted to replicate this for current local authorities, but have chosen broad groupings for ease of analysis across the whole of Great Britain. These are Black (i.e. Black-Caribbean, Black-African, Black-other) and South Asian (i.e. Indian, Pakistani, Bangladeshi). Table 3.1 gives the proportions of the population in the Black and South Asian minority ethnic groups for those authorities with more than 10 per cent of their population in either of these two groups at the time of the 1991 Census. This table confirms the regional picture presented above, but also shows that the geographic concentration of these groups differs. All of those authorities with more than 10 per cent of the population in Black minority ethnic groups were located in London, mostly concentrated in inner London boroughs. In the majority of outer London boroughs less than 5 per cent of the population belonged to Black minority ethnic groups.

Figure 3.7

Percentage of the population in all minority ethnic groups by country and region, persons all ages United Kingdom 1997

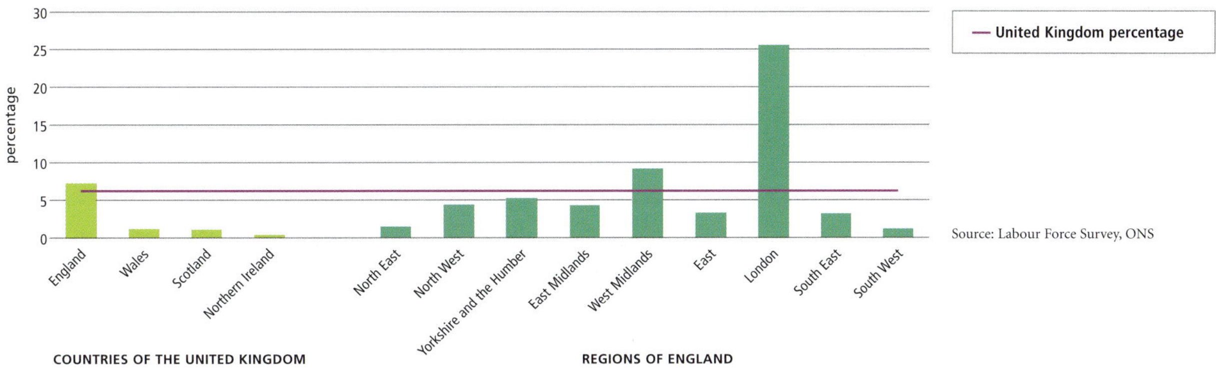

Figure 3.8

Percentage of the population in specific minority ethnic groups by region, persons all ages England 1997

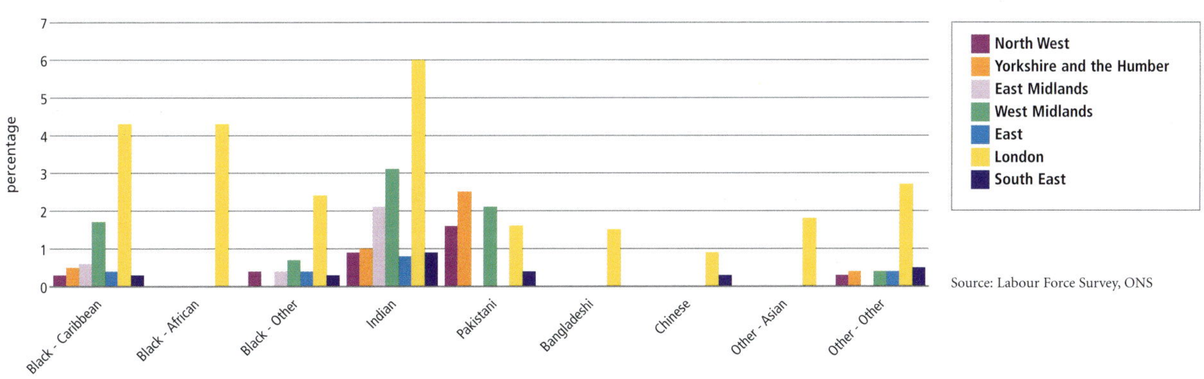

Table 3.1

Local authorities with the highest percentages of the population in Black and South Asian minority ethnic groups Great Britain 1991

LA Name	Black percentage	LA Name	South Asian percentage
Hackney	22	Tower Hamlets	25
Lambeth	22	Leicester	24
Southwark	18	Newham	23
Haringey	17	Slough	21
Brent	17	Brent	20
Lewisham	16	Ealing	19
Newham	14	Harrow	18
Waltham Forest	11	Hounslow	17
Wandsworth	11	Redbridge	14
Islington	11	Blackburn with Darwen	14
Hammersmith and Fulham	10	Birmingham	13
		Bradford	13
		Luton	13
		Wolverhampton	12
		Sandwell	11
		Waltham Forest	10

Source: 1991 Census

Although the South Asian population was more widely spread across England, the majority of local authorities with more than 10 per cent of their population in the South Asian minority ethnic groups were located in London. However, there were also a number in Lancashire, West Yorkshire and part of the Midlands including Birmingham and Leicester, which had the second largest percentage of the population in the South Asian minority ethnic group, 24 per cent. The distribution of the South Asian population in London was different to that of the Black populations, with two areas of concentration, boroughs in the east - Newham and Tower Hamlets, and a group of boroughs in the north west.

3.7 Country of birth

Country of birth is often used as a proxy for ethnicity in the analysis of health variations, largely because ethnicity is not available on the majority of datasets used for monitoring health status. However, analysis of health patterns by country of birth also enables the effects of international migration on health to be considered, for example the incidence of ovarian, cervical and lung cancer among women and prostate cancer among men has been found to be higher among Irish migrants than in the general population.[24]

It is in the study of mortality that most work has been carried out, however. Various studies have shown that the mortality position of international immigrants is not a clear one. For some groups mortality has been shown to be lower than those born in England and Wales, for example for all causes of death in Caribbean men[42] and Bangladeshi women,[43] for cancer in Bangladeshi men and women[43] and for suicide in men and women from Pakistan and Bangladesh.[44]

For others, however rates have been shown to be substantially higher. This is particularly apparent for Irish and Scottish first-generation male migrants who have been shown to have higher mortality than those born in England and Wales for all the main causes of death.[42] Men from the East African Commonwealth have been found to have higher mortality from ischaemic heart disease and respiratory diseases[42] and men from West and South Africa higher mortality from stroke.[42] Those from the Indian subcontinent,[42] Pakistan and Bangladesh[45] have been shown to have high mortality from cardiovascular disease. This was found to be most marked for Bangladeshis and least marked for Indians.[45] Bangladeshi men have also been shown to have higher mortality from diabetes[43] and liver disease.[43, 46] Higher suicide rates have been found in young Indian and East African men and women.[44] The relationships for cardiovascular disease were found to be independent of Social Class.[45] Others have suggested that poverty may account for at least some of the differences in mortality, particularly for tuberculosis.[47]

Differences by country of birth are also found in risk of childhood mortality. Children whose mothers were born in the New Commonwealth have been shown to have higher infant mortality rates than those whose mothers were born in the United Kingdom.[25, 14] However, children of mothers from the New Commonwealth have been found to have 42 per cent lower SIDS rates than those from the United Kingdom.[48] The mortality of children born to Irish migrants[24] and those born in the New Commonwealth[14] and living in England and Wales has been found to be higher than that of children born to all others in England and Wales. The association between infant mortality and country of birth across Wales and the regions of England is discussed in chapter 7.

At country and regional level the analysis in this chapter is restricted to those born in the Republic of Ireland, New Commonwealth, Europe and Rest of the World. Data for Northern Ireland only includes those born in the Republic of Ireland, as data for the other three groups would be unreliable. Box 3.3 shows the composition of these groups. Figure 3.9 shows the split of the population of the United Kingdom by country of birth in 1997 using data from the LFS. Those born in the New Commonwealth were the largest group born outside the United Kingdom in England. Northern Ireland had a larger percentage born in the Republic of Ireland than the other countries. Within England, all the regions except London had a similar proportion of their population born outside the United Kingdom, with the North East having the smallest. London had almost 25 per cent of its population born outside the United Kingdom, with a similar proportion born in the Republic of Ireland to that found in Northern Ireland. The largest proportion was from the New Commonwealth, over 10 per cent.

In order to ensure percentages were based on large enough numbers to present meaningful pictures the analysis at local authority level was restricted to the following groupings - outside the United Kingdom and Republic of Ireland. In the 1991 Census the majority of local authorities in the United Kingdom had less than 5 per cent of their population born outside the United Kingdom (Map 3.8). Most of the local authorities with more than 15 per cent of their population born outside the United Kingdom were located in London. Authorities in inner and west London had the highest proportions born outside the United Kingdom. The majority of authorities in Northern Ireland had a large percentage of the population born in the Republic of Ireland; those with the largest percentages were in the south and west of the country (Map 3.9). Within England, local authorities with high proportions of residents born in the Republic of Ireland were mainly found in London, Manchester and the Birmingham area.

3.8 Living alone

Living alone also seems to be associated with health. Contact rates with GPs appear to be increased for elderly people living alone, about 8 per cent higher than those living with others but not in institutions,[49] and pensioners living alone are more likely to attend accident and emergency centres.[50] Lack of social support, including living alone, also has been found to be associated with an increased risk of mortality after myocardial

Box 3.3 Country of birth categories

United Kingdom
England
Wales
Scotland
Northern Ireland
United Kingdom (part not stated)
Isle of Man
Channel Islands

Republic of Ireland
Republic of Ireland
Ireland (part not stated)

New Commonwealth
Kenya
Malawi
Tanzania
Uganda
Zambia
Zimbabwe
Botswana
Lesotho and Swaziland
Gambia
Ghana
Nigeria
Sierra Leone
Barbados
Jamaica
Trinidad and Tobago
Other Independent States
Caribbean Dependent Territories
West Indies (so stated)
Belize
Guyana
Bangladesh
Pakistan

India
Sri Lanka
Hong Kong
Malaysia
Singapore
Cyprus
Malta and Gozo
Mauritius
Seychelles
other New Commonwealth

Europe
Belgium
Denmark
France
Netherlands
Germany
Austria
Luxembourg
Finland
Sweden
Italy
Greece
Portugal
Spain
Norway
Switzerland
USSR
Albania
Bulgaria
Czechoslovakia
Hungary
Poland
Romania
Yugoslavia
other Europe

Rest of the World
Australia
New Zealand
Canada
Turkey
Iran
Iraq
Israel
Jordan
Lebanon
Saudi Arabia
Syria
other Middle East
Myanmar
China
Japan
Philippines
Taiwan
Thailand
Vietnam
other Asia
Algeria
Egypt
Libya
Morocco
Tunisia
Republic of South Africa
other Africa
USA
Central America
Brazil
Colombia
other South America
Caribbean non-New Commonwealth
Rest of World
At sea/In air

Figure 3.9

**Percentage of the population by country of birth, excluding United Kingdom, by country and region, persons all ages
United Kingdom 1997**

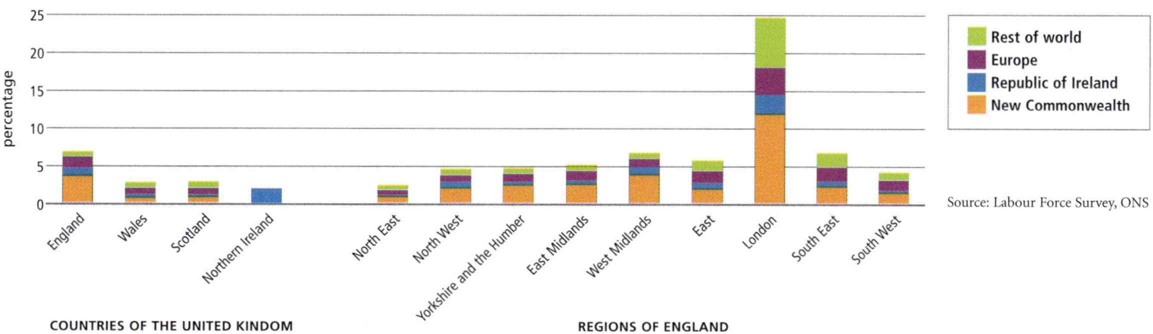

Source: Labour Force Survey, ONS

Map 3.8

Percentage of the population born outside the United Kingdom at the 1991 Census by local authority
United Kingdom 1991

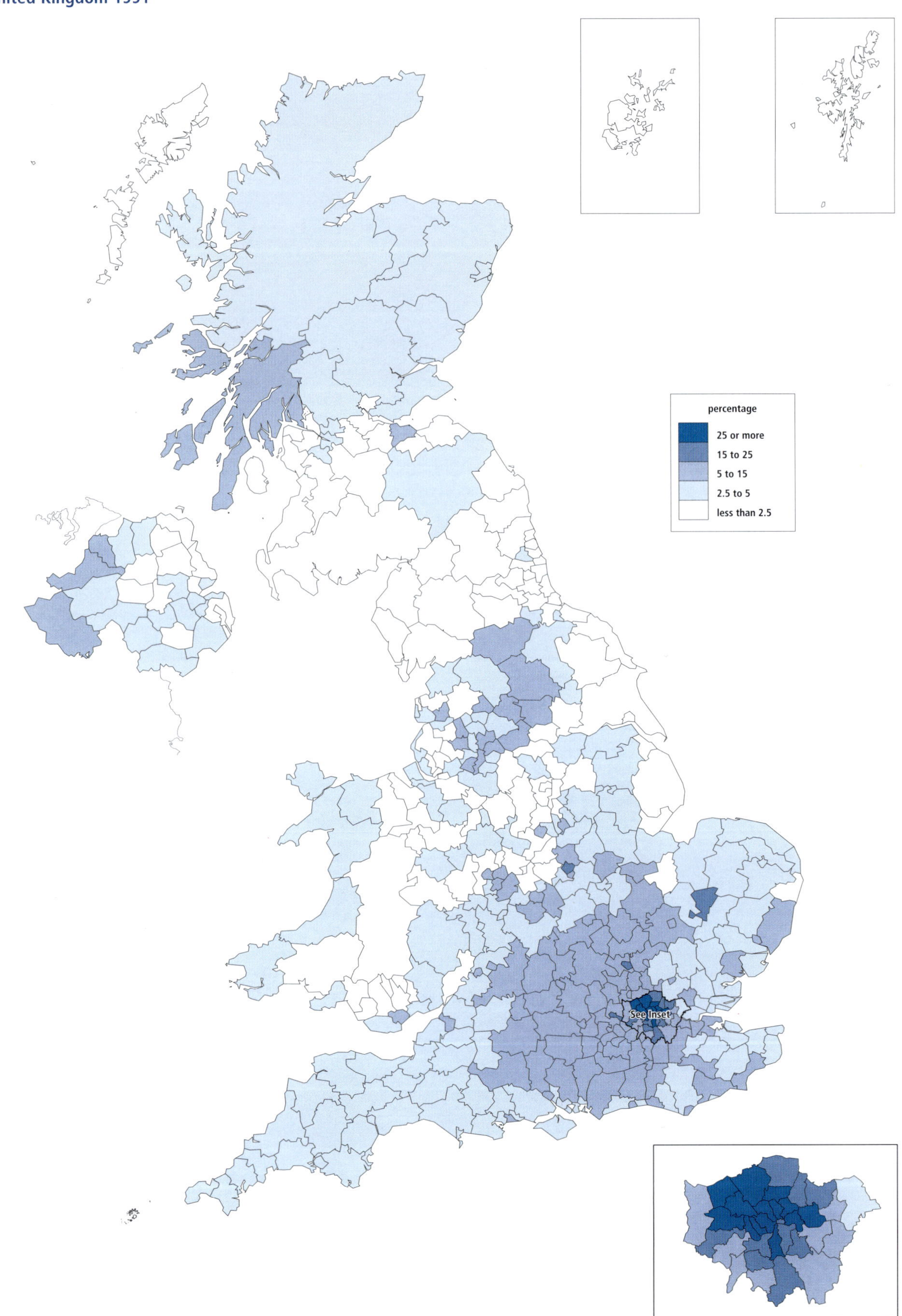

source: 1991 Census

Map 3.9

**Percentage of the population born in the Republic of Ireland at the 1991 Census by local authority
United Kingdom 1991**

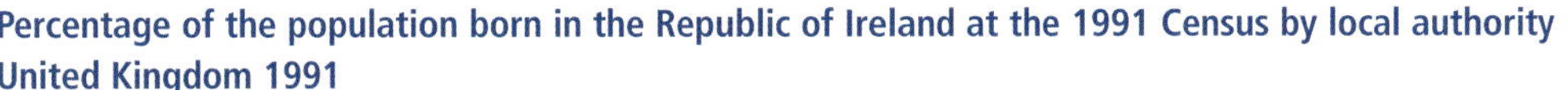

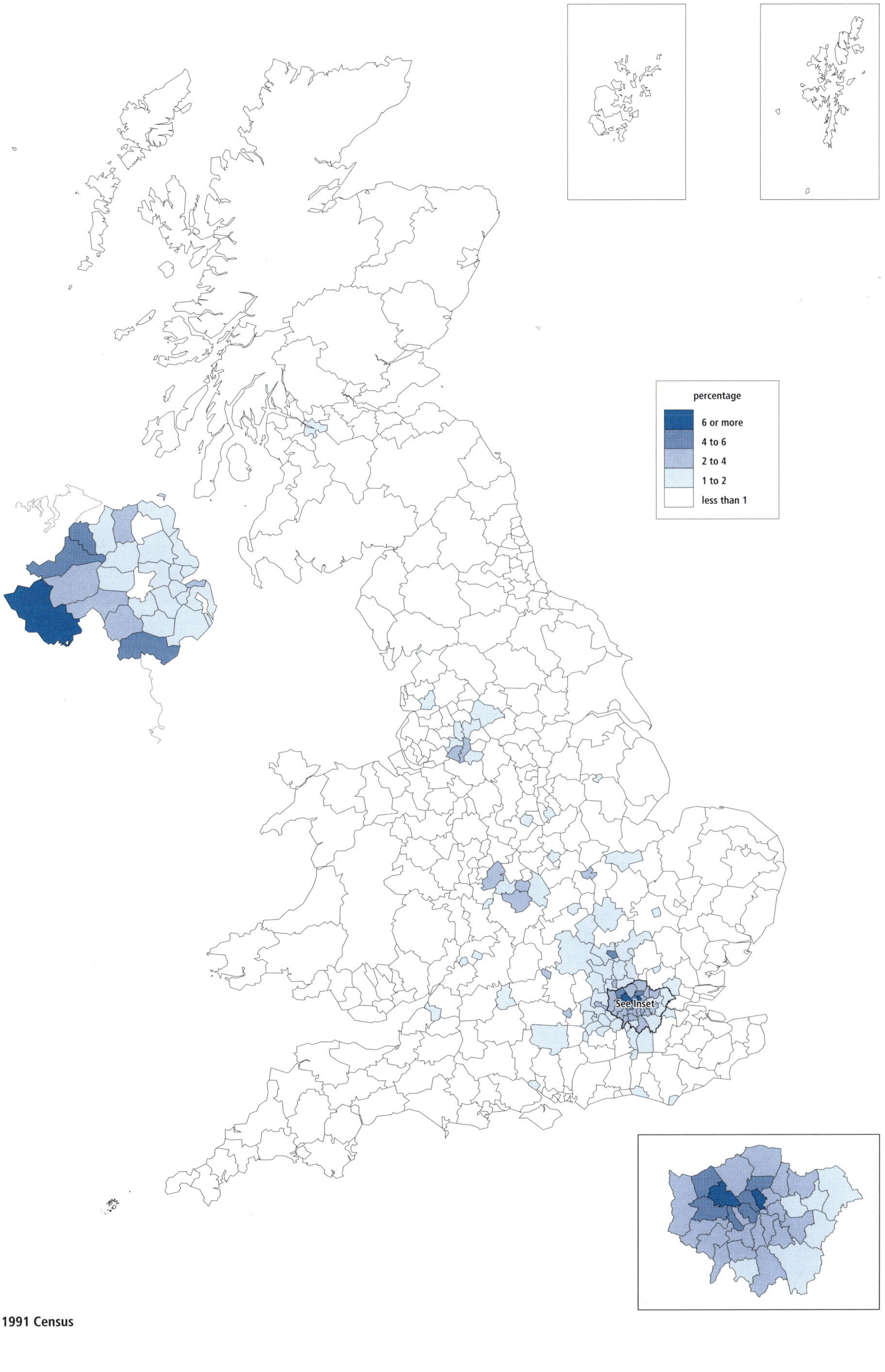

source: 1991 Census

Figure 3.10

**Percentage of people in one person households by country and region, persons all ages
United Kingdom 1997**

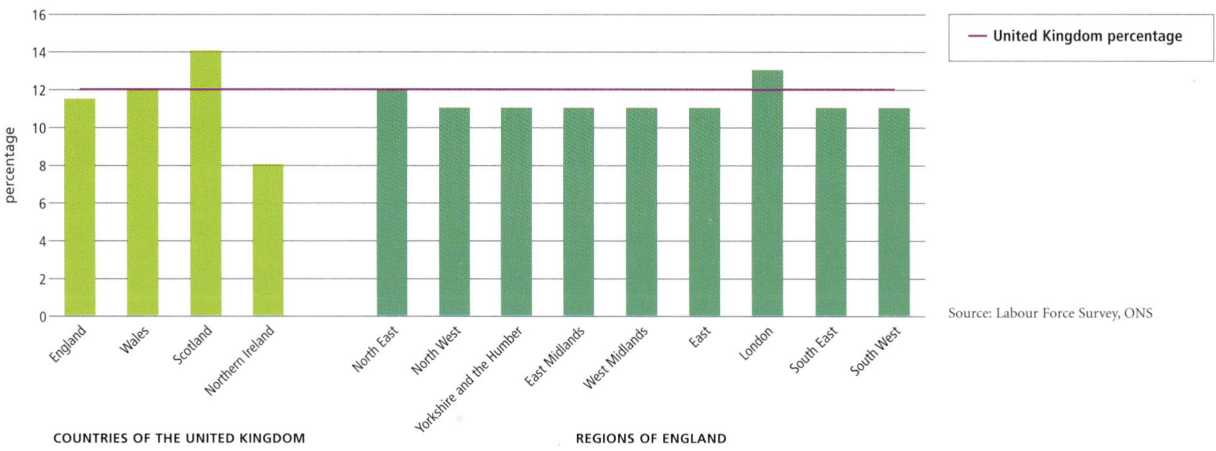

infarction. The risk for those with little or no social support seems to be over twice the risk for those with good social support over the first ten years after myocardial infarction.[51] Those living alone also seem likely to choose a worse diet than those living with others, which can lead to increased risk of poorer health outcomes.[52, 53]

Figure 3.10 shows the proportion of people who lived in one person households in 1997, using data from the Labour Force Survey. Of the countries of the United Kingdom, Scotland had the highest proportion of people living in a one person household and Northern Ireland had a substantially lower proportion than the other countries. Within England, all the regions had similar proportions of people living in one person households, except for London and the North East which had larger proportions.

At the time of the 1991 Census, in most local authorities in the United Kingdom, there was only a small proportion (under 10 per cent) of households containing one person. Like the patterns by region, the exception to this was again in London, where the inner authorities had larger proportions of households of this type (Map 3.10). Larger proportions were also seen in other major centres of population, coastal authorities and rural authorities within Scotland and the north of England. Small proportions of people living alone were seen in the majority of authorities in Northern Ireland, as would be expected from the pattern for the country as a whole.

Examining separately the proportion of pensioners in each area that live alone gives an idea of the potential effect on provision of health and social services and retirement accommodation. Figure 3.11 shows that in 1997, Scotland had the highest proportion of pensioners living alone. Forty per cent of pensioners were living alone compared with just over thirty per cent in Northern Ireland, the country with the lowest proportion of pensioners living alone. Across the regions of England, the North East and London had the highest

proportion of pensioners living alone, and the South West had the lowest.

At local authority level, high proportions of pensioners living alone were found in inner London, the Pennine area, the North East and Scotland, and also in towns and cities scattered throughout the United Kingdom. Low proportions were found in more remote rural areas and in Northern Ireland (Map 3.11).

3.9 Lone parent families

A number of studies have shown risks to health for lone parents and also for the children of lone parents. Lone mothers have been found to have high rates of depression compared to the general population, even after controlling for age, income and education.[54] Higher rates of illness[55] and poor self-reported general health[56] have also been found among lone mothers, compared to other mothers and to the general population. Lone parenthood has also been found to be an independent risk factor for lower rates of childhood immunisation,[57] putting children at increased risk of infectious disease. An increased risk of infant and childhood mortality has been found for children born to lone mothers.[14]

However, most children live in couple family households. In 1997 just over four fifths of children lived in this household type and the majority of the remainder lived in lone parent family households. There was little variation at country level in the percentage of children living in lone parent families, with the main features being the smaller percentage in Northern Ireland, and slightly higher proportion in Wales. There was more variation at regional level within England. The percentage of children living in lone parent family households was greatest in London; a fifth of children compared with just over a tenth in the East of England region, the region with the lowest proportion of children living in lone parent households (Figure 3.12).

Figure 3.11

**Percentage of pensioners in one person households by country and region
United Kingdom 1997**

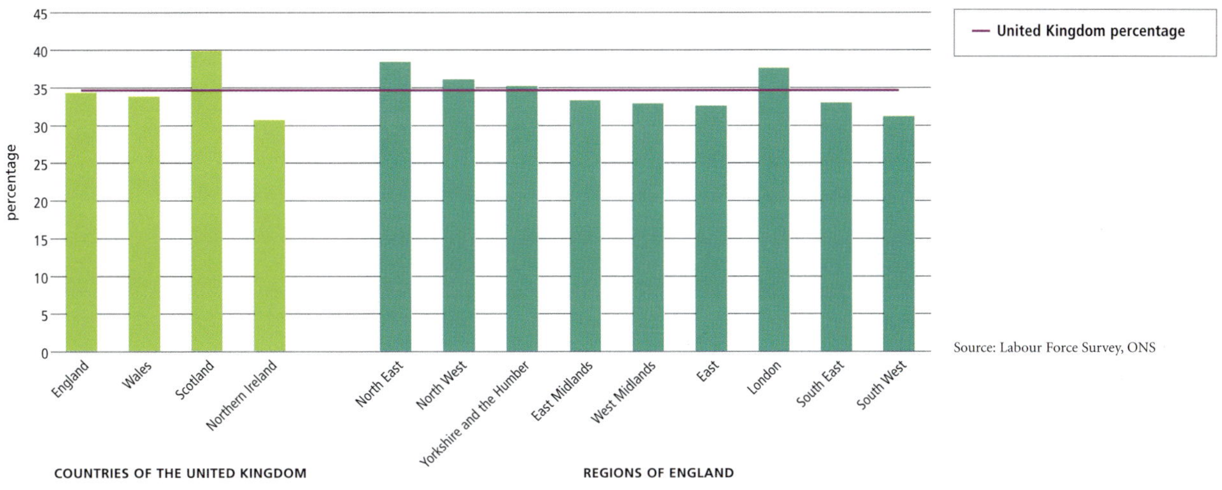

Figure 3.12

**Percentage of dependent children living in lone parent families by country and region
United Kingdom 1997**

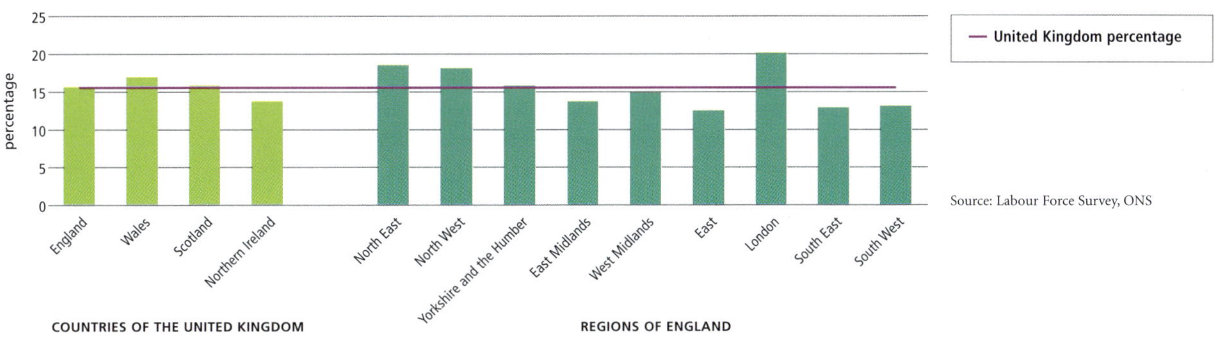

At local authority level, variation was wider and in 1991 there were high proportions of children living in lone parent households in major centres of population and low proportions in the surrounding suburban and rural areas (Map 3.12).

3.10 Housing tenure and access to cars

Over recent years there has been increasing interest in the analysis of patterns in health by housing characteristics and access to cars as an alternative to using Social Class or income. Both are thought to be a useful indicator of household assets and resources and useful in defining variations in health.

Early studies found that mortality in the 1970s and 1980s was higher among people in local authority housing, or without access to a car and lower among owner-occupiers or those with access to a car.[58] The same study also found that mortality differentials between those who had access to cars and were owner occupiers and those who did not have these characteristics had increased between the 1970s and the 1980s, and that the greatest differentials were found for lung cancer and respiratory disease mortality.

Analysis using 25 years of data from the ONS Longitudinal Study found that both childhood and adult circumstances (defined using housing tenure, car access and Social Class) were important predictors of limiting long term illness and premature mortality in adulthood, although the association with current socio-economic position appeared strongest. Accidents and injuries accounted for most of the premature deaths. Persisting disadvantage throughout the 25 years was significantly associated with worse health and survival.[59]

Being in rented accommodation and in a household with no access to a car in 1971 and 1981 has been shown to give an increased risk of mortality of 35-45 per cent over 21 years to

Map 3.10

**Percentage of people living in one person households at the 1991 Census by local authority
United Kingdom 1991**

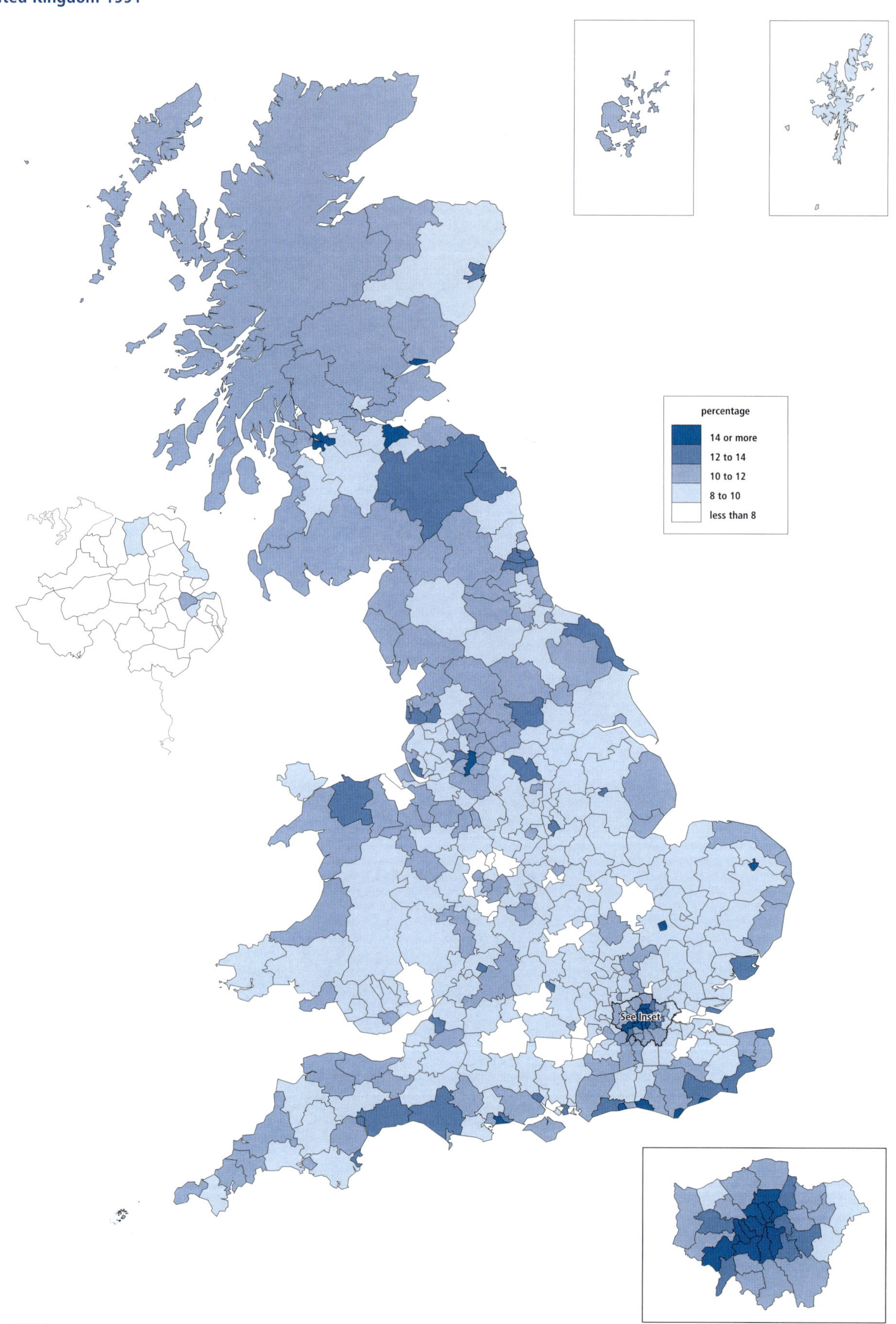

source: 1991 Census

Map 3.11

**Percentage of pensioners living in one person households at the 1991 Census by local authority
United Kingdom 1991**

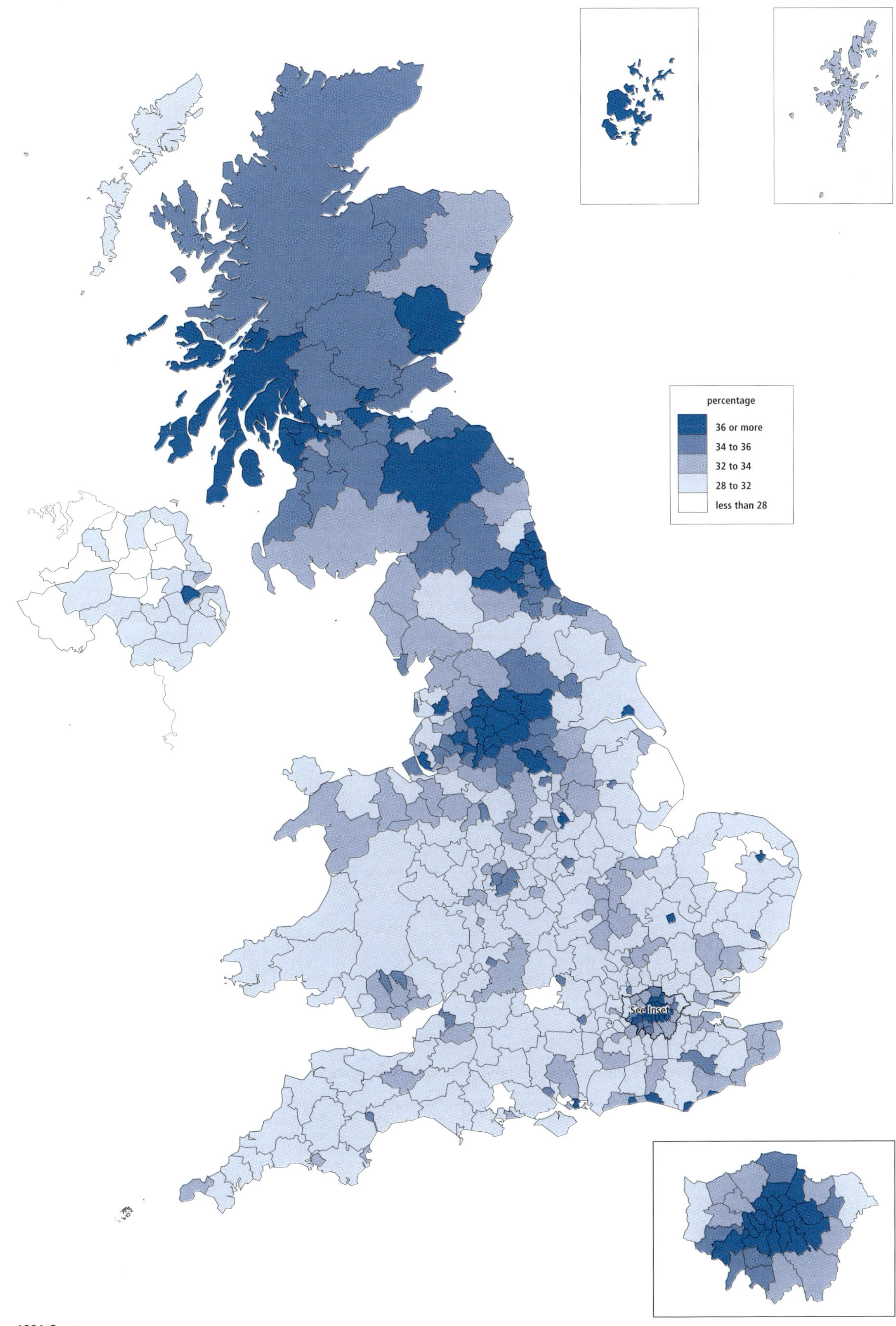

source: 1991 Census

Map 3.12

Percentage of dependent children living in lone parent households at the 1991 Census by local authority
United Kingdom 1991

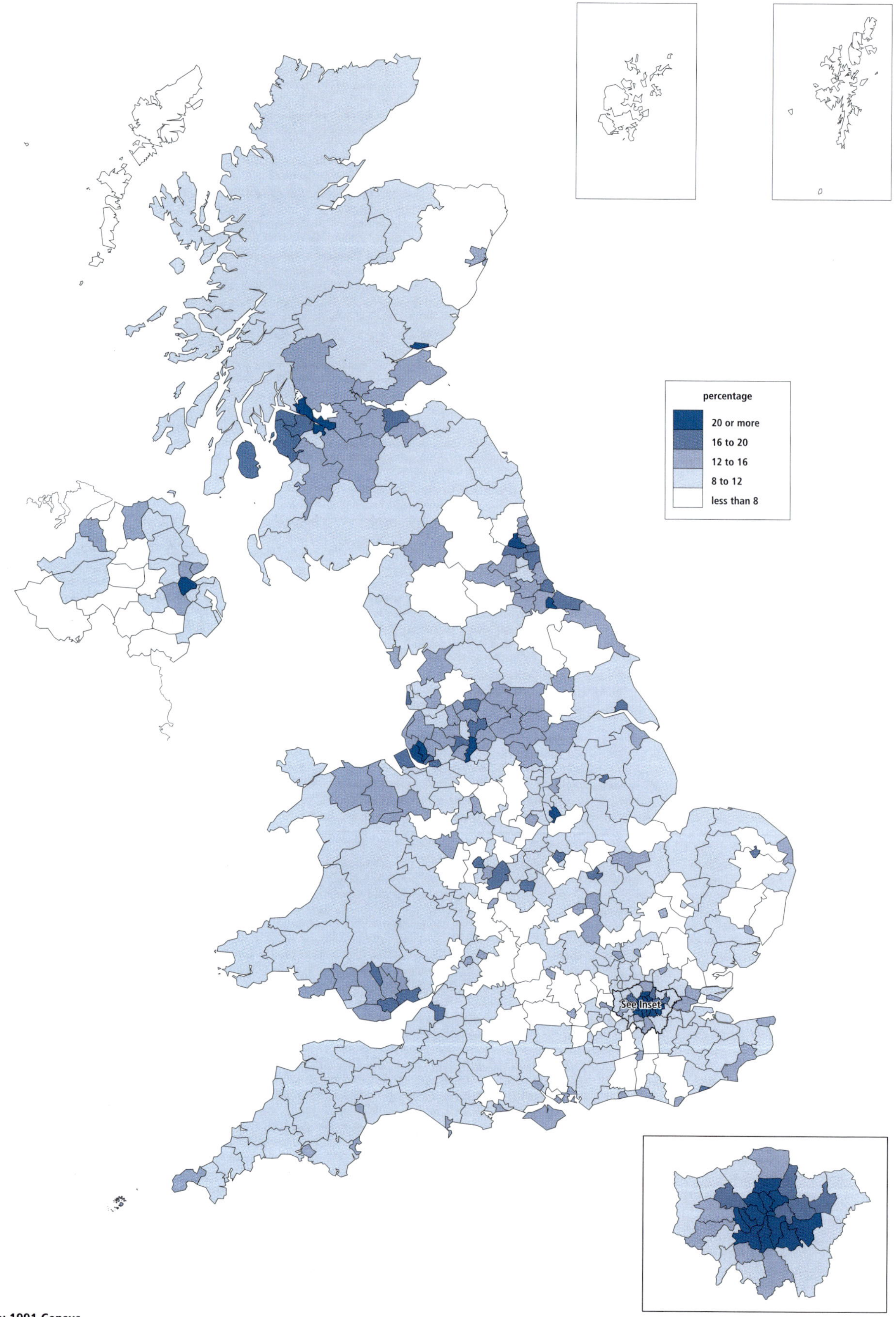

source: 1991 Census

Figure 3.13

**Percentage of households by tenure, country and region
United Kingdom 1997**

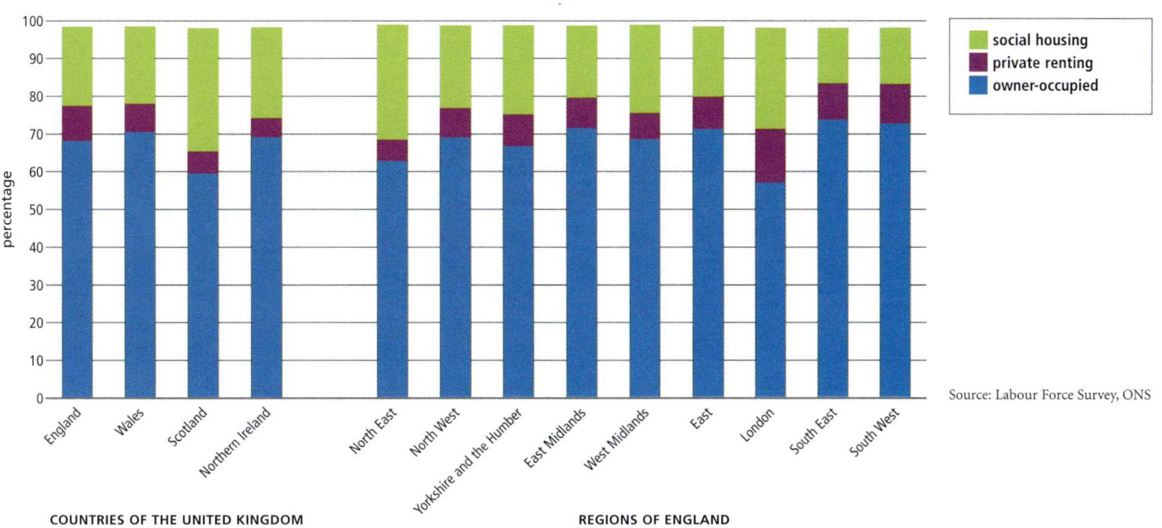

1992, and was also associated with an increased risk of living in an institution by 1991. Losing access to a car or moving into rented accommodation between 1971 and 1981 was also an important factor in increased mortality by 1992 and increased risk of being in an institution by 1991.[60]

Incidence of breast cancer has been found to be higher among women who were owner-occupiers compared to renters at ages 65 and over. At younger ages, incidence was higher among renters and survival poorer. Prostate cancer incidence was also found to be higher among men who were owner-occupiers, but no differences by tenure were found in six-year survival.[24]

Disadvantaged social circumstances, defined by living in rented housing, are not only associated with mortality but also teenage motherhood, with teenagers living in rented accommodation being more likely to become teenage mothers than those living in owner-occupied accommodation. This was found to be independent of whether or not the teenager's own mother had herself been a teenage mother.[24]

Analysis of the relationship between car access, housing tenure and mortality across Wales and the regions of England is described in chapter 12.

Figure 3.13 shows the breakdown of households by tenure in countries and regions of the United Kingdom for the three main types of tenure. At country level, Scotland had a different tenure profile to the other countries of the United Kingdom with a smaller than average proportion of households living in owner-occupied housing and a larger than average proportion living in social housing. Northern Ireland also had a higher percentage of households living in social housing than England or Wales, although it had similar levels of owner occupancy. At regional level within England, London and the North East had the lowest

percentages of households living in owner-occupied accommodation and the highest percentages living in social housing. London also had the highest proportion of households living in private-rented accommodation. The South East had the highest proportion living in owner-occupied accommodation.

At local authority level in 1991, high proportions of owner occupancy were found within England and Wales in suburban and rural areas. Major towns and cities had a low proportion of people living in owner-occupied housing (Map 3.13). This is especially true of inner London, where the very lowest levels of owner occupancy were found.

Private renting was common in the majority of authorities in London, the South West and Wales (Map 3.14). In addition, the map also shows that areas with large numbers of students such as Manchester, Liverpool, Oxford, Cambridge and Brighton had higher levels of private renting. Low proportions of people lived in privately rented accommodation in clusters of authorities in the North West, south Wales, Tyne and Wear and central Scotland.

Map 3.15 shows that most authorities in Scotland and Northern Ireland had over 20 per cent of the population living in social housing, as might be expected from the discussions of patterns at country level. However, some authorities in England and Wales had proportions very similar to this, for example parts of east inner London, Tyne and Wear, south Yorkshire and the West Midlands, and Torfaen and Wrexham in Wales.

Figure 3.14 shows that in all countries of the United Kingdom and regions of England in 1997 it was most common for households to have access to one car, except for the North East of England where it was more common to have no access to a car. In Scotland a high proportion of households had no access

Figure 3.14

Percentage of households by car access level, country and region United Kingdom 1997

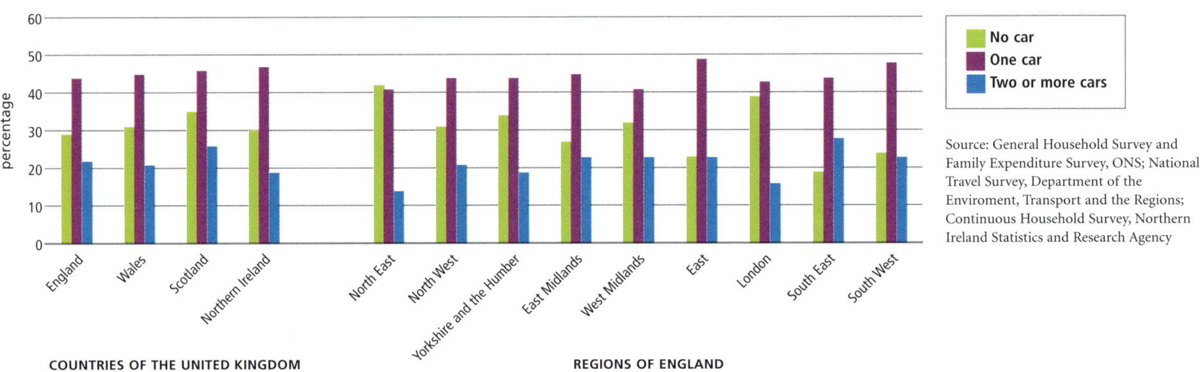

Source: General Household Survey and Family Expenditure Survey, ONS; National Travel Survey, Department of the Enviroment, Transport and the Regions; Continuous Household Survey, Northern Ireland Statistics and Research Agency

to a car, as did households in London. The South East region had the largest percentage of households with access to two or more cars and the smallest percentage of households with no access to a car.

There was wide variation between local authorities across the United Kingdom in the proportion of people in households without access to a car, ranging from 59.8 per cent in Glasgow City to 6.3 per cent in Hart. The area around Glasgow had a number of local authorities with high proportion of residents having no access to a car, as did Belfast, Liverpool, Knowsley, Manchester, authorities around Birmingham, inner London and most other major towns and cities. Authorities with low proportions of the population without car access were found in rural and suburban areas, largely in England and Wales (Map 3.16).

3.11 Migration

The health status of those who move within the country compared to those who do not has been much examined and the patterns seen are complex. Analysis in the previous Decennial Supplement on geography found that generally migrants had higher mortality than non-migrants. However, movers into areas of high status tended to have similar or lower mortality rates than the mortality rate for the area they moved into.[61] Fox and Goldblatt found that migrants who moved short distances had higher mortality rates than those who moved long distance.[6] Migrants had lower mortality from stroke and ischaemic heart disease than non-migrants, about 10 per cent lower after adjusting for housing tenure, access to cars and area of original residence and destination.[62]

The data on migration in this section come from the ONS Longitudinal Study (LS). The study is a 1 per cent sample of residents of England and Wales and is described in Appendix A. The base population used in this section is those LS members present at both the 1981 and 1991 Census. Data are analysed for regions within England and for Wales. The following populations are excluded: international migrants (including those moving to/from Scotland, Northern Ireland and the

Republic of Ireland in the period 1981-1991); those born after 1981; those from the 1981 Census who died before the 1991 Census and those who were not included on a relevant Census form. Only moves between regions and/or Wales are considered in the analysis and no information was available on moves that may have taken place in the intercensal period.

Using analysis of the LS, between 1981 and 1991, 89.3 per cent of people remained within the same region, that is they did not move, or only moved within the same region. There was very little sex difference between those who moved and those who did not. Figures 3.15 and 3.16 describe where inter-regional migrants had moved from in terms of their 1991 region and where they moved to in terms of their 1981 region respectively, as a proxy for distance moved in that time.

Figure 3.15 shows the percentage coming from contiguous counties. These figures reflect both the "pull" of the destination region to attract long distance internal migrants, and the juxtaposition of the regions. The North East region is contiguous to just two English counties, whereas the East Midlands is contiguous to 12. The North East had the lowest percentage of internal migrants from neighbouring counties at 14 per cent, with the South East receiving 57 per cent from neighbouring counties.

Figure 3.16 shows the percentage of those migrating to contiguous counties by 1991 by their region in 1981. Fifty-one per cent of those migrating out from London moved to one of the six neighbouring counties (compared with 35 per cent of in-migrants from contiguous counties reported in Figure 3.15), with only 15 per cent of those moving out of the North East recorded in the two neighbouring counties.

Figures 3.17-3.19 look at the effect that migration has had on the populations of different areas between 1981 and 1991. Figure 3.17 shows the change in the population of the regions caused by these patterns of migration. London experienced a decline of just over 8 per cent, while the South West experienced an increase of just under 8 per cent. Higher proportions of the population of the southern regions of England, including London, had moved

Map 3.13

**Percentage of people in owner-occupied accommodation at the 1991 Census by local authority
United Kingdom 1991**

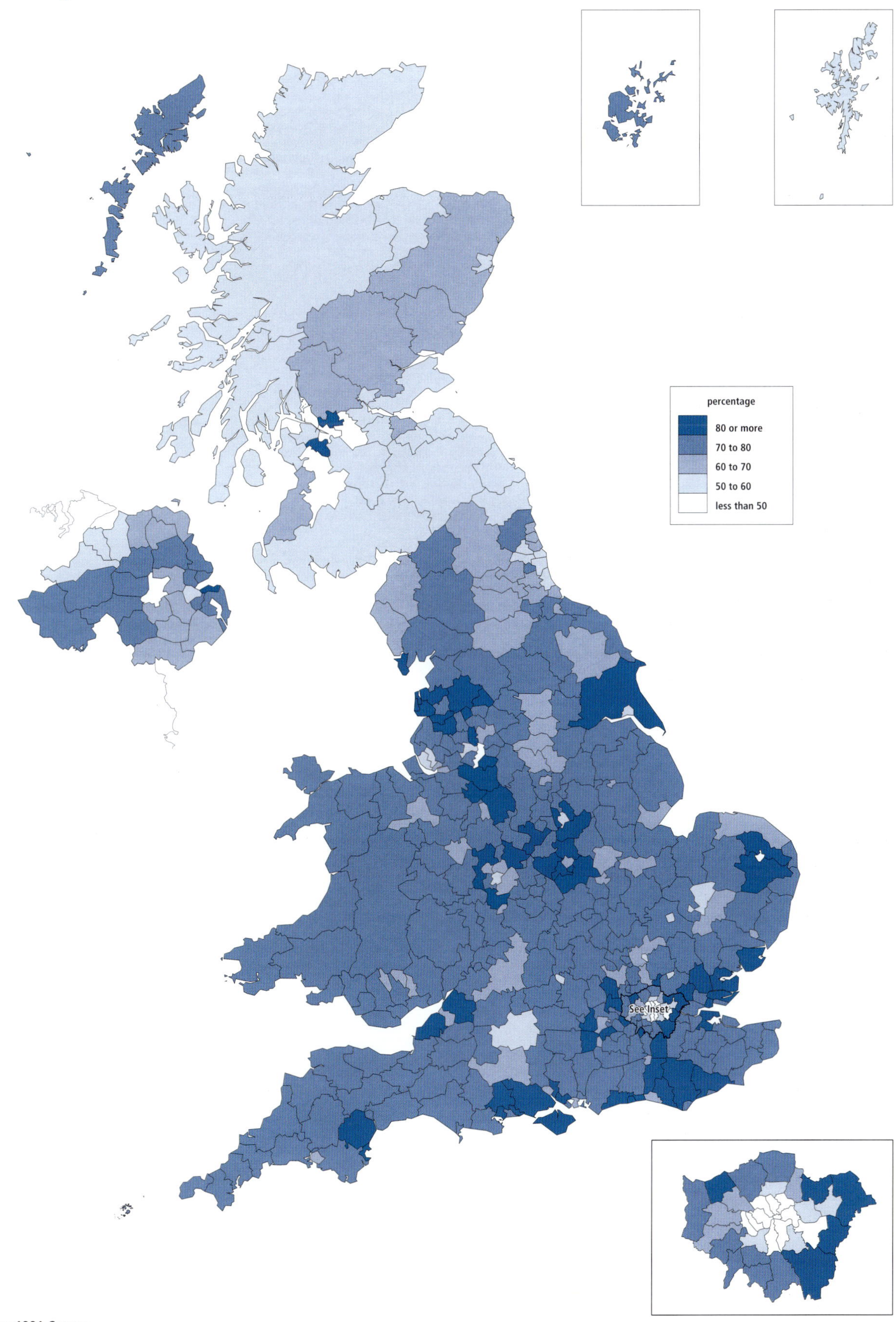

source: 1991 Census

Map 3.14

**Percentage of people in private-rented accommodation at the 1991 Census by local authority
United Kingdom 1991**

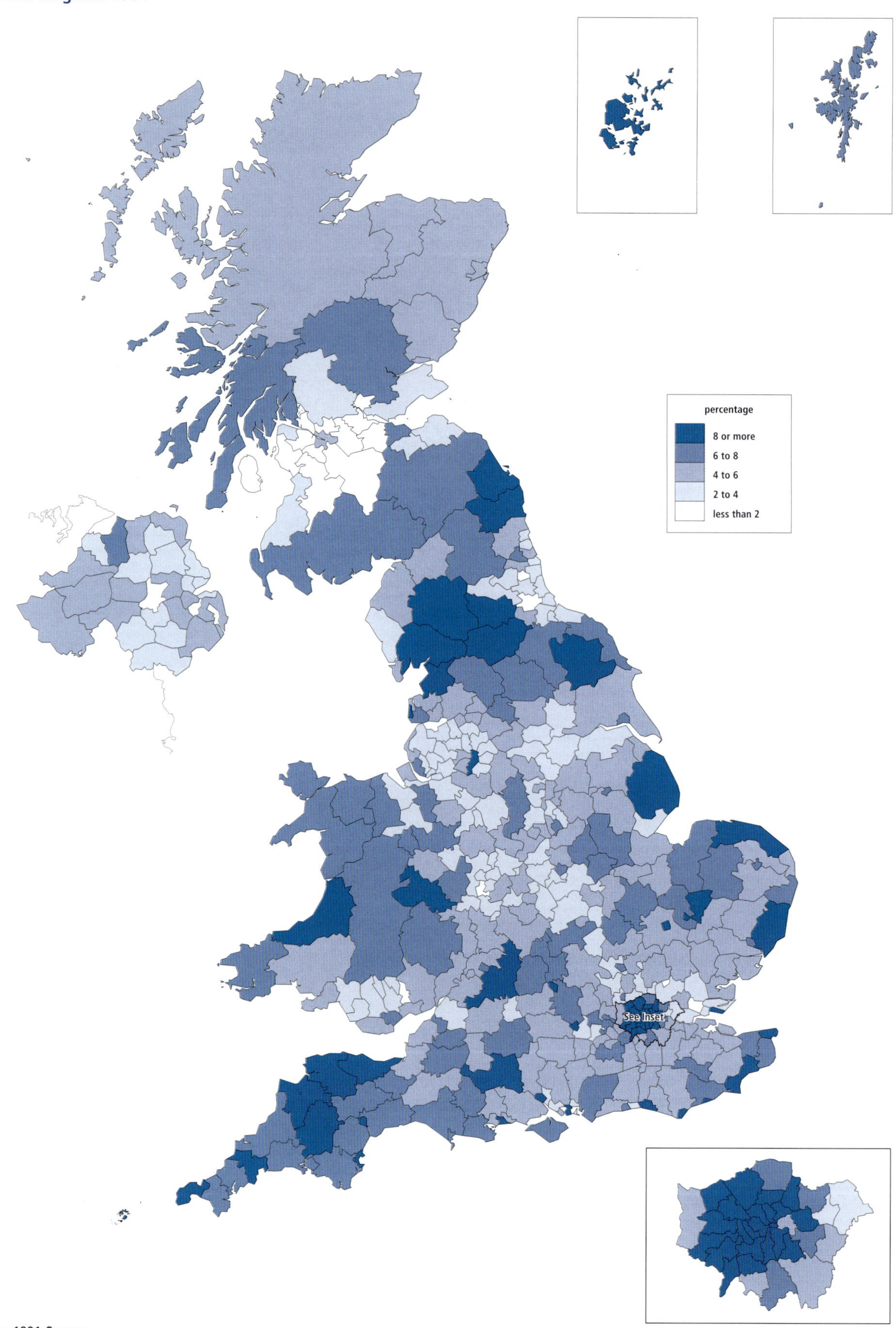

source: 1991 Census

Map 3.15

**Percentage of people in social housing at the 1991 Census by local authority
United Kingdom 1991**

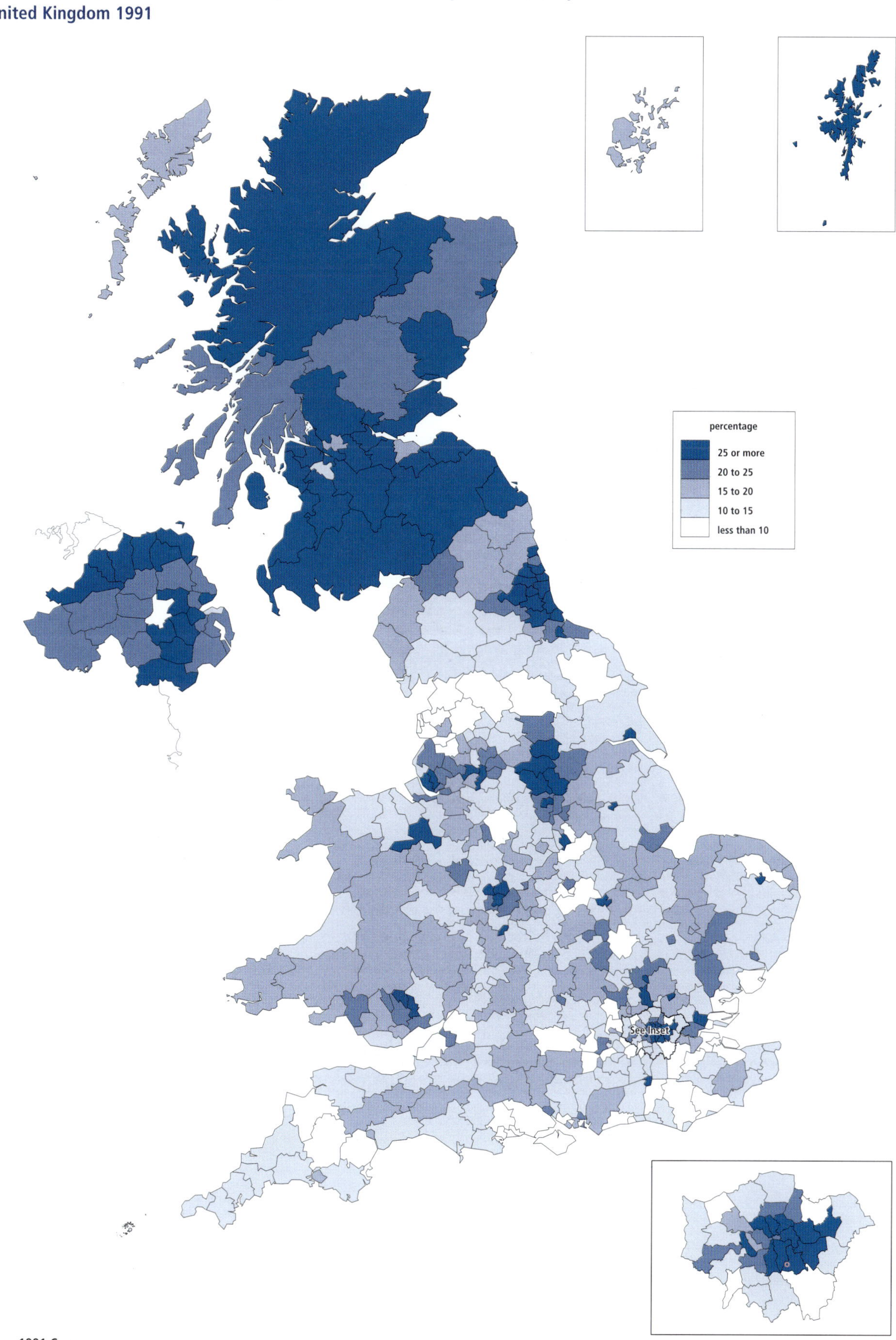

source: 1991 Census

Map 3.16

**Percentage of people in households with no access to a car at the 1991 Census by local authority
United Kingdom 1991**

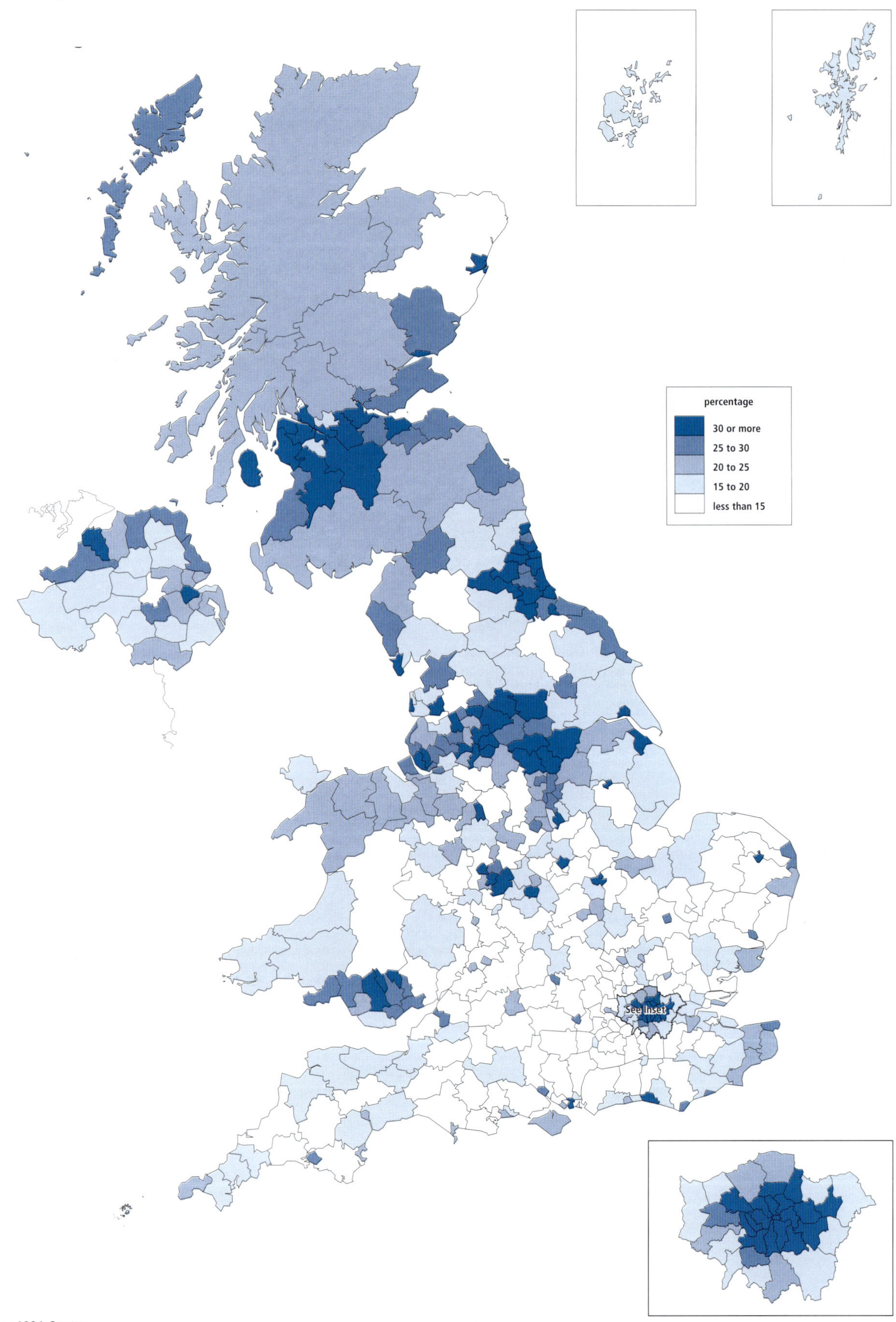

source: 1991 Census

Figure 3.15

Where inter-regional migrants were in 1981 by country or region in 1991
England and Wales 1991

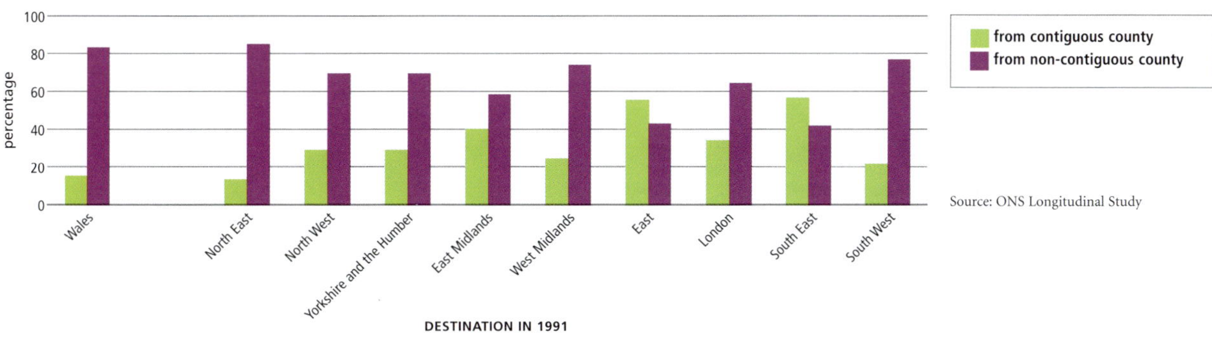

Figure 3.16

Where inter-regional migrants went to in 1991 by their 1981 country or region
England and Wales 1991

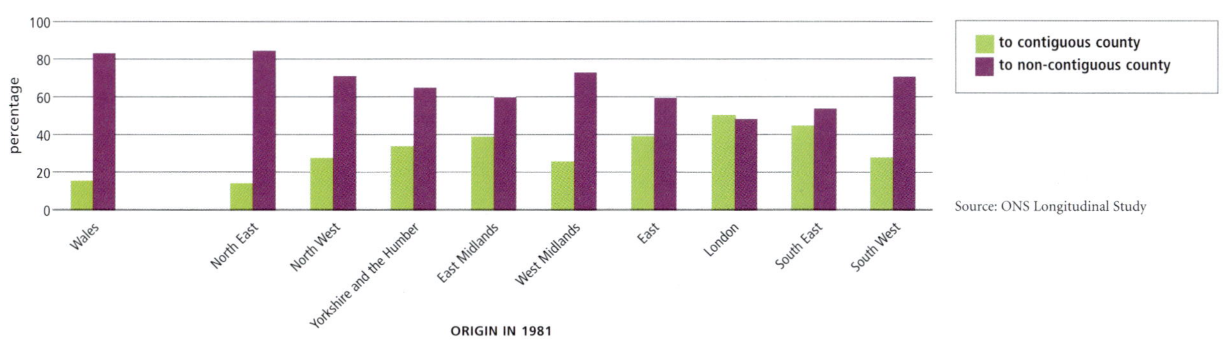

between 1981 and 1991 compared to the northern regions or Wales (Figure 3.18). The southern regions had a greater proportion of their 1991 population made up of people who had been in a different region 10 years earlier (Figure 3.19).

Figures 3.20 and 3.21 look at the age distribution of people who moved, by broad age band. People who moved were generally likely to be aged between 15 and 44, with over half of movers being in this age group. Of the remaining age groups, Figure 3.20 shows that people leaving their 1981 region were more likely to be under 15 in all areas except London, where people leaving were more likely to be aged 45-64. The northern regions had higher proportions of movers aged under 15 than the southern regions. Figure 3.21 shows the age profile at 1991 of those who had moved since 1981. In all regions those who had moved were most likely to be in the 45-64 age group, after the 15-44 age group. The South West and Wales had larger proportions of people arriving who were in the 65 and over age group than other parts of England and Wales.

More detail on migration can be found in the *Key Population and Vital Statistics*[63] publications and elsewhere,[64, 65] but more detailed analysis is beyond the scope of this volume.

3.12 Health-related behaviour

There is a large literature relating to certain behaviours and health or mortality. These include smoking, diet and alcohol consumption, which are the behaviours focused on in this section. Smoking has long been known to cause lung cancer[66, 67, 68, 69] and it is also related to ischaemic heart disease.[70] Research has also found smoking to be linked to other cancers, such as oesophageal cancer.[71] Oesophageal cancer has also been linked to alcohol consumption[72], as has general excess mortality.[72] Poor diet has also been linked to breast cancer[73] and ischaemic heart disease.[70, 74, 75]

People in all countries of the United Kingdom had a similar proportion of energy derived from fat, at around 40 per cent. Of the regions of England, London residents had the smallest percentage of energy derived from fat and the East Midlands the largest, although all were similar. Those in the London region also had a higher percentage of energy derived from cereals than those in other regions, higher than the percentage derived from fat (a pattern not seen in any other region). Those in Scotland had a higher proportion of energy coming from meat products (Figure 3.22).

Figure 3.17

Change in the population due to migration between 1981 and 1991
England and Wales 1991

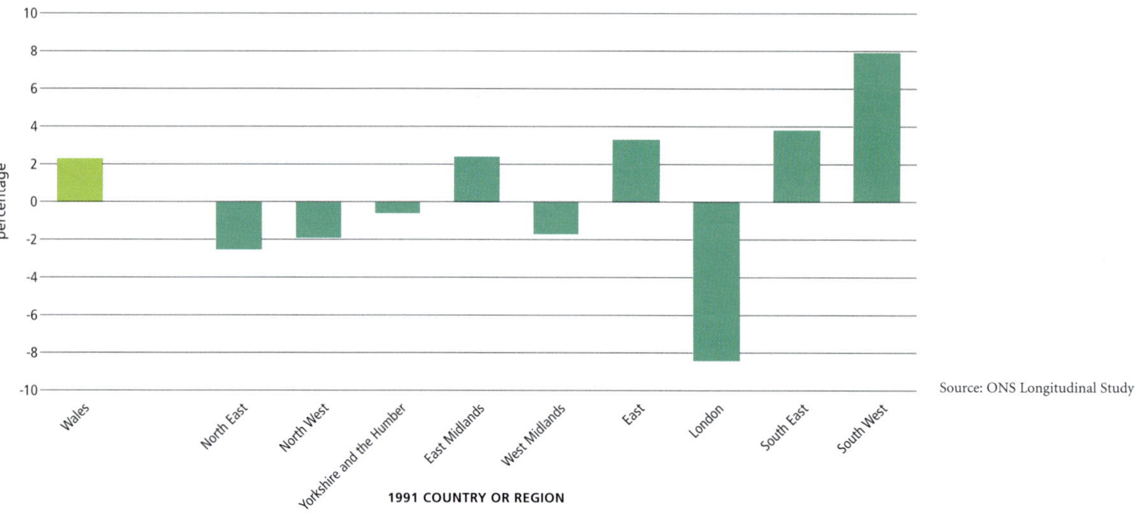

Source: ONS Longitudinal Study

Figure 3.18

Percentage of 1981 population who had left their 1981 region by 1991
England and Wales 1991

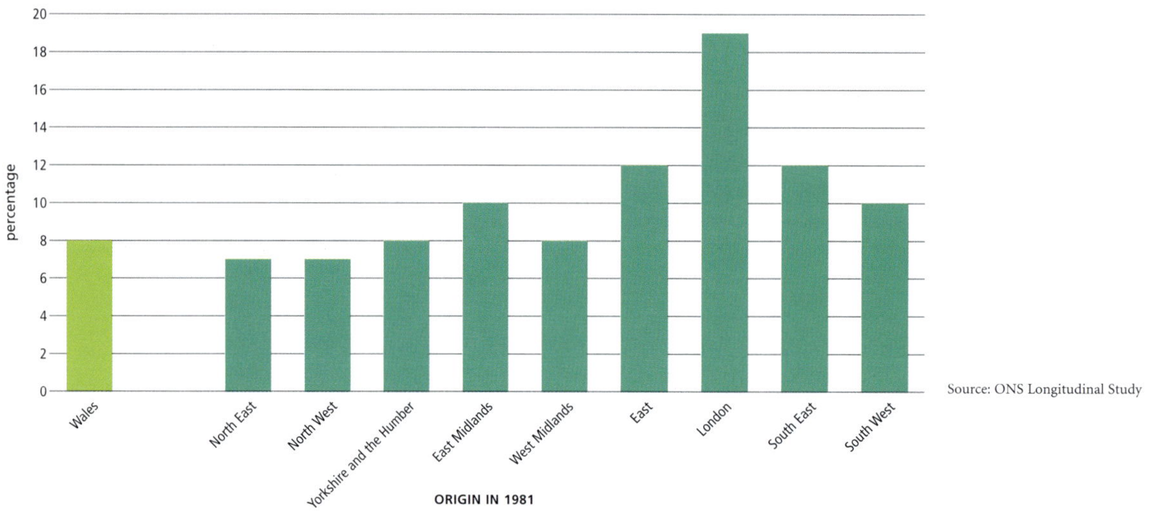

Source: ONS Longitudinal Study

Figure 3.19

Percentage of 1991 population who had been in a different region in 1981
England and Wales 1991

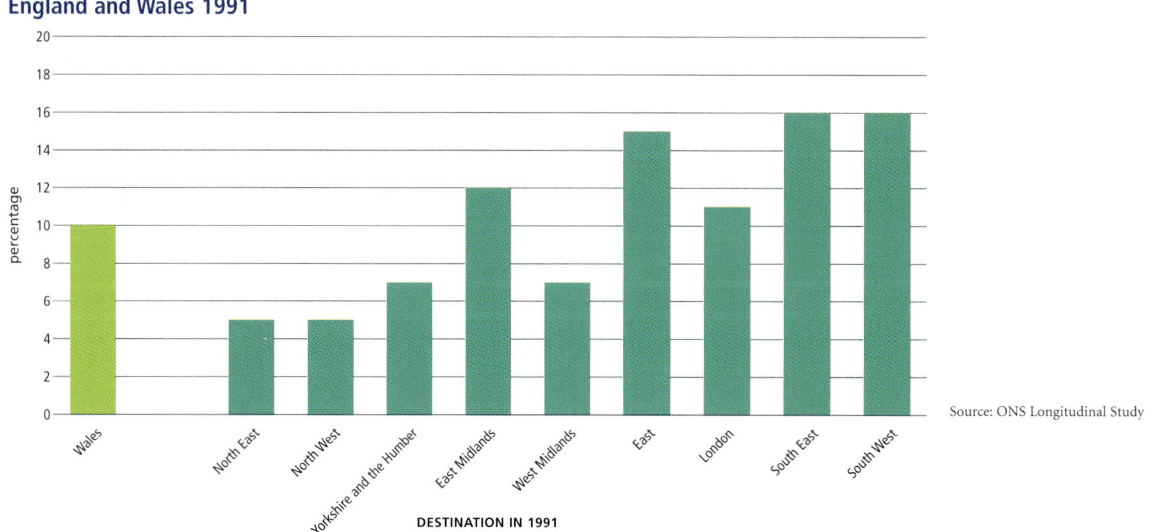

Source: ONS Longitudinal Study

Figure 3.20

Age profile of those who had left their 1981 region by 1991, age at 1981*
England and Wales 1991

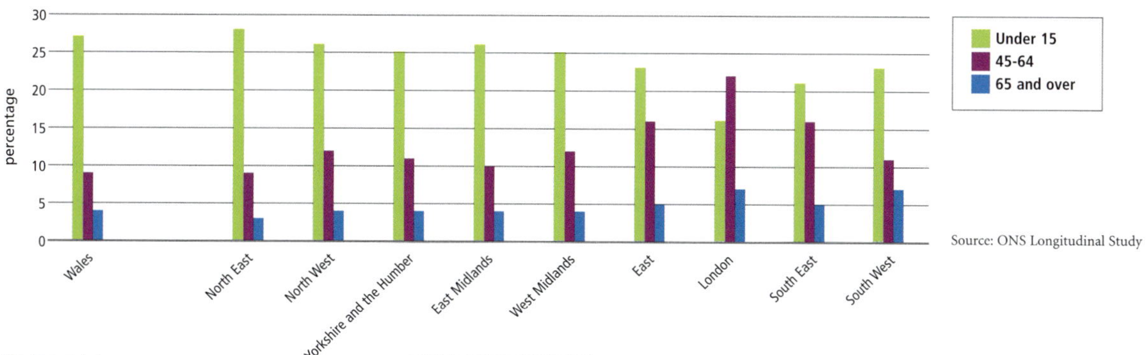

Figure 3.21

Age profile of those who had moved from other regions by 1991, age at 1991*
England and Wales 1991

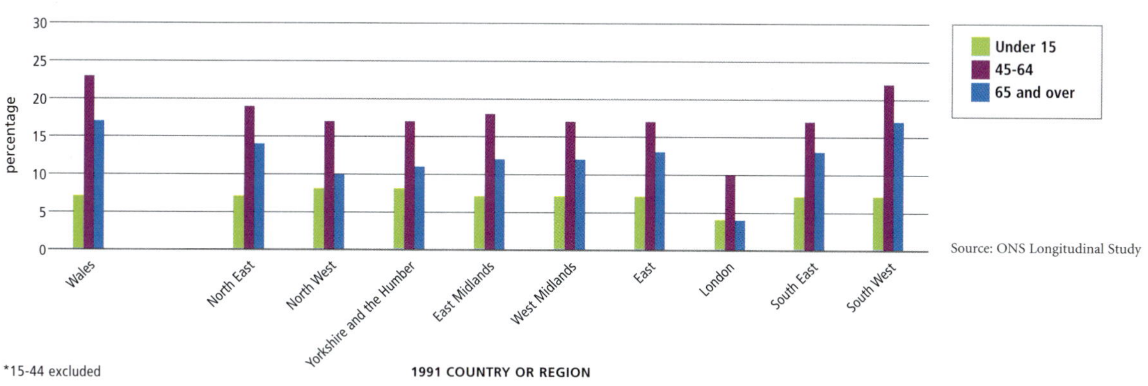

Figure 3.23 shows that in 1996-7 Scotland had the highest proportion of cigarette smokers of the countries in the United Kingdom and Wales the smallest. Within England, the North East and North West had the highest proportions and the South East the lowest. Alcohol consumption also varied, with both males and females in Northern Ireland consuming the least average number of units per week (Figure 3.24). Women in Wales consumed more units than women in other countries, while for men those in England and Scotland consumed the most. It was also men in England and women in Wales who were more likely to be heavy drinkers (21 plus and 14 plus units per week). Within England, men in the northern regions consumed more alcohol per week than those in the south, and were more likely to be heavy drinkers. Women in the North West stood out as consuming the most alcohol per week and were also most likely to be heavy drinkers. There was less variation across the other regions, and no indication of a north-south divide.

In addition, physical activity and participation in sports varies across Great Britain, according to the General Household Survey. Those in the northern regions of England were less likely to take part in physical activities and sports than those in the southern regions of England in 1996. Those in Scotland had levels of participation similar to those of people in the southern regions of England.[76]

Figure 3.22

Contribution of selected foods to nutritional intakes by country and region
United Kingdom 1996-1997

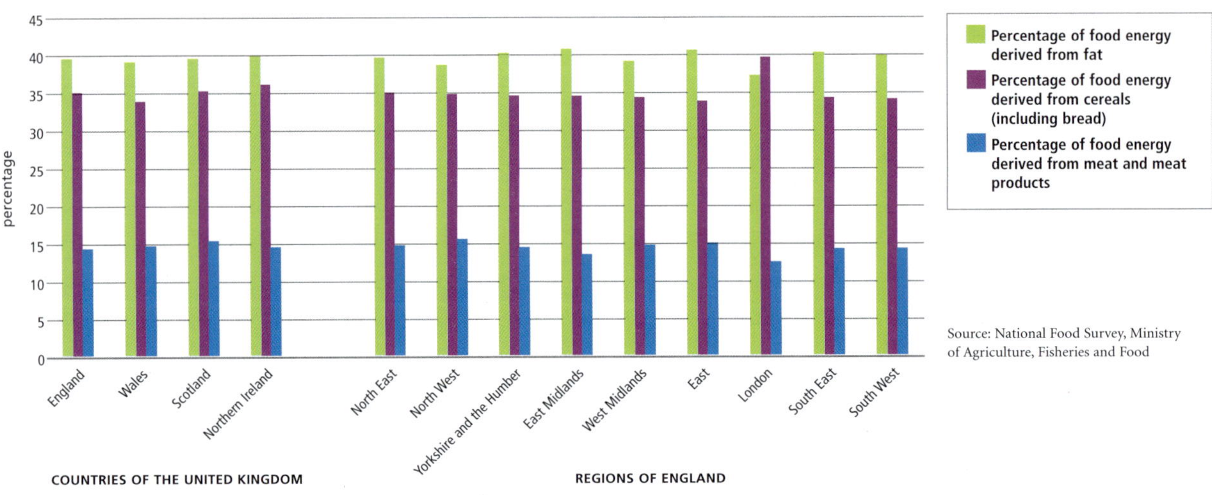

Source: National Food Survey, Ministry of Agriculture, Fisheries and Food

Figure 3.23

Proportion of people aged 16 or over who are cigarette smokers by country and region
United Kingdom 1996-1997

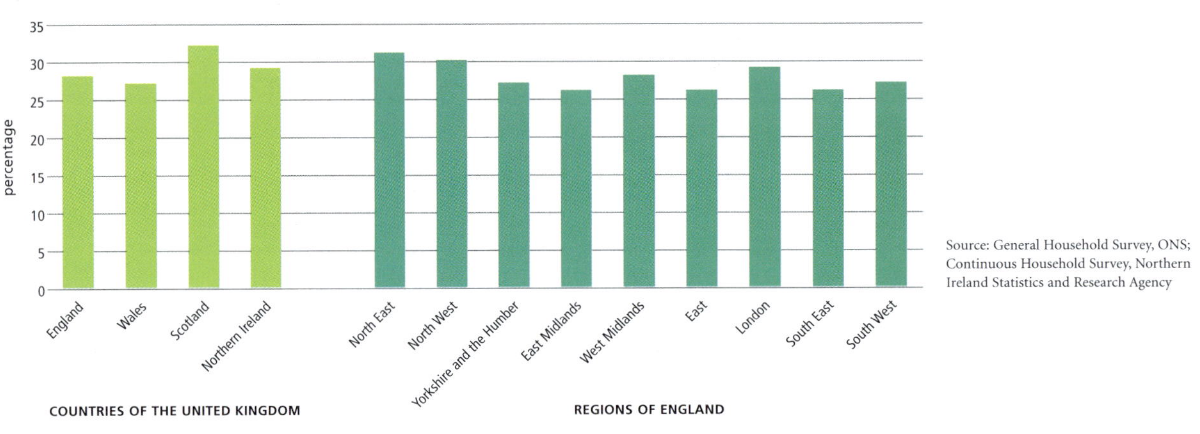

Source: General Household Survey, ONS; Continuous Household Survey, Northern Ireland Statistics and Research Agency

Figure 3.24

Alcohol consumption among people aged 16 or over by country and region
United Kingdom 1996-1997

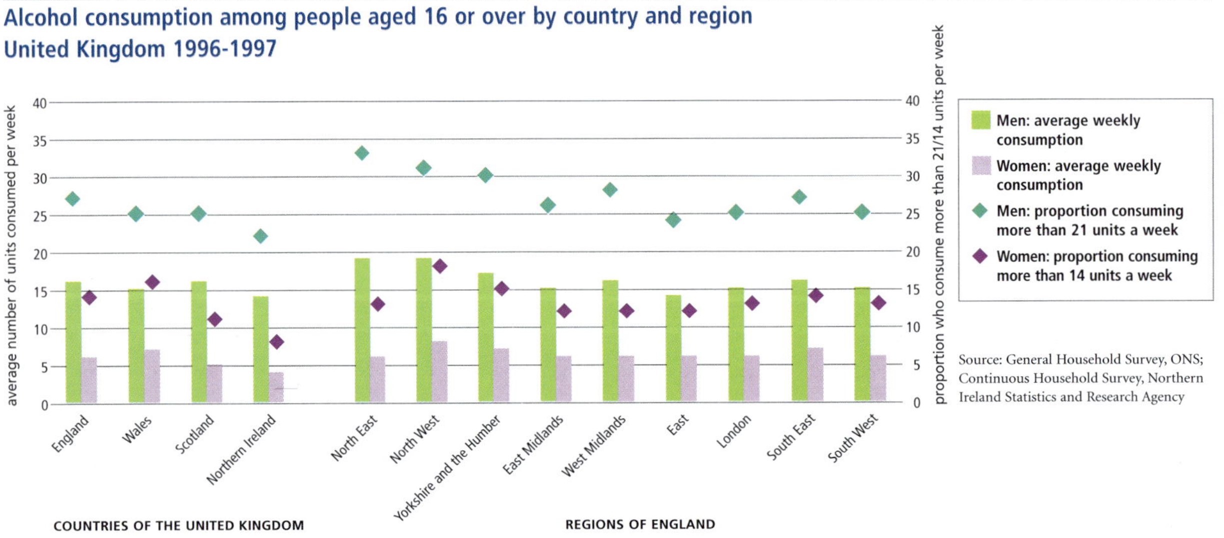

Source: General Household Survey, ONS; Continuous Household Survey, Northern Ireland Statistics and Research Agency

References

1 Dahlgren G and Whitehead M. *Policies and strategies to promote social equity in health. Institute for Future Studies* (Stockholm: 1991).

2 Farr W. Influence of marriage on the mortality of the French people. Savill and Edwards. (London: 1859).

3 Durkeim E. (1897) *Le Suicide.* Translated by Spaulding JA and Simpson G. *Suicide. A study in sociology.* Routledge and Kegan Paul (London: 1979).

4 General Register Office. *Registrar General's Statistical Review. Part III Commentary.* HMSO (London: 1967).

5 Charlton J. Trends and patterns in suicide in England and Wales. *International Journal of Epidemiology* 24 suppl. (1995), S45-S52.

6 Johnson NJ, Backlund E, Sorlie PD and Loveless CA. Marital status and mortality: the National Longitudinal Mortality Study. *Annals of Epidemiology* 10 (2000), 224-238.

7 Fox J and Goldblatt PO OPCS *Longitudinal Study, 1971-1975, Socio-demographic Mortality Differentials*, Series LS, No 1, HMSO (London: 1982).

8 Maxwell R and Harding S. Mortality of migrants from outside England and Wales by marital status. *Population Trends* 91 (1998), 15-22.

9 Ebrahim S, Wannamethee G, McCallum A, Walker M and Shaper AG. Marital Status, change in marital status and mortality in middle-aged British men. *American Journal of Epidemiology* 142 (1995), 834-842.

10 Kposowa AJ. Marital status and suicide in the National Longitudinal Mortality Study. *Journal of Epidemiology and Community Health* 54 (2000), 254-261.

11 Davies JM. Is testicular cancer incidence related to marital status? *International Journal of Cancer* 28 (1981), 721-724.

12 Cliff D and Deery R. Too much like school: Social Class, age, marital status and attendance/non-attendance at antenatal classes. *Midwifery* 13 (1997), 139-145.

13 Feldman PJ, Dunkel-Schetter C, Sandman CA and Wadhwa PD. Maternal social support predicts birth weight and foetal growth in human pregnancy. *Psychosomatic Medicine* 62 (2000), 715-725.

14 Dattani N. Mortality in children aged under 4. *Health Statistics Quarterly* 2 (1999), 41-49.

15 Bunting J. *Sources and Methods* in Drever F and Whitehead M. (Eds.) *Health Inequalities.* The Stationery Office (London: 1997).

16 Rose D, O'Reilly K and Martin J. The ESRC review of Government Social Classifications. *Population Trends* 89 (1997), 49-59.

17 Rose D and O'Reilly K. *Constructing Classes - towards a new social classification for the UK.* ESRC/ONS (London/Swindon: 1997).

18 Rose D and O'Reilly K. *The ESRC Review of Government Social Classifications.* ESRC/ONS (London/Swindon: 1998).

19 General Register Office. *Registrar General's 75th Annual Report - 1911 Supplement.* HMSO (London: 1919).

20 Drever F and Bunting J. Patterns and trends in male mortality. In Drever F and Whitehead M. (Eds.) *Health Inequalities.* The Stationery Office (London: 1997), 95-107.

21 Fitzpatrick J and Dollamore G. Examining adult mortality rates using the National Statistics Socio-Economic Classification. *Health Statistics Quarterly* 2 (1999), 33-40.

22 Hattersley L. Expectation of life by Social Class. In Drever F and Whitehead M. (Eds.) *Health Inequalities.* The Stationery Office (London: 1997), 73-82.

23 Hattersley L. Trends in life expectancy by Social Class - an update. *Health Statistics Quarterly* 2 (1999), 16-24.

24 Harding S, Brown J, Rosato M and Hattersley L. Socio-economic differentials in health: illustrations from the ONS Longitudinal Study. Health *Statistics Quarterly* 1 (1999), 5-15.

25 Botting B. Mortality in childhood. In Drever F and Whitehead M. (Eds.) *Health Inequalities.* The Stationery Office (London: 1997), 83-94.

26 Office for National Statistics. *Mortality statistics: perinatal and infant. Social and biological factors.* Series DH3. The Stationery Office (London).

27 Fear N, Roman E, Reeves G and Pannett B. Father's occupation and childhood mortality: analysis of routinely collected data. *Health Statistics Quarterly* 2 (1999), 7-15.

28 Botting B and Crawley R. Trends and patterns in childhood mortality. In Botting B (Ed.) *The Health of our Children.* HMSO (London: 1995).

29 Golding J, Paterson M and Kinlen LJ. Factors associated with childhood cancer in a national cohort study. *British Journal of Cancer* 62 (1990), 304-308.

30 Andersen R, Britton J, Esmail A, Hollowell J and Strachan D. Respiratory Disease and Sudden Infant Death Syndrome. In Botting B (Ed.) *The Health of our Children.* HMSO (London: 1995).

31 Bartley MJ, Ferrie J and Montgomery SM. Living in a high-unemployment economy: understanding the health consequences. In Marmot M and Wilkinson RG. (Eds.) *Social Determinants of Health.* Oxford University Press (Oxford: 1999), 81-104.

32 Moylan S and Davies R. The disadvantages of the unemployed. *Employment Gazette* 88 (1980), 830-832.

33 Moser KA, Fox AJ and Jones DR. Unemployment and mortality in the OPCS Longitudinal Study. *Lancet* 8415 (1984), 1324-1329.

34 Bethune A *Unemployment and mortality.* In Drever F and Whitehead M. (Eds.) *Health Inequalities.* The Stationery Office (London: 1997), 156-167.

35 Moser KA, Fox AJ, Jones DR and Goldblatt PO. Unemployment and mortality: further evidence from the OPCS Longitudinal Study 1971-1981. *Lancet* 8477 (1986), 365-367.

36 Moore A. Preventable childhood deaths in Wolverhampton. *British Medical Journal* 13 (1986), 656-658.

37 Leach CE, Blair PS, Fleming PJ, Smith IJ, Platt MW, Berry PJ and Golding J. Epidemiology of SIS and explained sudden infant deaths. CESDI SUDI Research Group. *Pediatrics* 104 (1999), 43.

38 Sly F. Economic activity results from the 1991 Labour Force Survey and Census of Population. *Employment Gazette* 102 (1994), 87-96.

39 Church J and Summerfield C. (Eds.) *Social Focus on Ethnic Minorities.* HMSO (London: 1996).

40 Schuman J. The ethnic minority populations of Great Britain - latest estimates. *Population Trends* 96 (1999), 33-42.

41 Ratcliffe P. *Ethnicity in the 1991 Census volume three. Social geography and ethnicity in Great Britain: geographical spread, spatial concentration and internal migration.* HMSO (London: 1996).

42 Harding S and Maxwell R. Differences in mortality of migrants. In Drever F and Whitehead M. (Eds.) *Health Inequalities.* The Stationery Office (London: 1997), 108-121.

43 Balarajan R and Raleigh VS. Patterns of mortality among Bangladeshis in England and Wales. *Ethnicity and Health* 2 (1997), 5-12.

44 Raleigh VS. Suicide patterns and trends in people of the Indian subcontinent and Caribbean origin in England and Wales. *Ethnicity and Health* 1 (1996), 55-63.

45 Harding S. Examining the contribution of Social Class to high cardiovascular disease mortality among Indian, Pakistani and Bangladeshi male migrants living in England and Wales. *Health Statistics Quarterly* 5 (2000), 26-29.

46 Haworth EA, Raleigh VS, Balarajan R. Cirrhosis and primary liver cancer amongst first generation migrants in England and Wales. *Ethnicity and Health* 4 (1999), 93-99.

47 Elender F, Bentham G and Langford I. Tuberculosis mortality in England and Wales during 1982-1992: its association with poverty, ethnicity and AIDS. *Social Science and Medicine* 46 (1998), 673-681.

48 Dattani N and Cooper N. Trends in cot deaths. *Health Statistics Quarterly* 5 (2000), 10-16.

49 McNiece R and Majeed A. Socio-economic differences in general practice consultation rates in patients aged 65 and over: prospective cohort study. *British Medical Journal* 319 (1999), 26-28.

50 Hull SA, Jones IR and Moser K. Factors influencing the attendance rate at accident and emergency departments in East London: the contributions of practice organisation, population characteristics and distance. *Journal of Health Services Research and Policy* 2 (1997), 6-13.

51 Welin C, Lappas G and Wilhelmsen L. Independent importance of psychosocial factors for prognosis after myocardial infarction. *Journal of International Medicine* 247 (2000), 629-639.

52 Davis MA, Murphy SP, Neuhaus JM, Gee L and Quiroga SS. Living arrangements affect dietary quality for US adults aged 50 years and older: NHANES III 1988-1994. *Journal of Nutrition* 130 (2000), 2256-2264.

53 Whichelow MJ and Prevost AT. Dietary patterns and their associations with demographic, lifestyle and health variables in a random sample of British adults. *British Journal of Nutrition* 76 (1996), 17-30.

54 Aneshensel C, Frerichs R and Clark V. Family roles and sex differences in depression. *Journal of Health and Social Behaviour* 22 (1981), 379-393.

55 Blaxter M. *Health and Lifestyles.* Tavistock/Routledge (London: 1990).

56 Benzeval M. The self-reported health status of lone parents. *Social Science and Medicine* 46 (1998), 1337-1353.

57 Sharland M, Atkinson P, Maguire H and Begg N. Lone parent families are an independent risk factor for lower rates of childhood immunisation in London. *Burisa* 17 (1997), 169-172.

58 Smith J and Harding S. Mortality of women and men using alternative social classifications. In Drever F and Whitehead M. (Eds.) *Health Inequalities.* The Stationery Office (London: 1997), 168-185.

59 Harding S, Rosato M, Brown J and Smith J. Social patterning of health and mortality: children, aged 6-15 years, followed up for 25 years in the ONS Longitudinal Study. *Health Statistics Quarterly* 3 (1999), 30-34.

60 Breeze E, Sloggett A and Fletcher A. Socio-economic and demographic predictors of mortality and institutional residence among middle-aged and older people: results from the Longitudinal Study. *Journal of Epidemiology and Community Health* 53 (1999), 765-774.

61 Britton M, Fox AJ, Goldblatt PO, Jones DR and Rosato M. The Influence of socio-economic and environmental factors on geographic variation in mortality. In Britton M. (Ed.) *Mortality and Geography: a review in the mid 1980s.* England and Wales. Series DS No. 9. HMSO (London: 1990), 58-78.

62 Strachan DP, Leon DA, Dodgeon B. mortality from cardiovascular disease among interregional migrants in England and Wales. *British Medical Journal* 310 (1995), 423-427.

63 Office for National Statistics. *Key Population and Vital Statistics 1998.* Series VS no. 25, PP1 no. 21. The Stationery Office (London: 2000).

64 Vickers L. Trends in migration in the UK. *Population Trends* 94 (1998), 25-34.

65 Champion T. Population review: (3) Migration to, from and within the United Kingdom. *Population Trends* 83 (1996), 5-16.

66 Doll R. Uncovering the effects of smoking: historical perspective. *Statistical Methods in Medical Research* 7 (1998), 87-117.

67 Doll R, Gray R, Hafner B, Peto R. Mortality in relation to smoking: 22 years' observations on female British doctors. *British Medical Journal* 280 (1980), 967-971.

68 Doll R. Risk from tobacco and potentials for health gain. *International Journal of Tuberculosis and Lung Diseases* 3 (1999), 90-99.

69 White C. Research on smoking and lung cancer: a landmark in the history of chronic disease epidemiology. *Yale Journal of Biology and Medicine* 63 (1990), 29-46.

70 Marmot MG. Life-style and national and international trends in coronary heart disease mortality. *Postgraduate Medical Journal* 60 (1984), 3-8.

71 Burch PR. Esophageal cancer in relation to cigarette and alcohol consumption. *Journal of Chronic Diseases* 37 (1984), 793-814.

72 Anderson P. Excess mortality associated with alcohol consumption. *British Medical Journal* 297 (1988), 824-826.

73 Ingram DM. Trends in diet and breast cancer mortality in England and Wales 1928-1977. *Nutrition and Cancer* 3 (1981), 75-80.

74 Barker DJ and Osmond C. Infant mortality, childhood nutrition and ischaemic heart disease in England and Wales. *Lancet* 8489 (1986), 1077-1081.

75 Mann JI, Appleby PN, Key TJ and Thorogood M. Dietary determinants of ischaemic heart disease in health conscious individuals. *Heart* 78 (1997), 450-455.

76 Office for National Statistics. *Living in Britain. Results from the 1996 General Household Survey.* The Stationery Office (London: 1998).

Classifications used in this volume

Justine Fitzpatrick

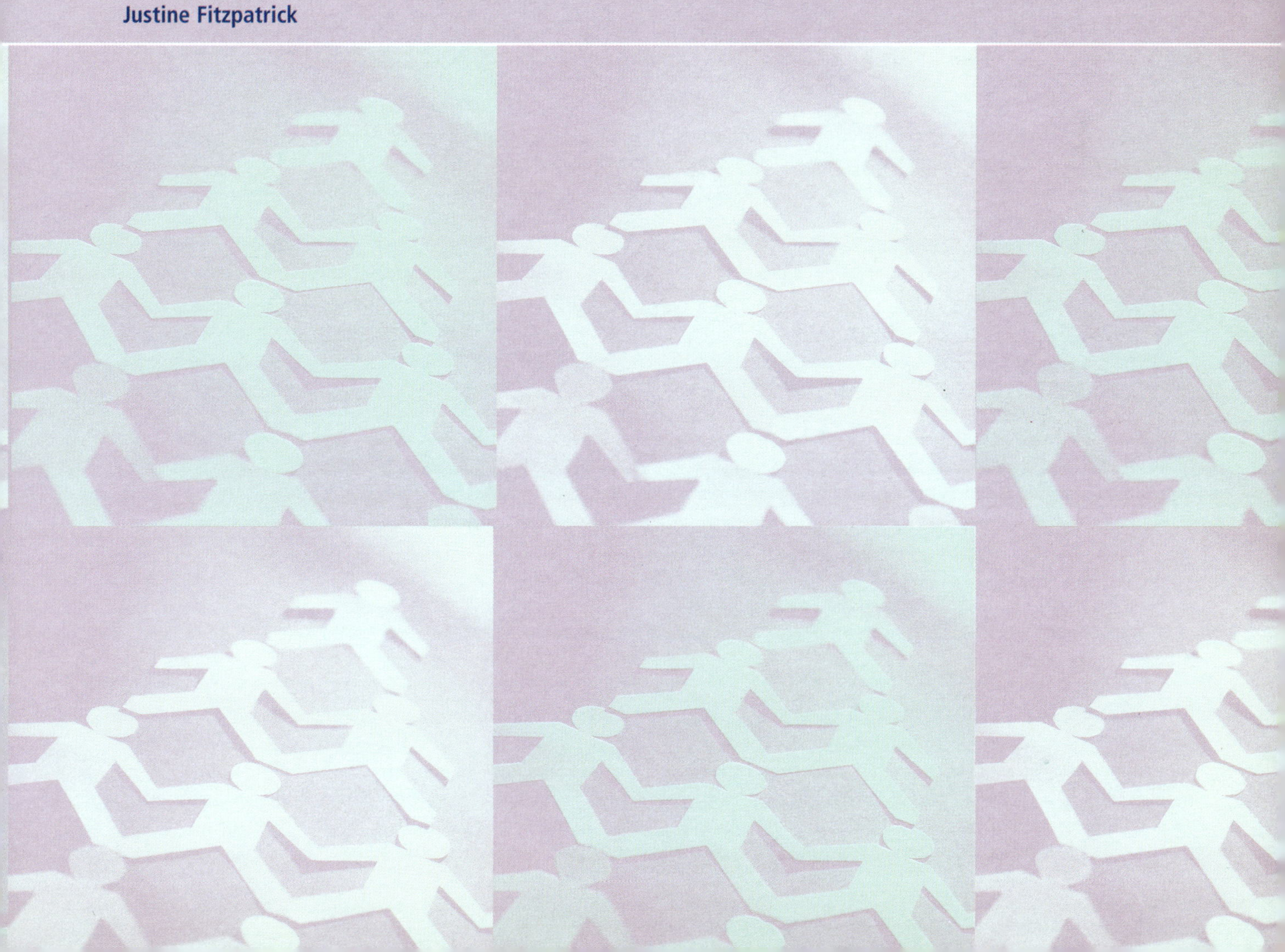

Chapter 4
Classifications used in this volume

This chapter is a description of the Carstairs and Morris deprivation index and the ONS classification of local authorities used in later chapters to explain geographic variations in health.

4.1 ONS classification of local and health authorities

Area classifications provide a simple and robust way of summarising information on the similarities and differences between geographic areas. They are used for a wide variety of purposes – to convey broad geographic patterns in the population, to categorise data for further analysis, to identify areas that are similar for comparative studies, to monitor performance and for marketing goods and services. A revised version of the ONS classification of local and health authorities of Great Britain was published in December 1999.[1] It provides an indication of the characteristics of the areas and the ways in which they differ from each other. ONS previously published a classification in 1996, based on 37 socio-economic and demographic variables from the 1991 Census.[2] Since the original classification was produced there have been substantial changes to the number and structure of boundaries of local and health authorities. The revised classification was produced for authorities as they existed at April 1999, using the same data and methodology as the original classification.

The aim of the classification is to place authorities into a hierarchy of mutually exclusive groups of authorities that share similar socio-economic and demographic profiles. Techniques that produce this type of classification are generally known as clustering techniques and the mutually exclusive groupings they produce are referred to as 'clusters'. In this case a three-tier hierarchy of clusters was produced known as Families, Groups and Clusters. Further details of the methods used are published elsewhere.[3]

Table 4.1 shows the hierarchy of Families, Groups and Clusters with their names and identifiers. The Families, Groups and Clusters were given names for ease of reference, based on the general characteristics of cluster members. These names reflect the socio-economic characteristics of cluster centroids, sometimes combined with geographic attributes of member authorities. They are not precise descriptions of all members of a cluster, particularly those that are statistically furthest from the cluster centroid. Clusters have also been identified by numbers 1 to 27, Groups with letters A to O and Families with Roman numerals I to VII.

Within this volume we have used the Group level to convey broad characteristics of the population living in local authorities within Great Britain and to examine patterns in fertility, congenital anomaly notifications, cancer incidence and mortality. Table 4.2 shows Group membership for all local authorities in Great Britain. Map 4.1 shows the fifteen Groups

by local authority. No geographic variables, such as regional location, were used in the classification. However it is clear from the map that many adjacent authorities lie within the same Group. The most geographically scattered Groups are the *New and Developing Areas* and the *Mixed Urban* Groups.

Profile of the Groups
This section provides a brief overview of the characteristics of each Group within their Families and the geographic location of authorities within each Group.

Rural Areas
Rural Amenity, Remoter Rural
Geographic location: authorities in this Family are located away from urban areas in the south west of England, central Wales, parts of eastern and northern England, and much of Scotland.
Key characteristics: a relatively mature population, predominance of employment in agriculture, high car ownership and large dwellings. *Remoter Rural* has the highest employment in agriculture whilst *Rural Amenity* has a slightly more prosperous profile.

Urban Fringe
Established Manufacturing Fringe, New and Developing Areas, Mixed Urban
Geographic location: authorities are generally on the edges of main urban centres and most are within England.
Key characteristics: this group of authorities falls most closely to the Great Britain average for the range of socio-economic and demographic variables used in the classification. *Established Manufacturing Fringe* has an employment profile characterised by mining and production and manufacturing. *New and Developing Areas* has a more mobile population with a very young age structure, while *Mixed Urban* is more prosperous than either of the other two Groups.

Coast and Services
Coast and Country Resorts, Established Service Centres
Geographic location: authorities are widely scattered across England and Wales only. The majority are in coastal locations.
Key characteristics: a relatively mature population with below average household size. Finance and services are the dominant forms of employment. *Coast and Country Resorts* has an older age structure, while *Established Service Centres* has higher unemployment.

Prosperous England
Growth Areas, Most Prosperous
Geographic location: all authorities in this Family are English, with a notable circle around central and south east England.
Key characteristics: higher than average values for all indicators of affluence including the proportion of the population where the household head is in Social Class I or II, households with two or more cars, households with two earners and no

Table 4.1

Structure of Families, Groups and Clusters

Family	Group	Cluster
I Rural Areas	A Rural Amenity	1 Rural Amenity
	B Remoter Rural	2 Rural England and Wales
		3 Rural Scotland
II Urban Fringe	C Established Manufacturing Fringe	4 Established Manufacturing Fringe
	D New and Developing Areas	5 New and Expanding Towns
		6 Developing Towns
	E Mixed Urban	7 Most Typical Towns and Cities
		8 London and Glasgow Periphery
III Coast and Services	F Coast and Country Resorts	9 Seaside Towns
		10 Traditional Rural Coast
	G Established Service Centres	11 Established Service Centres
IV Prosperous England	H Growth Areas	12 Town and Country Growth
		13 Prosperous Growth Areas
	I Most Prosperous	14 Most Prosperous
V Mining, Manufacturing and Industry	J Coalfields	15 Mining and Inner City
		16 Mining and Industry
		17 Former Mining Areas
	K Manufacturing Centres	18 Manufacturing Centres
	L Ports and Industry	19 Urban Industry
		20 Liverpool and Manchester
		21 Clydeside and Dundee
VI Education Centres and Outer London	M Education Centres and Outer London	22 Suburbs
		23 Cosmopolitan Outer London
		24 Education Centres
VII Inner London	N West Inner London	25 West Inner London
	O East Inner London	26 Inner City Boroughs
		27 Newham and Tower Hamlets

children, owner occupied housing and households with more than seven rooms. *Growth Areas* has a slightly younger population structure while the *Most Prosperous* Group has the most affluent profile of any Group.

Mining, Manufacturing and Industry
Coalfields, Manufacturing Centres, Ports and Industry
Geographic location: a strong link to all the former mining, primary production and early industrial areas of England, Wales and Scotland, including all major ports.
Key characteristics: a less affluent population with high proportions of the population in households where the household head is in Social Class IV or V, high unemployment and high employment in mining, primary production and manufacturing. *Coalfields* has the highest employment in mining and production, *Manufacturing Centres* has a slightly more affluent profile with higher employment in manufacturing, *Ports and Industry* has lower employment in all sectors and higher unemployment.

Education Centres and Outer London
Education Centres and Outer London
Geographic location: authorities are located entirely in outer London and a number of authorities containing university towns scattered across England and Scotland.
Key characteristics: a larger than average student population, high reliance on public transport to work, high proportions of the population in households where the households head is in Social Class IIIN.

Inner London
West Inner London, East Inner London
Geographic location: entirely within inner London.
Key characteristics: very diverse population characteristics including a large minority ethnic population, high unemployment, high employment in finance and services, a high proportion of the population that has moved in the last year and a high proportion of students. *West Inner London* is the more affluent of the two Groups.

Table 4.2

Group membership - local authorities
(local authorities in alphabetical order)

Local authority	Group	
Aberdeen City	M	Education Centres and Outer London
Aberdeenshire	B	Remoter Rural
Adur	F	Coast and Country Resorts
Allerdale	C	Established Manufacturing Fringe
Alnwick	B	Remoter Rural
Amber Valley	C	Established Manufacturing Fringe
Angus	B	Remoter Rural
Argyll and Bute	B	Remoter Rural
Arun	F	Coast and Country Resorts
Ashfield	C	Established Manufacturing Fringe
Ashford	E	Mixed Urban
Aylesbury Vale	H	Growth Areas
Babergh	H	Growth Areas
Barking and Dagenham	J	Coalfields
Barnet	M	Education Centres and Outer London
Barnsley	J	Coalfields
Barrow-in-Furness	K	Manufacturing Centres
Basildon	D	New and Developing Areas
Basingstoke and Deane	H	Growth Areas
Bassetlaw	C	Established Manufacturing Fringe
Bath and North East Somerset	A	Rural Amenity
Bedford	E	Mixed Urban
Berwick-upon-Tweed	B	Remoter Rural
Bexley	E	Mixed Urban
Birmingham	K	Manufacturing Centres
Blaby	H	Growth Areas
Blackburn with Darwen	K	Manufacturing Centres
Blackpool	F	Coast and Country Resorts
Blaenau Gwent	J	Coalfields
Blyth Valley	D	New and Developing Areas
Bolsover	J	Coalfields
Bolton	K	Manufacturing Centres
Boston	B	Remoter Rural
Bournemouth	F	Coast and Country Resorts
Bracknell Forest	D	New and Developing Areas
Bradford	K	Manufacturing Centres
Braintree	H	Growth Areas
Breckland	B	Remoter Rural
Brent	M	Education Centres and Outer London
Brentwood	I	Most Prosperous
Bridgend	J	Coalfields
Bridgnorth	A	Rural Amenity
Brighton and Hove	M	Education Centres and Outer London
Bristol, City of	G	Established Service Centres
Broadland	H	Growth Areas
Bromley	E	Mixed Urban
Bromsgrove	H	Growth Areas
Broxbourne	E	Mixed Urban
Broxtowe	E	Mixed Urban
Burnley	K	Manufacturing Centres

Table 4.2 - continued

Group membership - local authorities (local authorities in alphabetical order)

Local authority	Group		Local authority	Group	
Bury	E	Mixed Urban	Dundee City	L	Ports and Industry
Caerphilly	J	Coalfields	Durham	E	Mixed Urban
Calderdale	K	Manufacturing Centres	Ealing	M	Education Centres and Outer London
Cambridge	M	Education Centres and Outer London	Easington	J	Coalfields
Camden	N	West Inner London	East Ayrshire	L	Ports and Industry
Cannock Chase	C	Established Manufacturing Fringe	Eastbourne	F	Coast and Country Resorts
Canterbury	F	Coast and Country Resorts	East Cambridgeshire	H	Growth Areas
Caradon	F	Coast and Country Resorts	East Devon	F	Coast and Country Resorts
Cardiff	G	Established Service Centres	East Dorset	A	Rural Amenity
Carlisle	G	Established Service Centres	East Dunbartonshire	E	Mixed Urban
Carmarthenshire	F	Coast and Country Resorts	East Hampshire	H	Growth Areas
Carrick	F	Coast and Country Resorts	East Hertfordshire	H	Growth Areas
Castle Morpeth	A	Rural Amenity	Eastleigh	H	Growth Areas
Castle Point	E	Mixed Urban	East Lindsey	B	Remoter Rural
Ceredigion	B	Remoter Rural	East Lothian	E	Mixed Urban
Charnwood	H	Growth Areas	East Northamptonshire	H	Growth Areas
Chelmsford	H	Growth Areas	East Renfrewshire	E	Mixed Urban
Cheltenham	E	Mixed Urban	East Riding of Yorkshire	A	Rural Amenity
Cherwell	D	New and Developing Areas	East Staffordshire	C	Established Manufacturing Fringe
Chester	A	Rural Amenity	Eden	B	Remoter Rural
Chesterfield	J	Coalfields	Edinburgh, City of	M	Education Centres and Outer London
Chester-le-Street	J	Coalfields	Eilean Siar	B	Remoter Rural
Chichester	A	Rural Amenity	Ellesmere Port and Neston	C	Established Manufacturing Fringe
Chiltern	I	Most Prosperous	Elmbridge	I	Most Prosperous
Chorley	E	Mixed Urban	Enfield	M	Education Centres and Outer London
Christchurch	F	Coast and Country Resorts	Epping Forest	E	Mixed Urban
Clackmannanshire	L	Ports and Industry	Epsom and Ewell	I	Most Prosperous
Colchester	E	Mixed Urban	Erewash	C	Established Manufacturing Fringe
Congleton	H	Growth Areas	Exeter	G	Established Service Centres
Conwy	F	Coast and Country Resorts	Falkirk	L	Ports and Industry
Copeland	J	Coalfields	Fareham	H	Growth Areas
Corby	J	Coalfields	Fenland	C	Established Manufacturing Fringe
Cotswold	A	Rural Amenity	Fife	L	Ports and Industry
Coventry	K	Manufacturing Centres	Flintshire	C	Established Manufacturing Fringe
Craven	A	Rural Amenity	Forest Heath	D	New and Developing Areas
Crawley	D	New and Developing Areas	Forest of Dean	C	Established Manufacturing Fringe
Crewe and Nantwich	C	Established Manufacturing Fringe	Fylde	F	Coast and Country Resorts
Croydon	M	Education Centres and Outer London	Gateshead	L	Ports and Industry
Dacorum	H	Growth Areas	Gedling	E	Mixed Urban
Darlington	G	Established Service Centres	Glasgow City	L	Ports and Industry
Dartford	E	Mixed Urban	Gloucester	D	New and Developing Areas
Daventry	H	Growth Areas	Gosport	D	New and Developing Areas
Denbighshire	F	Coast and Country Resorts	Gravesham	D	New and Developing Areas
Derby	K	Manufacturing Centres	Great Yarmouth	F	Coast and Country Resorts
Derbyshire Dales	A	Rural Amenity	Greenwich	M	Education Centres and Outer London
Derwentside	J	Coalfields	Guildford	I	Most Prosperous
Doncaster	J	Coalfields	Gwynedd	F	Coast and Country Resorts
Dover	F	Coast and Country Resorts	Hackney	O	East Inner London
Dudley	C	Established Manufacturing Fringe	Halton	J	Coalfields
Dumfries and Galloway	B	Remoter Rural	Hambleton	A	Rural Amenity

Table 4.2 - continued

Group membership - local authorities (local authorities in alphabetical order)

Local authority		Group
Hammersmith and Fulham	N	West Inner London
Harborough	H	Growth Areas
Haringey	M	Education Centres and Outer London
Harlow	D	New and Developing Areas
Harrogate	A	Rural Amenity
Harrow	M	Education Centres and Outer London
Hart	H	Growth Areas
Hartlepool	J	Coalfields
Hastings	G	Established Service Centres
Havant	C	Established Manufacturing Fringe
Havering	E	Mixed Urban
Herefordshire, County of	B	Remoter Rural
Hertsmere	E	Mixed Urban
High Peak	E	Mixed Urban
Highland	B	Remoter Rural
Hillingdon	D	New and Developing Areas
Hinckley and Bosworth	H	Growth Areas
Horsham	I	Most Prosperous
Hounslow	M	Education Centres and Outer London
Huntingdonshire	H	Growth Areas
Hyndburn	K	Manufacturing Centres
Inverclyde	L	Ports and Industry
Ipswich	G	Established Service Centres
Isle of Anglesey	F	Coast and Country Resorts
Isle of Wight	F	Coast and Country Resorts
Islington	O	East Inner London
Kennet	H	Growth Areas
Kensington and Chelsea	N	West Inner London
Kerrier	F	Coast and Country Resorts
Kettering	E	Mixed Urban
King's Lynn and West Norfolk	B	Remoter Rural
Kingston upon Hull, City of	J	Coalfields
Kingston upon Thames	M	Education Centres and Outer London
Kirklees	K	Manufacturing Centres
Knowsley	L	Ports and Industry
Lambeth	O	East Inner London
Lancaster	F	Coast and Country Resorts
Leeds	G	Established Service Centres
Leicester	K	Manufacturing Centres
Lewes	F	Coast and Country Resorts
Lewisham	M	Education Centres and Outer London
Lichfield	H	Growth Areas
Lincoln	G	Established Service Centres
Liverpool	L	Ports and Industry
Luton	D	New and Developing Areas
Macclesfield	I	Most Prosperous
Maidstone	H	Growth Areas
Maldon	H	Growth Areas
Malvern Hills	A	Rural Amenity
Manchester	L	Ports and Industry

Local authority		Group
Mansfield	J	Coalfields
Medway	D	New and Developing Areas
Melton	H	Growth Areas
Mendip	H	Growth Areas
Merthyr Tydfil	J	Coalfields
Merton	M	Education Centres and Outer London
Mid Bedfordshire	H	Growth Areas
Mid Devon	B	Remoter Rural
Middlesbrough	J	Coalfields
Midlothian	D	New and Developing Areas
Mid Suffolk	H	Growth Areas
Mid Sussex	I	Most Prosperous
Milton Keynes	D	New and Developing Areas
Mole Valley	I	Most Prosperous
Monmouthshire	A	Rural Amenity
Moray	B	Remoter Rural
Neath Port Talbot	J	Coalfields
Newark and Sherwood	C	Established Manufacturing Fringe
Newcastle-under-Lyme	C	Established Manufacturing Fringe
Newcastle upon Tyne	L	Ports and Industry
New Forest	A	Rural Amenity
Newham	O	East Inner London
Newport	J	Coalfields
Northampton	D	New and Developing Areas
North Ayrshire	L	Ports and Industry
North Cornwall	B	Remoter Rural
North Devon	B	Remoter Rural
North Dorset	B	Remoter Rural
North East Derbyshire	C	Established Manufacturing Fringe
North East Lincolnshire	J	Coalfields
North Hertfordshire	H	Growth Areas
North Kesteven	A	Rural Amenity
North Lanarkshire	L	Ports and Industry
North Lincolnshire	C	Established Manufacturing Fringe
North Norfolk	B	Remoter Rural
North Shropshire	B	Remoter Rural
North Somerset	A	Rural Amenity
North Tyneside	L	Ports and Industry
North Warwickshire	C	Established Manufacturing Fringe
North West Leicestershire	C	Established Manufacturing Fringe
North Wiltshire	H	Growth Areas
Norwich	G	Established Service Centres
Nottingham	L	Ports and Industry
Nuneaton and Bedworth	C	Established Manufacturing Fringe
Oadby and Wigston	H	Growth Areas
Oldham	K	Manufacturing Centres
Orkney Islands	B	Remoter Rural
Oswestry	B	Remoter Rural
Oxford	M	Education Centres and Outer London
Pembrokeshire	F	Coast and Country Resorts

Table 4.2 - continued

Group membership - local authorities (local authorities in alphabetical order)

Local authority	Group		Local authority	Group	
Pendle	K	Manufacturing Centres	Solihull	H	Growth Areas
Penwith and Isles of Scilly	F	Coast and Country Resorts	Southampton	G	Established Service Centres
Perth and Kinross	B	Remoter Rural	South Ayrshire	B	Remoter Rural
Peterborough	D	New and Developing Areas	South Bedfordshire	H	Growth Areas
Plymouth	G	Established Service Centres	South Bucks	I	Most Prosperous
Poole	E	Mixed Urban	South Cambridgeshire	H	Growth Areas
Portsmouth	G	Established Service Centres	South Derbyshire	C	Established Manufacturing Fringe
Powys	B	Remoter Rural	Southend-on-Sea	F	Coast and Country Resorts
Preston	K	Manufacturing Centres	South Gloucestershire	H	Growth Areas
Purbeck	A	Rural Amenity	South Hams	A	Rural Amenity
Reading	D	New and Developing Areas	South Holland	B	Remoter Rural
Redbridge	M	Education Centres and Outer London	South Kesteven	H	Growth Areas
Redcar and Cleveland	J	Coalfields	South Lakeland	A	Rural Amenity
Redditch	D	New and Developing Areas	South Lanarkshire	L	Ports and Industry
Reigate and Banstead	I	Most Prosperous	South Norfolk	A	Rural Amenity
Renfrewshire	L	Ports and Industry	South Northamptonshire	H	Growth Areas
Restormel	F	Coast and Country Resorts	South Oxfordshire	H	Growth Areas
Rhondda, Cynon, Taff	J	Coalfields	South Ribble	H	Growth Areas
Ribble Valley	A	Rural Amenity	South Shropshire	B	Remoter Rural
Richmond upon Thames	M	Education Centres and Outer London	South Somerset	B	Remoter Rural
Richmondshire	B	Remoter Rural	South Staffordshire	H	Growth Areas
Rochdale	K	Manufacturing Centres	South Tyneside	L	Ports and Industry
Rochford	E	Mixed Urban	Southwark	O	East Inner London
Rossendale	D	New and Developing Areas	Spelthorne	E	Mixed Urban
Rother	F	Coast and Country Resorts	Stafford	H	Growth Areas
Rotherham	J	Coalfields	Staffordshire Moorlands	C	Established Manufacturing Fringe
Rugby	H	Growth Areas	Stevenage	D	New and Developing Areas
Runnymede	H	Growth Areas	Stirling	E	Mixed Urban
Rushcliffe	I	Most Prosperous	Stockport	E	Mixed Urban
Rushmoor	D	New and Developing Areas	Stockton-on-Tees	J	Coalfields
Rutland	H	Growth Areas	Stoke-on-Trent	J	Coalfields
Ryedale	B	Remoter Rural	Stratford-on-Avon	A	Rural Amenity
St. Albans	I	Most Prosperous	Stroud	H	Growth Areas
St. Edmundsbury	H	Growth Areas	Suffolk Coastal	A	Rural Amenity
St. Helens	J	Coalfields	Sunderland	L	Ports and Industry
Salford	L	Ports and Industry	Surrey Heath	H	Growth Areas
Salisbury	A	Rural Amenity	Sutton	E	Mixed Urban
Sandwell	K	Manufacturing Centres	Swale	C	Established Manufacturing Fringe
Scarborough	F	Coast and Country Resorts	Swansea	J	Coalfields
Scottish Borders	B	Remoter Rural	Swindon	D	New and Developing Areas
Sedgefield	J	Coalfields	Tameside	K	Manufacturing Centres
Sedgemoor	B	Remoter Rural	Tamworth	D	New and Developing Areas
Sefton	F	Coast and Country Resorts	Tandridge	I	Most Prosperous
Selby	H	Growth Areas	Taunton Deane	A	Rural Amenity
Sevenoaks	I	Most Prosperous	Teesdale	B	Remoter Rural
Sheffield	L	Ports and Industry	Teignbridge	A	Rural Amenity
Shepway	F	Coast and Country Resorts	Telford and Wrekin	D	New and Developing Areas
Shetland Islands	B	Remoter Rural	Tendring	F	Coast and Country Resorts
Shrewsbury and Atcham	E	Mixed Urban	Test Valley	H	Growth Areas
Slough	D	New and Developing Areas	Tewkesbury	H	Growth Areas

Table 4.2 - continued

Group membership - local authorities (local authorities in alphabetical order)

Local authority	Group	
Thanet	F	Coast and Country Resorts
Three Rivers	I	Most Prosperous
Thurrock	D	New and Developing Areas
Tonbridge and Malling	H	Growth Areas
Torbay	F	Coast and Country Resorts
Torfaen	J	Coalfields
Torridge	B	Remoter Rural
Tower Hamlets	O	East Inner London
Trafford	E	Mixed Urban
Tunbridge Wells	I	Most Prosperous
Tynedale	A	Rural Amenity
Uttlesford	H	Growth Areas
Vale of Glamorgan, The	E	Mixed Urban
Vale of White Horse	H	Growth Areas
Vale Royal	C	Established Manufacturing Fringe
Wakefield	J	Coalfields
Walsall	K	Manufacturing Centres
Waltham Forest	M	Education Centres and Outer London
Wandsworth	N	West Inner London
Wansbeck	J	Coalfields
Warrington	E	Mixed Urban
Warwick	E	Mixed Urban
Watford	D	New and Developing Areas
Waveney	F	Coast and Country Resorts
Waverley	I	Most Prosperous
Wealden	A	Rural Amenity
Wear Valley	J	Coalfields
Wellingborough	D	New and Developing Areas
Welwyn Hatfield	E	Mixed Urban
West Berkshire	H	Growth Areas
West Devon	B	Remoter Rural
West Dorset	B	Remoter Rural
West Dunbartonshire	L	Ports and Industry
West Lancashire	E	Mixed Urban
West Lindsey	B	Remoter Rural
West Lothian	D	New and Developing Areas
Westminster and City of London	N	West Inner London
West Oxfordshire	H	Growth Areas
West Somerset	B	Remoter Rural
West Wiltshire	H	Growth Areas
Weymouth and Portland	G	Established Service Centres
Wigan	J	Coalfields
Winchester	I	Most Prosperous
Windsor and Maidenhead	I	Most Prosperous
Wirral	G	Established Service Centres

Local authority	Group	
Woking	H	Growth Areas
Wokingham	H	Growth Areas
Wolverhampton	K	Manufacturing Centres
Worcester	D	New and Developing Areas
Worthing	F	Coast and Country Resorts
Wrexham	J	Coalfields
Wychavon	H	Growth Areas
Wycombe	H	Growth Areas
Wyre	F	Coast and Country Resorts
Wyre Forest	C	Established Manufacturing Fringe
York	E	Mixed Urban

Footnote: The City of London and the Isles of Scilly were combined with neighbouring authorities for the purposes of analysis and are listed with Westminster, City of and Penwith respectively

Map 4.1

The ONS classification of local authorities: the fifteen Groups

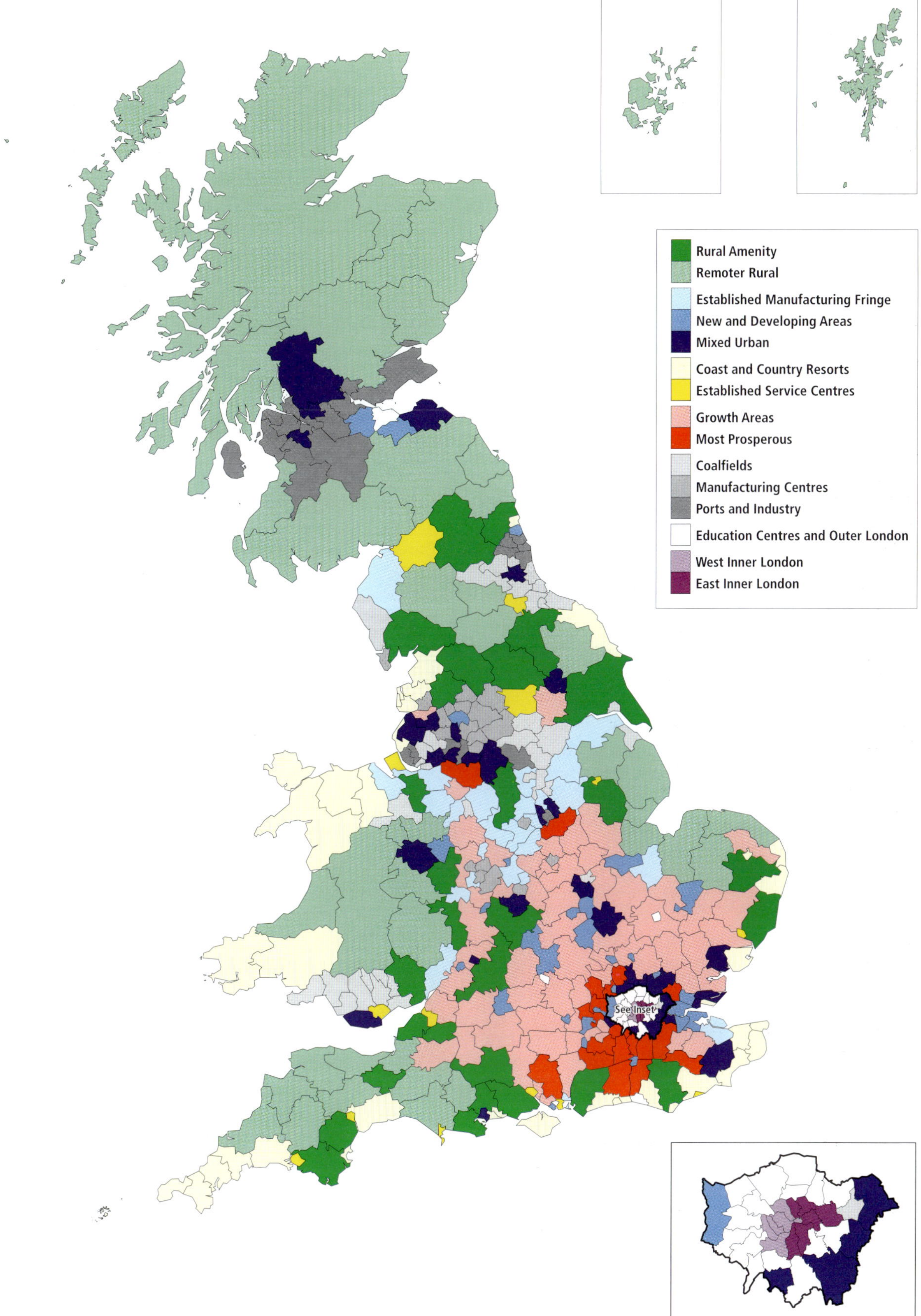

4.2 The Carstairs and Morris index of deprivation

There are various ways of measuring the level of deprivation within an area. In this volume we have used the Carstairs and Morris index of deprivation which was developed to explain variations in health data.[4,5] It is a measure of material rather than social deprivation. Townsend[6] states that material disadvantage involves 'the material apparatus, goods, services, resources, amenities and physical environment and location of life' and social deprivation 'access to ordinary social customs, activities and relationships'.

The Carstairs and Morris index of deprivation is calculated using the following variables:

- The proportion of economically active men who are unemployed
- The proportion of individuals in overcrowded accommodation (more than one person per room)
- The proportion of the population (excluding those who are retired) where the head of the household is in Social Class IV or V
- The proportion of individuals with no access to a car

The overall index is calculated by first standardising the variables listed above and then combining them, treating each variable with equal weight.

This index has been calculated for all 1991 Census wards in England and Wales and 1991 postcode sectors in Scotland using data from the 1991 Census. Northern Ireland has been excluded due to differences in Census definitions. We have divided wards and postcode sectors in Great Britain into twentieths according to the value of their Carstairs and Morris index, that is 5 per cent of areas in Great Britain will be classified to each category according to the level of deprivation. These are called deprivation twentieths, with twentieth 1 being the least deprived and twentieth 20 the most. Wards and postcode sectors in Great Britain have also been divided into quintiles,

that is, 20 per cent of areas in Great Britain will be classified to each category according to the level of deprivation. These are called deprivation quintiles, with quintile 1 being the least deprived and quintile 5 the most. Twentieths 1 to 4 are grouped to form quintile 1, 5 to 8 are grouped to form quintile 2 and so on until twentieths 17 to 20 form quintile 5.

Maps 4.2 to 4.12 show the distribution of deprivation quintiles by ward within regions and local authorities in England, by ward and local authority within Wales and by postcode sector and local authority within Scotland. The data presented and the ward and postcode sector boundaries used are from the 1991 Census, however 1999 local authority boundaries have been added to the maps for information. In 1991, all countries and regions within Great Britain had areas allocated to all 5 deprivation categories. Indeed the majority of local authorities had areas allocated to all 5 deprivation categories. However, there were a number of noticeable exceptions to this general pattern. For example, in the North East region a number of local authorities, for example, Easington, Sunderland and Wear Valley, had no wards in the least deprived quintile, quintile 1. Of these local authorities, only Sunderland had any wards in quintile 2. Within the North West region, Eden, Ribble Valley and Macclesfield had no wards in quintile 5. Within London, Newham, Tower Hamlets, Islington and Hackney had all their wards in quintile 5.

Population living in deprived areas

Figure 4.1 shows the proportion of the population living in wards by quintile for countries and regions within Great Britain in 1991. Almost half of the population of the North East were living in wards in quintile 5 (49 per cent). Other areas with large populations in this quintile were Scotland (47 per cent) and London (45 per cent). Four areas had fewer than 10 per cent of the population living in wards in quintile 1: Scotland (6 per cent), the North East (7 per cent), Yorkshire and the Humber (7 per cent) and London (7 per cent). Just over one quarter of the population of the South East was living in wards in quintile 1.

Figure 4.1

Percentage of the population of wards by deprivation quintile, country and region Great Britain 1991

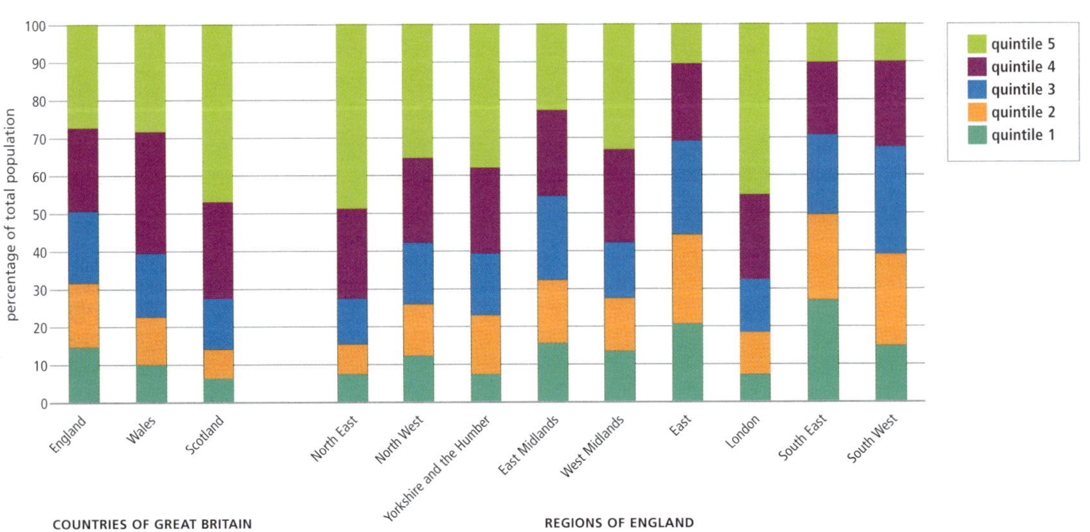

Map 4.2

**Deprivation by ward in 1991 showing local authorities in 1999
North East region**

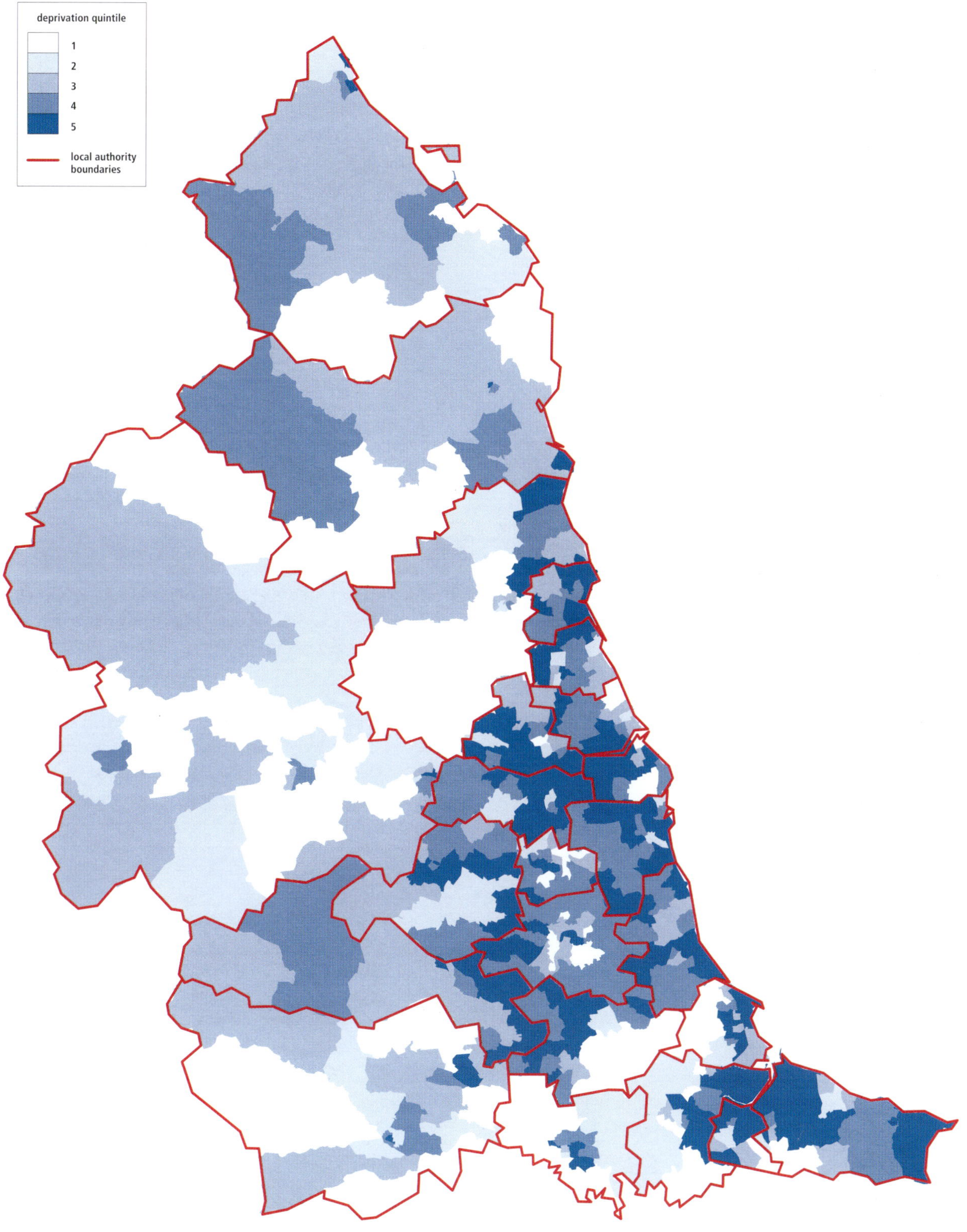

Map 4.3

**Deprivation by ward in 1991 showing local authorities in 1999
North West region**

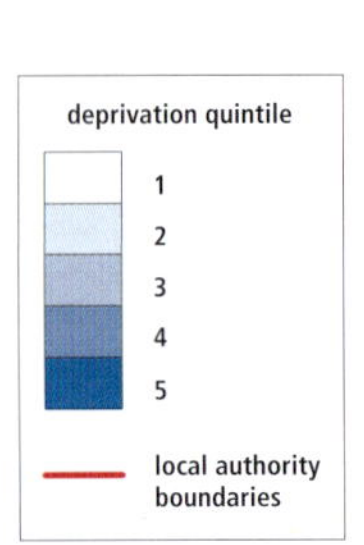

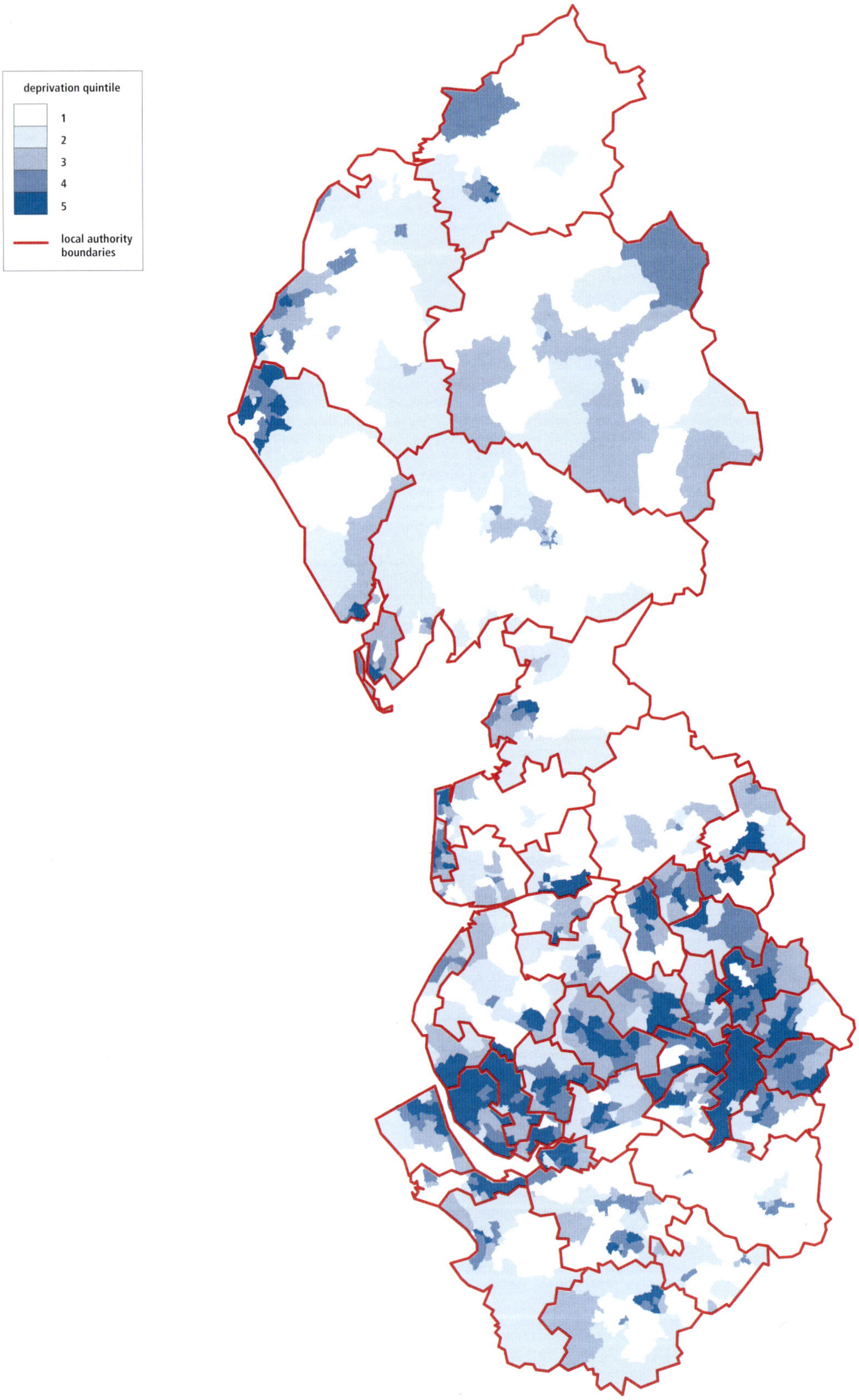

Map 4.4

**Deprivation by ward in 1991 showing local authorities in 1999
Yorkshire and the Humber region**

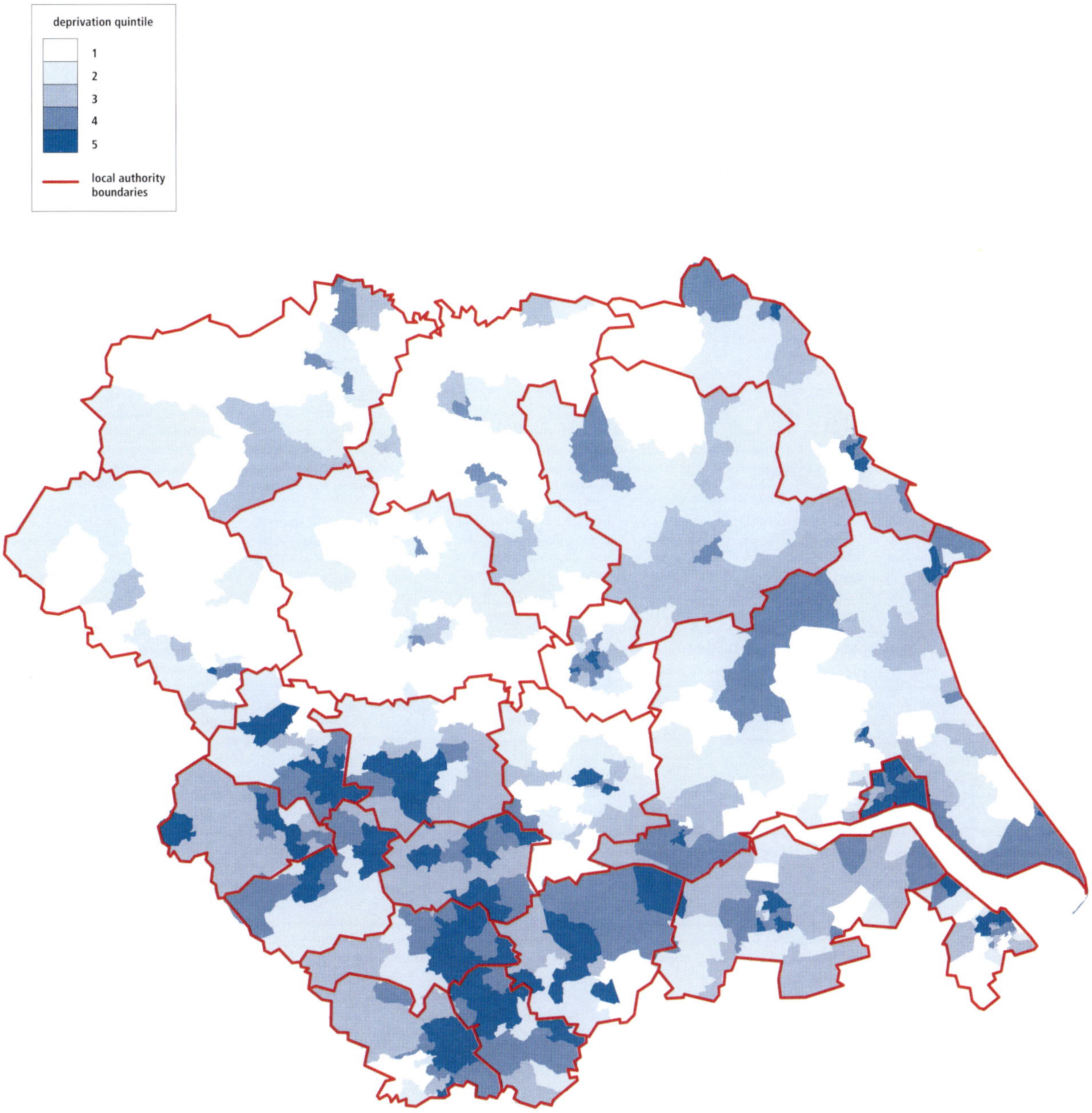

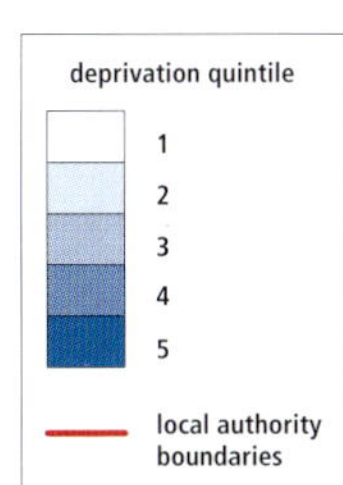

Map 4.5

**Deprivation by ward in 1991 showing local authorities in 1999
East Midlands region**

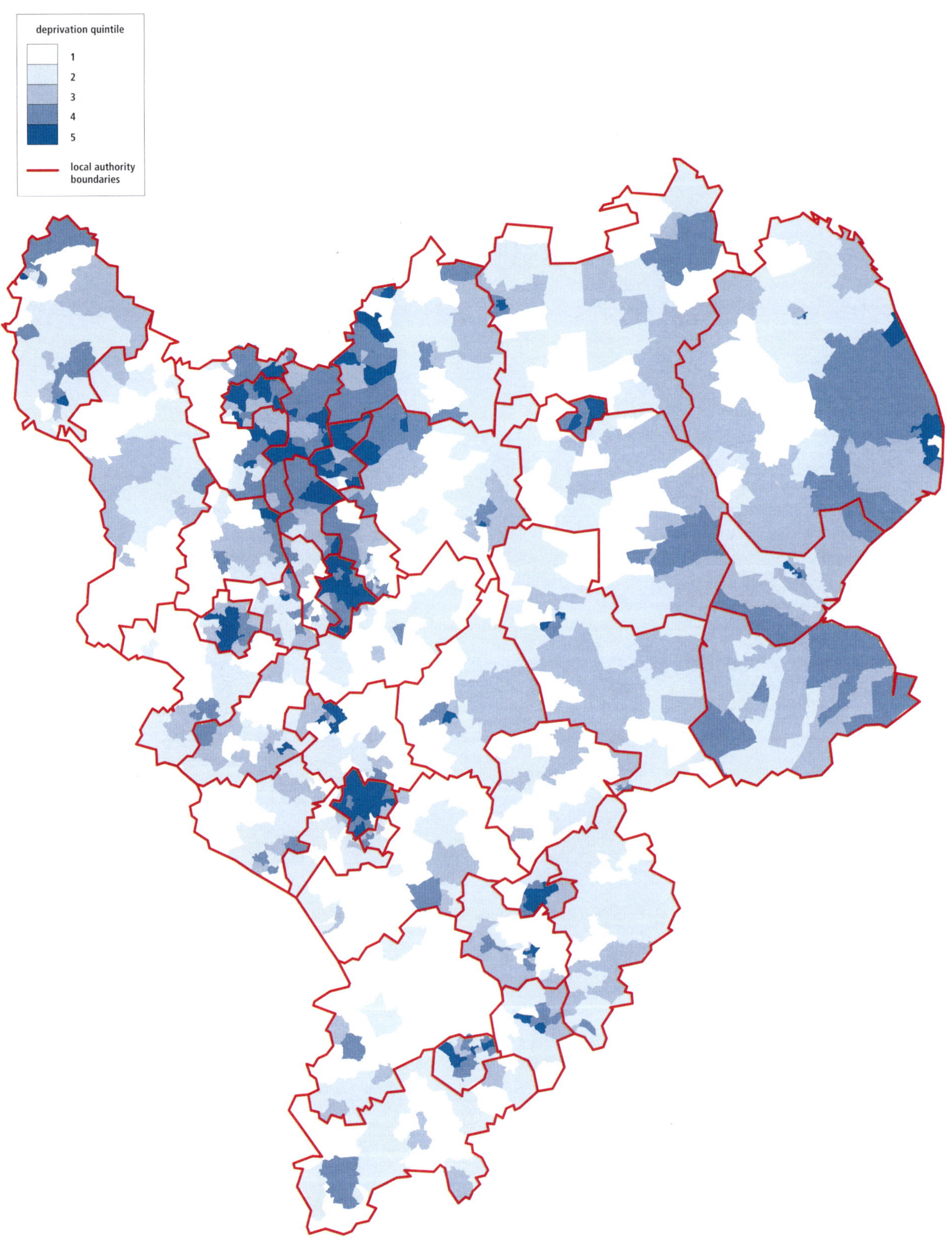

Map 4.6

Deprivation by ward in 1991 showing local authorities in 1999
West Midlands region

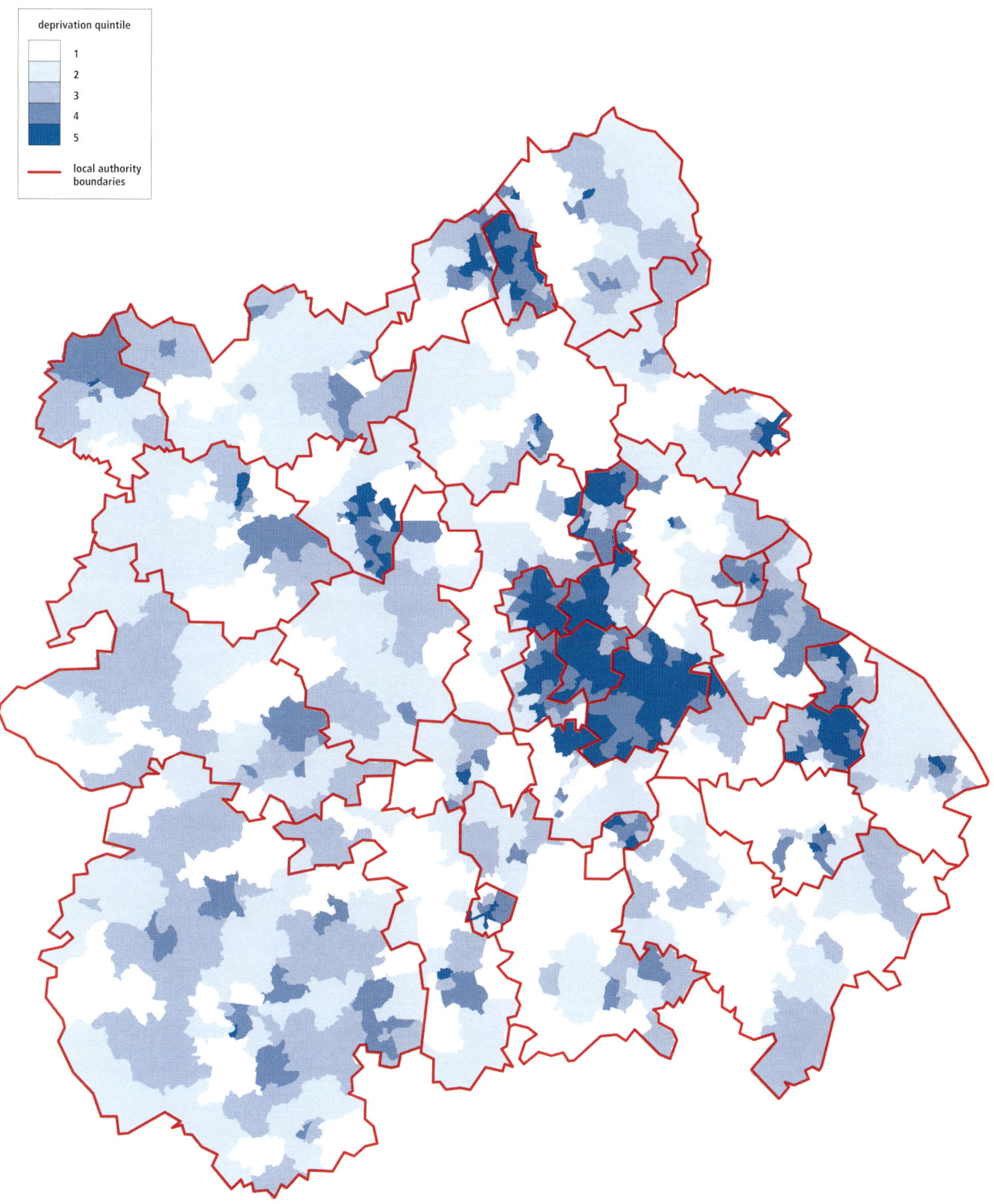

Map 4.7

**Deprivation by ward in 1991 showing local authorities in 1999
East of England region**

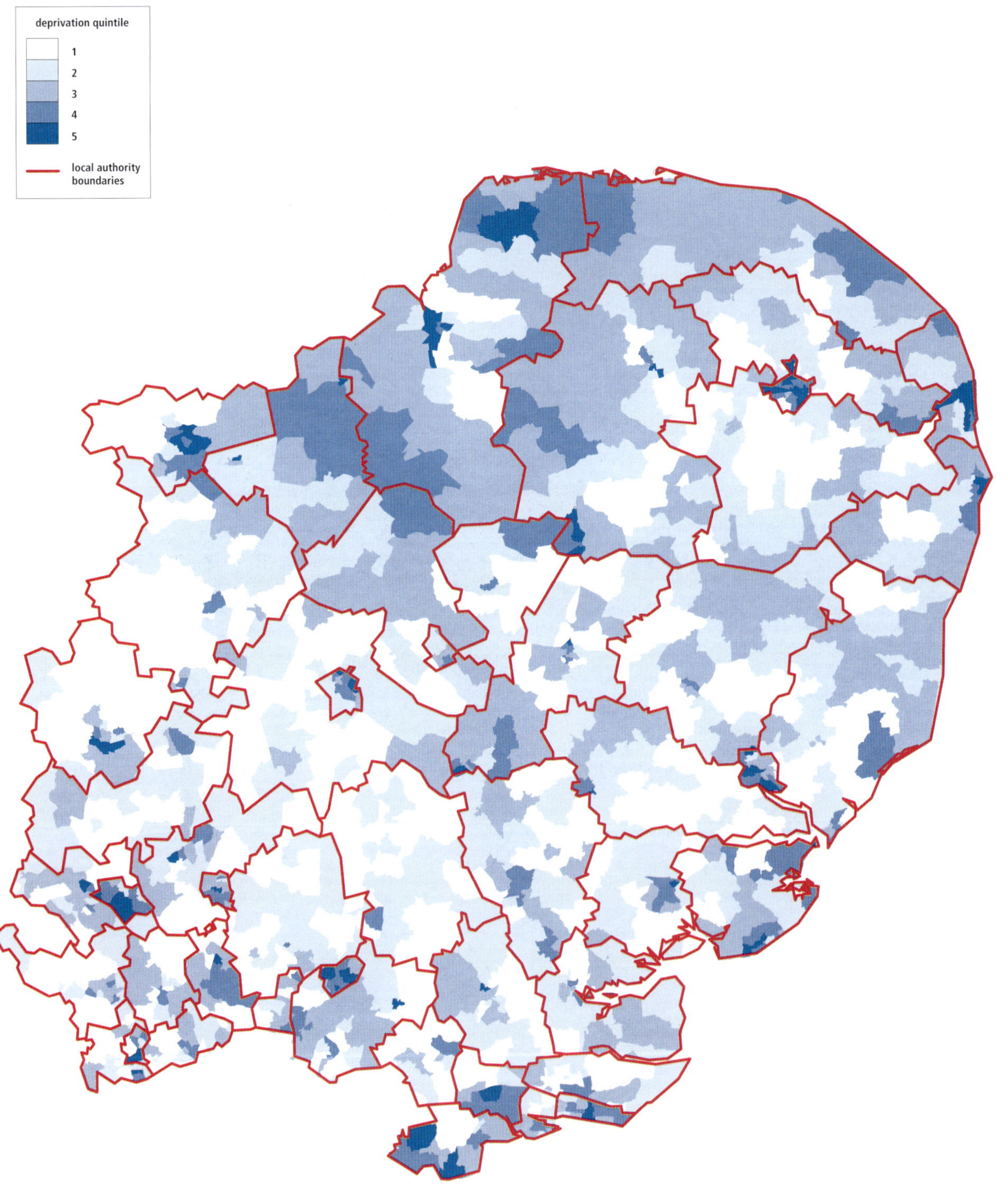

Map 4.8

Deprivation by ward in 1991 showing local authorities in 1999
London region

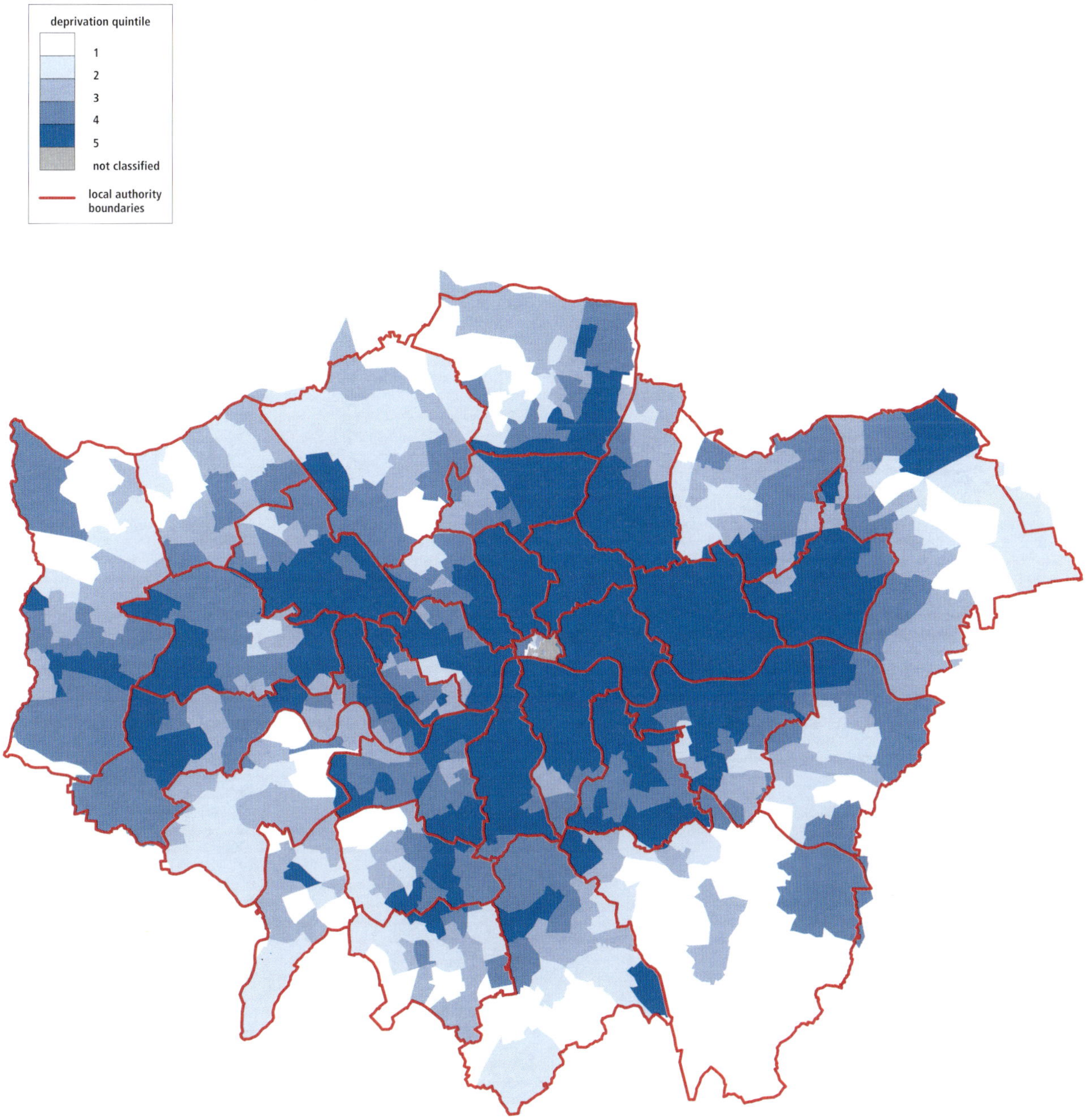

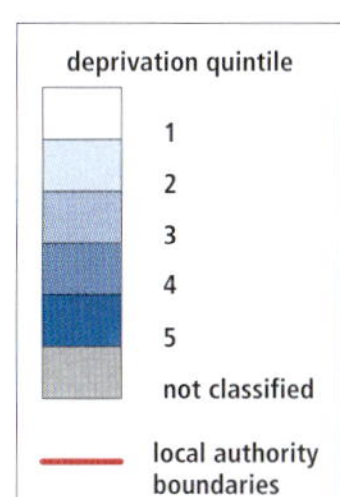

Map 4.9

**Deprivation by ward in 1991 showing local authorities in 1999
South East region**

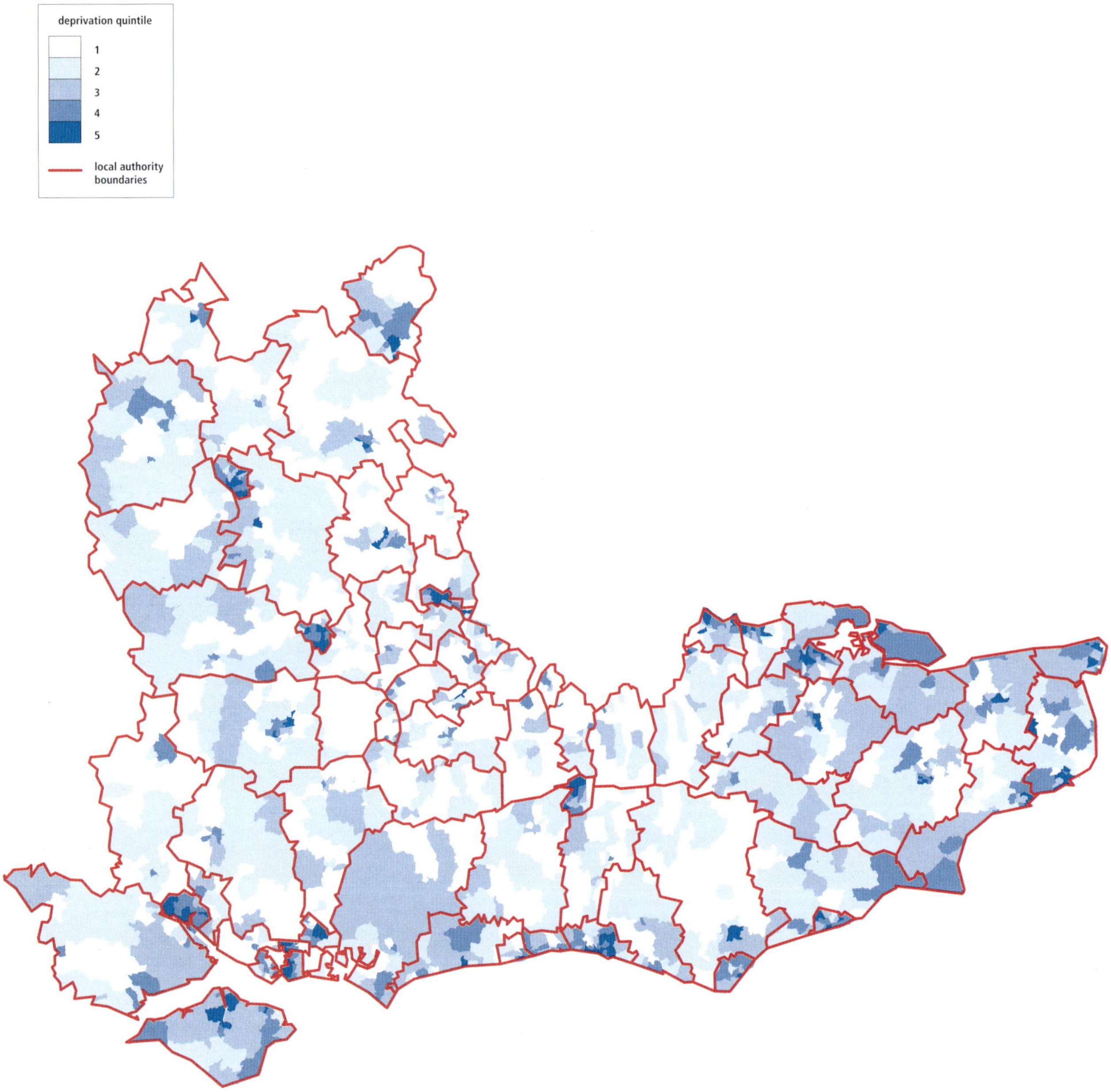

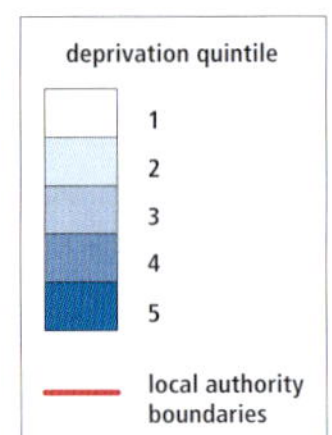

Map 4.10

**Deprivation by ward in 1991 showing local authorities in 1999
South West region**

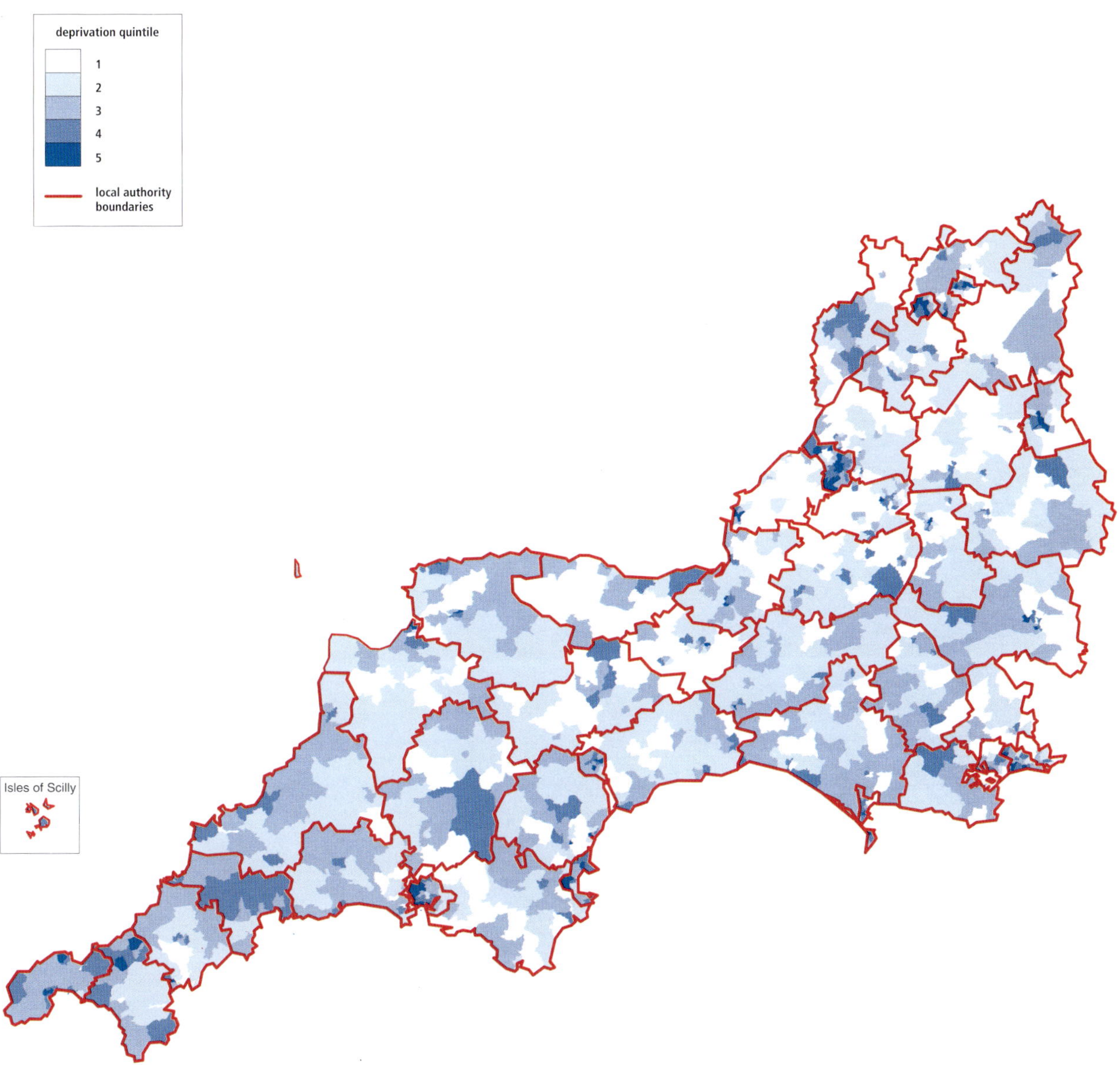

Map 4.11

Deprivation by ward in 1991 showing local authorities in 1999
Wales

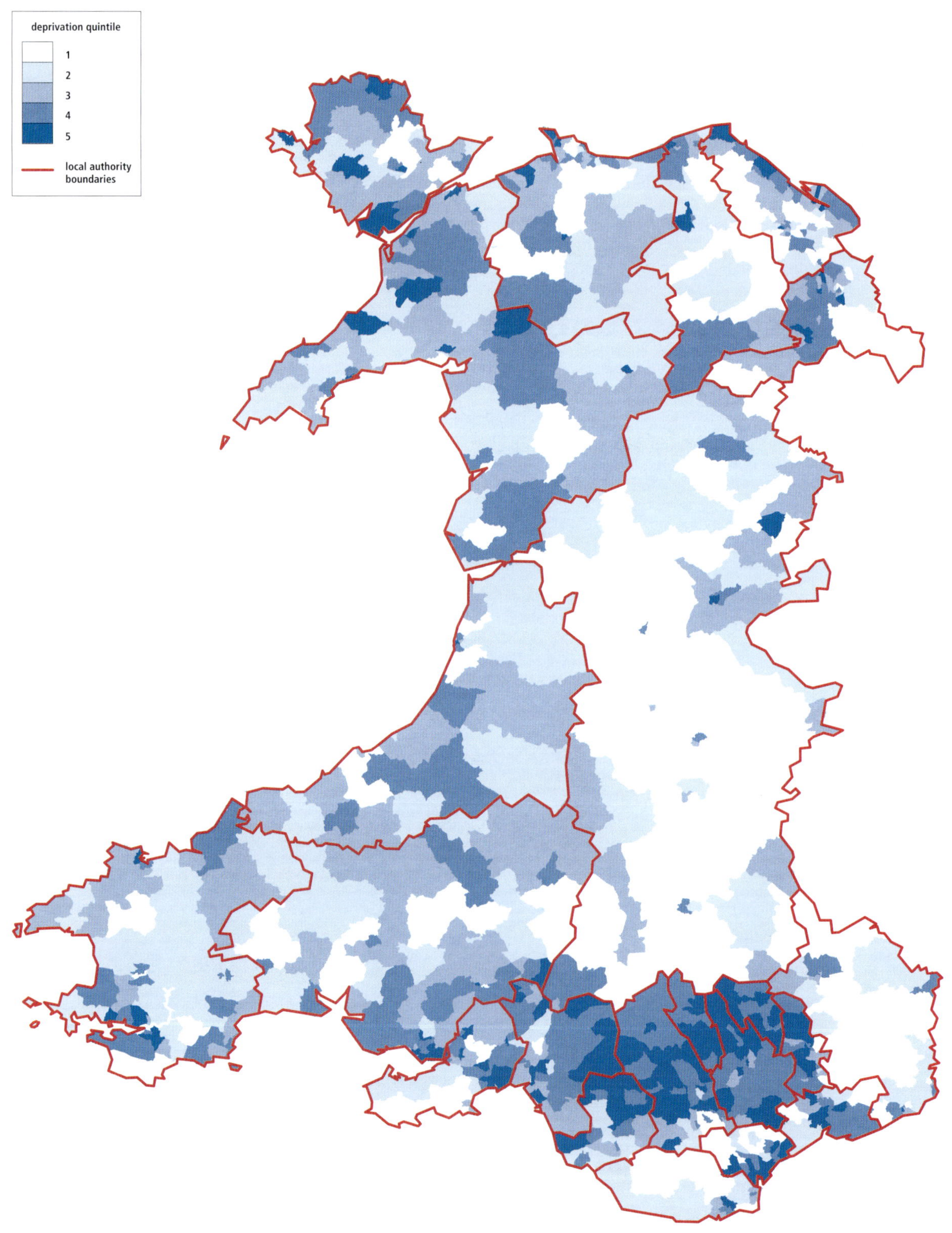

Map 4.12

**Deprivation by postcode sector in 1991 showing local authorities in 1999
Scotland**

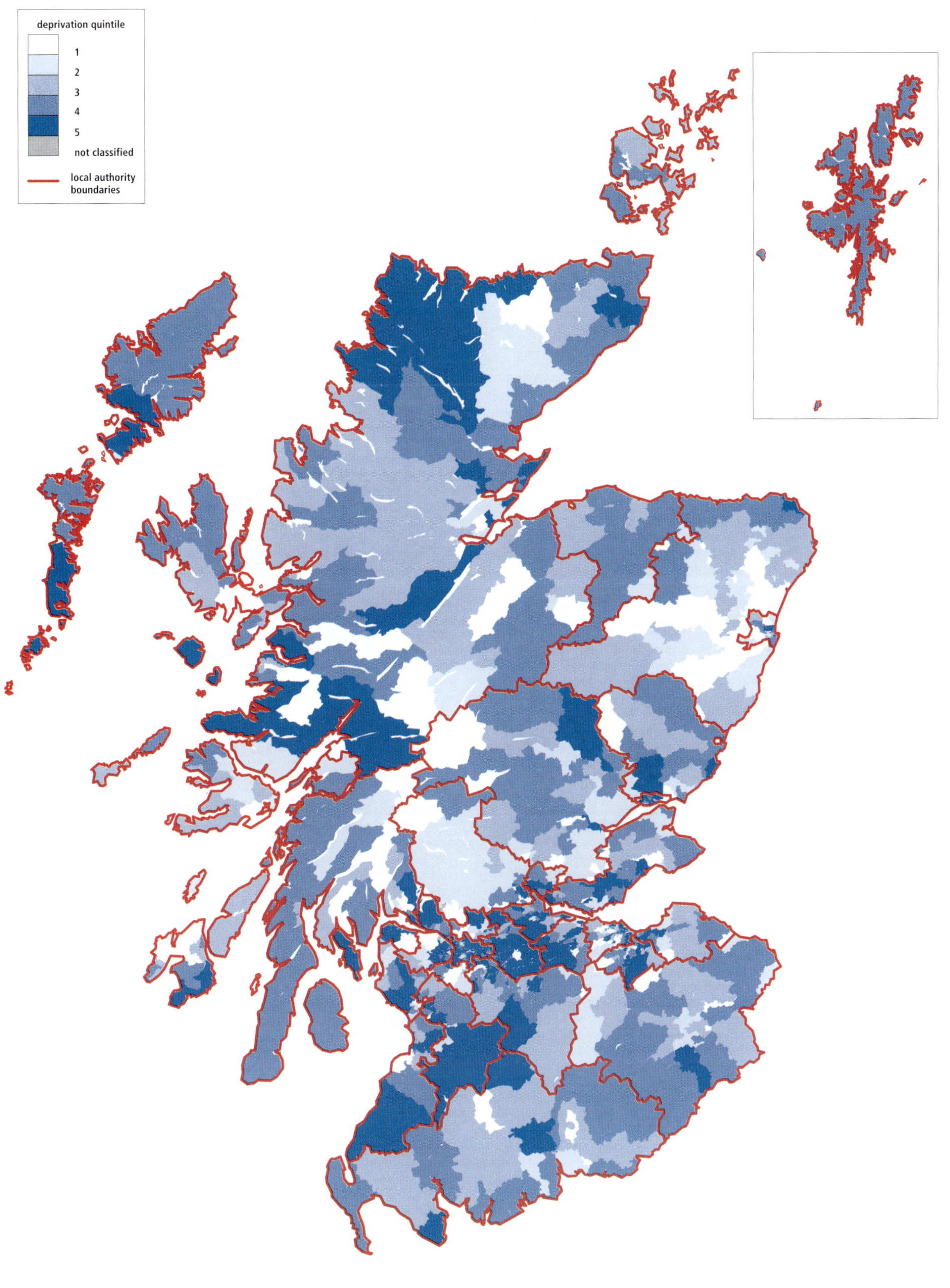

References

1 Office for National Statistics. *The ONS classification of local and health authorities of Great Britain: revised for authorities in 1999*. Series SMPS 63. Office for National Statistics (London: 1999).

2 Wallace M and Denham C. *The ONS classification of local and health authorities of Great Britain*. Series SMPS 59. HMSO (London: 1996).

3 Bailey S, Charlton J, Dollamore G and Fitzpatrick J. Families, Groups and Clusters of local and health authorities: revised for authorities in 1999. *Population Trends* 99 (2000), 37-52.

4 Morris R and Carstairs V. Which deprivation? A comparison of selected deprivation indices. *Journal of Public Health Medicine* 13 (1989), 318-326.

5 Carstairs V and Morris R. *Deprivation and health in Scotland*. Aberdeen University Press (Aberdeen: 1991).

6 Townsend P. Deprivation. *Journal of Social Policy* 16 (1987), 125-146.

Patterns and trends in fertility

Clare Griffiths and Liz Kirby

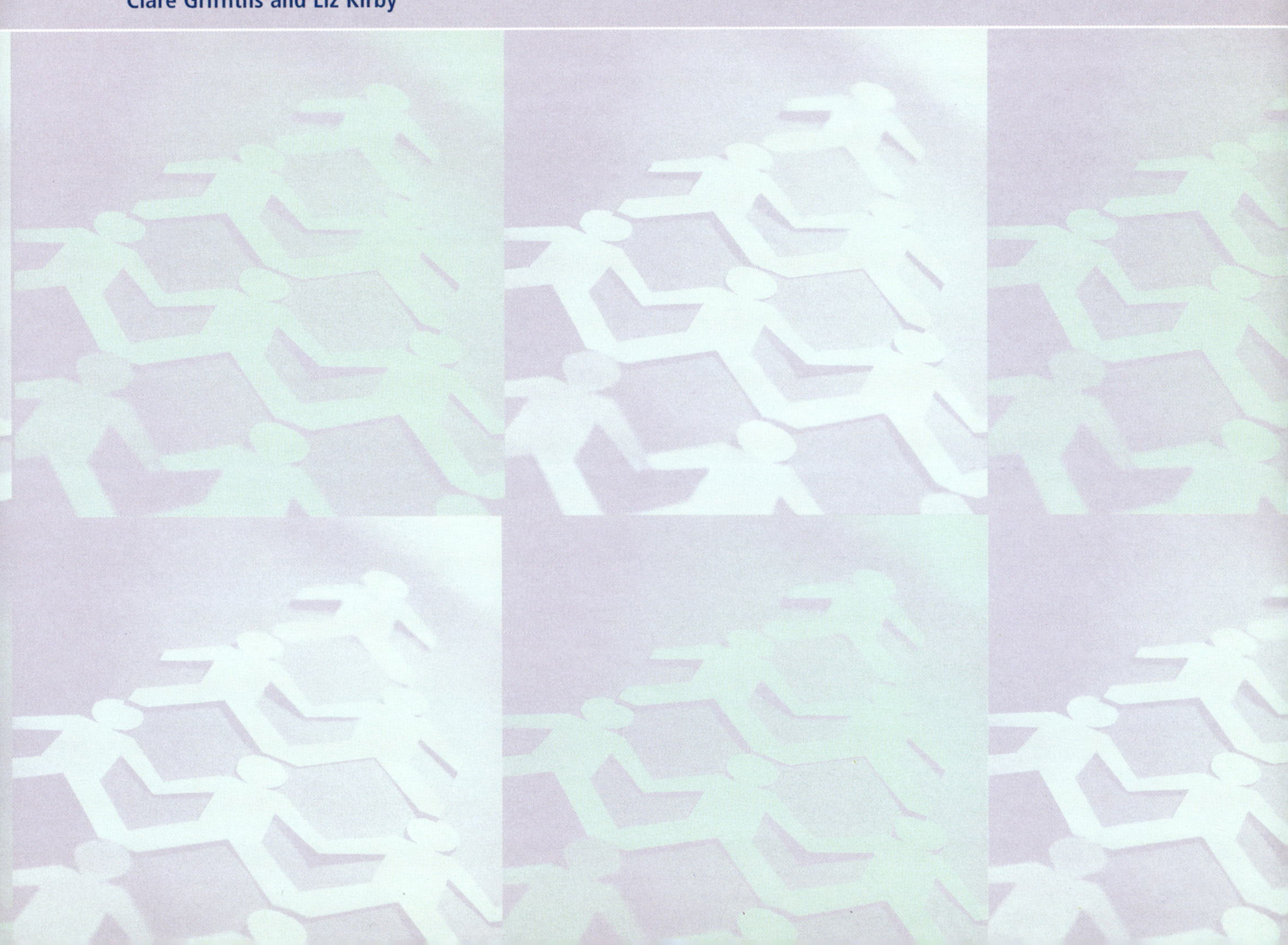

Chapter 5

Patterns and trends in fertility

Summary

• The Total Fertility Rate was highest in Northern Ireland and lowest in Scotland and has declined steadily throughout the 1990s in all countries of the United Kingdom. Within England, it was highest in the West Midlands and has been declining in all regions, except London.

• All-age conception and abortion rates were highest in England and lowest in Scotland. Within England, all-age conception and abortion rates were highest in London throughout the 1990s. Rates were stable in the early part of the 1990s and increased in 1996 following the 1995 pill scare in all countries of Great Britain and regions of England.

• The percentage of conceptions leading to abortion was highest in England and lowest in Scotland of the countries of Great Britain. Within England, London had the highest percentage of conceptions leading to abortion.

• Scotland had the lowest conception and abortion rates in every age group. Wales had high conception and birth rates at younger ages; England had high conception rates at older ages. Northern Ireland had high birth rates at older ages. England had the highest abortion rate and percentage of conceptions leading to abortion in all age groups.

• Within England, there was a marked north-south divide in conception and birth rates, with northern regions having higher rates at younger ages and southern regions at older ages. London had a different pattern, having high conception rates in all age groups over age 20, high birth rates over age 30 and the highest abortion rates in every age group.

• The mean age of mother at live birth showed a north-south divide within England with low mean ages in the northern regions and high mean ages in the south. The mean age at live birth has been steadily increasing throughout the 1990s.

• The highest teenage fertility was found in urban and industrial areas and the lowest in prosperous areas. Teenage birth rates were seven times higher in the most deprived areas of Great Britain than in the least deprived.

• Teenage conception and birth rates declined in the early part of the 1990s but increased in the later part following the 1995 pill scare.

• Fertility in women aged 35-39 has increased substantially throughout the 1990s. The highest rates were found in London and its surrounding area and also in prosperous areas.

• High percentages of abortions performed in 13 or more weeks gestation were found in local authorities in east London, parts of the West Midlands, south Wales, Bristol and Pennine areas. Low proportions were found in East Anglia, outer London, the rural north of England and the south and west of Scotland.

• About a third of all abortions in England were performed privately, compared to a quarter in Wales. Authorities with low proportions performed privately tended to be in the north, South West and East Anglia, whereas those with high proportions were found in London and the South East, as well as parts of Shropshire, Staffordshire and the North West.

• Northern Ireland had higher proportions of live births registered inside marriage than the rest of the United Kingdom at older ages, and higher proportions registered solely by the mother at younger ages.

5.1 Introduction

There is interest in the geographic distribution of fertility within the United Kingdom for a number of reasons. The main areas of interest that we consider in this chapter are in teenage pregnancy, delayed childbearing, the effect of the 1995 pill scare and the decline in births inside marriage.

Teenage pregnancy is an issue that has been high on the policy agenda for some time. There have been concerns both at the number of conceptions, the links with deprivation and the range of adverse outcomes for both mother and child. There are health risks known to be associated with teenage motherhood, including increased risk of infant mortality.[1] This is mainly due to the fact that teenage mothers are more likely to have low birthweight babies.[2] Increased rates of cardiovascular

and central nervous system anomalies have also been found among the children of younger mothers.[3] The children of teenage mothers are also at higher risk of sudden infant death syndrome[4] and of being admitted to hospital as a result of an accident than the children of older mothers.[5] However, it is also thought that the increased risk of maternal complications from pregnancy and childbirth in teenagers is more associated with socio-economic factors than with the biological effects of age and also the fact that teenagers are more likely to seek care late in pregnancy, or not at all.[3]

The longer-term outcomes also appear to be generally poorer for teenage mothers and their children, with 41 per cent of teenage mothers having an episode of depression within one year of childbirth, higher than for teenage girls in general,[6] an increased likelihood of the child experiencing the divorce or separation of its parents[7] and an increased likelihood of the daughters of teenage mothers becoming teenage mothers themselves.[8] In June 1999 the Social Exclusion Unit published a report[9] examining the scale of and trends in teenage pregnancy and looking at approaches to tackle the issue. Following the report a Teenage Pregnancy Unit was established at the Department of Health to co-ordinate action across Government.

Delayed childbearing is also an issue that has been increasing in importance during recent years. The pattern of age-specific fertility is becoming older over time, with several factors influencing this trend. There is perceived to be a need for women to establish their career before having children, indicated by the fact that a disproportionate number of older mothers are in Social Classes I or II. There is also the increasing contribution of remarriages (about one in four marriages) and the desire to have a family in the new partnership.[10] Infant death rates appear to be lower for older mothers.[4] However, there are concerns that later childbearing may bring other risks for both mother and child. Older mothers are known to be at increased risk of having a child with Down syndrome.[11] There is debate as to whether there is an increased risk of diabetes in the children of older mothers with some studies finding a link[12, 13] and others not.[14] A further study found that the risk was highest in the first born,[15] so that delaying childbearing would have an even bigger effect.

In October 1995, the Committee on Safety of Medicines issued a warning that seven brands of the contraceptive pill, known as third-generation contraceptives, carried a relatively higher risk of thrombosis. This received much attention from the media, and there was concern that this scare would result in an increase in unplanned pregnancies, as women stopped taking the pill. The effect of this on fertility rates, especially conception and abortion rates, has been examined at a national level[16] and it is also important to look at a possible variation in the effect in different parts of the country. This has been examined in a number of studies at local level, for example in Oxford a 10 per cent increase in terminations of pregnancy was noted, 8 per cent of which was due to women having stopped taking third-generation oral contraceptives.[17] However, in other studies no effect on the number of abortions or deliveries was found, for example in Grampian.[18] This is examined across Great Britain particularly in sections 5.2 and 5.3 of this chapter.

Another issue that has a high profile is the decline of births inside marriage and increasing numbers of births born to cohabiting couples.[19] We examine how this varies geographically within the United Kingdom in section 5.4 of this chapter. The proportion of births born to lone mothers has remained relatively stable, but there is an increased risk of infant mortality associated with the sole registration of births,[1] although this is strongly related to birthweight and for normal weight babies lone mothers are not at increased risk. This is examined in more detail in chapter 7 of this volume.

Previous studies examining geographic variations in fertility have found that the areas which covered most of London had high conception rates and a higher than average percentage

leading to abortion, an exceptional pattern. The urban and industrial areas had the highest percentages of conceptions leading to a maternity. The most prosperous areas had high conception rates at older ages and lower at younger ages. Suburban areas of London and university towns had high conception rates in the over 30s, and urban and industrial areas had higher rates at younger ages.[20] These areas also had the same pattern in birth rates.[21] The proportion of live births within marriage has also been found to be highest in former manufacturing areas of the north and Midlands, and in most of London.[21] In this chapter we examine variations in fertility using the ONS classification of local authorities throughout the sections on conceptions, abortions and live births (5.2-5.4).

A substantial amount of research on the relationship between fertility and deprivation has focused on the relationship for teenagers, finding a strong association between high teenage fertility and high levels of deprivation.[22, 23, 24] In this chapter we examine the relationship between fertility and deprivation in section 5.5.

This chapter adds to previous research by examining conceptions, abortions and live births data together for the 1990s - conceptions and abortions data for Great Britain for 1992-1997 and births data for the United Kingdom for 1991-1997, in sections 5.2-5.4. The sections have been taken in chronological order of event to aid understanding. The chapter includes analysis not just of rates, but of the percentage of conceptions leading to abortion, the percentage of abortions by gestation length and purchaser and births by the marital status of the mother. The age-specific analysis covers all age groups, but we have focused on the patterns for under 18s and 35-39 year old women, as these are the areas where most interest lies. Throughout the chapter we use 'fertility' as a general term to cover all the topics for ease of discussion. When specific topics are discussed, they are referred to by name, that is conceptions, abortions or live births. Stillbirths are discussed in chapter 6.

Within each topic we first consider variations at constituent country level (England, Wales and Scotland for conceptions and abortions and England, Wales, Scotland and Northern Ireland for live births). We then examine variations between the Government Office Regions within England. Finally, we examine variations at local authority level, using the revised ONS classification of local authorities[25] as an indicator of the characteristics of areas. We also use the Carstairs and Morris index of deprivation as a possible explanatory variable for some of the patterns observed in section 5.5. Other possible explanations for the patterns seen are discussed in section 5.6.

Maps are used to describe the patterns at local authority level, and details of how these were constructed can be found in Appendix A. All rates presented in this chapter, with the exception of the Total Fertility Rate, are expressed per 1,000 women in the age group under discussion. For all-age rates the population of women aged 15-44 is used. For rates that are under 18 and 40 plus, the populations of women aged 15-17 and 40-44 respectively are used.

5.2 Conceptions

In this section we examine geographic variation across Great Britain in the conception rate and the percentage of conceptions leading to abortion between 1992 and 1997. The conceptions data used are compiled from:

- live or still births (*maternities*), and

- legal abortions under the Abortion Act 1967 (*abortions*).

Miscarriages and illegal abortions are not included; therefore the figures will be an underestimate of the true number of conceptions.

Data for Scotland have been compiled by the Information and Statistics Division (ISD). ISD routinely produce data on pregnancies which usually include data on miscarriages, but these have been excluded for the purposes of this analysis, to achieve comparability across Great Britain. The conceptions data for Scotland in this chapter are derived from maternity discharge records and abortion notifications, whereas in England and Wales birth registrations and abortion notifications are used. Therefore, any births to Scottish residents which occur at home are excluded. This accounts for about 0.5 per cent of all births.

For England and Wales data, the date of conception is estimated using recorded gestation for abortions and stillbirths, and assuming 40 weeks gestation for live births.

For Scottish maternities, date of conception is estimated from recorded gestation in 99.8 per cent of cases and estimated gestation of 40 weeks is used in 0.2 per cent. Age at conception is then estimated from this date. This will lead to an underestimation of the age at conception in England and Wales compared to Scotland. For Scottish abortions data, date of conception is estimated from recorded gestation.

Conceptions and abortions data for Northern Ireland are not included, as the Abortion Act 1967 does not apply to Northern Ireland. Less than 100 legal abortions are performed there each year on medical grounds in health service hospitals under case law, as was the legal situation in the rest of the United Kingdom before the 1967 Act. Data on abortions to residents of Northern Ireland performed in the rest of the United Kingdom are not analysed in this chapter, as it would be impossible to obtain a dataset that was of comparable quality to those for England, Wales and Scotland and that would allow analysis by district council area and by age group. This is partly because some of those women from Northern Ireland who attend for abortion in the rest of the United Kingdom may state a temporary residence in England, Wales or Scotland. This also means that conception figures calculated for local authorities may be inflated in areas where any non-residents attend for abortion giving a temporary address as their address of usual residence.[26]

Prior to 1992, the postcode of usual residence was not retained for analysis of abortions once the administrative area information such as local authority or health authority applicable at the time were derived. These data cannot, therefore, be recast to the latest boundaries. Analysis in this volume is based on boundaries in 1999 and has therefore been restricted to 1992 onwards for the conceptions and abortions sections of this chapter.

Conception rates
All-age patterns
Country and regional level variation
The overall conception rate in Great Britain was 74.1 over the period 1992 to 1997. Wales and Scotland had significantly lower conception rates than Great Britain (Figure 5.1). Scotland had the lowest conception rate and England the highest rate. Two regions within England had higher conception rates than the Great Britain rate for 1992 to 1997, the West Midlands and

Figure 5.1

Conception rates by country and region, women all ages Great Britain 1992-1997

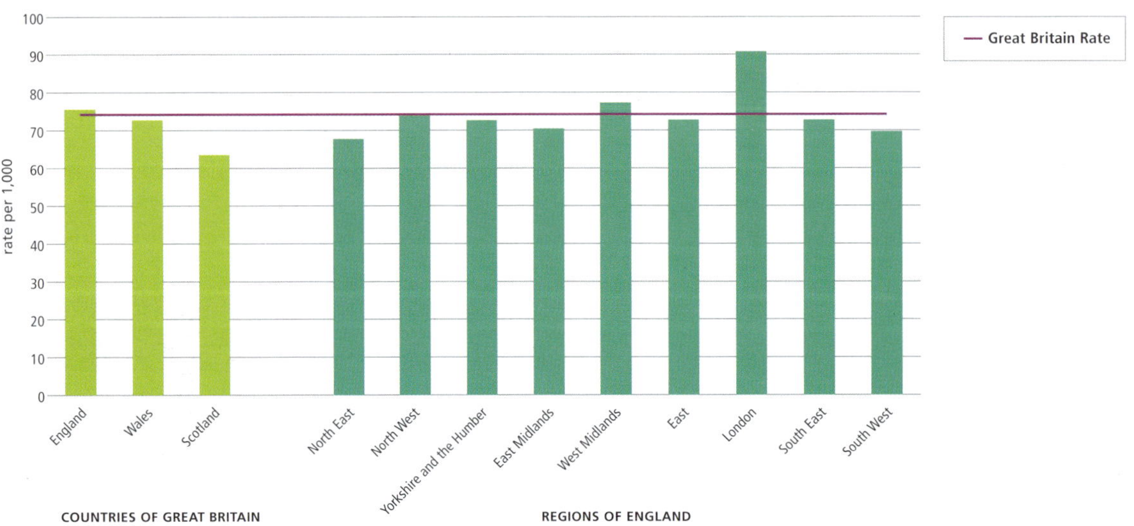

Map 5.1

**Conception rates by local authority, women all ages
Great Britain 1992-1997**

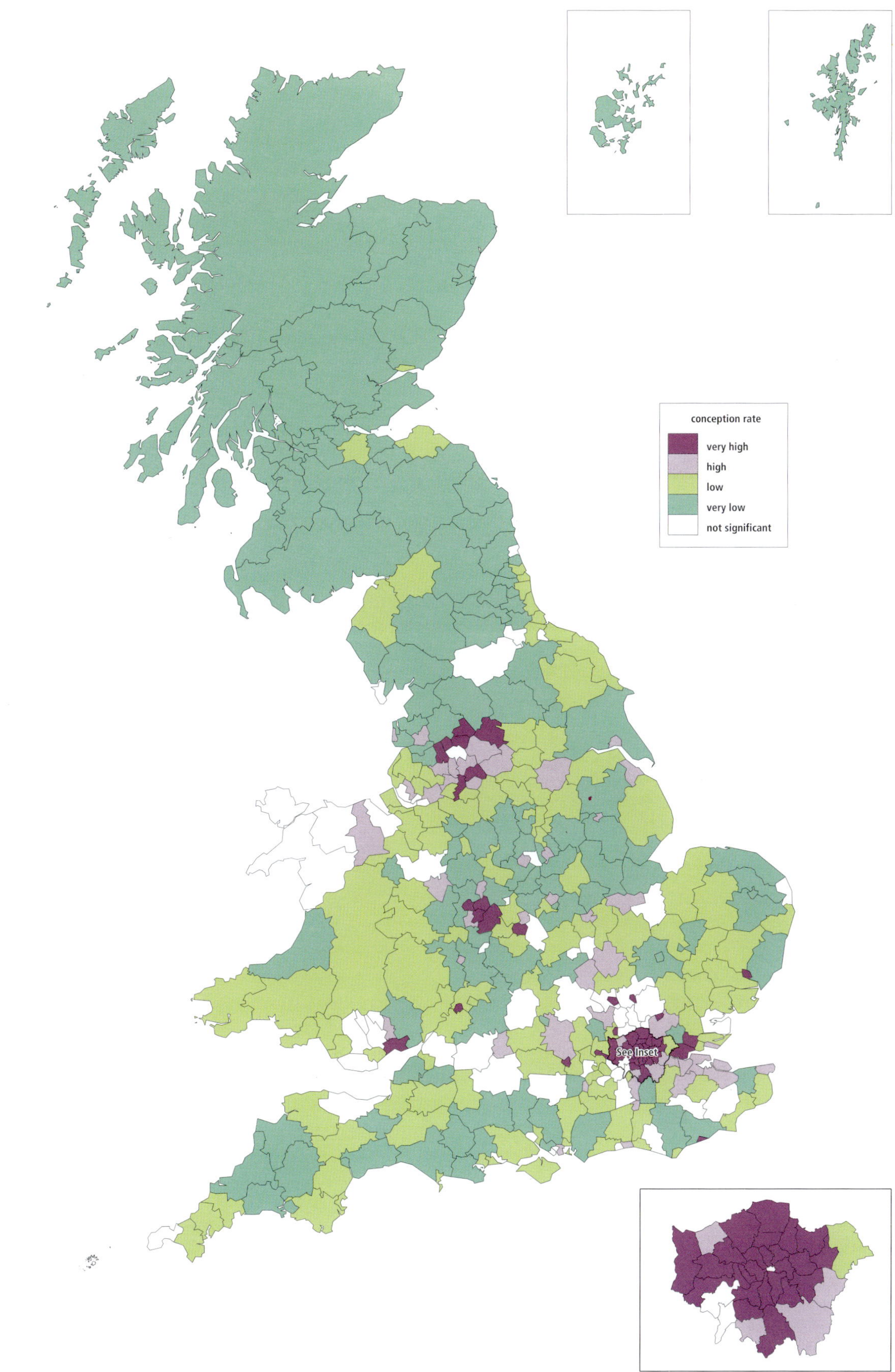

Figure 5.2

**Conception rates by country and age group
Great Britain 1992-1997**

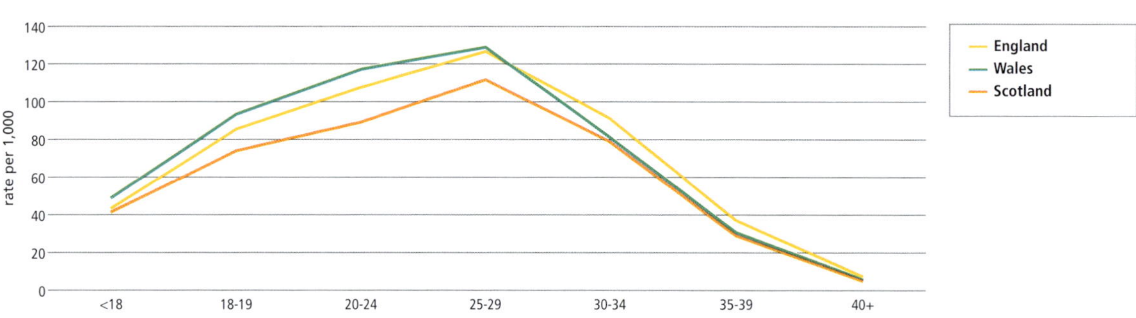

Figure 5.3

**Trends in conception rates by country, women aged under 18
Great Britain 1992-1997**

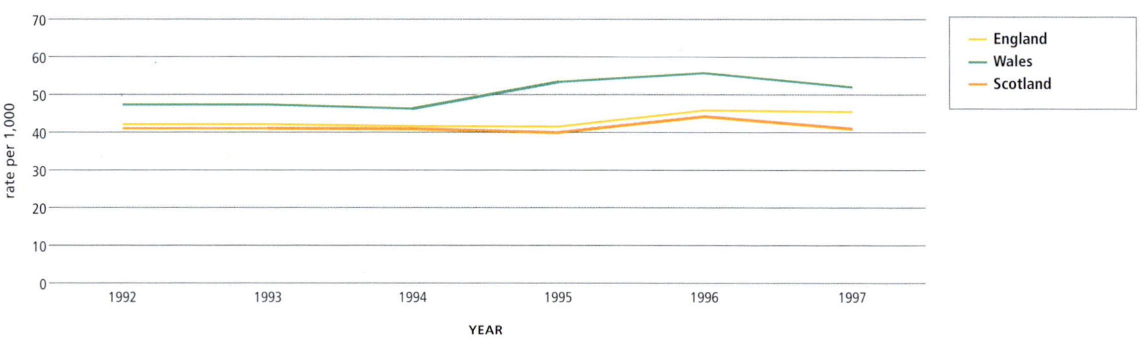

London. The rate in London was substantially higher than the Great Britain rate. All other regions had significantly lower conception rates than Great Britain, with the lowest rate being in the North East (Figure 5.1).

Local authority level variation
The pattern described for countries and regions masks variation that is apparent at local authority level. Rather than rates simply being much higher in London than elsewhere, there were in fact small clusters of local authorities with very high conception rates around London, Birmingham and Manchester (Map 5.1). However, the local authorities with the highest conception rates were mainly found in London, with Newham having the highest rate.

Map 5.1 also shows that all local authorities in Scotland had an all-age conception rate that was significantly lower than in Great Britain as a whole, as did a substantial number of rural areas in England and Wales. No local authorities in the North East or South West regions had higher conception rates than Great Britain as a whole. In London, only Havering had a lower conception rate than Great Britain.

Age-specific patterns
Patterns in the all-age rate can be partly explained by the age distribution in the population. Areas with a high proportion of

women aged 20-34 will tend to have higher conception rates than areas with lower proportions in this age group, as these are the peak ages for conception.[19] In order to take this into account it is important to examine age-specific rates.

Country and regional level variation
The conception rate in all the countries of Great Britain increases with age to a peak in the 25-29 age group and then declines steadily with age. In our analysis, Scotland had the lowest rates in every age group, but the difference was more marked for women in their late teens to late twenties. Wales had the highest rates up to the late twenties; at older ages the highest rates were found in England (Figure 5.2).

All the countries had steady conception rates for under 18s until 1995. A substantial increase occurred in 1996, followed by a decline in 1997 in all the countries, most markedly in Scotland (Figure 5.3). The increase in conception rate in 1996 followed the pill scare in 1995, with most of the excess conceptions occurring in the first half of 1996.[16] However, Figure 5.4 shows that for women in their late thirties, conception rates in England and Wales did not fall after the increase in 1996.

Within England, the northern regions and the West Midlands generally had high conception rates in the younger age groups,

Figure 5.4

Trends in conception rates by country, women aged 35-39
Great Britain 1992-1997

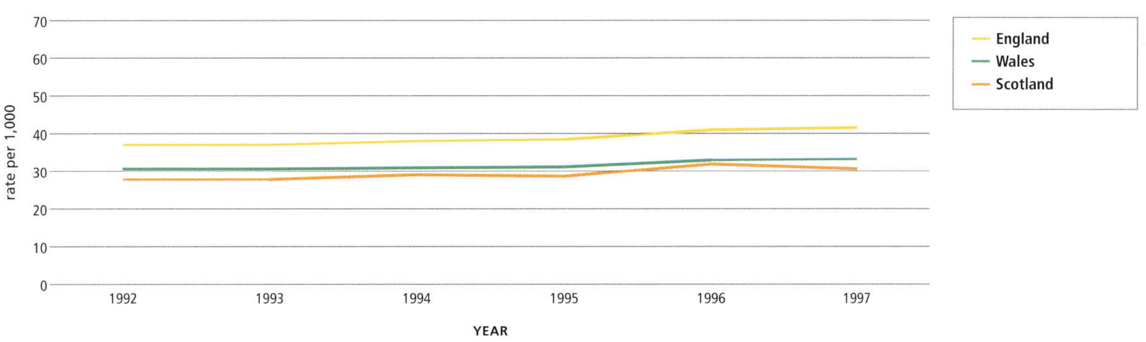

Figure 5.5

Conception rates by region and age group
England 1992-1997

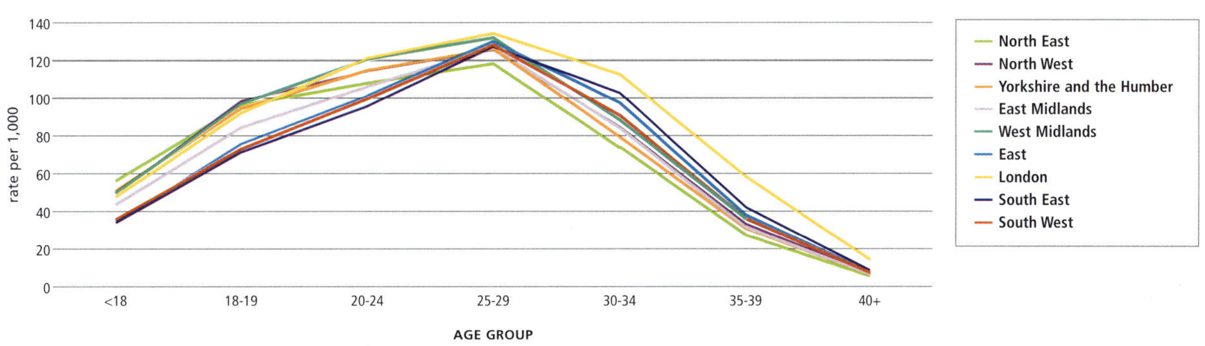

Figure 5.6

Trends in conception rates by region, women aged under 18
England 1992-1997

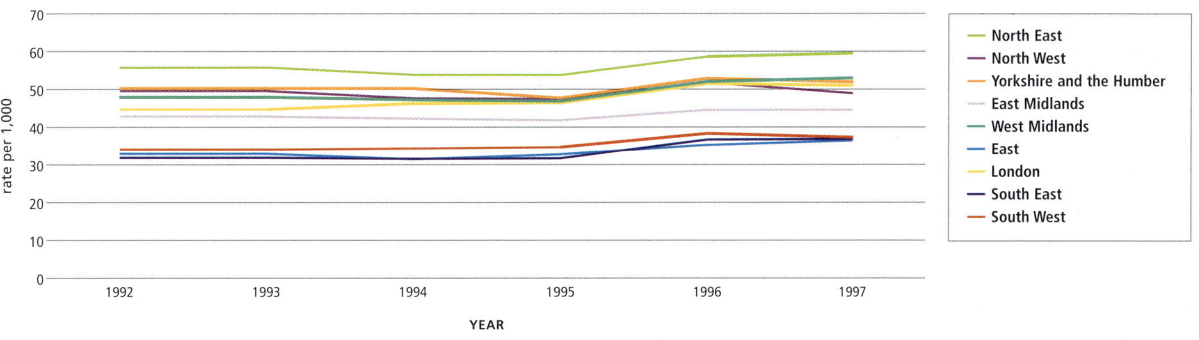

Figure 5.7

Trends in conception rates by region, women aged 35-39
England 1992-1997

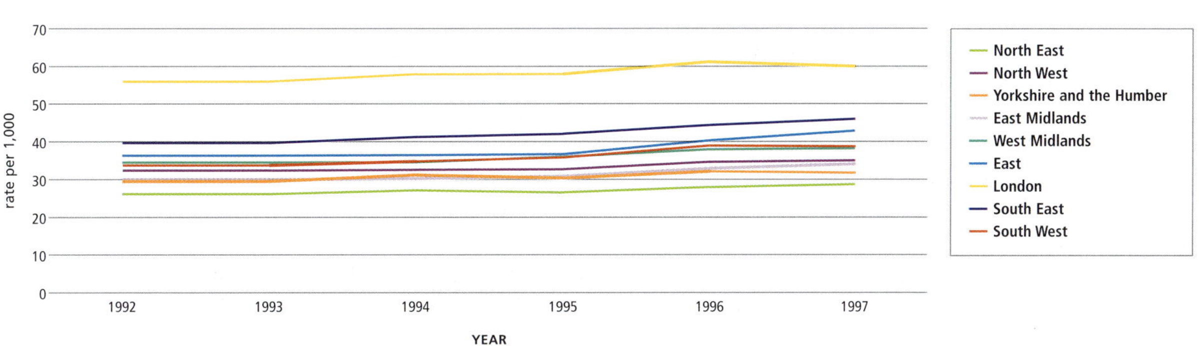

but low rates in the older age groups, in contrast to the South East and East of England regions, which showed a reverse pattern. The East Midlands, however, had lower rates than Great Britain in every age group. The South West had lower rates than Great Britain in every age group except 25-29. In London, rates were higher than the other regions in every age group over age 20 (Figure 5.5).

As seen for the countries of Great Britain, age-specific conception rates in the regions of England were also stable until 1995 and increased in 1996. Main differences to this pattern were seen in the North West, which had no overall increase in its under 18 conception rate between 1992 and 1997 (Figure 5.6) and in London and the South East, where conception rates had been increasing in 35-39 year old women since 1993 (Figure 5.7).

Local authority level variation
As with the all-age patterns, analysis at the country and regional level masks variations at the local authority level in each age group. High teenage conception rates seen in the northern regions of England and in Wales mask the fact that the high rates in Wales were due primarily to a cluster of authorities with high rates in south Wales, for both under 18s and those aged 18-19, and that there were also high rates in authorities in inner London and scattered urban authorities across Britain (Maps 5.2, 5.3). Areas with very low rates were mainly rural areas across Great Britain.

When examining under 18 rates using ONS Classification Groups, the majority of authorities with highest rates were found in the *Coalfields, Manufacturing Centres* and *Ports and Industry* Groups (62 per cent of authorities with very high rates on Map 5.2). These areas have characteristics generally associated with disadvantage, such as high unemployment, a high proportion of the population in Social Classes IV and V and high levels of social housing. This finding backs up the results of previous studies showing that teenage pregnancy is associated with material deprivation.

Authorities with the lowest teenage conception rates were mainly in the *Most Prosperous, Growth Areas, Rural Amenity* and *Remoter Rural* Groups (89 per cent of authorities with very low rates on Map 5.2). Three of these four Groups have a number of socio-demographic characteristics associated with affluence, for example low unemployment, a high proportion of the population in Social Classes I or II, low levels of local authority-rented accommodation and high levels of car access. The fourth Group, *Remoter Rural,* does not share all these characteristics, but still had low teenage conception rates.

At Group level, *East Inner London* had the highest teenage conception rate, and *Coalfields, Manufacturing Centres* and *Ports and Industry* also had high rates. The *Most Prosperous, Growth Areas, Rural Amenity* and *Remoter Rural* Groups had the lowest rates (Figure 5.8).

The geographic pattern in conception rates changes with age (Maps 5.4-5.8). The pattern for women in their early twenties was similar to teenagers, with clusters of authorities with higher rates in broadly the same areas. A large number of local authorities in the South East and Scotland had significantly lower rates than Great Britain, (Map 5.4). For women aged 25-29 rates were generally lower than average in local authorities in Scotland and the North East (Map 5.5). Higher rates were mainly found in England and Wales, with the local authorities with the highest rates being in London and the Home Counties.

For women in their thirties there was a large concentration of local authorities with significantly higher conception rates in the south central and eastern areas of England (Maps 5.6, 5.7) and, for women aged 35-39, local authorities with very high rates were only found in three regions - the East of England, London and the South East. A large number of local authorities in south Wales, Scotland, the East Midlands and the north of England had lower conception rates than Great Britain as a whole. London had no local authorities that had very low conception rates for women aged 35-39. For women aged over 40 the local authorities with high rates were again concentrated around London, with a few other areas with high rates scattered around the country. The lowest rates were found in local authorities in Scotland, the North East and North West, Yorkshire and the Humber, Wales and the East Midlands, a pattern also clearly seen in the regional figures (Map 5.8).

For women in their late thirties a different pattern by ONS classification Group to teenagers was seen. The *Most Prosperous* Group had high conception rates, but it was in London (*West Inner London* and *East Inner London*) where the highest rates were seen (Figure 5.9). Low rates for women in their late thirties were found in the *Coalfields, Manufacturing Centres* and *Ports and Industry* Groups and about half of all those authorities with very low rates are classified to these three groups. Low rates were also found in the *Remoter Rural* and *Established Manufacturing Fringe* Groups. In this age group there seems to be a clustering of high rates around London and in the South East, rather than a substantial pattern using ONS classification Groups.

The age-specific pattern of conception differed for local authorities in London compared to those in the rest of the country. In local authorities in other parts of Great Britain that had high teenage conception rates, low conception rates were found at older ages. However, in London there were high conception rates throughout each age group. These were found in central London authorities only for the age groups under twenty and throughout most of London for women in their twenties, and the whole of London for women aged thirty and over. This leads to the regional pattern described earlier with London having higher conception rates than the rest of the regions of England in all the age groups over age twenty.

Map 5.2

**Conception rates by local authority, women aged under 18
Great Britain 1992-1997**

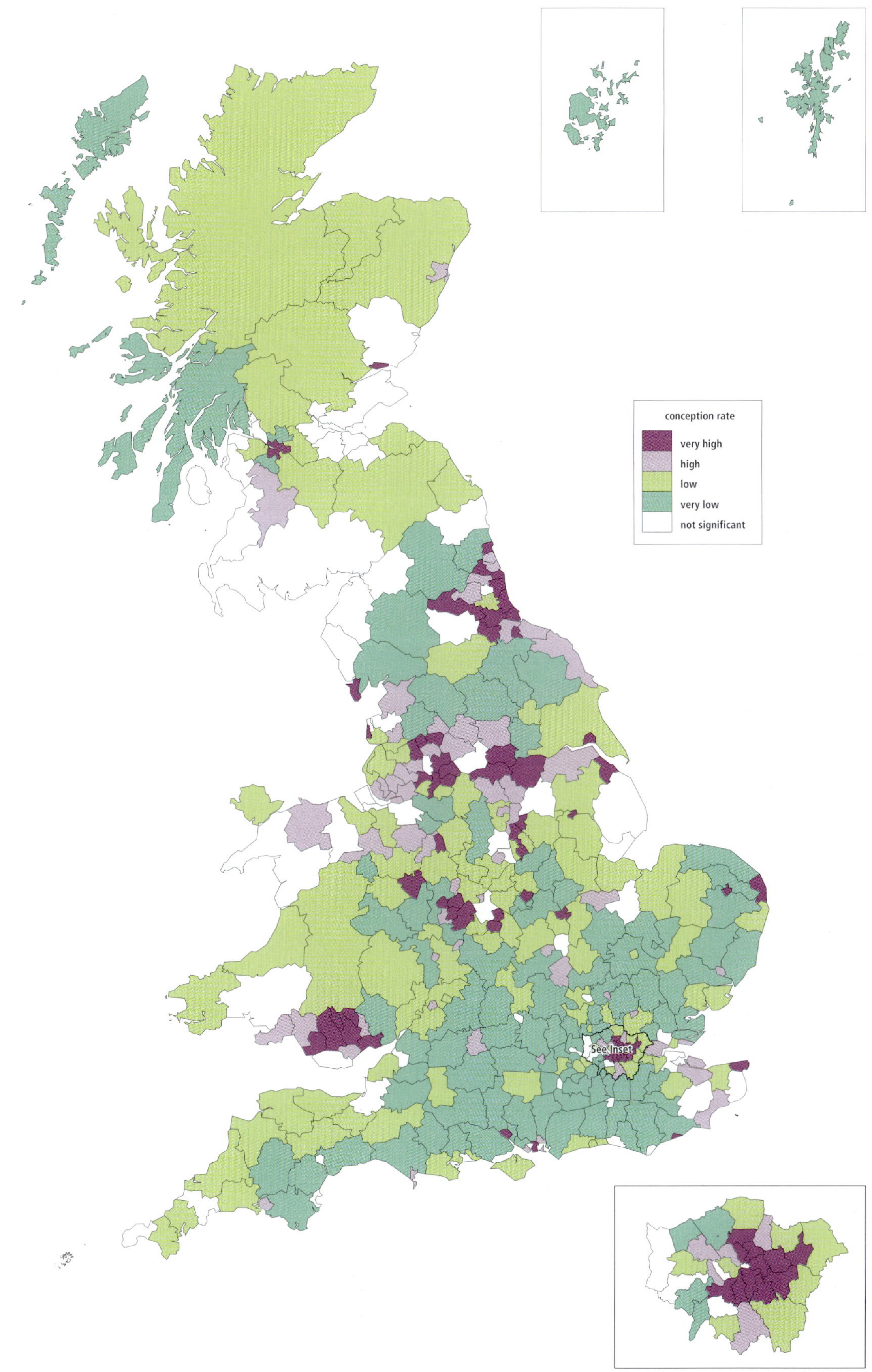

Map 5.3

**Conception rates by local authority, women aged 18-19
Great Britain 1992-1997**

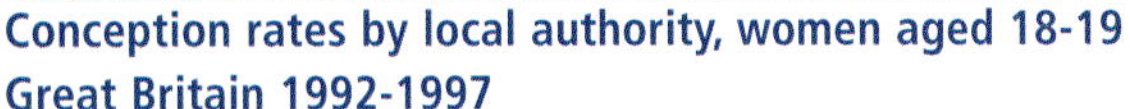

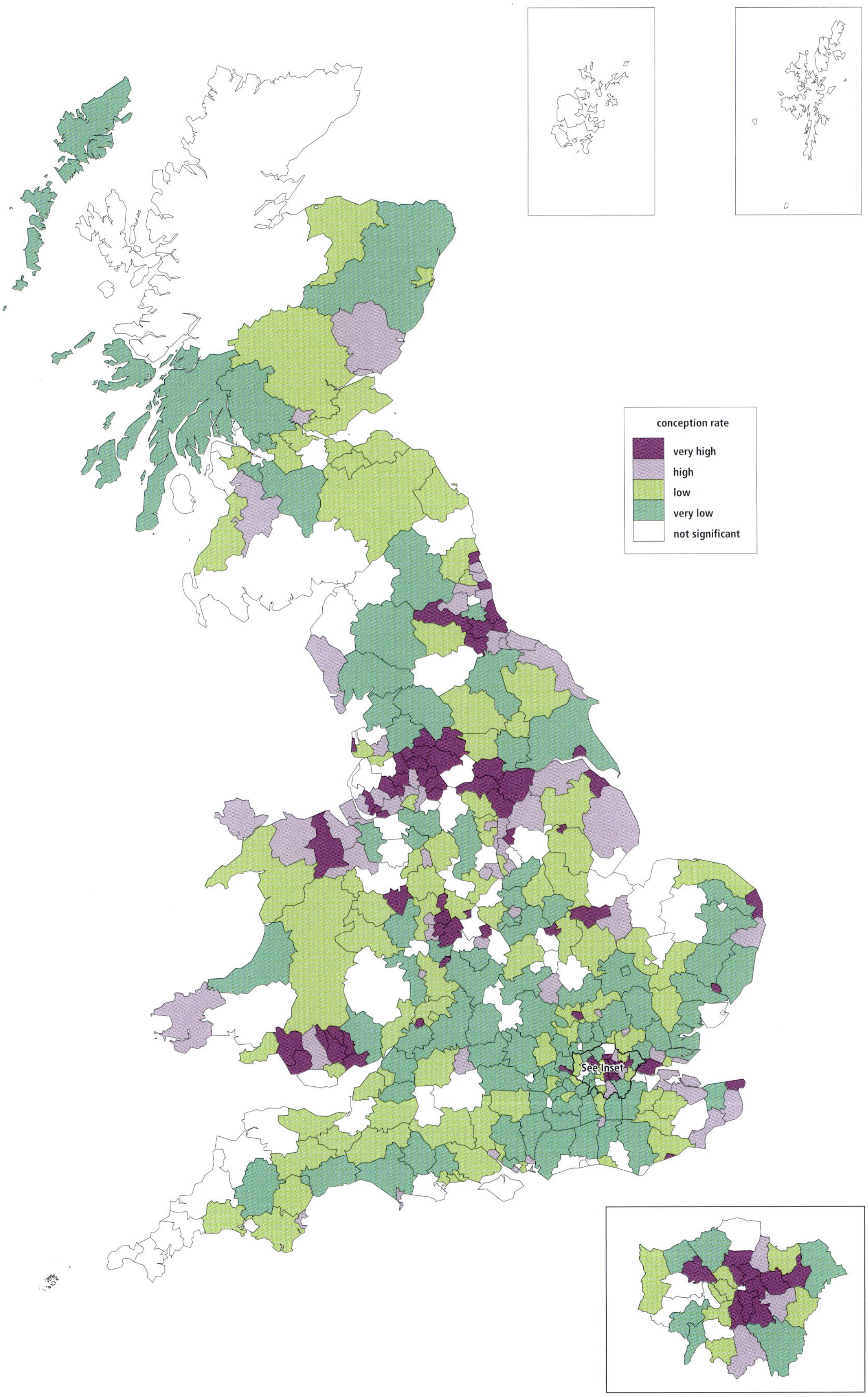

Map 5.4

**Conception rates by local authority, women aged 20-24
Great Britain 1992-1997**

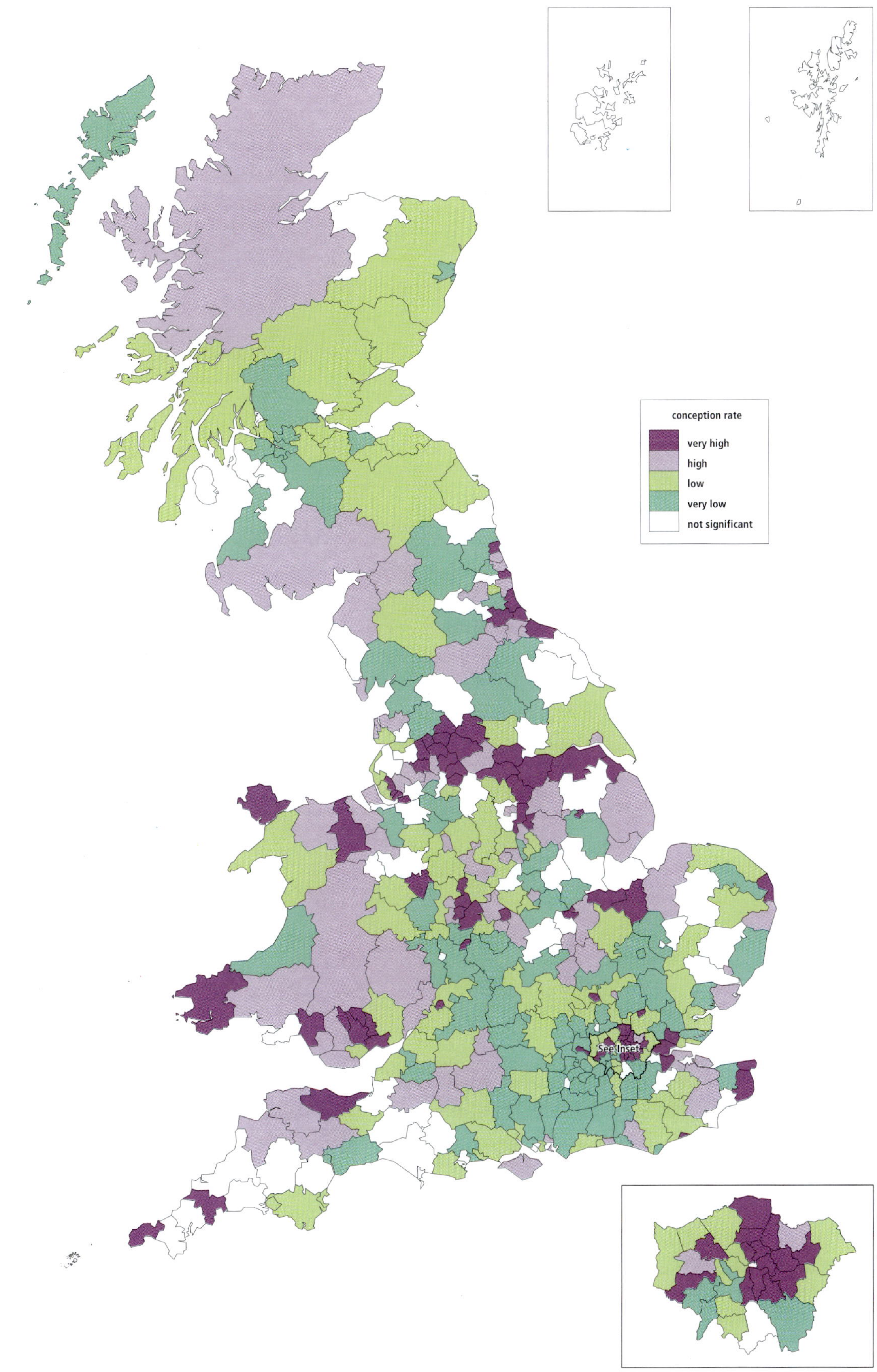

Map 5.5

**Conception rates by local authority, women aged 25-29
Great Britain 1992-1997**

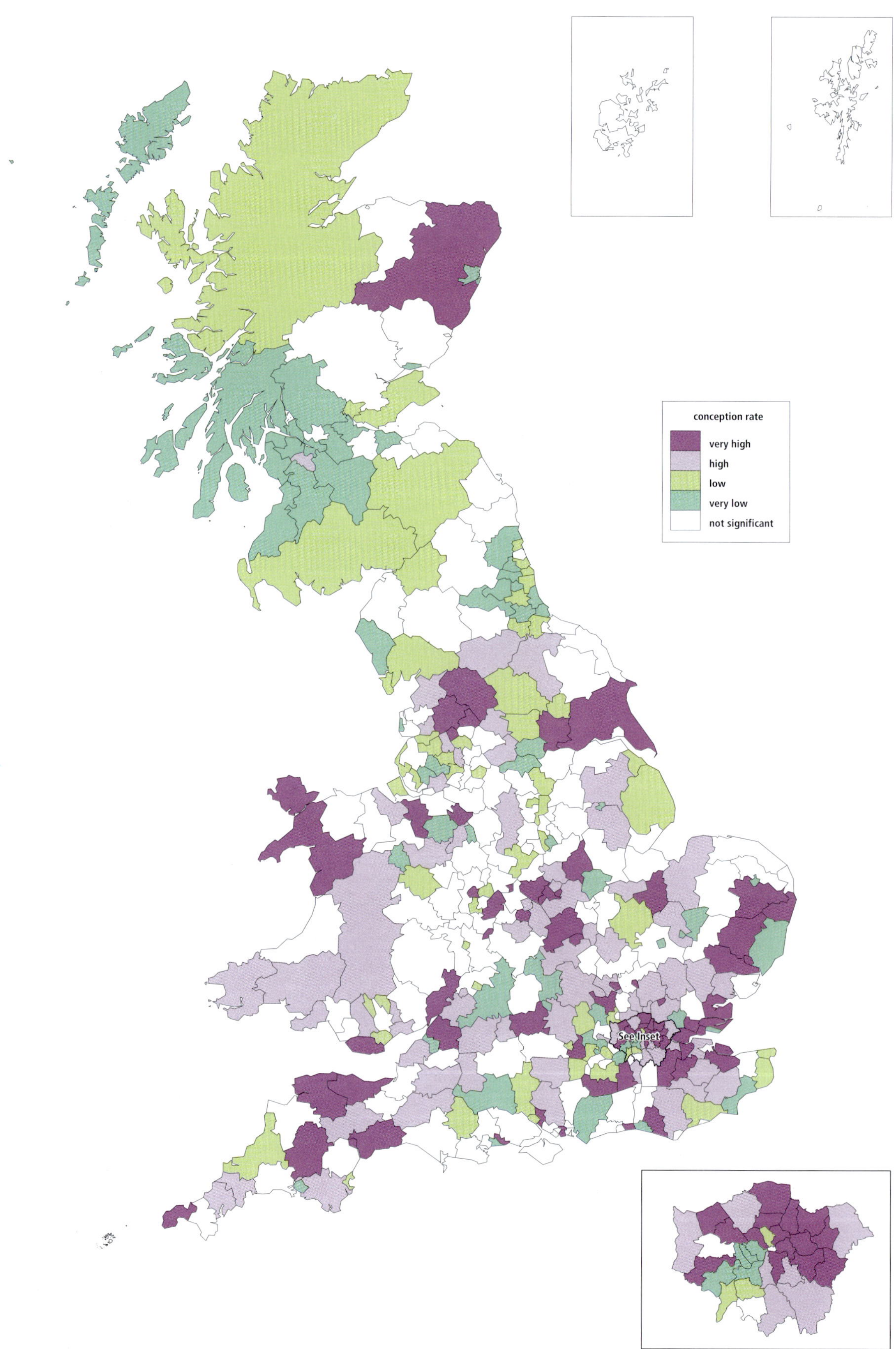

Map 5.6

Conception rates by local authority, women aged 30-34
Great Britain 1992-1997

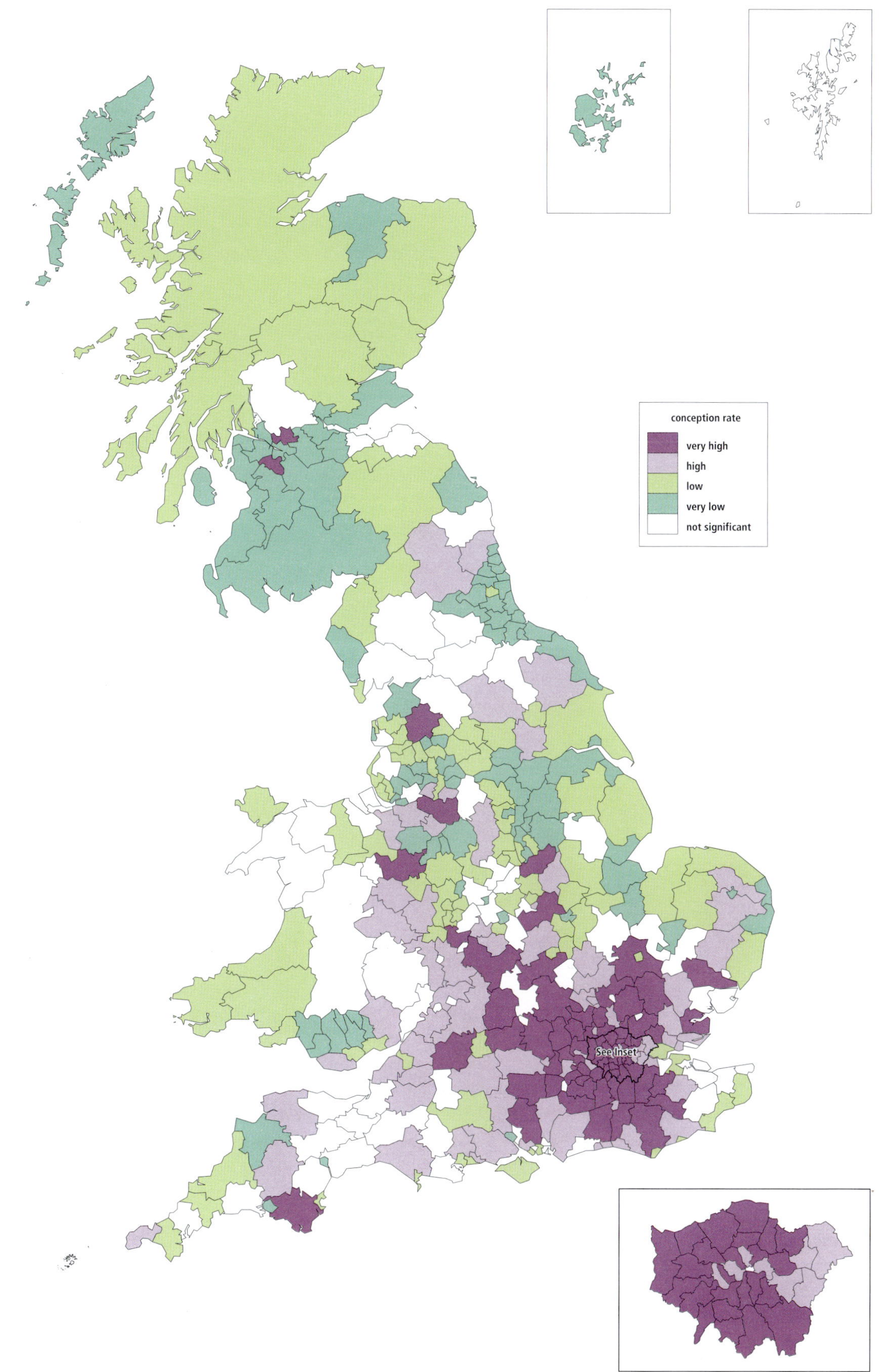

Map 5.7

**Conception rates by local authority, women aged 35-39
Great Britain 1992-1997**

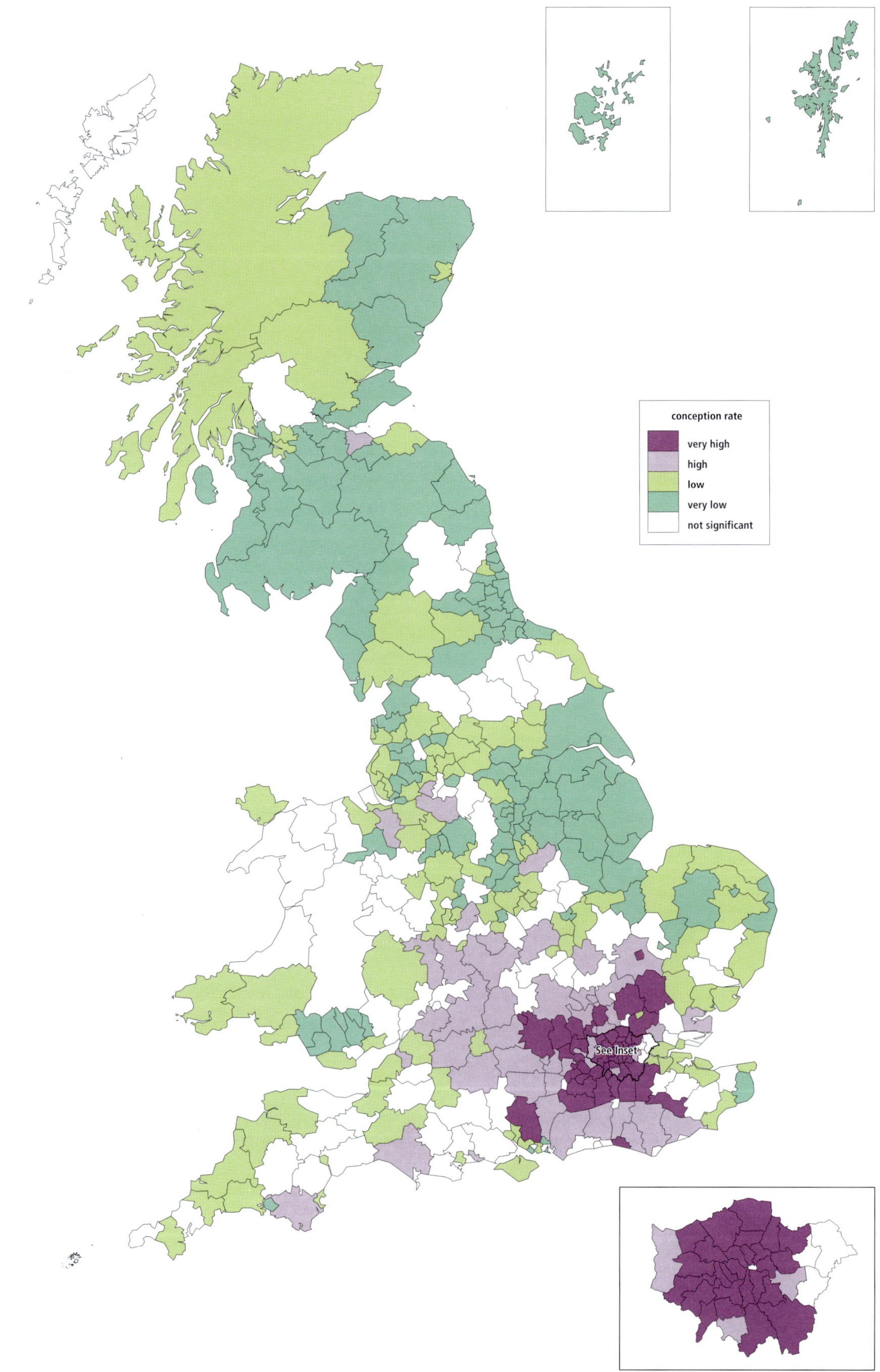

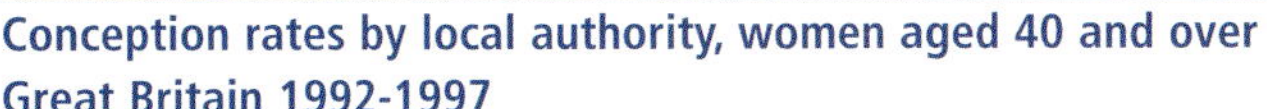

Map 5.8

**Conception rates by local authority, women aged 40 and over
Great Britain 1992-1997**

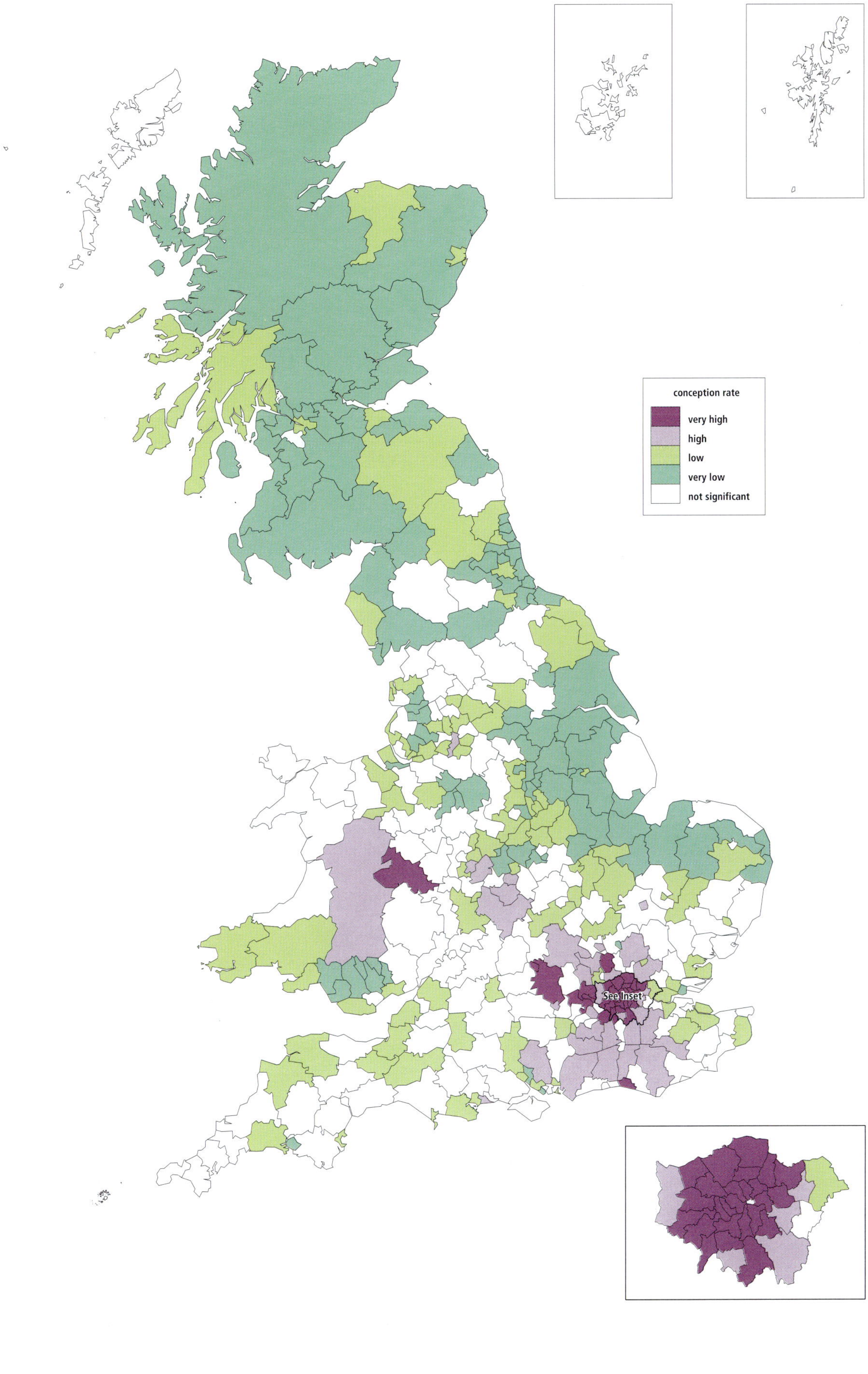

Figure 5.8

Conception rates by ONS classification Group, women aged under 18
Great Britain 1992-1997

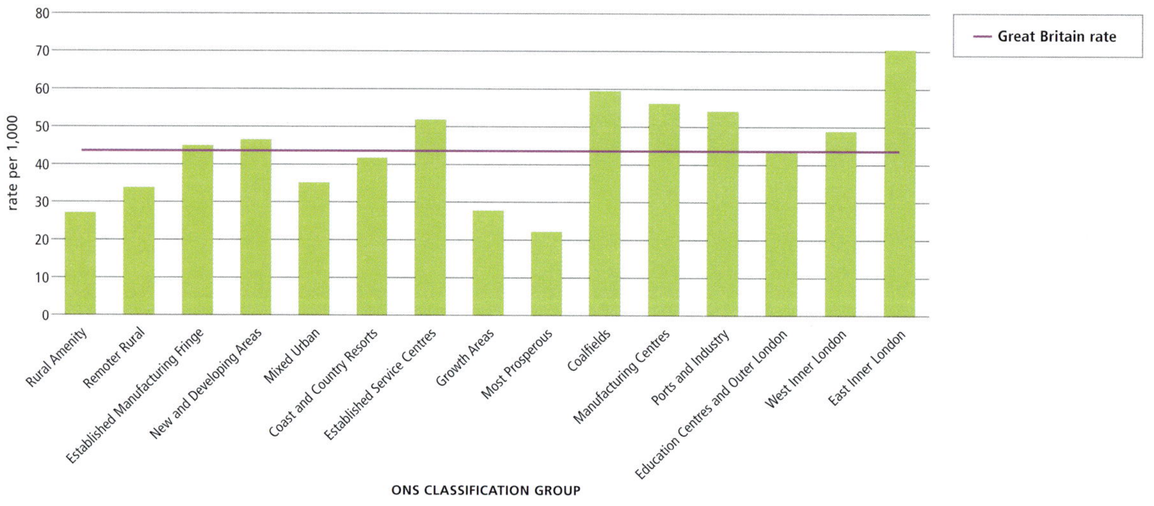

Figure 5.9

Conception rates by ONS classification Group, women aged 35-39
Great Britain 1992-1997

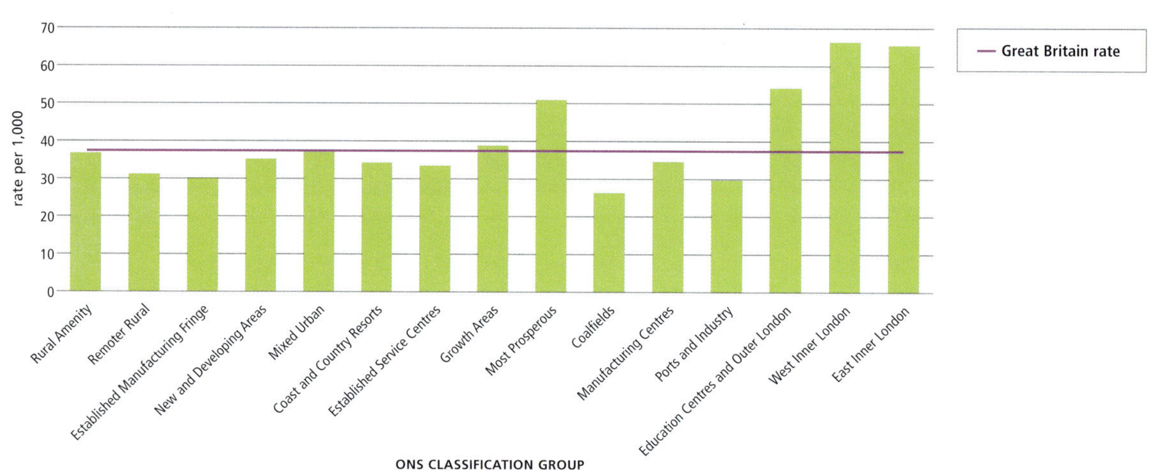

Percentage of conceptions leading to a legal abortion

All-age patterns

Country and regional level variation

Nearly 20 per cent of conceptions in Great Britain between 1992 and 1997 led to an abortion. As for conception rates, Wales and Scotland had lower percentages of conceptions leading to abortion than Great Britain, with England having the highest percentage (Figure 5.10). In London, between 1992 and 1997, just under 30 per cent of conceptions led to abortion, much higher than in any other region of England (Figure 5.10). As for the conception rate, every other region, except the West Midlands, had a lower percentage than Great Britain. The North East and South West had the lowest percentage of conceptions leading to abortion.

Local authority level variation

This pattern masks variation at the local authority level, where the areas with the highest percentage of conceptions leading to

abortion were not just in London, but also in local authorities around Birmingham and other major centres of population. Areas with low percentages of conceptions leading to abortion were found in more rural areas, with especially low percentages found in local authorities in Scotland (Map 5.9).

Age-specific patterns

The overall percentage of conceptions leading to abortion is affected by differences in the age-structure of the population in different areas. The relationship between age and the percentage of conceptions leading to an abortion is u-shaped, with the lowest percentages in the 25-29 and 30-34 age groups. Areas with high proportions of women in these age groups (when many women are having families) are likely to have lower proportions of conceptions leading to abortion than those with lots of teenagers or older women. For this reason it is important to examine the percentage of conceptions leading to abortion by age.

Figure 5.10

**Percentage of conceptions leading to abortion by country and region, women all ages
Great Britain 1992-1997**

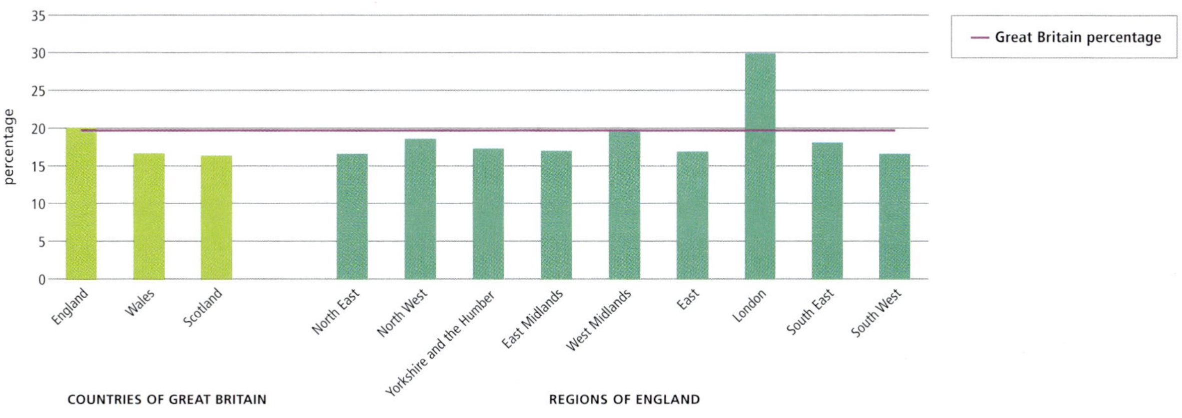

Figure 5.11

**Percentage of conceptions leading to abortion by country and age group
Great Britain 1992-1997**

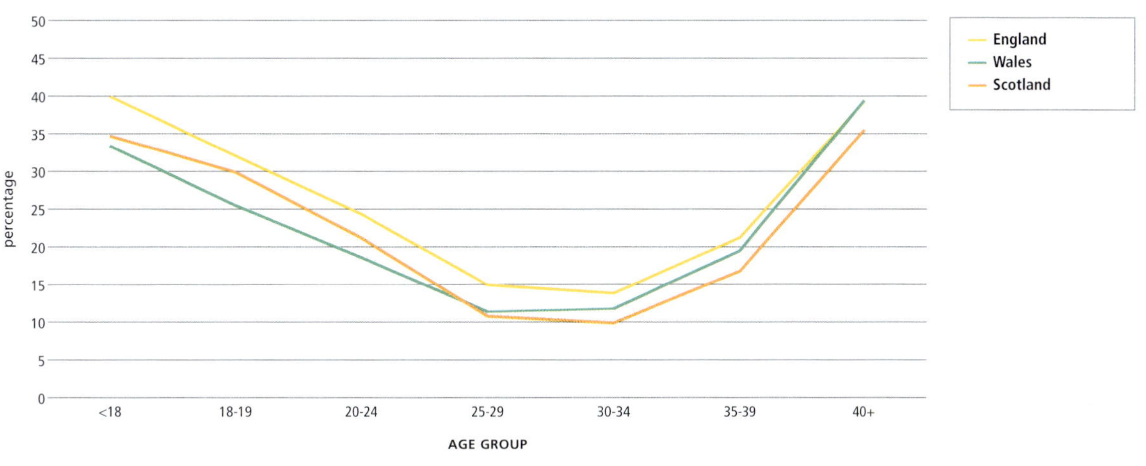

Figure 5.12

**Trends in the percentage of conceptions leading to abortion by country, women aged under 18
Great Britain 1992-1997**

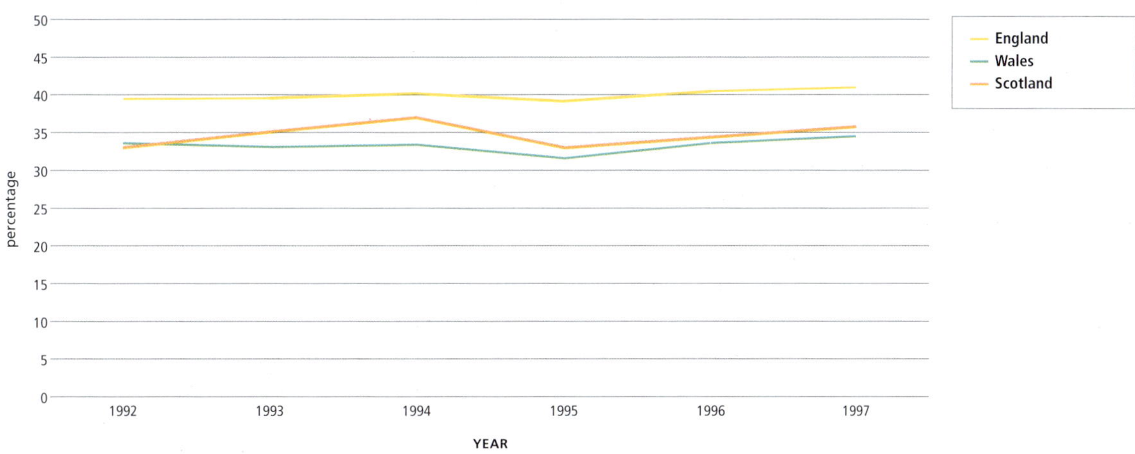

Map 5.9

**Percentage of conceptions leading to abortion by local authority, women all ages
Great Britain 1992-1997**

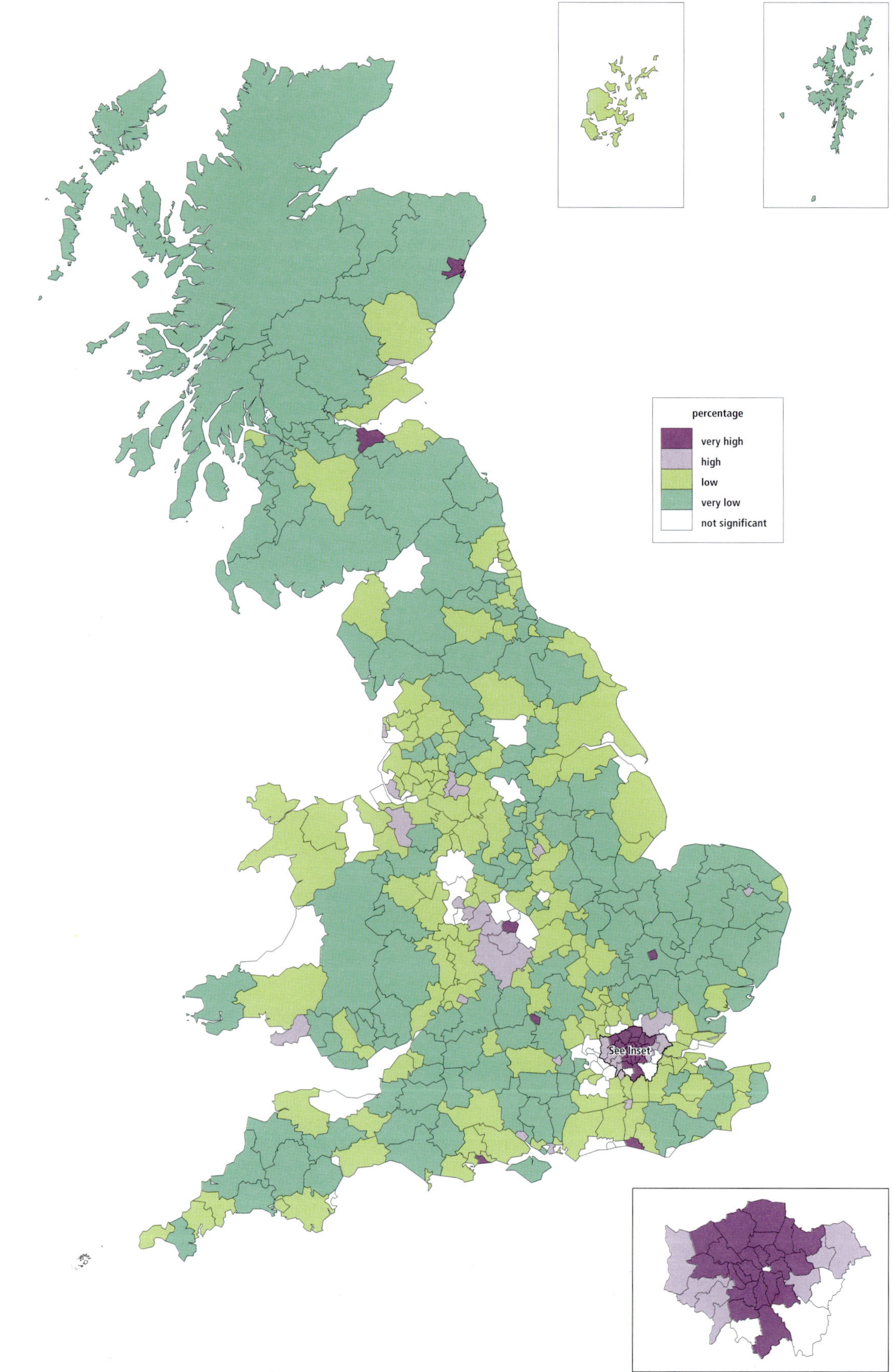

Figure 5.13

**Percentage of conceptions leading to abortion by region and age group
England 1992-1997**

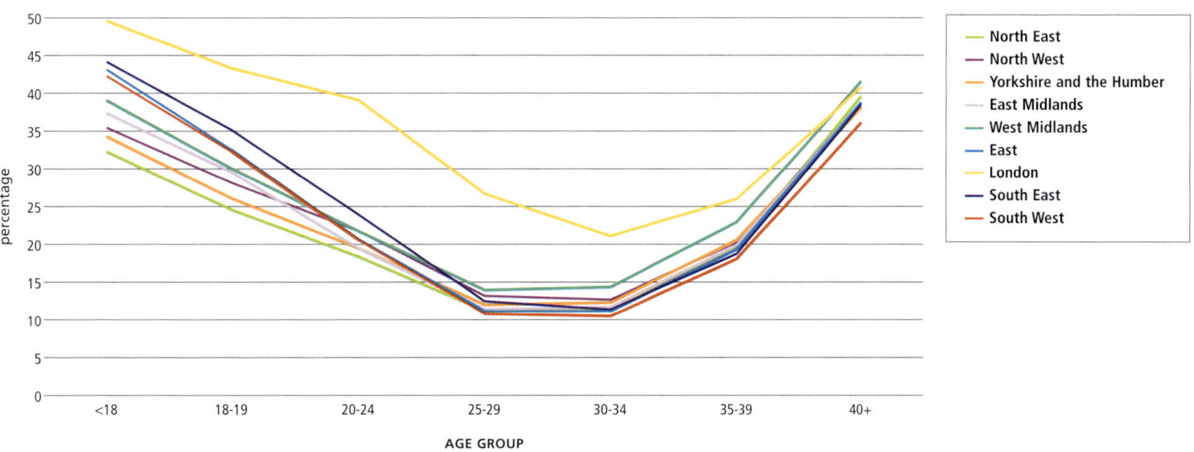

Figure 5.14

**Trends in the percentage of conceptions leading to abortion by region, women aged under 18
England 1992-1997**

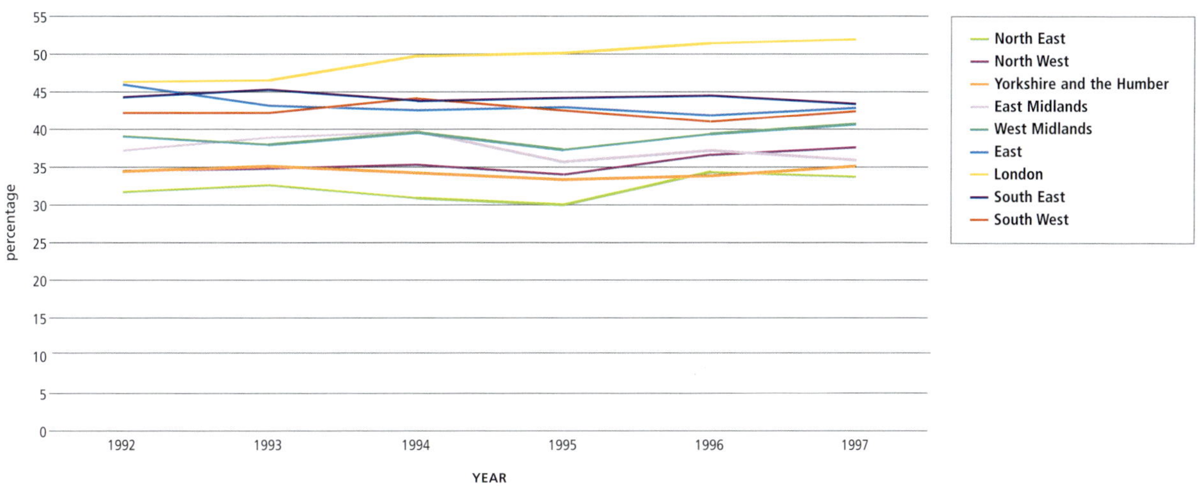

Country and regional level variation
England had the highest percentage of conceptions leading to abortion in every age group except 40 plus, where it was equal with Wales. Wales had the lowest percentage in the younger age groups and Scotland the lowest in the older age groups (Figure 5.11). Between 1992 and 1997, all of the countries of Great Britain experienced an increase in the percentage of conceptions leading to abortion in women aged under 18 (Figure 5.12). For women aged 35-39 there were no major changes in the percentage of conceptions leading to abortion in any of the countries.

London had markedly higher percentages of conceptions leading to abortion than the other regions in the younger and middle age groups (Figure 5.13). For women aged under 20, the East of England, South East and South West also had a percentage of conceptions leading to abortion higher than Great Britain. There was greater variation in percentages between regions at younger ages than in older age groups.

Between 1992 and 1997, for women aged under 18, the percentage leading to abortion remained fairly stable, with a slight increase in 1996, in all regions except London. In London the increase began in 1993 not 1996 (Figure 5.14).
The pattern for older women over time is very different to what is seen at younger ages - where the percentage of conceptions leading to abortion, and the conception rate increased between 1992 and 1997. In older women, the conception rate increased, but with little change in the percentage leading to abortion.

Local authority level variation
For women aged under 20, the areas with percentages of conceptions leading to abortion higher than the Great Britain level were spread around the country and especially concentrated in the areas around London and south central England, as would be expected given the pattern seen at regional level. The areas with lower percentages were

Figure 5.15

**Percentage of conceptions leading to abortion by ONS classification Group, women aged under 18
Great Britain 1992-1997**

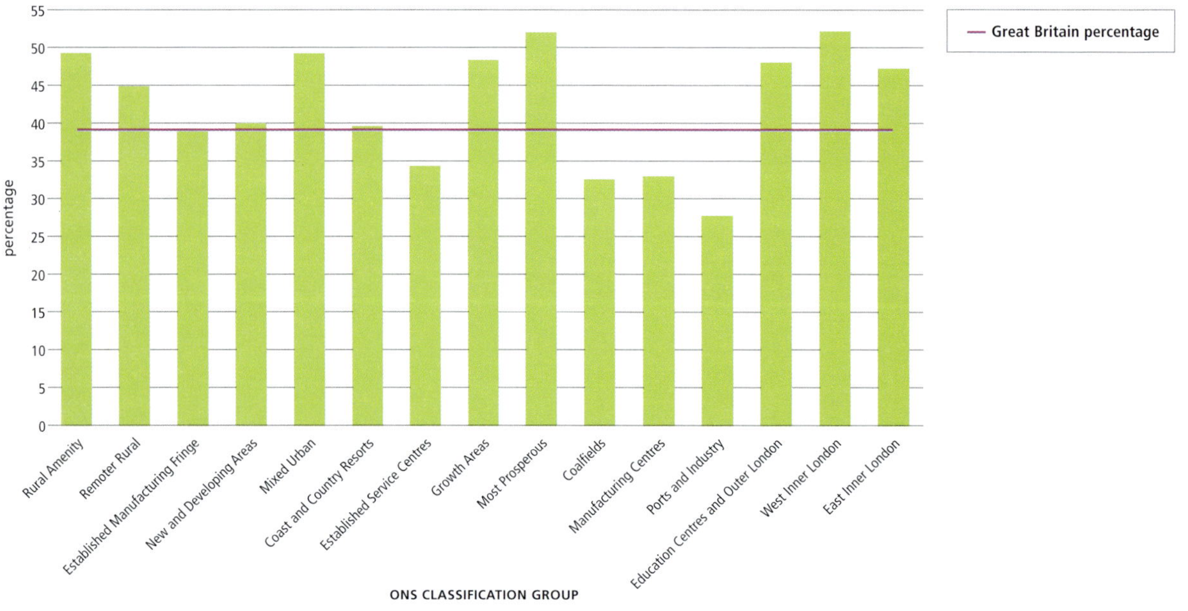

Figure 5.16

**Percentage of conceptions leading to abortion by ONS classification Group, women aged 35-39
Great Britain 1992-1997**

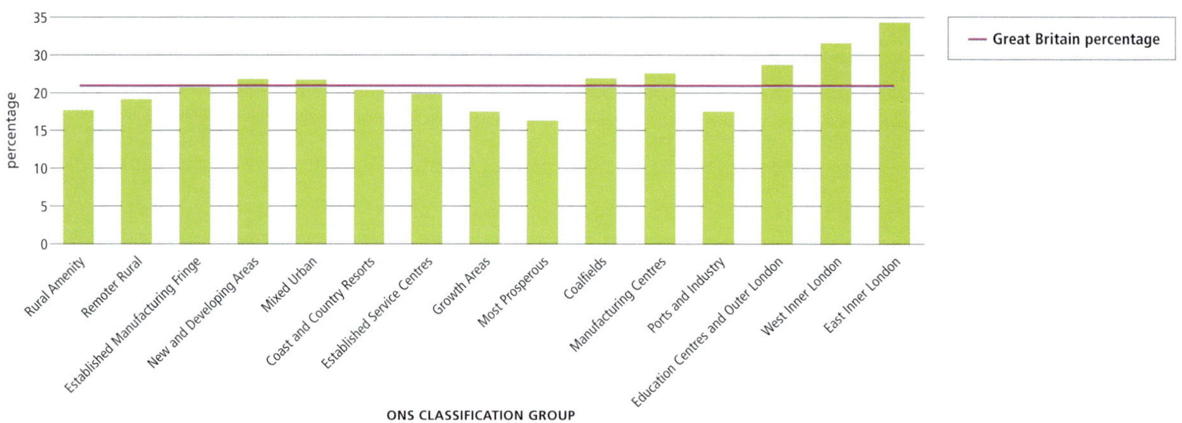

consistently found in south Wales, the North East and in a band across the country from the North West to Yorkshire and the Humber. Areas south of Glasgow also had consistently low percentages (Maps 5.10, 5.11). This is almost a reversal of the pattern seen for the conception rate.

When examining this pattern using the ONS Classification Groups, the *Most Prosperous* Group had the highest percentage of under 18 conceptions leading to abortion (Figure 5.15), with all the local authorities within this Group having higher percentages than the Great Britain percentage, whereas it had a low under 18 conception rate. The *West Inner London* Group also had a very high percentage of teenage conceptions leading to abortion. The *Coalfields, Manufacturing Centres* and *Ports and Industry* Groups had substantially lower percentages than the Great Britain percentage, compared to their high under 18 conception rates.

For women in their twenties and thirties the percentage of conceptions leading to abortion was generally lower than the Great Britain level in areas outside the major centres of population. The areas with higher percentages of conceptions leading to abortion were consistently around London, Birmingham, Liverpool, Manchester and major cities in Scotland (Maps 5.12-5.15).

For women in their late thirties, the highest percentages were really only found in Groups containing authorities within London, most noticeably *East Inner London* and *West Inner London* (Figure 5.16). In this case the location of local authorities appears to explain more of the patterns than the socio-demographic characteristics of these local authorities. Areas that have very different characteristics had similar percentages of conceptions leading to abortion, for example *Most Prosperous* and *Ports and Industry*.

Map 5.10

**Percentage of conceptions leading to abortion by local authority, women aged under 18
Great Britain 1992-1997**

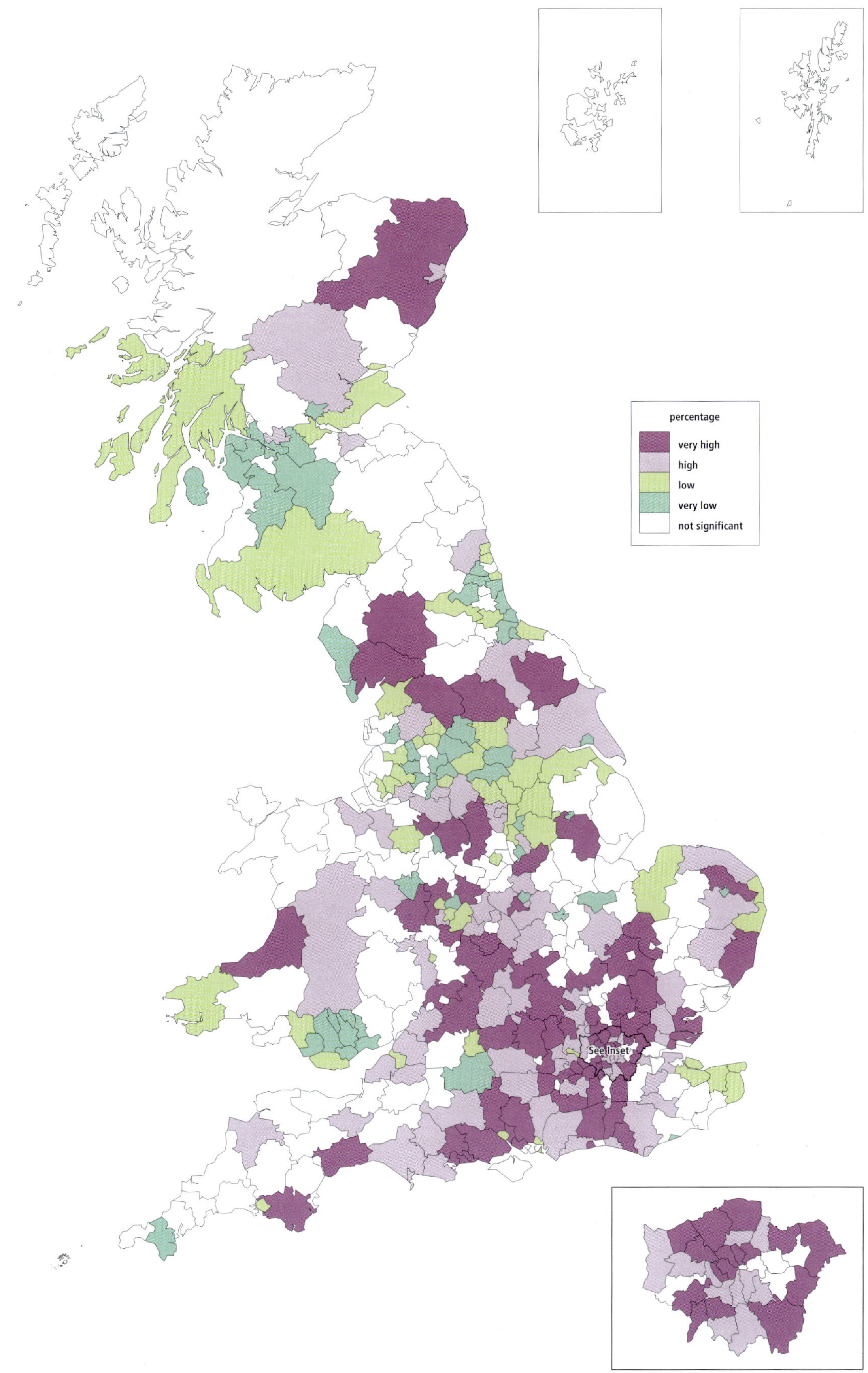

Map 5.11

Percentage of conceptions leading to abortion by local authority, women aged 18-19
Great Britain 1992-1997

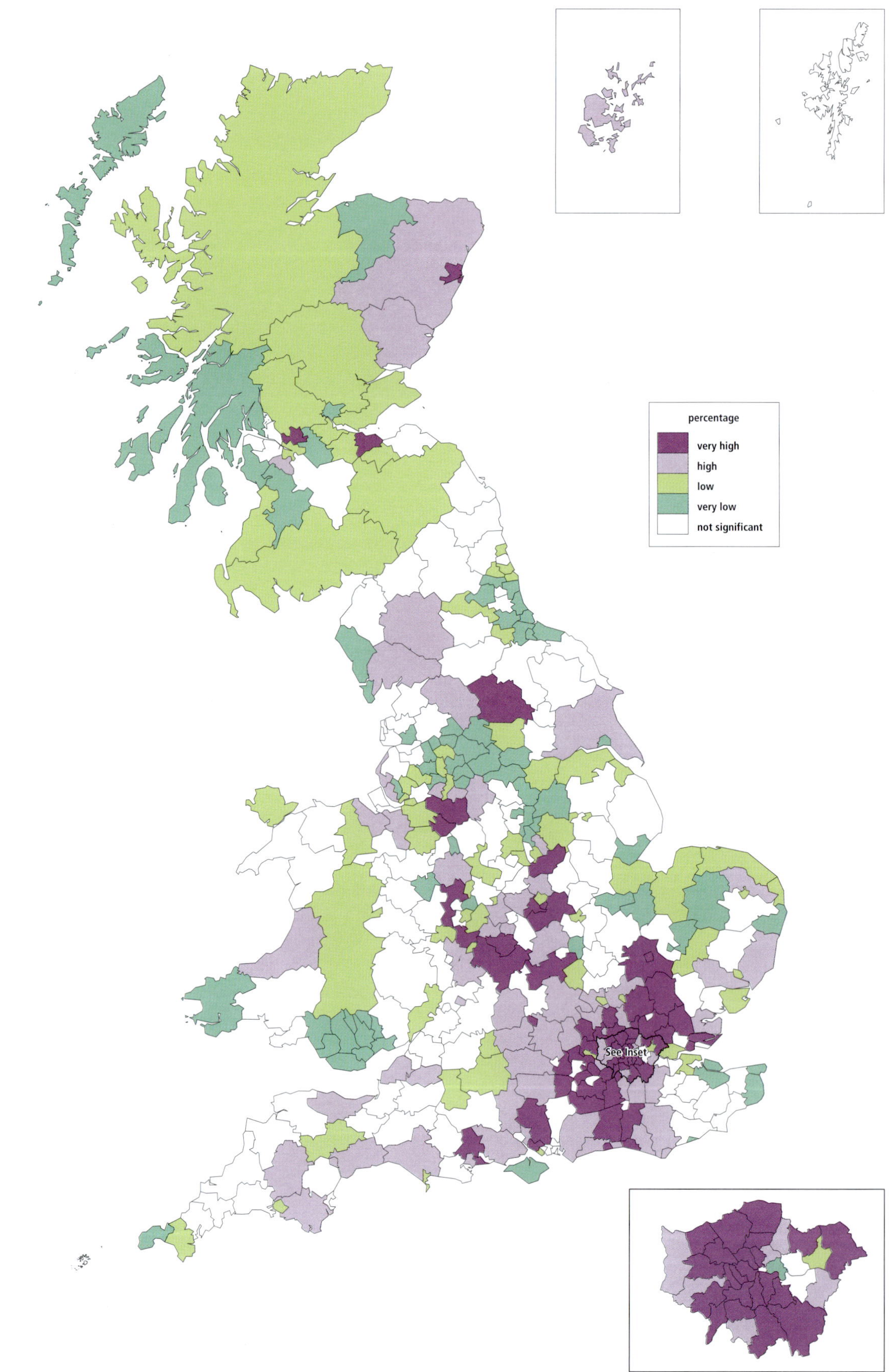

Map 5.12

**Percentage of conceptions leading to abortion by local authority, women aged 20-24
Great Britain 1992-1997**

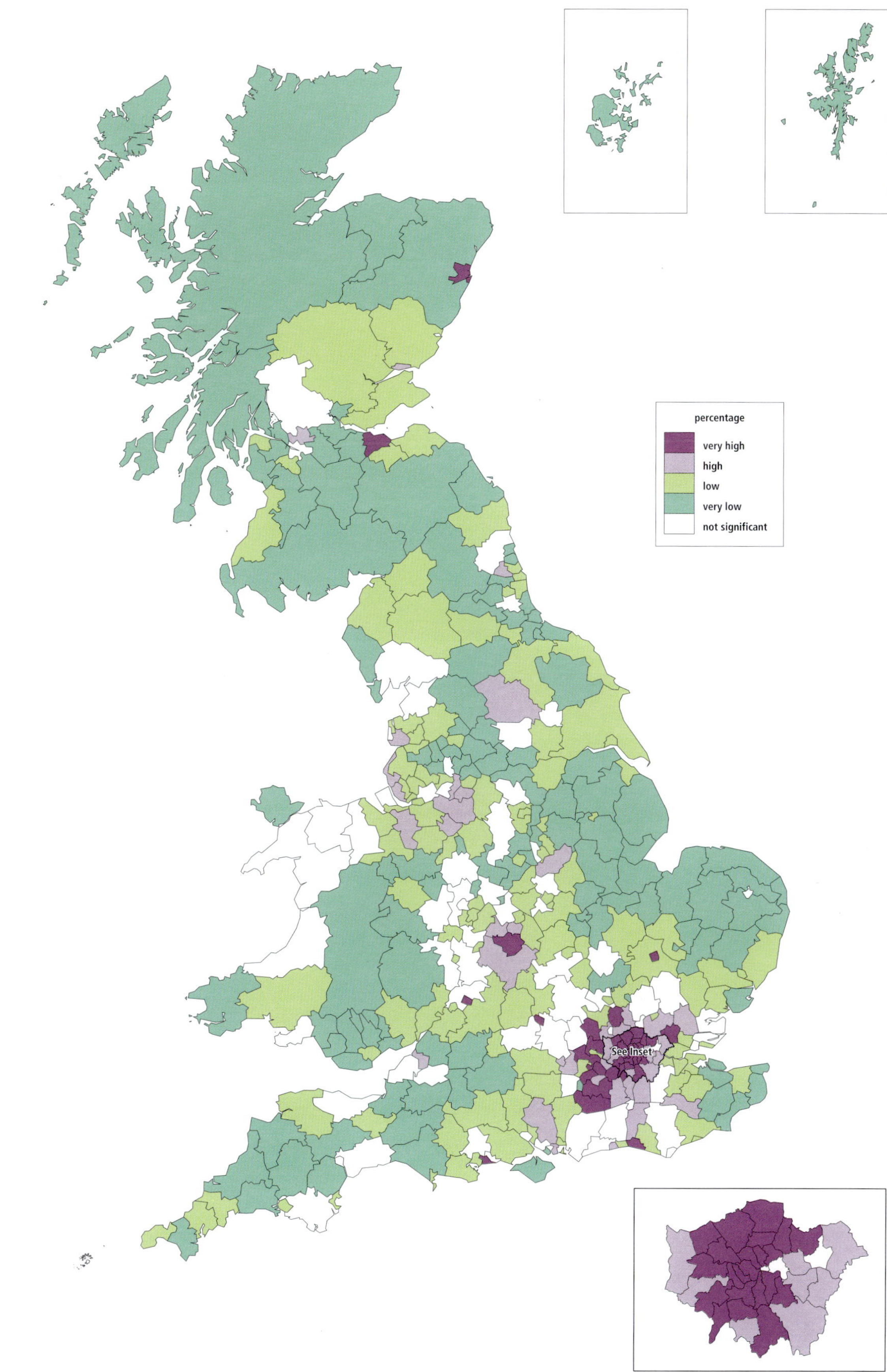

Map 5.13

**Percentage of conceptions leading to abortion by local authority, women aged 25-29
Great Britain 1992-1997**

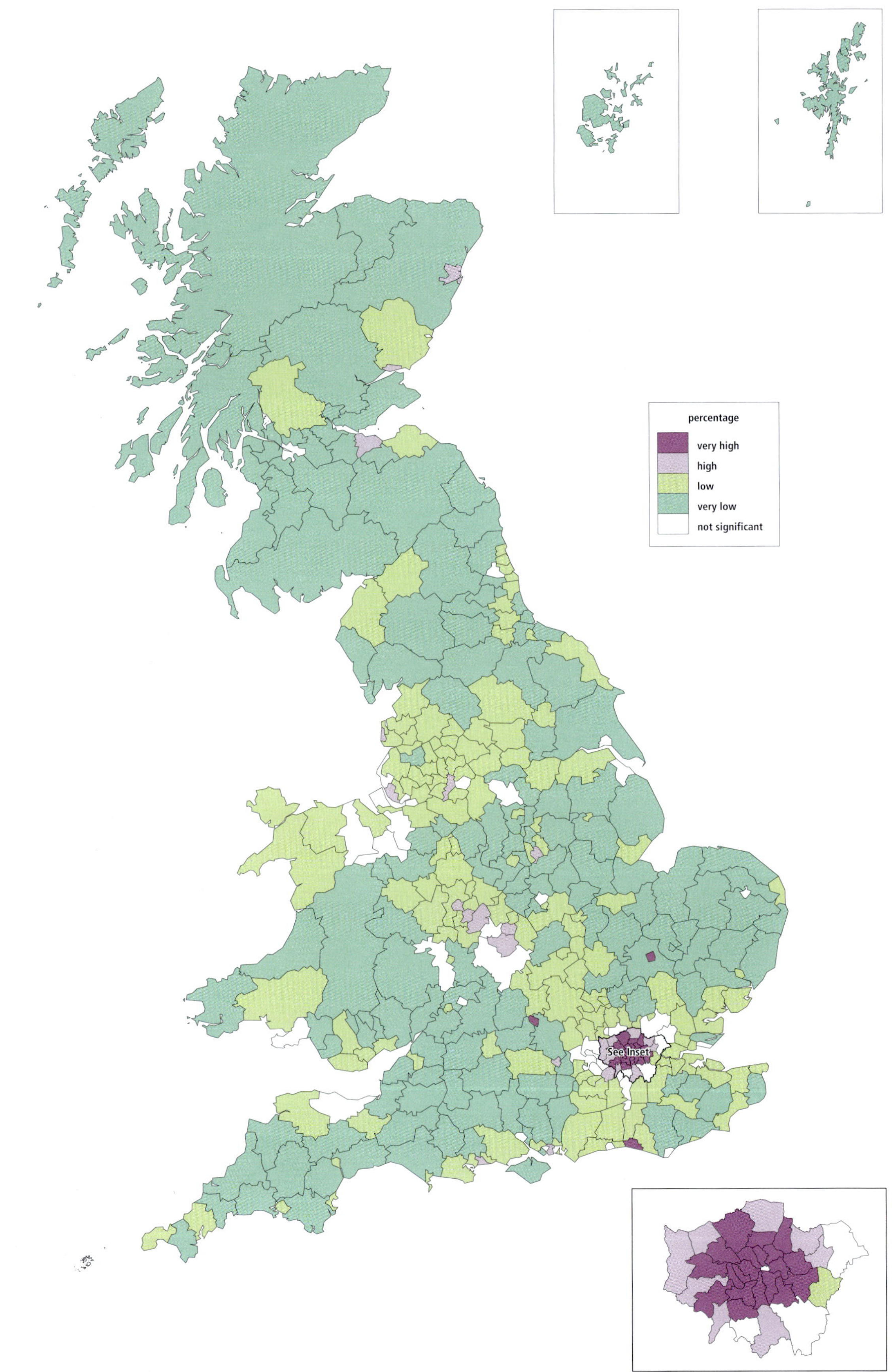

Map 5.14

**Percentage of conceptions leading to abortion by local authority, women aged 30-34
Great Britain 1992-1997**

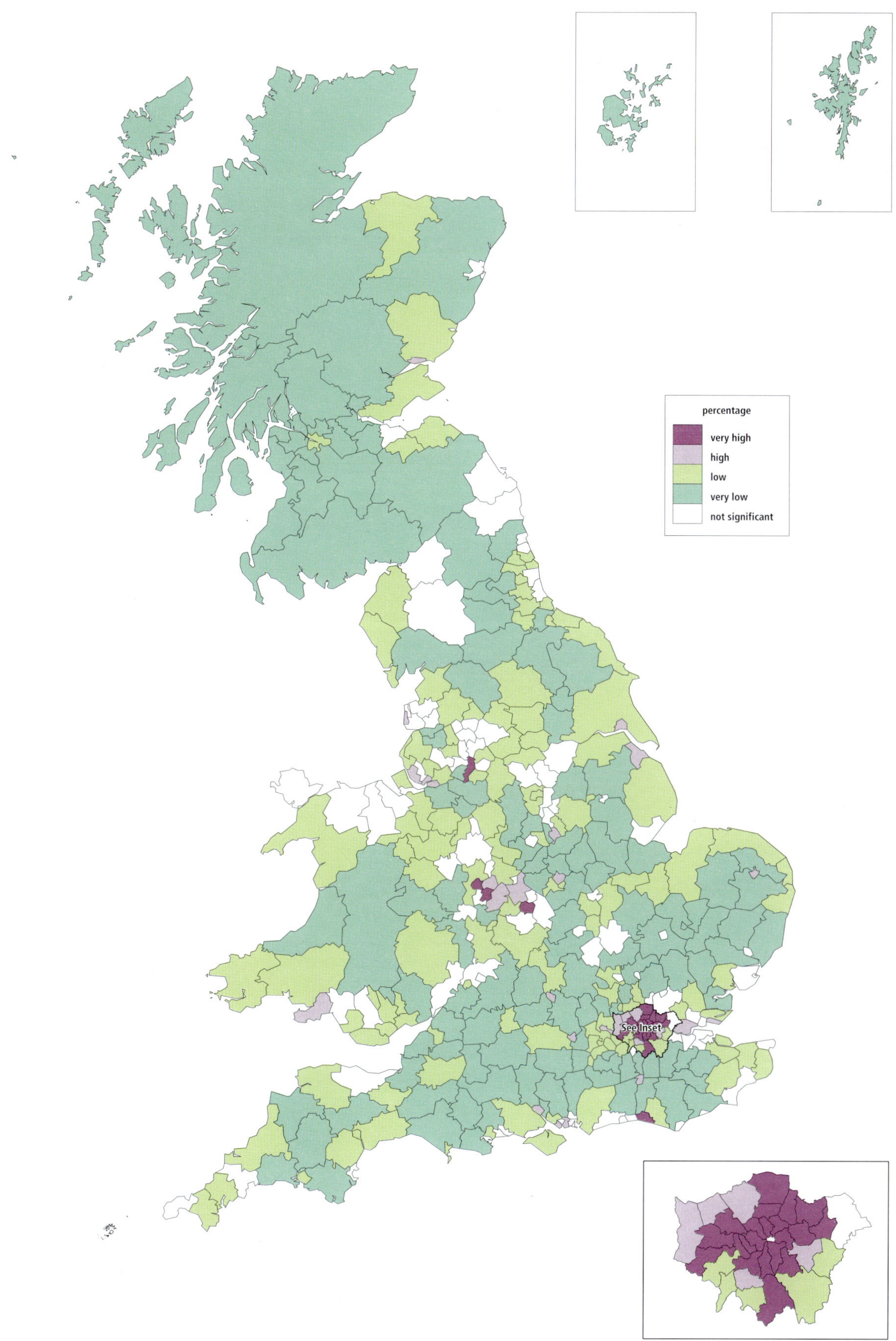

Map 5.15

**Percentage of conceptions leading to abortion by local authority, women aged 35-39
Great Britain 1992-1997**

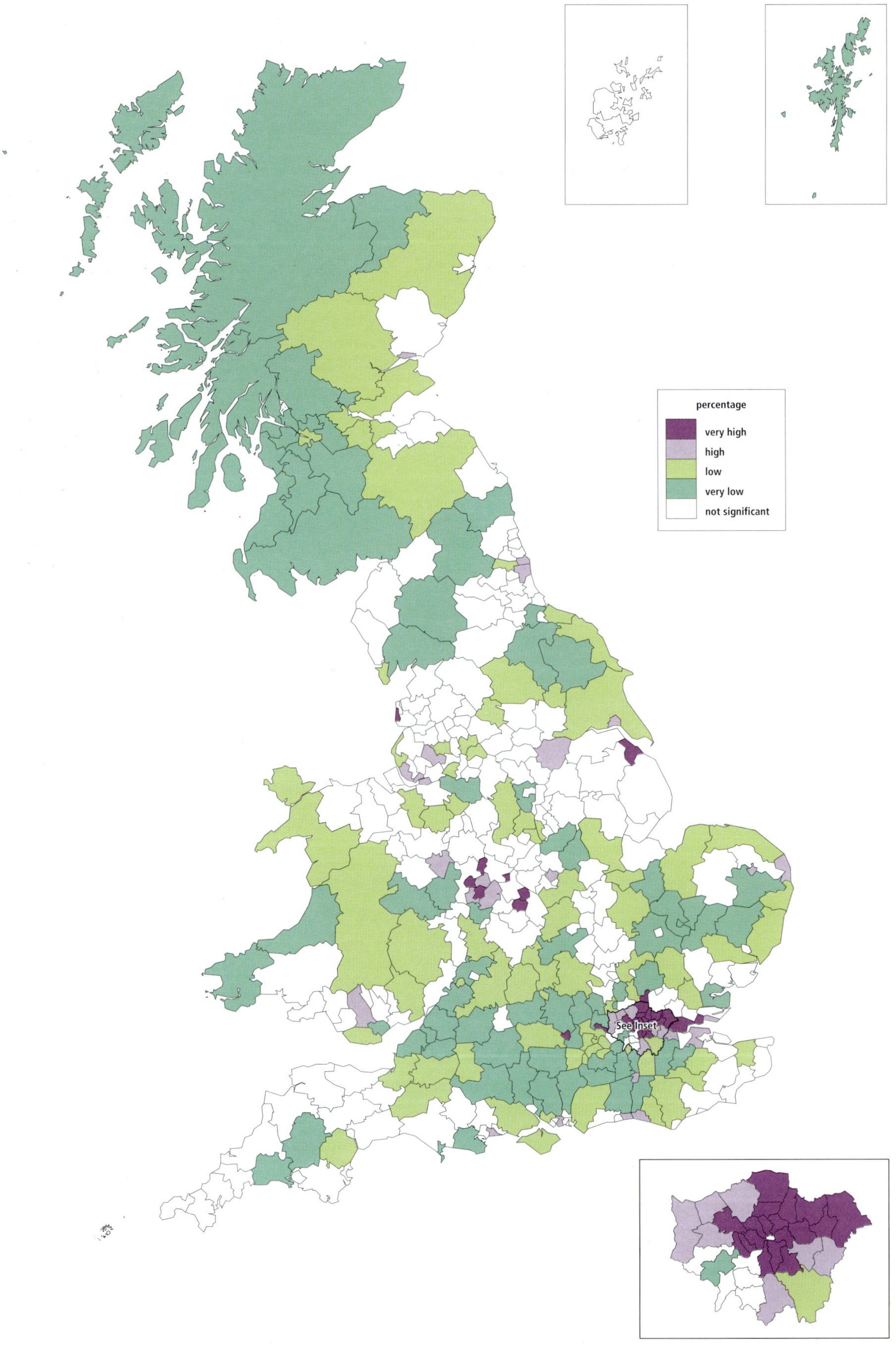

5.3 Abortions

This section examines geographic variation in abortion rates and the percentage of abortions by gestation weeks and purchaser across Great Britain between 1992 and 1997. Data is not available for Northern Ireland, or for 1991 (see section 5.2).

Abortion rates
All-age patterns
Country and regional level variation
As for the conception rate, and the percentage leading to abortion, the abortion rate in England was substantially higher than in Wales or Scotland, with Scotland having the lowest rate of the countries of Great Britain (Figure 5.17). Two regions in England had higher abortion rates than Great Britain - the West Midlands and London. All the other regions had lower abortion rates than Great Britain, with the lowest rate being in the North East. This pattern was also seen for the conception rate and percentage leading to abortion. This geographic pattern was maintained throughout 1992 to 1997, with each country and region having an increase in the abortion rate in 1996, following the 1995 pill scare (Figures 5.18, 5.19).

Local authority level variation
Map 5.16 shows clearly the high rates in the West Midlands and London, with all authorities bar two in London having higher abortion rates than Great Britain as a whole and almost all of

those having very high rates. The high rates in the West Midlands appeared to be confined to Birmingham and authorities close by. High rates were also found in Manchester, Liverpool and other scattered authorities throughout Great Britain, although no authorities in Wales had higher abortion rates than Great Britain as a whole. Low rates were distributed throughout the rest of the country.

Age-specific patterns
Patterns in the overall rate can be partly explained by the age distribution of the population, areas with a high proportion of women aged 18-19 will tend to have higher all-age abortion rates than areas with lower proportions in this age group, as this is the age group in which the abortion rate is highest. In order to take this into account it is important to examine age-specific rates.

Country and regional level variation
The abortion rate peaks in the 18-19 age group, remains high in 20-24 year olds and then declines steadily with age. England had the highest and Scotland the lowest rate in each age group (Figure 5.20). Trends by age group for the countries of Great Britain showed the same pattern and trend as the all-age trends.

All the regions except London showed a similar pattern to the countries with rates peaking in the 18-19 age group (Figure 5.21). London had higher rates than the rest of England in all the age groups. The West Midlands had the next highest rates.

Figure 5.17

Abortion rates by country and region, women all ages
Great Britain 1992-1997

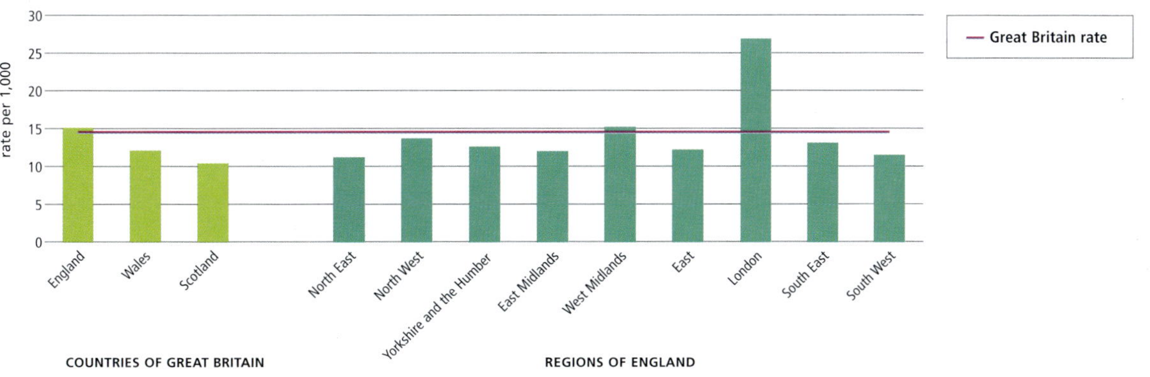

Figure 5.18

Trends in abortion rates by country, women all ages
Great Britain 1992-1997

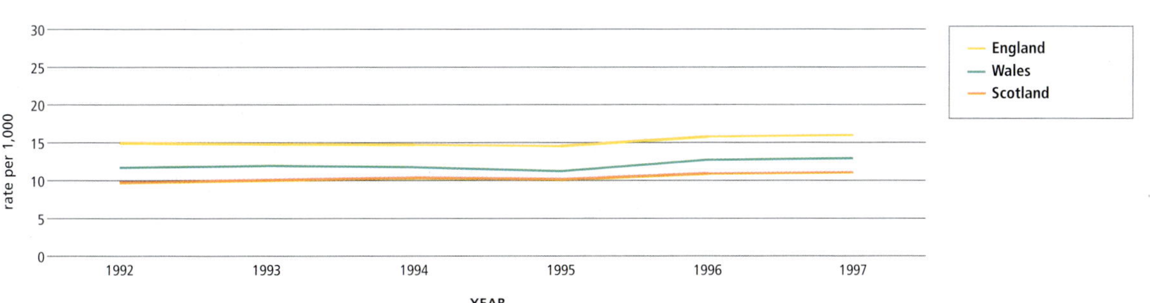

Map 5.16

Abortion rates by local authority, women all ages
Great Britain 1992-1997

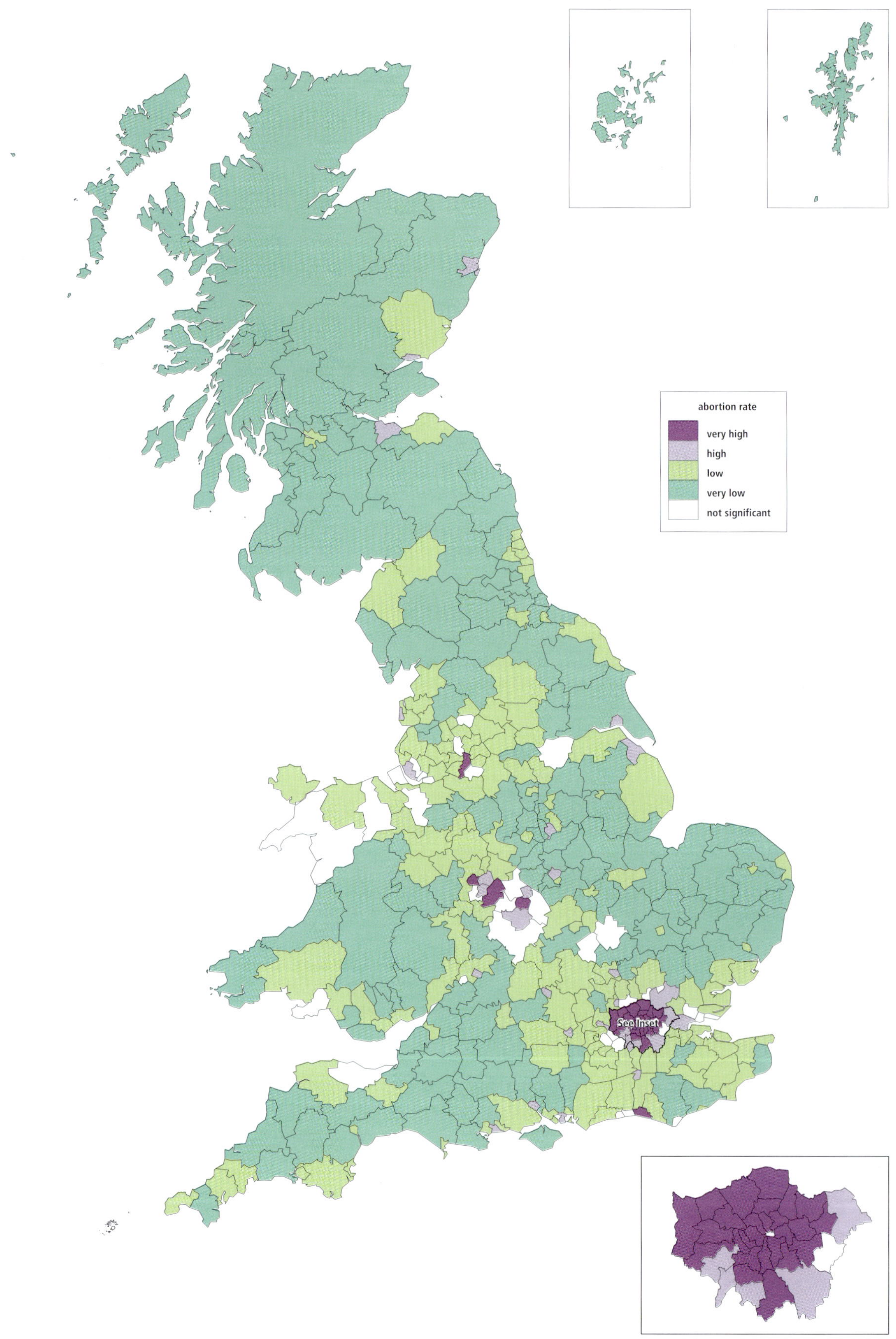

Figure 5.19

Trends in abortion rates by region, women all ages
England 1992-1997

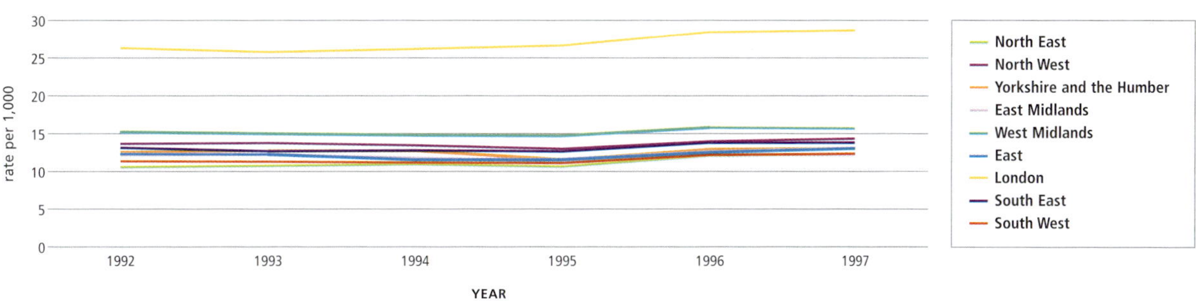

Figure 5.20

Abortion rates by country and age group
Great Britain 1992-1997

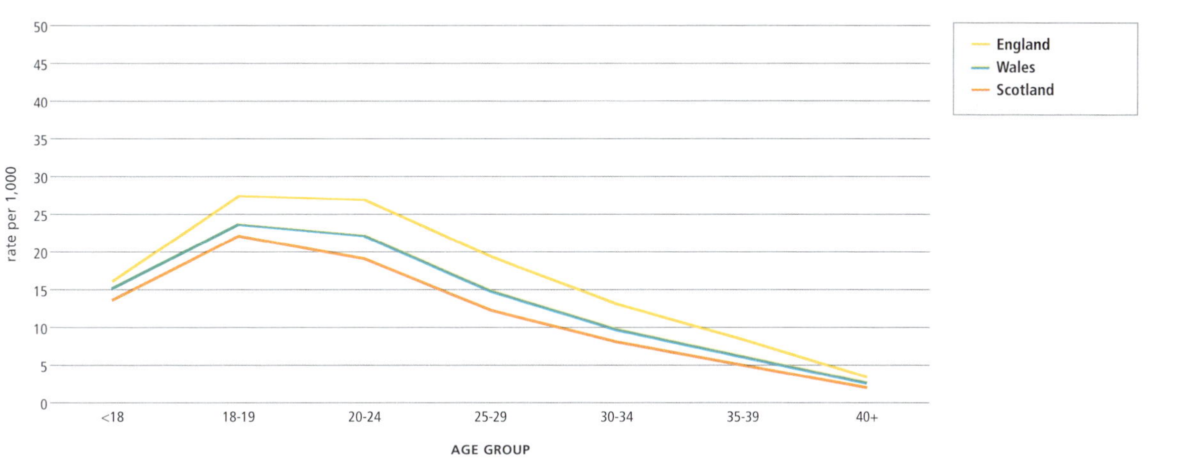

Figure 5.21

Abortion rates by region and age group
England 1992-1997

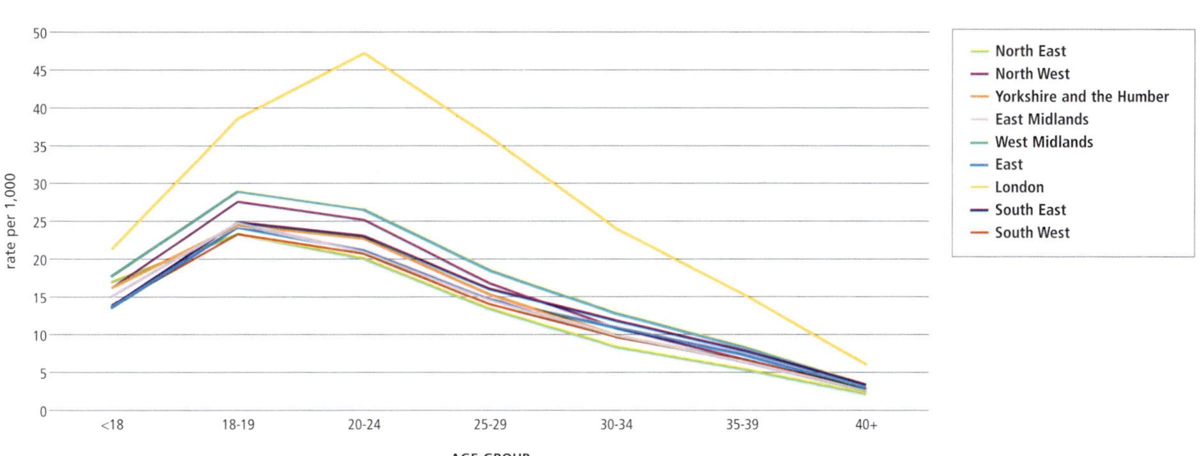

Map 5.17

Abortion rates by local authority, women aged under 18
Great Britain 1992-1997

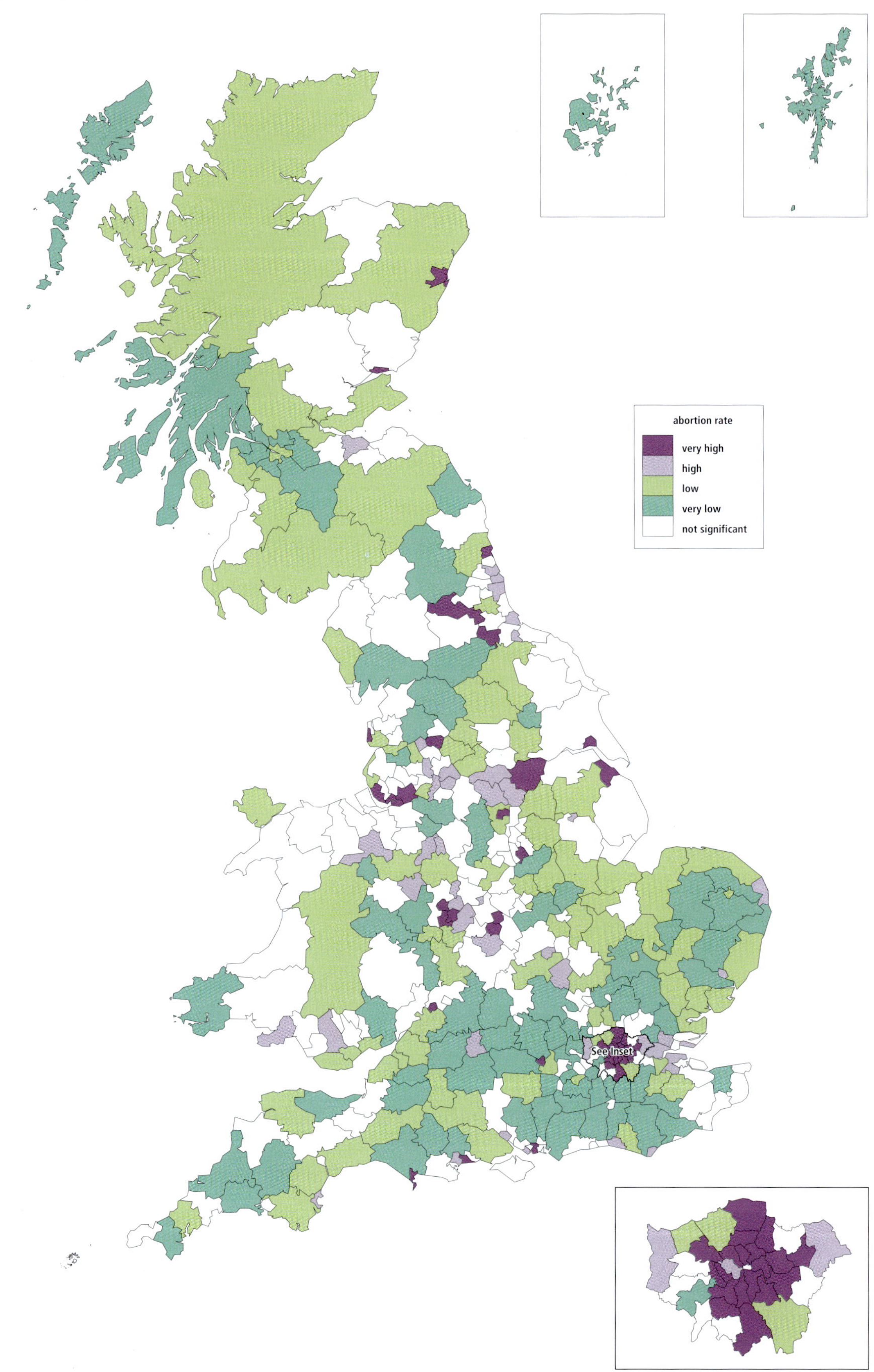

Map 5.18

Abortion rates by local authority, women aged 18-19
Great Britain 1992-1997

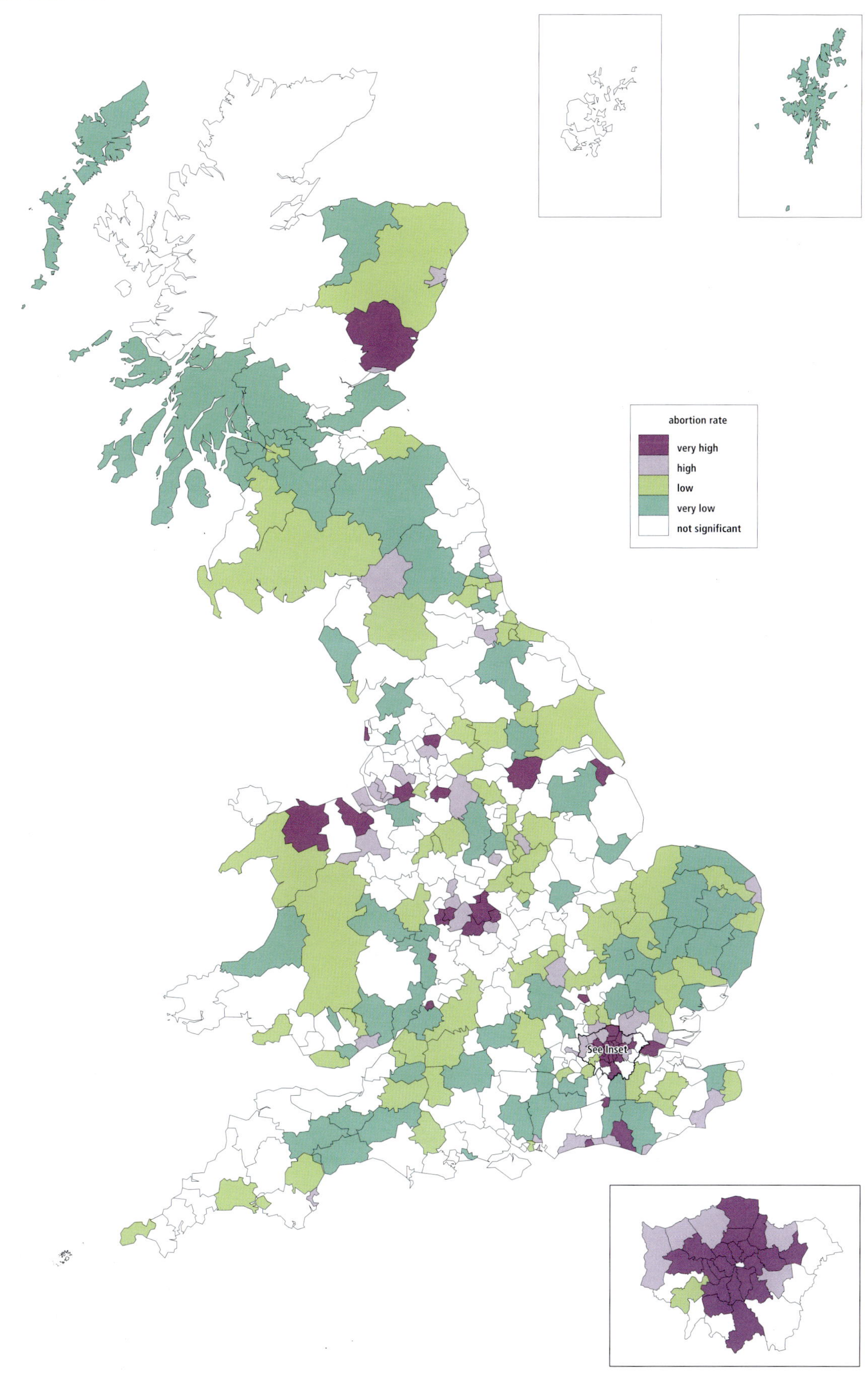

Map 5.19

Abortion rates by local authority, women aged 20-24
Great Britain 1992-1997

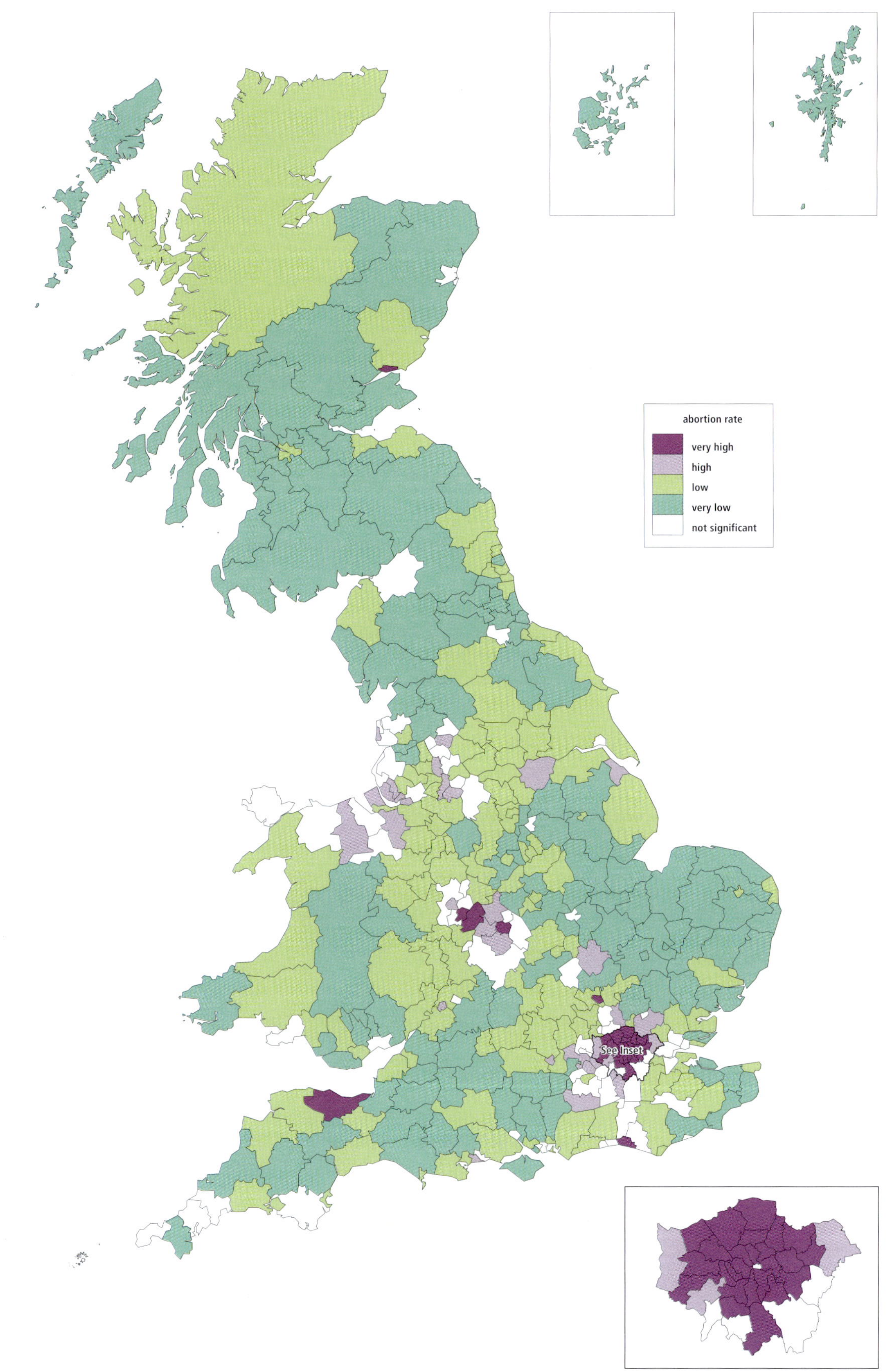

Map 5.20

Abortion rates by local authority, women aged 25-29
Great Britain 1992-1997

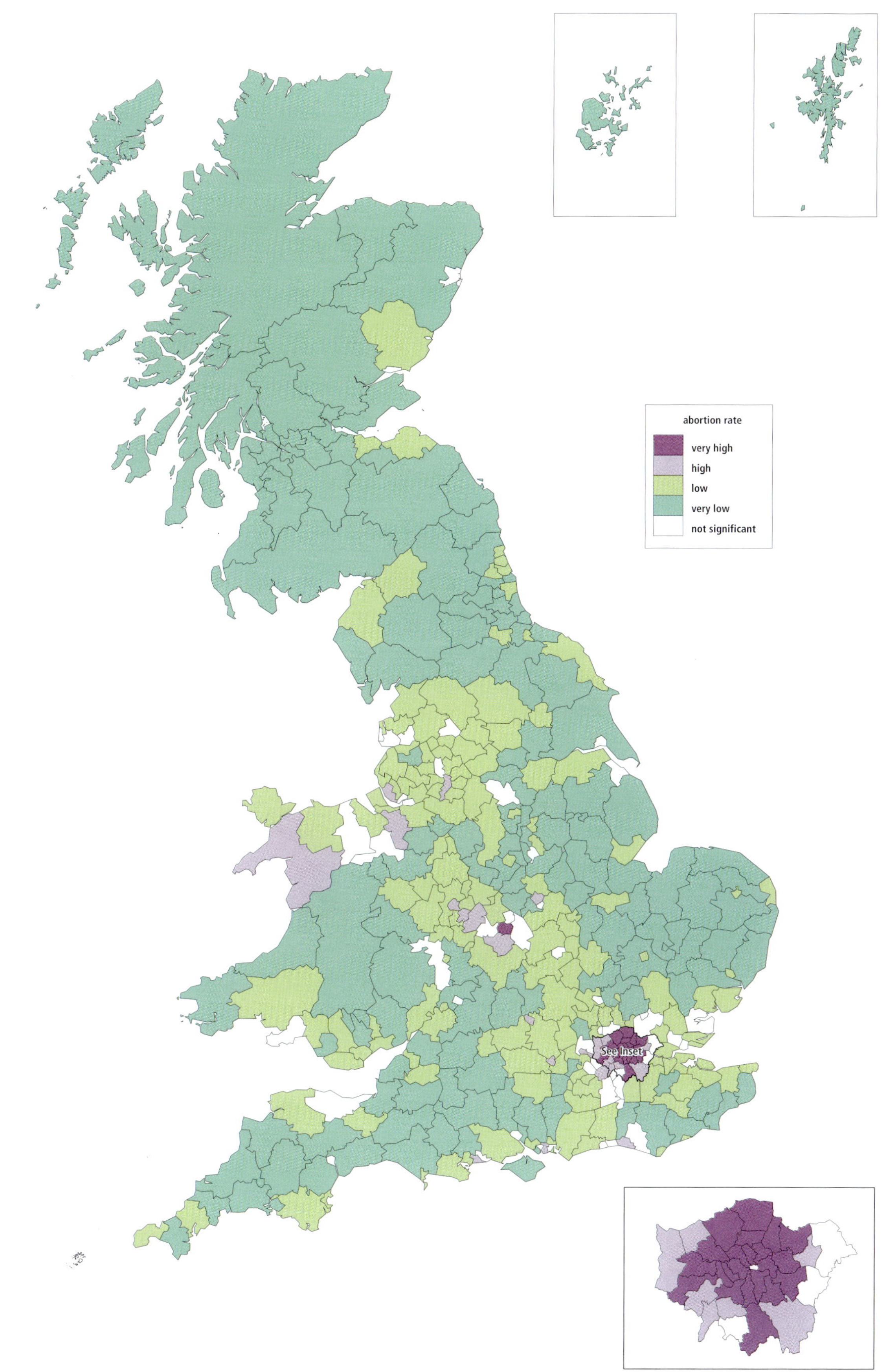

Map 5.21

**Abortion rates by local authority, women aged 30-34
Great Britain 1992-1997**

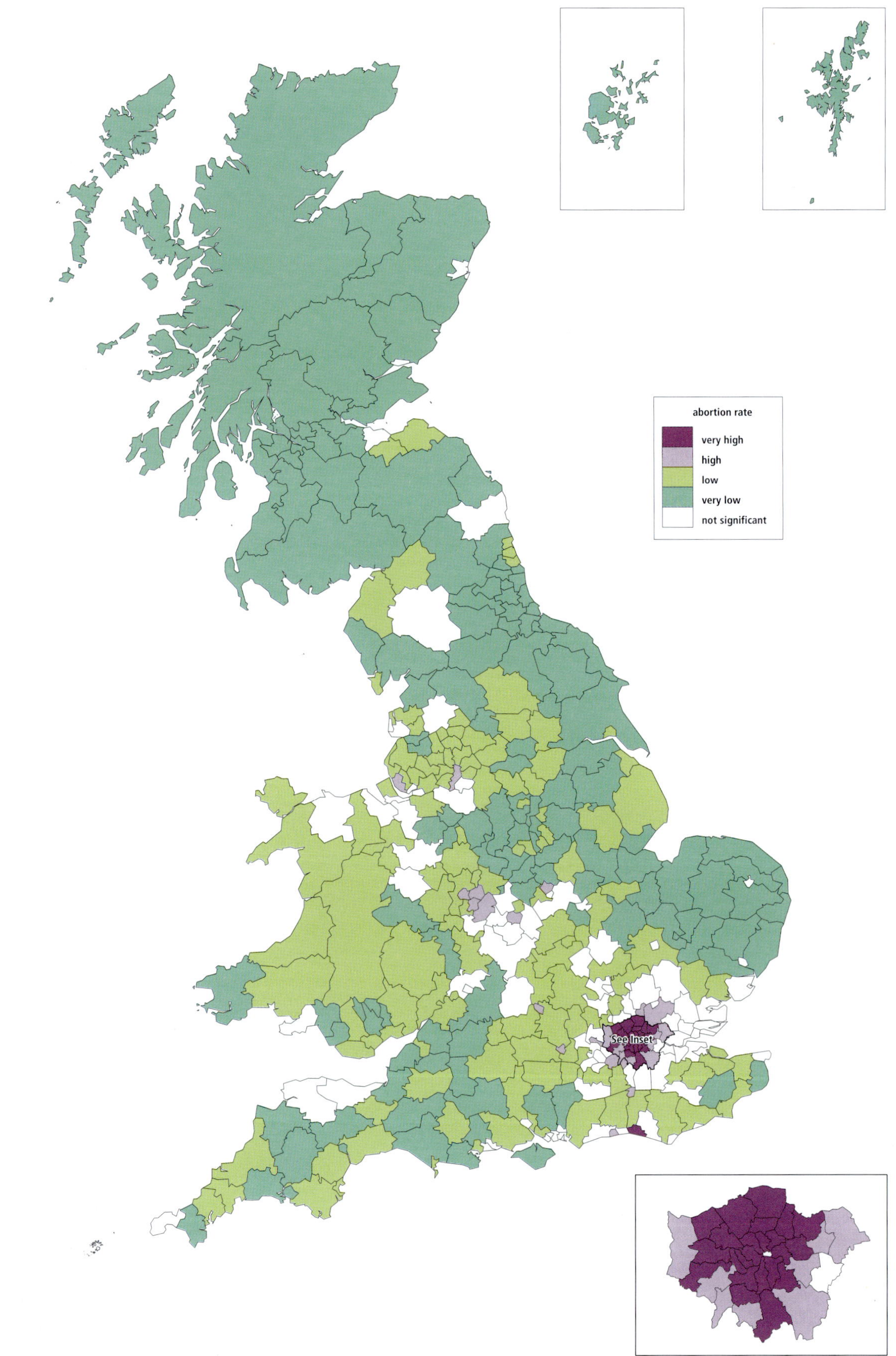

Map 5.22

**Abortion rates by local authority, women aged 35-39
Great Britain 1992-1997**

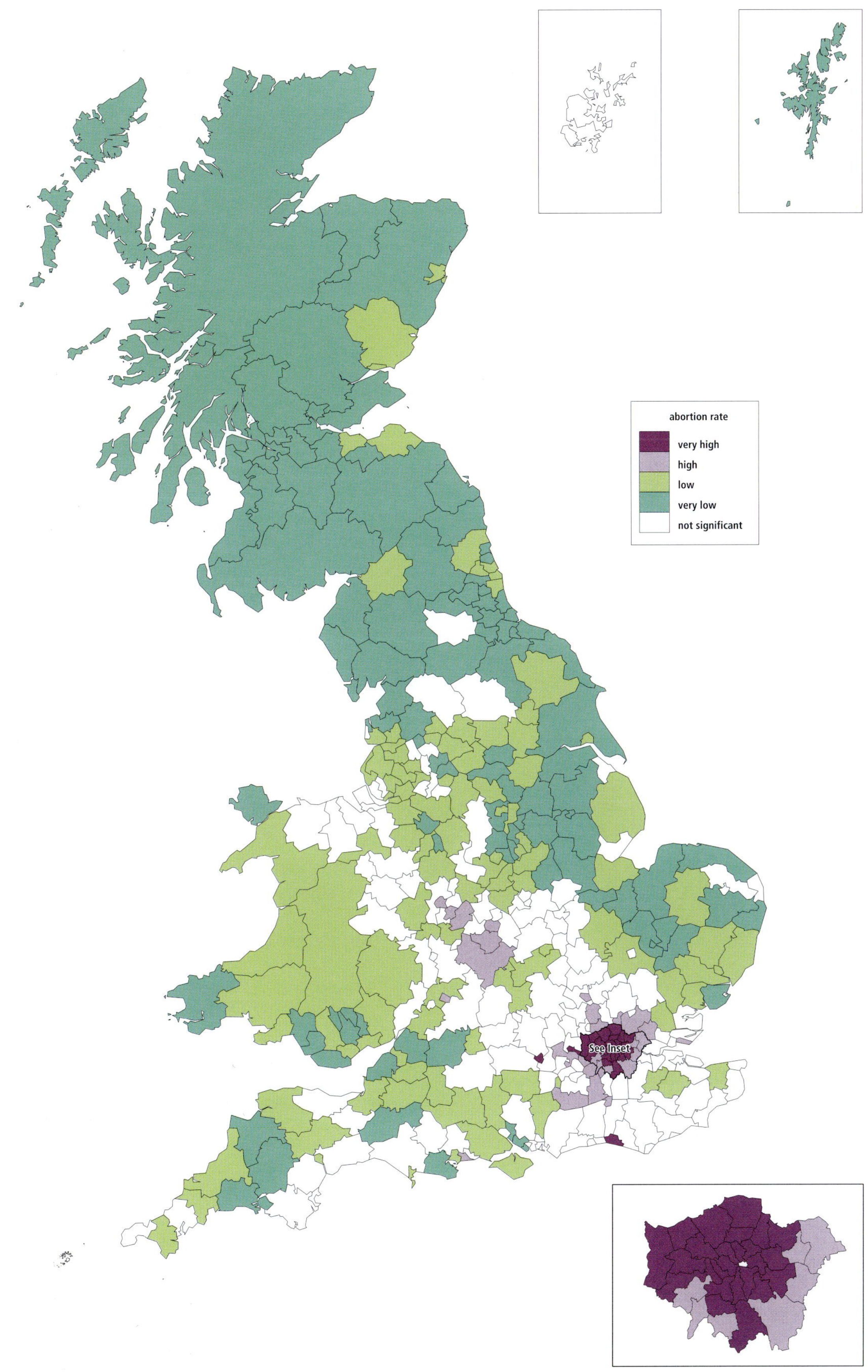

Figure 5.22

**Abortion rates by ONS classification Group, women aged under 18
Great Britain 1992-1997**

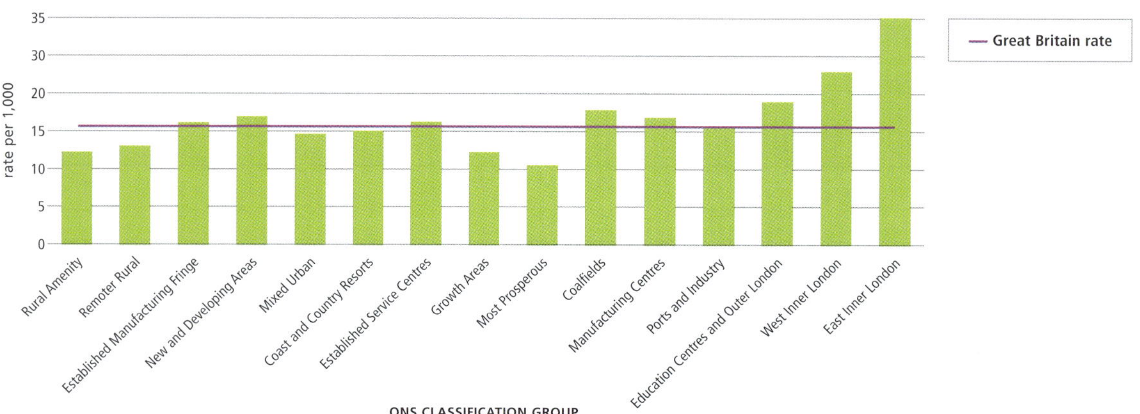

Figure 5.23

**Abortion rates by ONS classification Group, women aged 35-39
Great Britain 1992-1997**

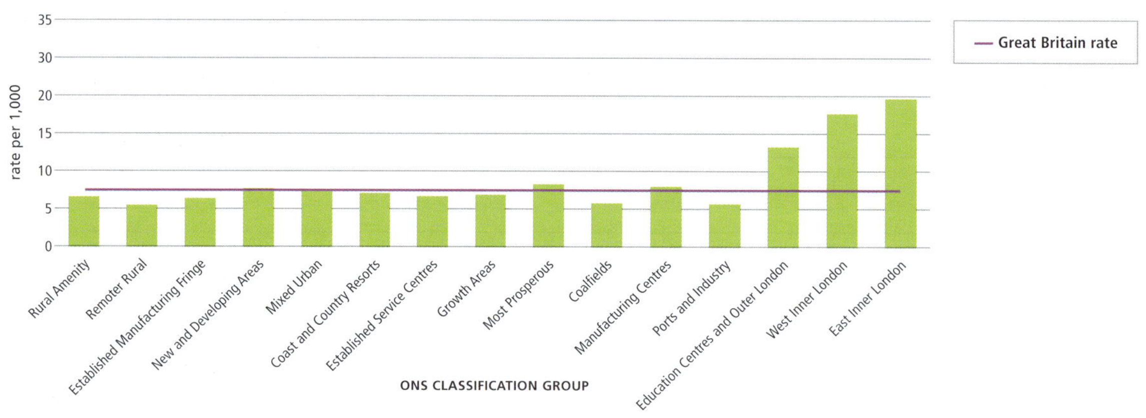

The North East had a high rate in the youngest age group, but the lowest rate in the older age groups. The North West had high rates up to age 30.

In London the abortion rate peaked in the 20-24 age group. It was in this age group that the differential between the rate in London and the rate in the other regions was greatest. The rate in London in this age group was over 75 per cent greater than the rate in the West Midlands, the region with the next highest rate, and over twice as high as the rate in the North East, the region with the lowest rate. Trends between 1992 and 1997 were similar in each age group to the all-age trends.

Local authority level variation
Variation at local authority level in teenagers followed that of the countries and regions. However, although authorities with high rates were found throughout Great Britain, the majority were in London and the West Midlands regions. Other authorities with higher rates than Great Britain were found in the Liverpool, Manchester and Pennine areas, as well as the North East and north Wales in 18-19 year olds (Maps 5.17 and 5.18).

When looking at the variation for women aged under 18 using ONS classification Groups, it was those Groups which were solely or mostly located within London which had the highest abortion rates, with the highest rate being in *East Inner London*. The *Most Prosperous* and *Growth Areas* Groups had the lowest under 18 abortion rates within Great Britain (Figure 5.22).

At ages 20 and over the pattern of variation at local authority level more closely matched that of the all-age pattern described earlier, with high rates concentrated in London and the West Midlands, around Birmingham. For those aged 20-24 high rates were also found in the Liverpool and Manchester areas and scattered other urban local authorities (Map 5.19). For women aged 25-29 high rates were also found in Liverpool and Manchester, but in few other local authorities outside London and the Birmingham area (Map 5.20). For women in their early thirties the very highest rates were concentrated in London, and also in Brighton and Hove, and high rates were found in Liverpool, Manchester and the Birmingham area (Map 5.21). For women aged 35-39, Liverpool and Manchester did not have high rates (Map 5.22).

Figure 5.24

**Percentage of abortions by gestation weeks, country and region, women all ages
Great Britain 1992-1997**

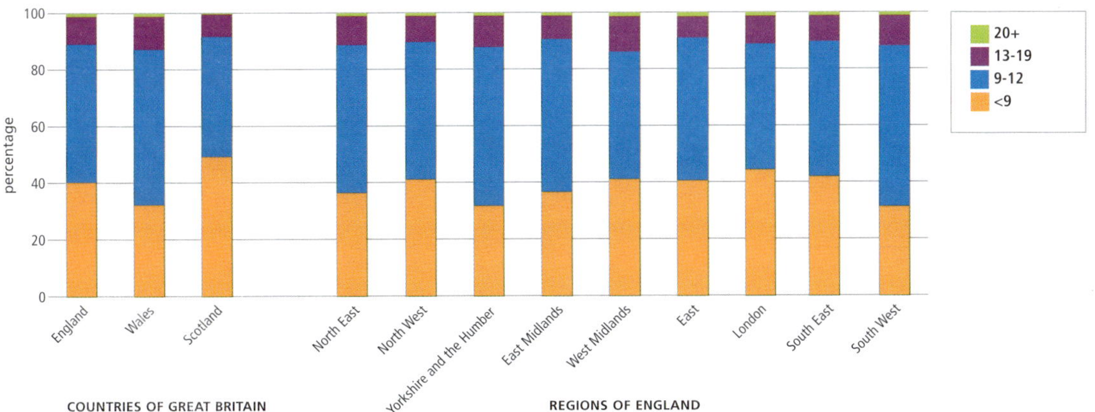

For women aged 35-39 the local authority rates in London were more markedly greater than the rates in the rest of Great Britain (Figure 5.23). The pattern for ONS classification Groups was similar, but not identical to the pattern described above for teenagers. The Groups located in London again had the highest rates and contained local authorities with substantially higher rates than the rest of the local authorities in Great Britain. There was very little variation by ONS classification Group outside of London, although the *Most Prosperous* Group had a rate higher than Great Britain in this age group, whereas it had the lowest rate for teenagers.

Percentage of abortions by gestation weeks

This section looks at the percentage of abortions performed by the duration of pregnancy (in weeks) before abortion. It is important to examine gestation length as the procedures that can be used to carry out an abortion vary depending on the length of gestation, and the grounds for carrying out the termination also depend on gestation length.[26]

In our analysis abortion data are grouped into four categories as follows: less than 9 weeks gestation, 9 to 12 weeks, 13 to 19 weeks and 20 or more weeks gestation. For the all-age country and regional level analysis we used these four categories of gestation length. At local authority level three categories are used, with 13 or more weeks gestation combining 13-19 and 20 plus. Small numbers in the 20 plus category preclude further disaggregation. For each age group, at all geographic levels, only the percentage of abortions performed at 13 or more weeks gestation is examined.

Almost nine out of ten abortions take place during the first 12 weeks of pregnancy, and this has not changed dramatically over the 1990s.[27] Here we examine variations by area in this general pattern.

All-age patterns

Country and regional level variation
In Great Britain between 1992 and 1997 41 per cent of abortions were performed under 9 weeks of gestation, 48 per

cent between 9 and 12 weeks, 10 per cent between 13 and 19 weeks and 1 per cent over 20 weeks. Scotland had more abortions performed under 9 weeks than England or Wales and in contrast had a smaller proportion of abortions performed between 9 and 12 weeks of gestation. The percentage of abortions performed between 13 and 19 weeks of gestation was lowest in Scotland and highest in Wales. There was a very low percentage of abortions performed after 20 weeks of gestation in all the countries (Figure 5.24).

London had a high proportion of abortions performed under 9 weeks of gestation. The South West and Yorkshire and the Humber had the lowest proportions performed under 9 weeks and the highest proportions performed between 9 and 12 weeks. The proportion of abortions performed between 13 and 19 weeks was highest in the East Midlands and lowest in the West Midlands. The proportion performed after 20 weeks was low in all the regions (Figure 5.24).

Local authority level variation
As would be expected from the country and regional pattern described above, areas with high percentages of abortions performed in less than 9 weeks were found in the South East, west London, West Midlands and Scotland. Areas with lower percentages were found on the east coast, Wales, Cornwall, south Devon and east London (Map 5.23). This geographic pattern was reversed for 9-12 weeks of gestation.

For 13 and over weeks gestation the picture is less clear, with areas that had high percentages of abortions performed at 13 weeks or over scattered throughout Great Britain. A major concentration was in the South Wales/Bristol areas, and also in the east of inner London and parts of the West Midlands. The North West and Pennine areas also had areas with high percentages of abortions performed at 13 weeks or over whereas East Anglia, outer London, the rural north of England and south and west Scotland had lower percentages of abortions performed in this gestation period (Map 5.24).

Figure 5.25

**Percentage of abortions performed in 13 or more weeks gestation by country and age group
Great Britain 1992-1997**

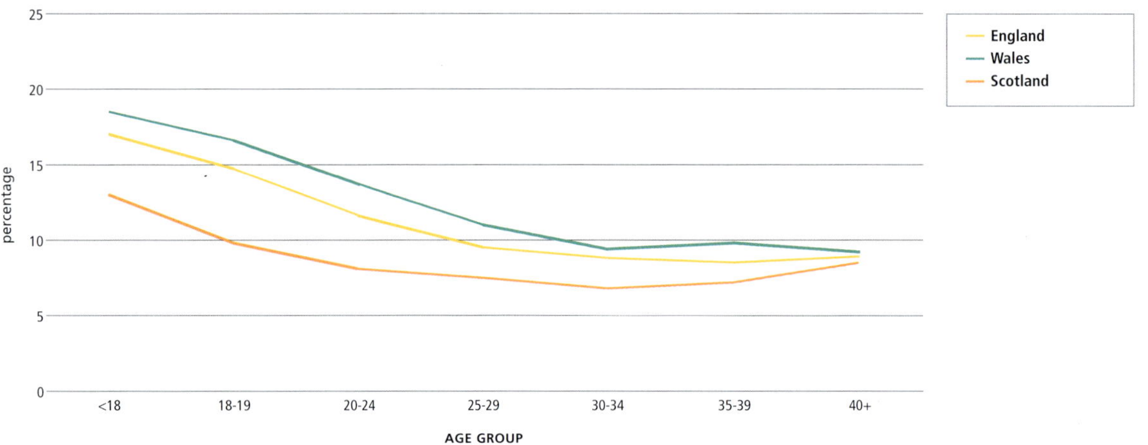

Figure 5.26

**Percentage of abortions performed in 13 or more weeks gestation by region and age group
England 1992-1997**

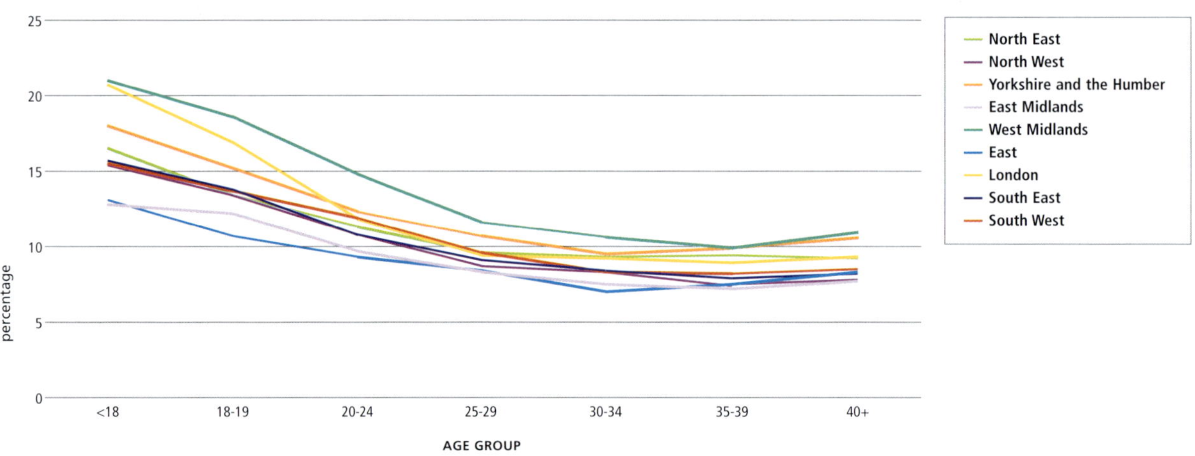

Age-specific patterns

Country and regional level variation

The percentage of abortions performed at 13 or more weeks of
gestation showed a decrease with age in all the countries of
Great Britain. It was highest in the under 18s (17 per cent in
Great Britain) and levelled off for women aged over 30 at about
9 per cent (Figure 5.25). Wales had the highest proportion of
abortions performed at 13 or more weeks in all the age groups,
and Scotland had the lowest.

The highest proportion of abortions performed at 13 or more
weeks in the regions of England was found in the West
Midlands in every age group. London had a high proportion of
abortions performed at 13 or more weeks at younger ages and
an average proportion at older ages. The East of England and
East Midlands had the lowest proportions of abortions
performed at 13 or more weeks gestation in all the age groups
(Figure 5.26).

Local authority level variation

The pattern of variation within Great Britain was not a clear
cut one, with areas that had high percentages of abortions
performed at 13 or more weeks being scattered throughout
Great Britain in under 18s (Map 5.25). Areas with low
proportions were mainly rural areas.

Percentage of abortions by purchaser

The information on the purchaser of an abortion reflects
changes in health care provision and funding in England and
Wales over the last decade. Abortions may be purchased and
carried out by the NHS, purchased by the NHS but performed
in private clinics or paid for privately. For Scotland, data on the
premises where the abortion was performed is available, but
not on who funded the abortion, therefore the analysis by
purchaser is restricted to England and Wales only. This section
looks at the percentage of abortions purchased privately, firstly
for all women and then by age group.

Map 5.23

**Percentage of abortions performed in under 9 weeks gestation by local authority, women all ages
Great Britain 1992-1997**

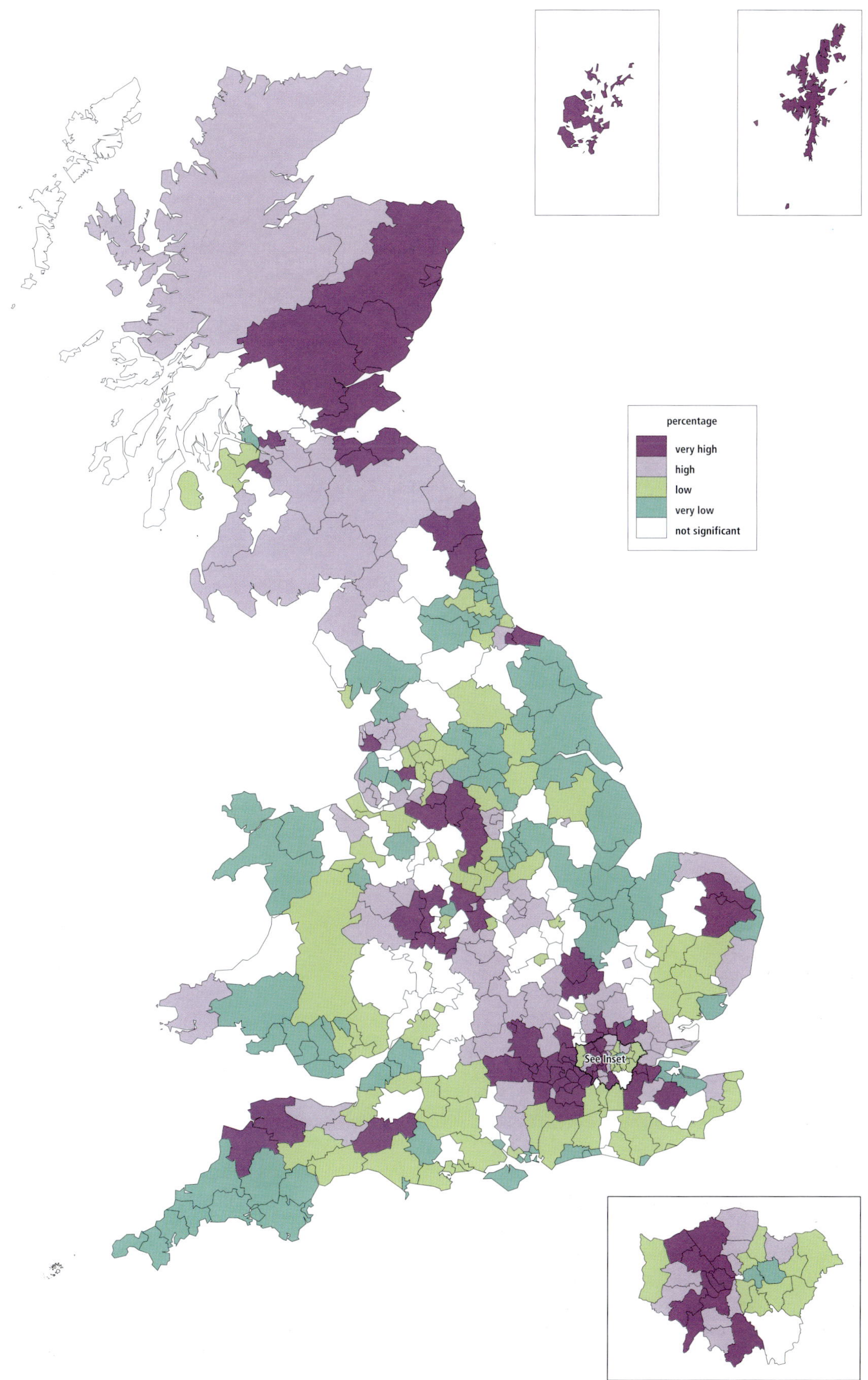

Map 5.24

Percentage of abortions performed in 13 or more weeks gestation by local authority, women all ages
Great Britain 1992-1997

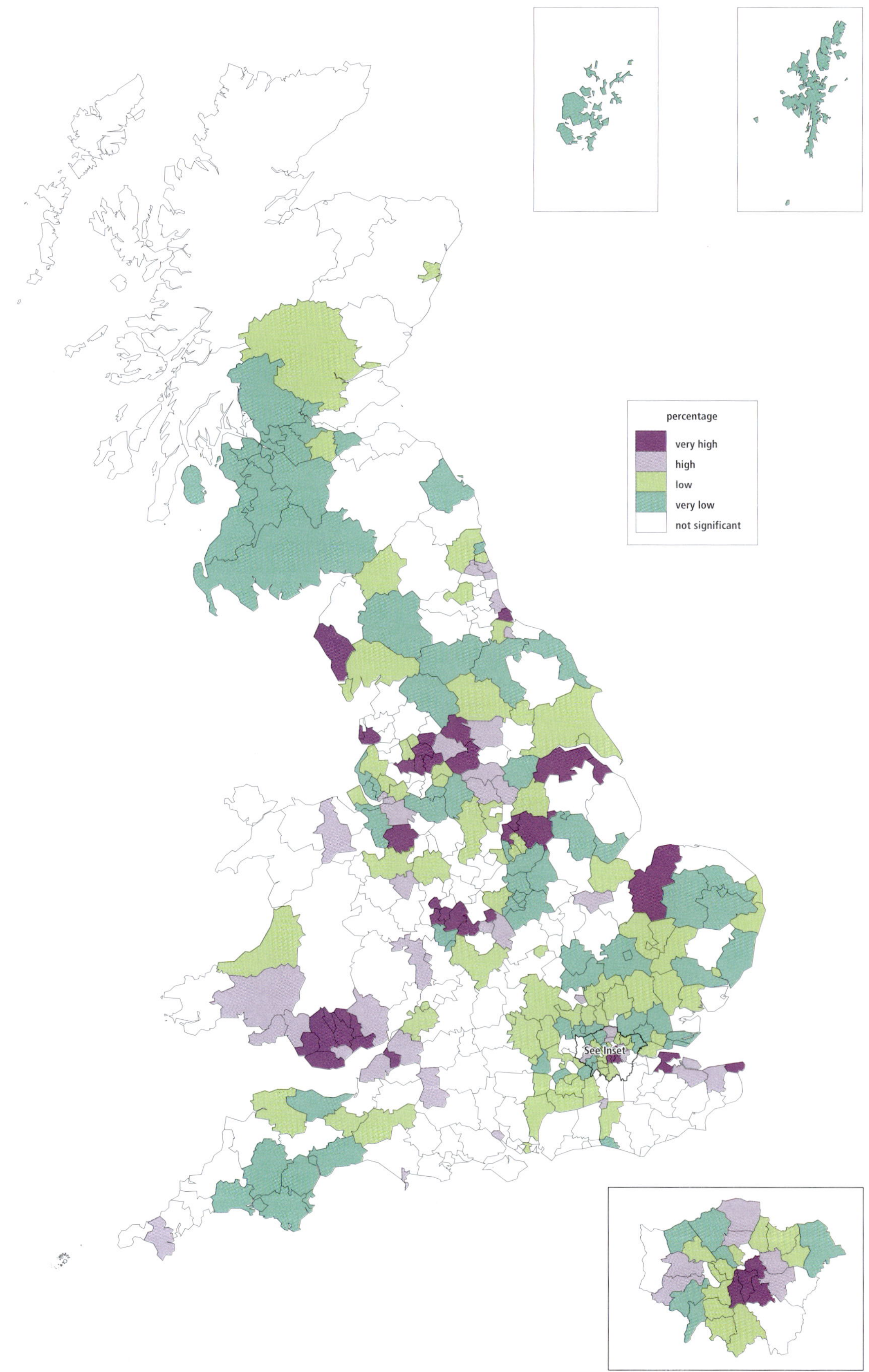

Map 5.25

**Percentage of abortions performed in 13 or more weeks gestation by local authority, women aged under 18
Great Britain 1992-1997**

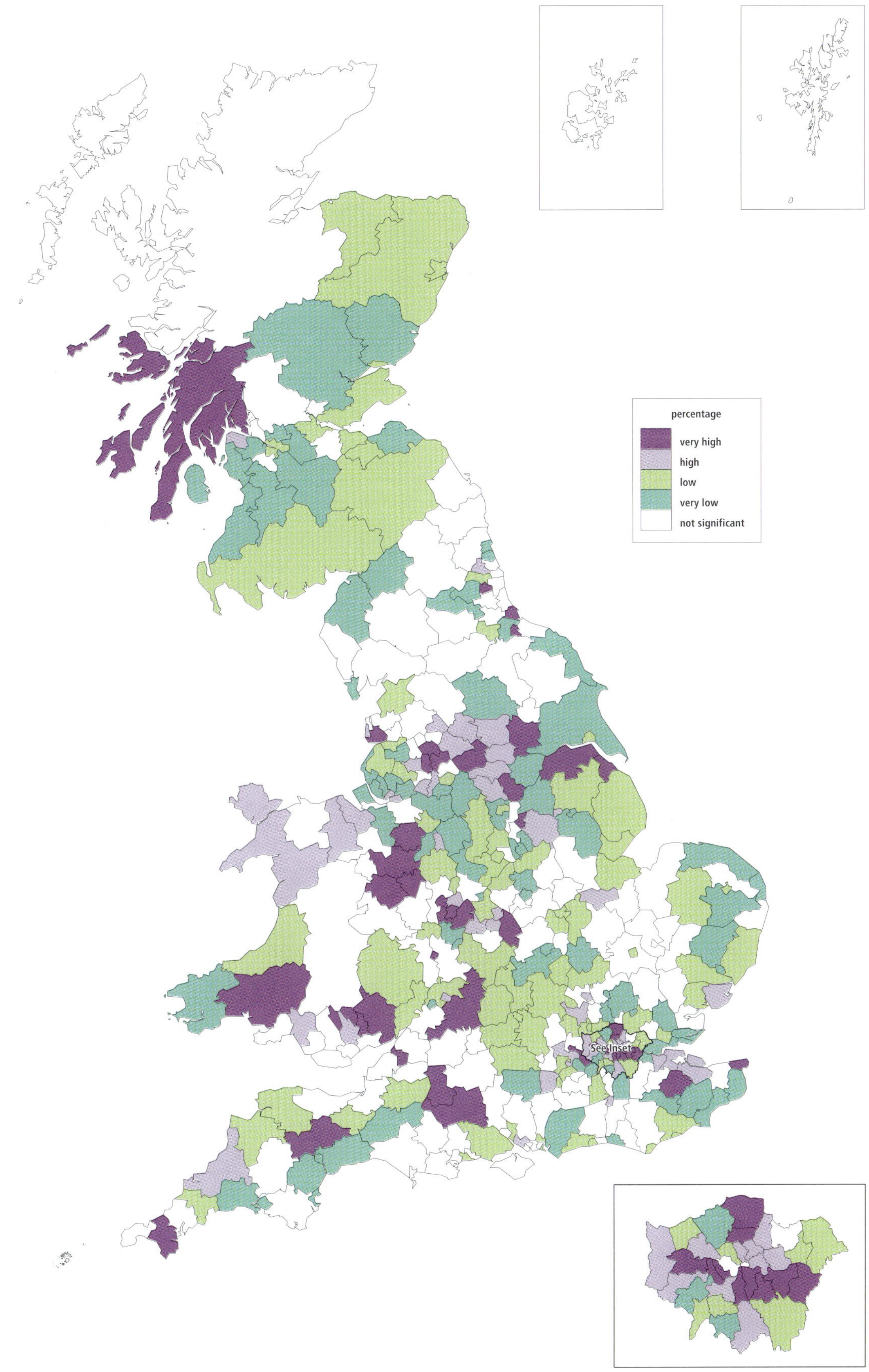

Figure 5.27

Percentage of abortions that are privately purchased by country and region, women all ages England and Wales 1992-1997

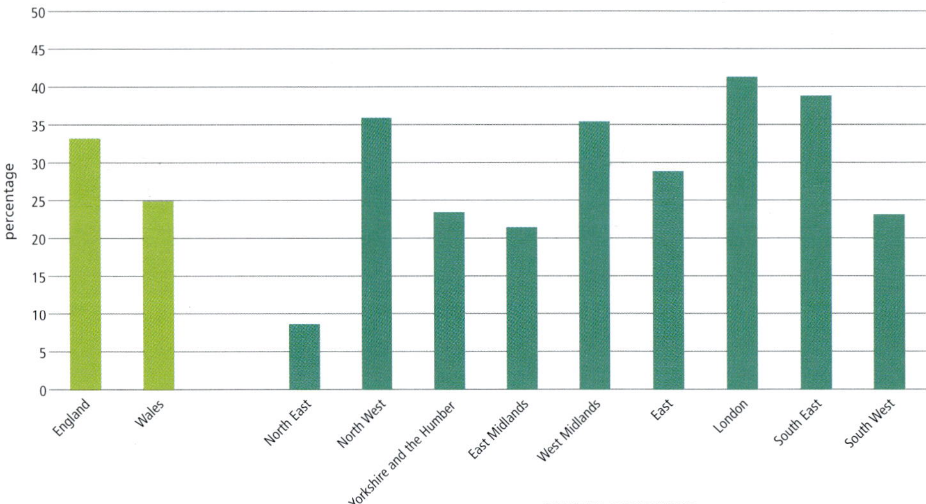

Figure 5.28

Percentage of abortions that are privately purchased by age group, country and region, women all ages England and Wales 1992-1997

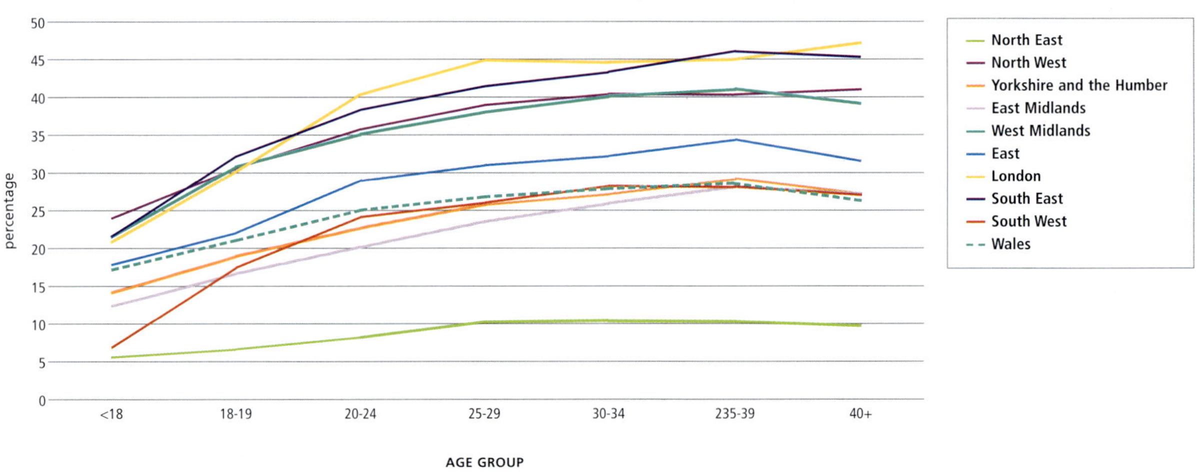

All-age patterns

Country and regional level variation

There were large variations in how services are purchased within England and Wales. Comparing England as a whole with Wales, the proportion of abortions purchased privately was greater in England, about a third compared to a quarter in Wales.

Within England, London and the South East had the highest percentages of abortions purchased privately. The North West and West Midlands also had higher proportions of abortions purchased privately than in England and Wales as a whole. In contrast the North East had the lowest percentage (Figure 5.27).

Local authority level variation

The pattern of local authority level variation within England and Wales was very clear cut. Clusters of authorities in the South East, London, Shropshire and Staffordshire and parts of the North West had high proportions of privately purchased abortions, and clusters of authorities in the South West, far North, Wales, Lincolnshire and East Anglia had low proportions (Map 5.26).

Age-specific patterns

Country and regional level variation

When we look at variation by age we can see that the geographic pattern seen for all ages largely holds throughout the age groups (Figure 5.28). The percentage of abortions purchased privately increased with age up to the 25-29 age group and then levelled off. This increase was far less substantial in the North East than the other regions, meaning that the difference between the percentage of privately purchased abortions in the other regions and the North East was more marked with increasing age. Age-specific patterns by local authority were very similar to the all-age patterns and are therefore not discussed here.

Map 5.26

**Percentage of abortions that are privately purchased by local authority, women all ages
England and Wales 1992-1997**

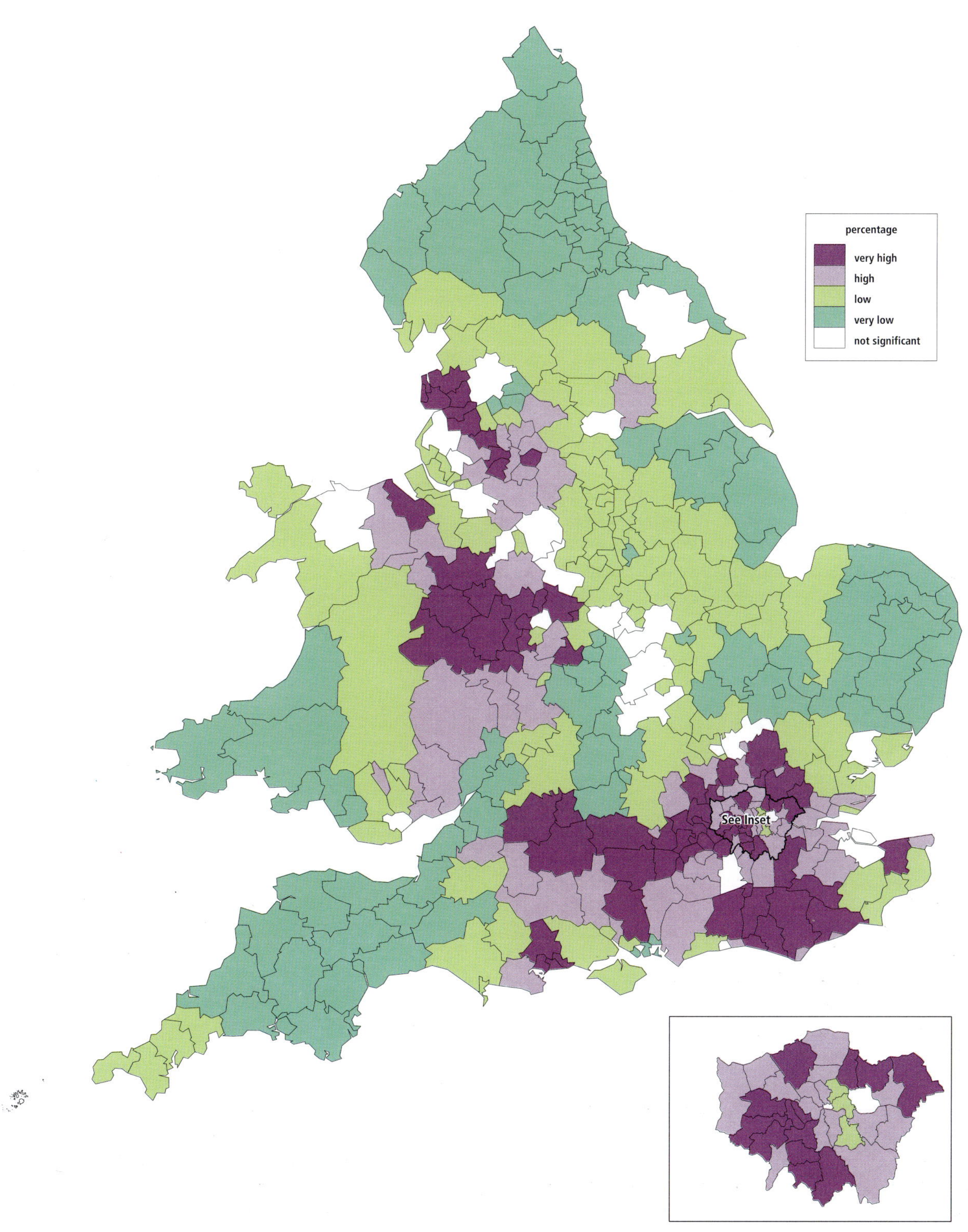

5.4 Live births

In this section we examine geographic variations in live birth rates and also the marital status of the mother at birth registration across the United Kingdom for 1991 to 1997. Still births are not discussed in this section, but are examined in chapter 6.

Live birth rates

All-age patterns

Country and regional level variation

Table 5.1 shows Total Fertility Rates (TFR) for the countries of the United Kingdom and regions of England for the period 1991 to 1997. Box 5.1 describes the method of calculation for the TFR. In the United Kingdom as a whole the TFR was 1.76 births per woman. Scotland had a lower TFR than the United Kingdom as a whole and Wales and Northern Ireland both had higher rates. All of the countries experienced a decline in their TFR between 1991 and 1997 (Figure 5.29). Northern Ireland's TFR remained about 25 per cent greater than the TFR in Scotland throughout 1991 to 1997.

The variation between the regions of England was not as great as the variation between the countries of the United Kingdom. The region with the lowest TFR was the North East and the region with the highest TFR the West Midlands, a similar but not identical pattern to the conception and abortion rates, where London had the highest rates, but the West Midlands also had high rates. All of the regions of England apart from London had a decline in fertility between 1991 and 1997. London's TFR was the lowest in England in 1991, but by 1997 it had the second highest TFR, behind the West Midlands which had consistently the highest TFR (Figure 5.30).

Box 5.1 Total Fertility Rate

The Total Fertility Rate (TFR) provides us with a single measure of the level of fertility in an area which takes into account the age structure of the population, as it is calculated using age-specific fertility rates. In this volume we have used the following age-specific rates - under 20, 20-24, 25-29, 30-34, 35-39 and 40 plus. For those aged under 20 the population denominator used is women aged 15-19, for those aged 40 and over the population denominator used is women aged 40-44. In calculating confidence intervals for the TFR we have used the method described by Breslow and Day.[28]

The TFR is usually interpreted as the number of children a woman would have in her lifetime if she survived to the end of her reproductive period and experienced, throughout that period, the current age-specific fertility rates.[29] Calot[30] provides another definition of the TFR, showing that it can be interpreted on a period basis as the ratio of the number of children born in a year to the weighted average size of female cohorts of childbearing age in that year, using the age-specific fertility rates as the weights.

Table 5.1

Total Fertility Rates by country and region United Kingdom 1991-1997

United Kingdom	1.76
England	1.76
North East	1.72 ~
North West	1.80 *
Yorkshire and the Humber	1.78 *
East Midlands	1.74 ~
West Midlands	1.84 *
East	1.77
London	1.74 ~
South East	1.74 ~
South West	1.73 ~
Wales	1.84 *
Scotland	1.62 ~
Northern Ireland	2.02 *

* significantly higher than the United Kingdom rate

~ signifcantly lower than the United Kingdom rate

Local authority level variation

When we examined rates for local authorities a more varied distribution was found and areas with high TFRs were scattered throughout the United Kingdom, although there was a concentration in Northern Ireland, as might be expected given the substantially higher TFR for Northern Ireland as a whole. Within Northern Ireland, Newry and Mourne had the highest TFR; at 2.44 it was the highest of any local authority in the United Kingdom. Outside Northern Ireland, local authorities in the Birmingham area, south Lancashire, west Yorkshire and east London had high TFRs. Local authorities in the east of London tended to have higher TFRs than those in the west of London (Map 5.27).

When TFRs are analysed by ONS Classification Group we see that *East Inner London* had the highest TFR in Great Britain, along with *Manufacturing Centres* (Figure 5.31). Characteristics of both these Groups include high unemployment, high proportions of social housing, a high percentage of lone parent families and high proportions of the population in Social Classes IV and V. The *East Inner London* Group has a large minority ethnic population in both the Black and Asian minority ethnic groups. *Manufacturing Centres* has a large population in the Asian minority ethnic groups. Additionally *East Inner London* has large families and the *Manufacturing Centres* Group has a high proportion of terraced housing.

Map 5.27 shows that local authorities in Scotland generally had low TFRs, a similar pattern to conception and abortion rates, although Highland, Moray, Shetland Islands and Orkney Islands had higher rates than the United Kingdom as a whole. Cambridge had the lowest TFR in the United Kingdom, 1.19.

Using ONS classification Groups, the *West Inner London* Group had the lowest TFR. Characteristics of this Group include a high level of employment in finance and services and low levels of manufacturing and production, a large proportion of single person of working-age households, a mobile and relatively affluent population and a high proportion of people living in privately rented accommodation.

Local authorities with very low TFRs, including Cambridge, were also found in the *Education Centres and Outer London* Group, but the value for the Group as a whole was raised by local authorities within the Group that had relatively high

TFRs. The characteristics of these areas are large numbers of students, high levels of employment in finance and services and higher than average levels of private renting, purpose-built flats and terraced houses.

None of the local authorities within the *Manufacturing Centres* Group had a TFR below 1.80; in contrast the *Rural Amenity* Group had no local authorities which have a TFR above 1.80. Characteristics of the *Rural Amenity* Group include a mature population, high employment in agriculture, low unemployment and low levels of local authority renting.

Figure 5.29

**Trends in Total Fertility Rates by country
United Kingdom 1991-1997**

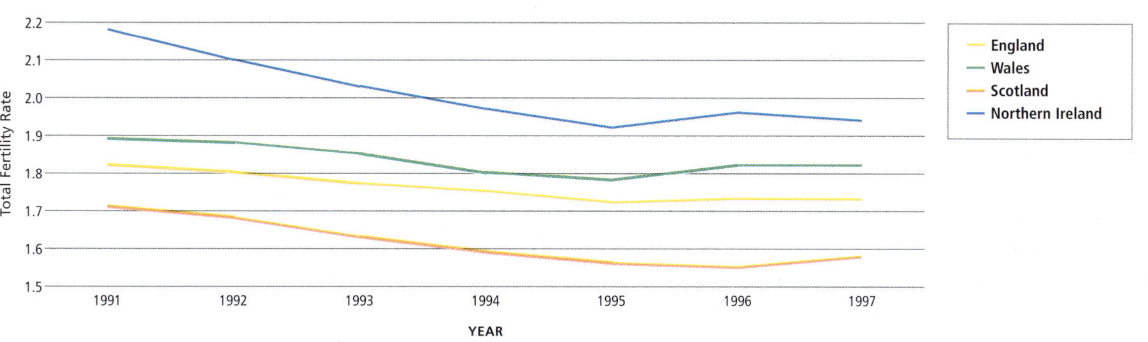

Figure 5.30

**Trends in Total Fertility Rates by region
England 1991-1997**

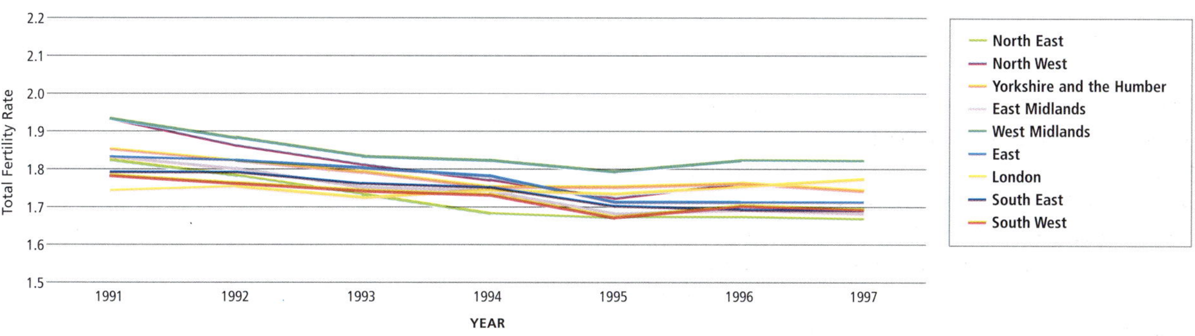

Figure 5.31

**Total Fertility Rates by ONS classification Group
Great Britain 1991-1997**

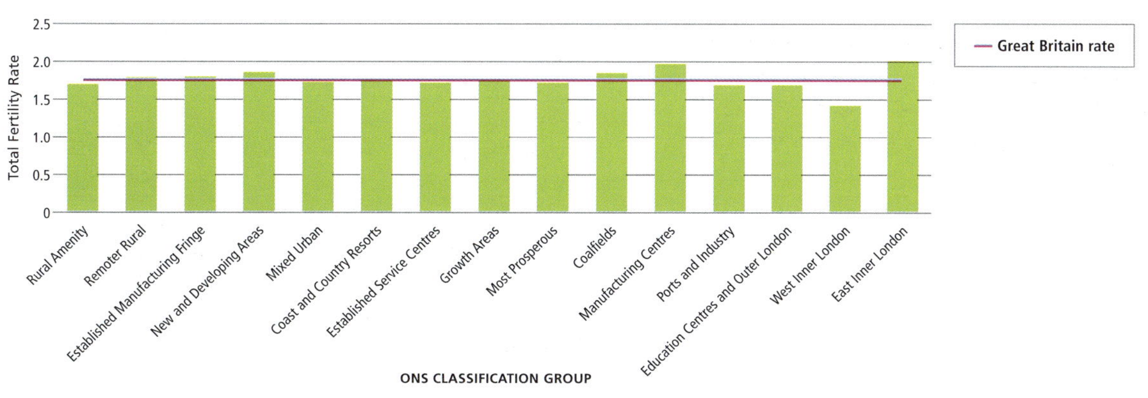

Map 5.27

Total Fertility Rates by local authority
United Kingdom 1991-1997

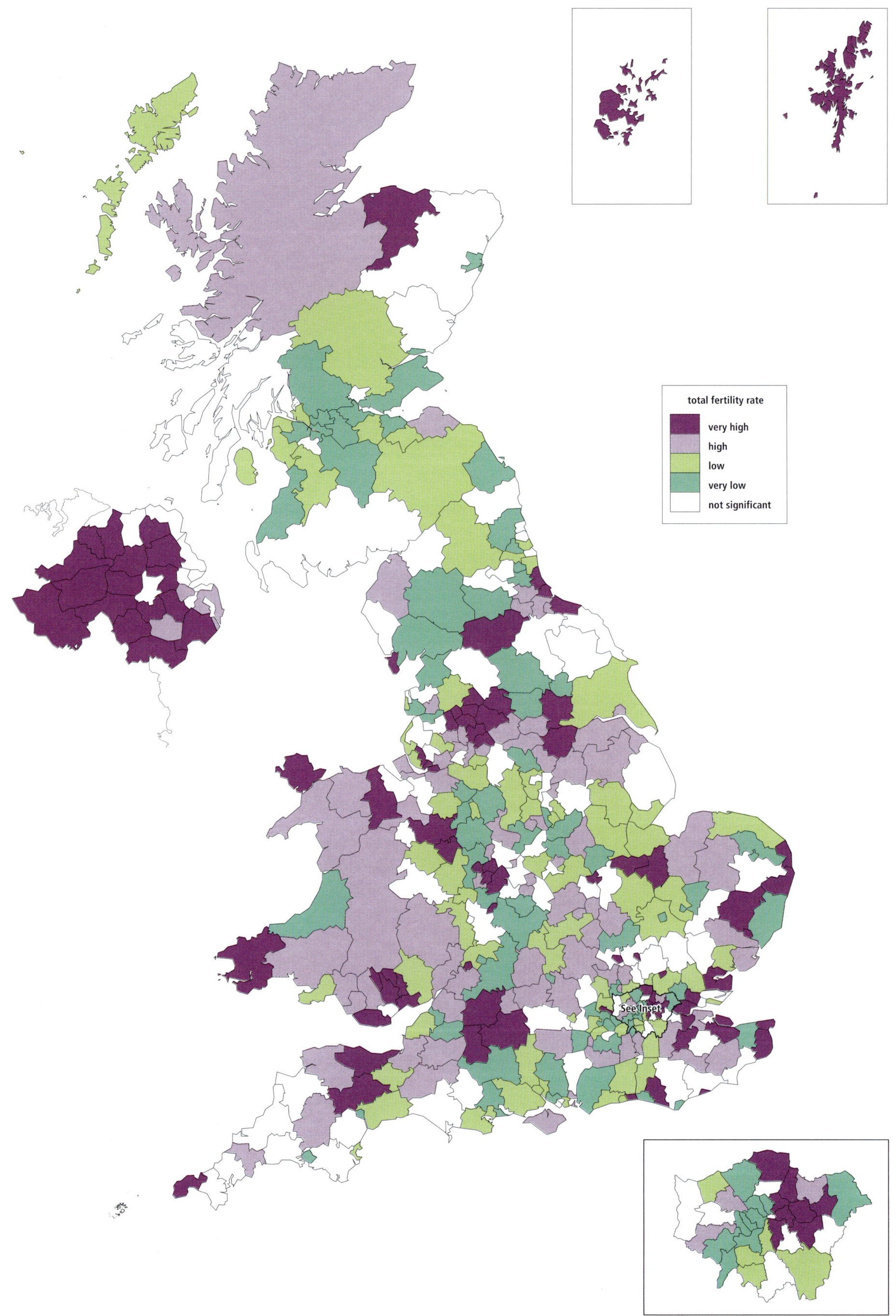

Figure 5.32

Live birth rates by country and age group
United Kingdom 1991-1997

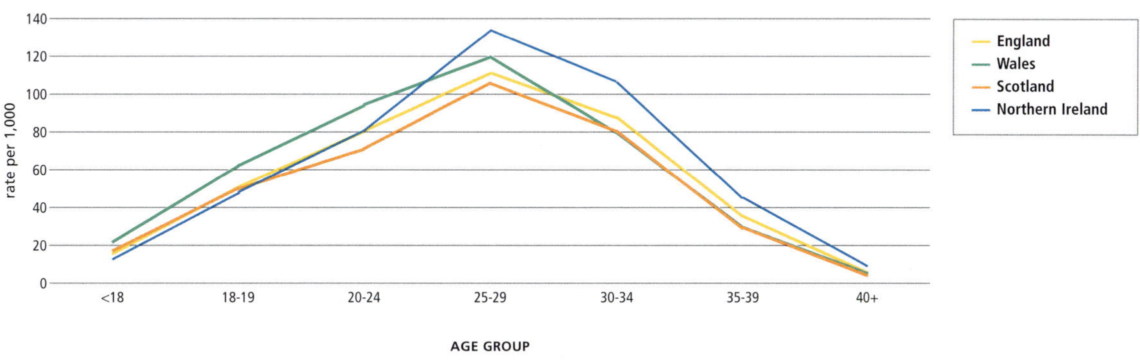

Figure 5.33

Trends in live birth rates by country, women aged under 18
United Kingdom 1991-1997

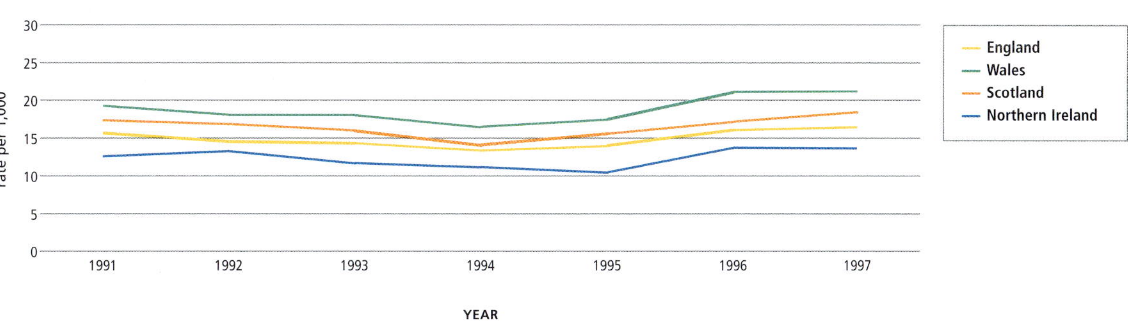

Figure 5.34

Trends in live birth rates by country, women aged 20-24
United Kingdom 1991-1997

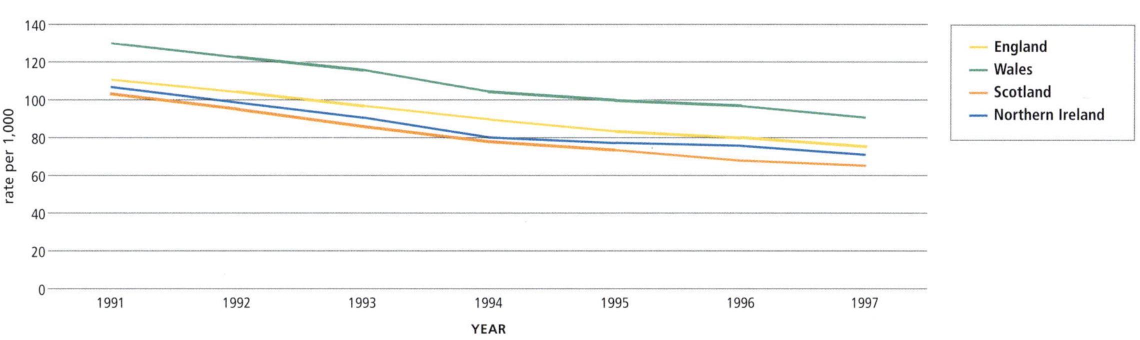

Figure 5.35

Trends in live birth rates by country, women aged 35-39
United Kingdom 1991-1997

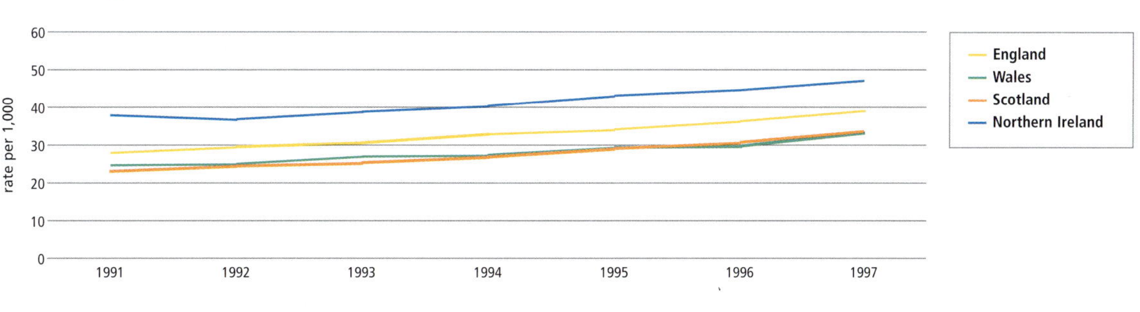

Figure 5.36

**Mean age of mother at live birth by country and region
United Kingdom 1991-1997**

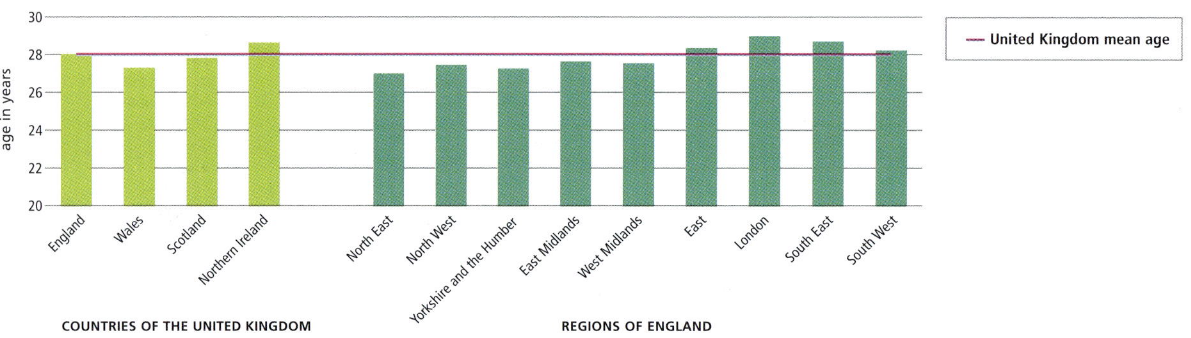

Figure 5.37

**Trends in the mean age of mother at live birth by country
United Kingdom 1991-1997**

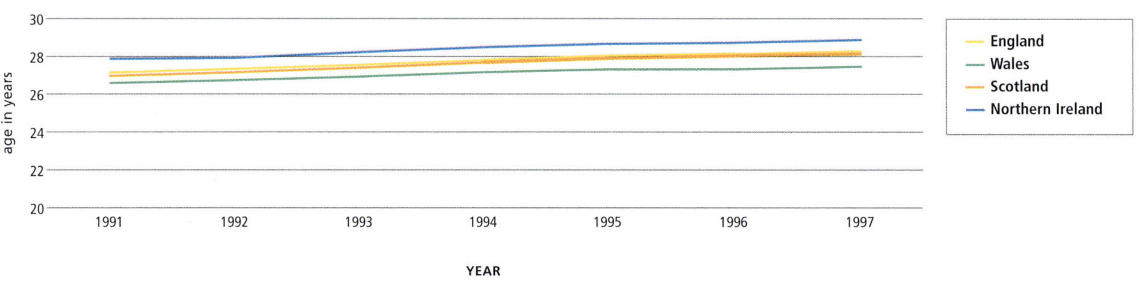

Age-specific patterns

Country and regional level variation

In all countries of the United Kingdom, women aged 25-29 had the highest birth rates (Figure 5.32). Under 18s in Scotland had higher birth rates than under 18s in England but those aged over 20 had lower rates in Scotland than in England. Wales had the highest teenage birth rates and higher rates than England up to the age of 30. After this age Wales had lower birth rates than England. Teenagers in Northern Ireland had lower birth rates than teenagers in the other countries, but in older women rates were much higher and the peak birth rate was substantially higher. Women aged 30-34 in Northern Ireland had higher birth rates than women aged 25-29 in Scotland.

The most dramatic change in fertility over the last 20 years has been a shift towards later childbearing, with fertility in women in their thirties and forties increasing and fertility in women in their twenties decreasing.[31] Between 1991 and 1997 birth rates for teenagers increased overall in all countries of the United Kingdom, after a fall in the early part of the 1990s (Figure 5.33). All countries showed a decline in birth rates in women in their twenties throughout the period, continuing the long term trend. This decline was more marked for 20-24 year olds than 25-29s (Figure 5.34). Birth rates for women in their thirties increased substantially, both in the early and late thirties, also continuing long term trends (Figure 5.35).

Figure 5.38

**Live birth rates by region and age group
England 1991-1997**

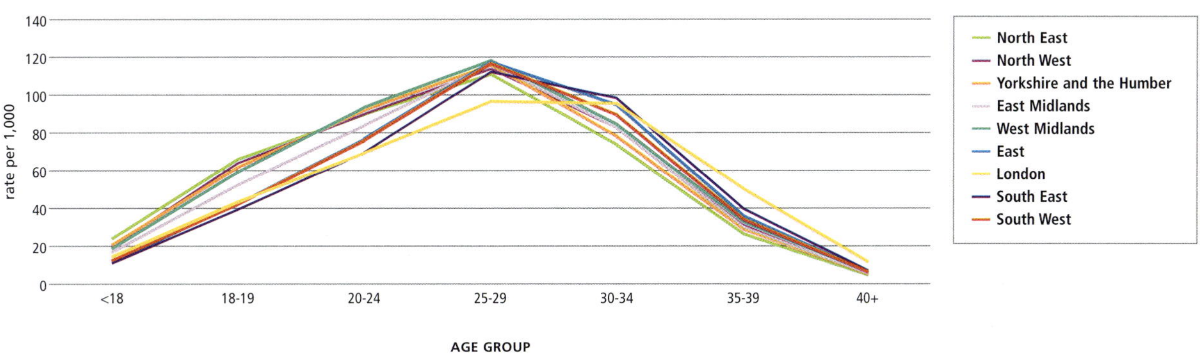

Figure 5.39

**Trends in live birth rates by region, women aged under 18
England 1991-1997**

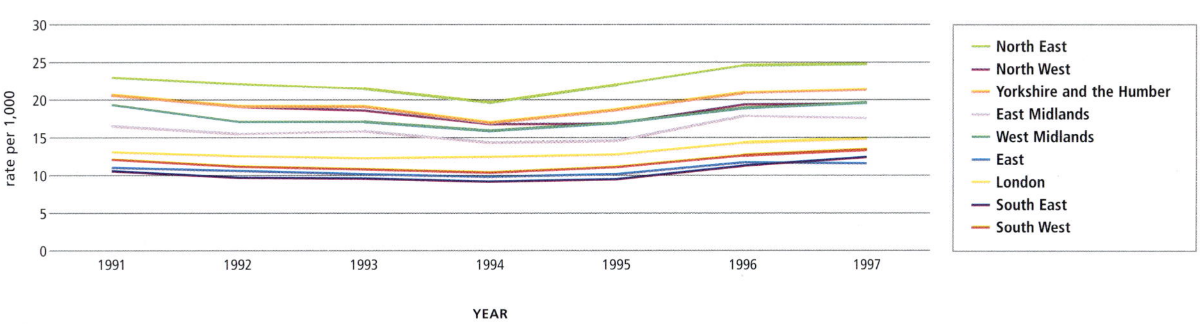

Figure 5.40

**Trends in live birth rates by region, women aged 20-24
England 1991-1997**

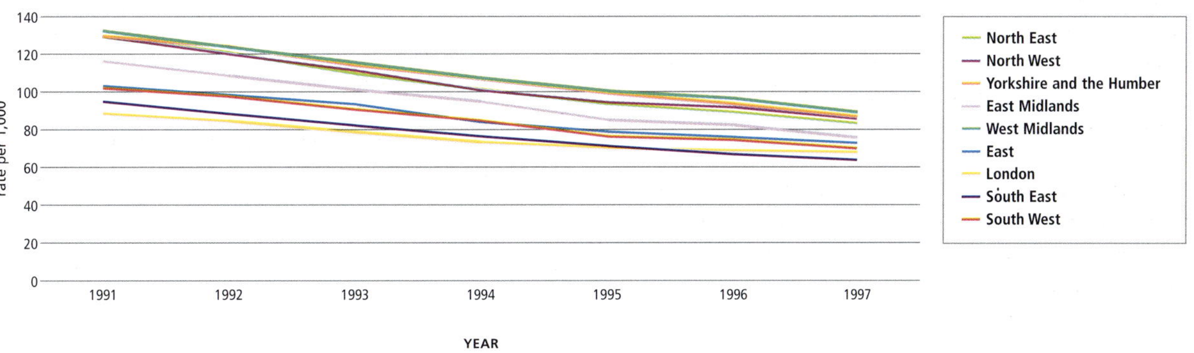

Figure 5.41

**Trends in live birth rates by region, women aged 35-39
England 1991-1997**

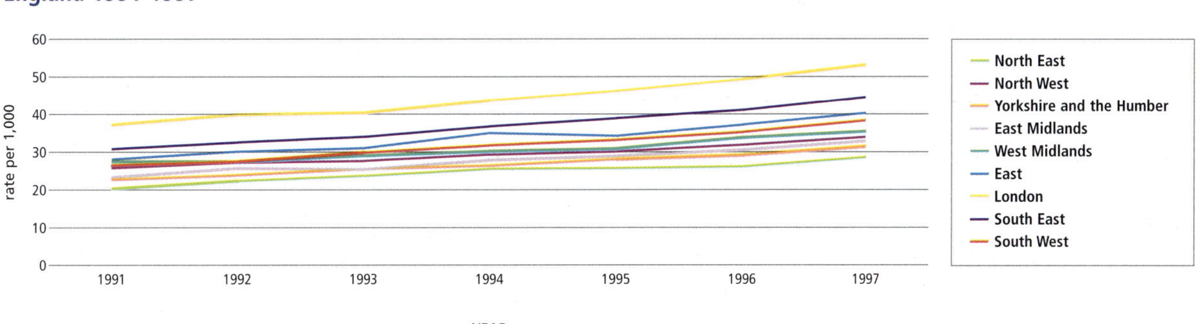

Figure 5.42

Trends in the mean age of mother at live birth by region England 1991-1997

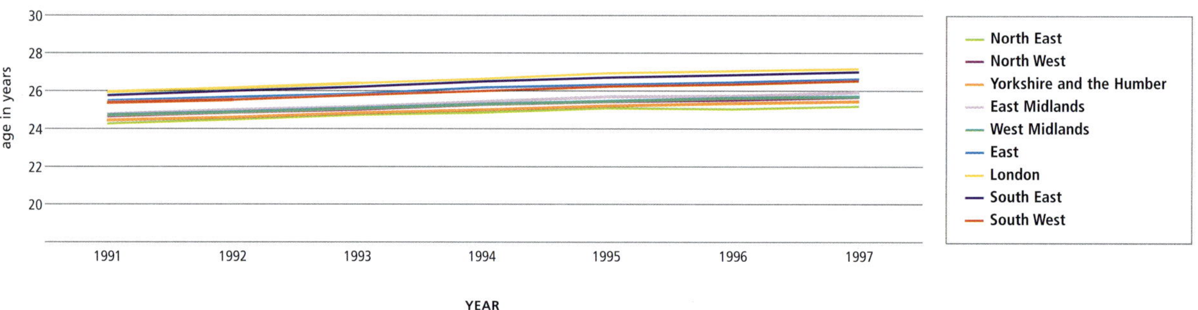

Figure 5.43

Mean age of mother at first to fourth births by country and region England and Wales 1991-1997

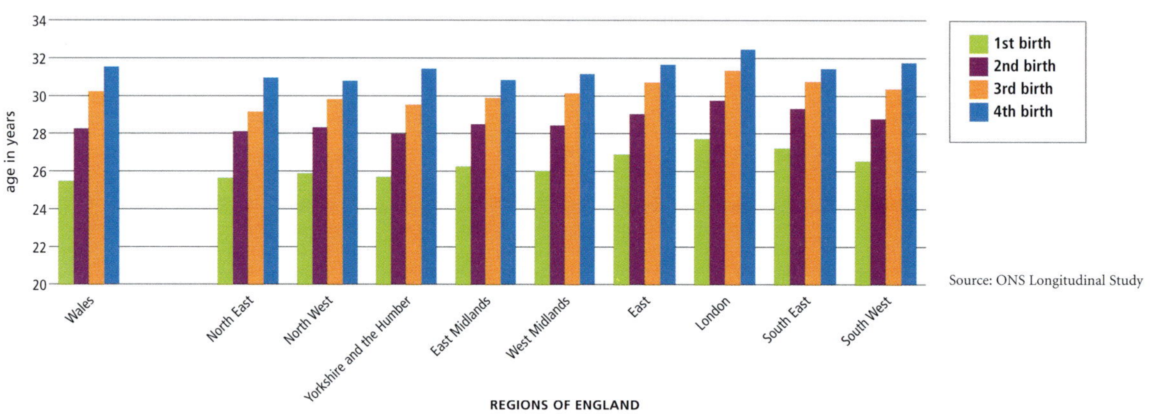

This age-specific pattern can be summarised in a single measure - the mean age at live birth. The method of calculating this measure is described in Box 5.2. Women in Northern Ireland had the highest mean age at live birth and women in Wales the lowest, 28.6 years compared to 27.3 years (Figure 5.36). In each of the countries, between 1991 and 1997, there was an increase of about one year in the mean age of mother at live birth (Figure 5.37). The difference of just over one year was therefore maintained between women in Northern Ireland and Wales.

The northern and Midlands regions showed a much younger pattern of age-specific birth rates than regions in the south, with higher rates in the age groups under age 25 (Figure 5.38). At older ages their rates were generally lower than in the southern regions. The East of England and South West had similar patterns of age-specific birth rates to each other. Women in the South East had lower rates than women in these two regions up to and including the 25-29 age group, but they had the highest rates in the 30-34 age group. London had a different pattern. It had much lower rates in the 25-29 age group, almost the same as the 30-34 rate, so the curve does not show the traditional peak. Rates in women aged over 35 were much higher in London than in the other regions.

All the regions of England had an increase in birth rates in women aged under 18, following an initial decline (Figure 5.39). For women in their twenties, a marked decline in rates was experienced in all regions, although only 20-24 year olds are shown (Figure 5.40). Women in their thirties in each region experienced an increase in their birth rates, data are shown for those aged 35-39 (Figure 5.41).

These age-specific patterns mean that within England there was a marked split between the regions in the mean age of mother at live birth. Women in the south of England were, on average, older when they gave birth than women in the north and Midlands. The four southern regions had higher mean ages at live birth than the United Kingdom as a whole and the other five regions had lower mean ages. Mean age at live birth varied between 27.0 years in the North East and 29.0 years in London (Figure 5.36). This pattern is similar to that seen for mean age at conception. Each region also had an increase of about one year in its mean age at live birth between 1991 and 1997 (Figure 5.42).

The results of analysis using the ONS Longitudinal Study, described in Appendix A, to calculate mean age at the first to fourth births also showed this north-south pattern (Figure

Figure 5.44

**Live birth rates by ONS classification Group, women aged under 18
Great Britain 1991-1997**

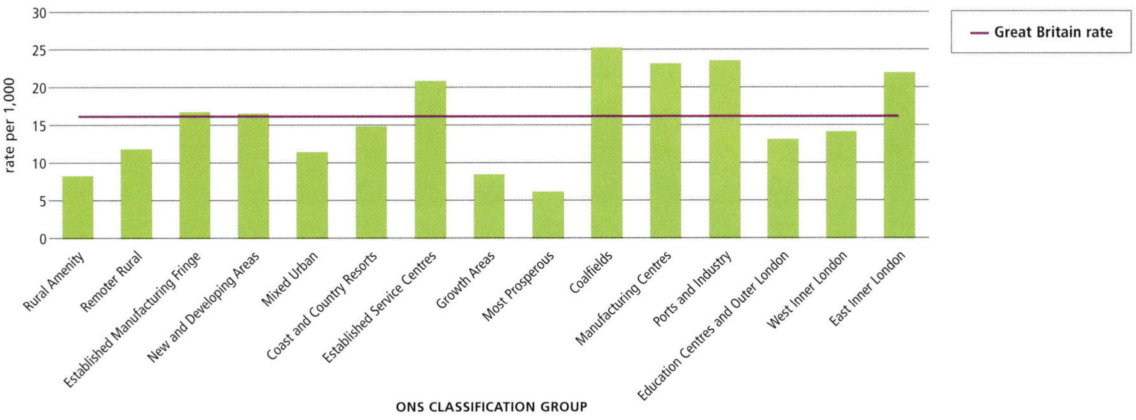

Figure 5.45

**Live birth rates by ONS classification Group, women aged 35-39
Great Britain 1991-1997**

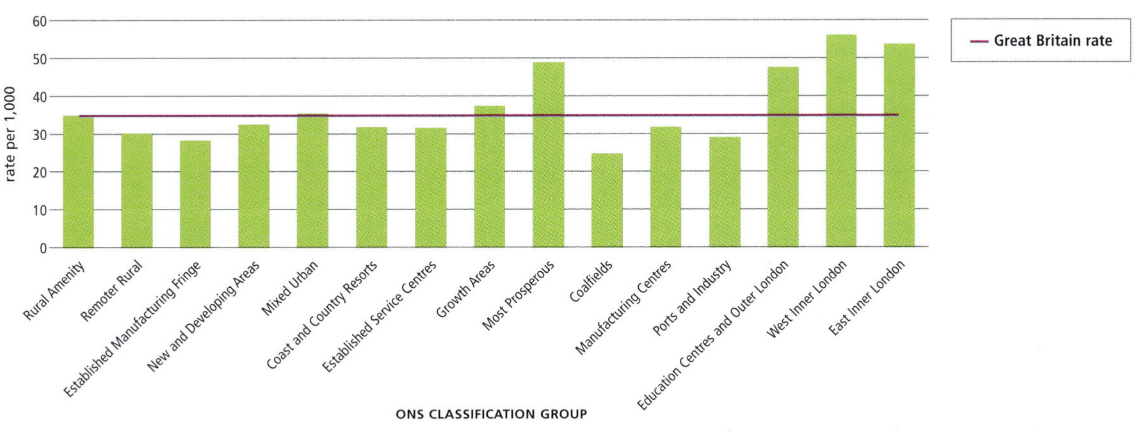

5.43). At each of the first to third births women in the north of England, and also in Wales had lower mean ages than women in the south. This pattern was not clear for the fourth birth. Women in London and the South East had a higher mean age at second birth than women in the North East's mean age at third birth.

Local authority level variation
The geographic pattern of birth rates across the United Kingdom was more varied at the local authority level and also changed very clearly with age. The pattern for teenagers was similar in both the under 18 and 18-19 age groups, although there were slightly more areas with high 18-19 rates. Areas with high teenage birth rates were clustered together in the North East region, south Wales, in a band across the country from Greater Manchester to Humberside, inner London, West Midlands and the large urban centres in Scotland. The lowest birth rates in teenagers were spread across rural and southern England and Northern Ireland (Maps 5.28, 5.29).

The lowest local authority rates for under 18s within Great Britain were found in those authorities classified as *Most Prosperous, Growth Areas, Rural Amenity* or *Remoter Rural* using the ONS Classification, with 75 per cent of authorities with very low rates on Map 5.28 being from these four Groups. All the authorities in *Most Prosperous* and *Growth Areas* Groups had teenage birth rates classified as very low on Map 5.28.

The highest local authority rates were found in those classified as *Coalfields, Manufacturing Centres* and *Ports and Industry.* The local authorities within the *Established Service Centres* Group also had high teenage birth rates; this was due to them having average conception rates, but a low percentage leading to abortion in general. These four groups accounted for 85 per cent of authorities with very high rates on Map 5.28 and also just over half of those with high rates. The *Coalfields* Group as a whole was the Group with the highest teenage birth rates and the *Most Prosperous* substantially the lowest, a difference of almost 5 times in the rate (Figure 5.44). The pattern in London showed a divide between *East Inner London* and *West Inner London,* with high rates in the East and low rates in the West.

Figure 5.46

**Mean age of mother at live birth by ONS classification Group
Great Britain 1991-1997**

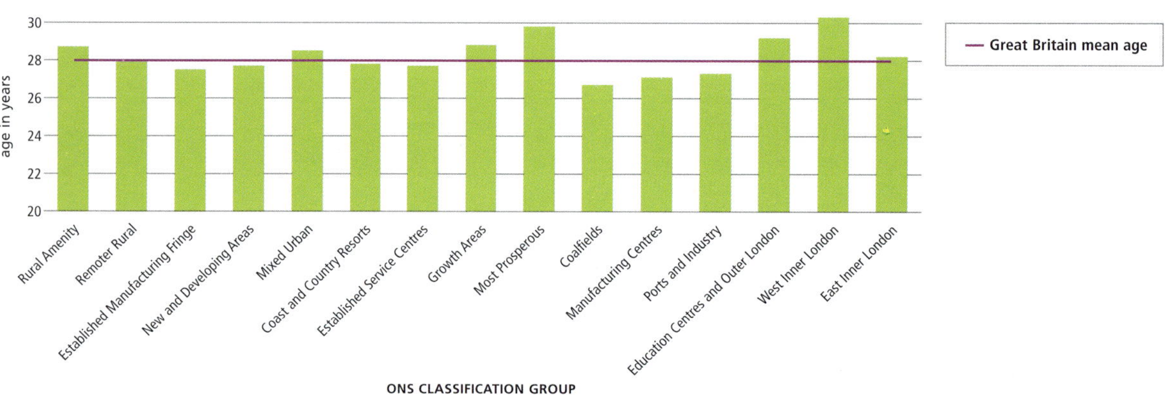

For women aged 20-24, the areas with the lowest birth rates were found mainly in the Home Counties (Map 5.30). Areas with high rates in women aged 20-24 were similar to those seen for teenagers. The pattern of fertility across the country changes for older women. For the 25-29 age group the majority of local authorities in Northern Ireland had higher rates than the United Kingdom, whereas in younger age groups they had lower rates. Outside Northern Ireland, local authorities with high fertility rates were concentrated in rural areas such as Devon and Cornwall and Wales. Areas with low birth rates were located around London, Gloucestershire, Warwickshire and parts of the North West (Map 5.31).

The geographic pattern was again different for women aged over 30 (Maps 5.32-5.34), with the opposite pattern to that at younger ages. Areas with high birth rates were concentrated in Northern Ireland and the south of England. Lower rates were now seen in the North East, south Wales, Scotland, and in a band across the country from the North West to the East Midlands. The 35-39 and over 40 age groups tended to show an accentuation of the pattern seen for women aged 30-34.

For women aged 35-39, examining the rates by ONS classification Group showed that, within Great Britain, high rates were found in those Groups located solely or primarily in London and also in the *Most Prosperous* Group. Low rates were found in the *Coalfields, Manufacturing Centres* and *Ports and Industry* Groups, as well as the *Remoter Rural* and *Established Manufacturing Fringe* (Figure 5.45).

The north-south divide in mean age of mother at live birth discussed above at regional level was clearly apparent at local authority level within the United Kingdom, with lower mean ages at birth being found in many local authorities in Wales, North East, North West and Yorkshire and the Humber and the higher mean ages in local authorities in London, excluding the east of inner London, and the South East. High mean ages at live birth were also found in authorities in Northern Ireland. The higher mean ages at birth in the East of England and South East were found in the areas bordering London (Map 5.35). The average age of women giving birth in the United Kingdom varied from 25.7 in Blaenau Gwent to 31.3 in Richmond-upon-Thames, a range of 5.6 years. However, there were only two local authorities in the United Kingdom with a mean age at birth lower than 26 - Blaenau Gwent and Merthyr Tydfil - and only two with a mean age at birth higher than 31 years - Richmond-upon-Thames and Kensington and Chelsea.

When we examine this using ONS classification Groups we can see that the Groups which are concentrated in more northern areas, such as *Coalfields, Manufacturing Centres, Ports and Industry* and *Established Manufacturing Fringe* had the lowest mean ages at birth in Great Britain (Figure 5.46). The highest mean ages were found in Groups that are mainly concentrated in the south and London - *West Inner London, Education Centres and Outer London* and *Most Prosperous*. Authorities within these Groups that are located outside London and the South East, for example Cambridge, Edinburgh, Macclesfield and Rushcliffe also had high mean ages at live birth, suggesting that it is the characteristics of those living in and moving into these areas that are creating the fertility pattern, rather than simply the location of the area. The characteristics of the *Most Prosperous* Group include low unemployment, high employment in finance and service occupations, a high proportion of the population in Social Class I or II and a high proportion of owner occupied housing.

Map 5.28

Live birth rates by local authority, women aged under 18
United Kingdom 1991-1997

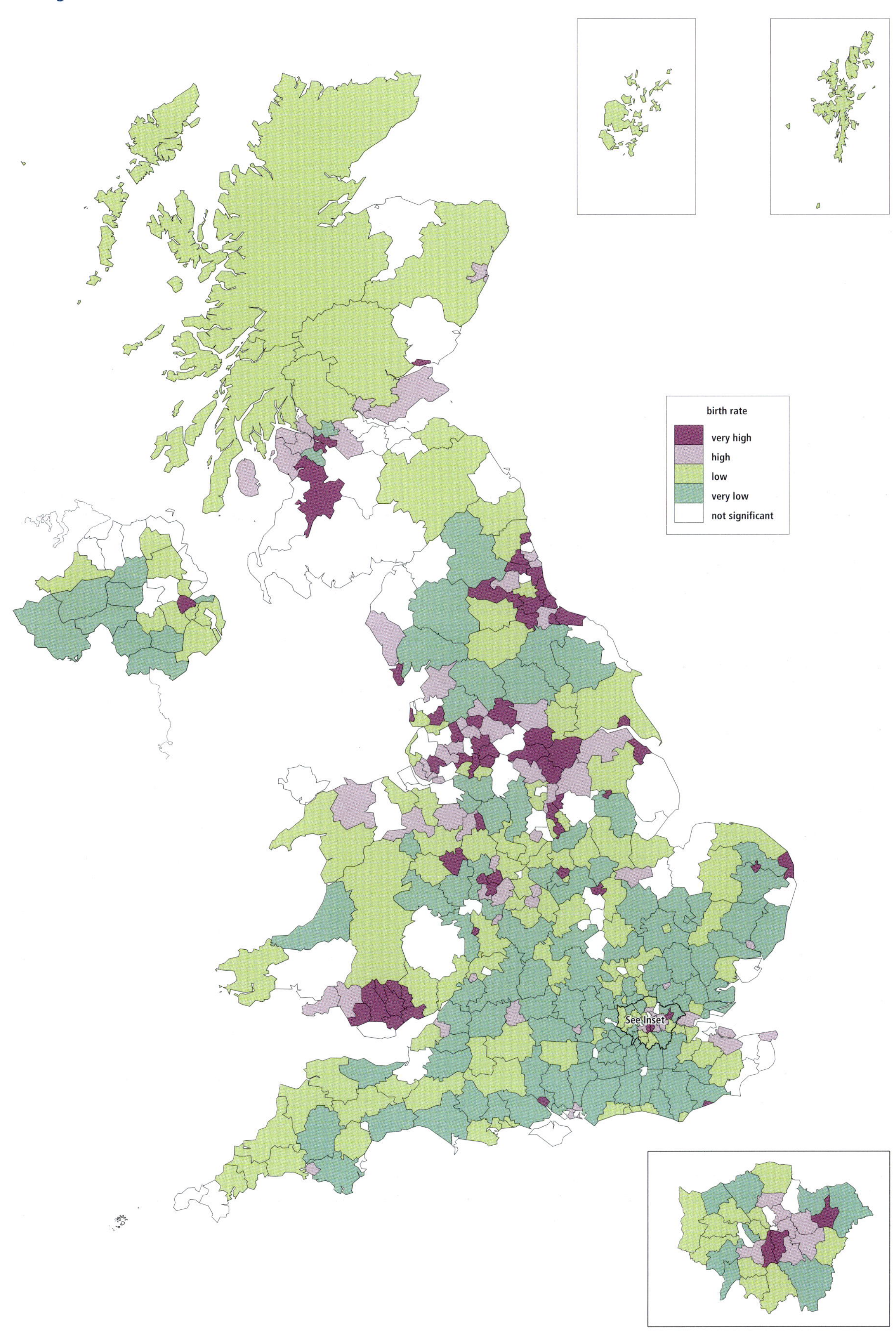

Map 5.29

Live birth rates by local authority, women aged 18-19
United Kingdom 1991-1997

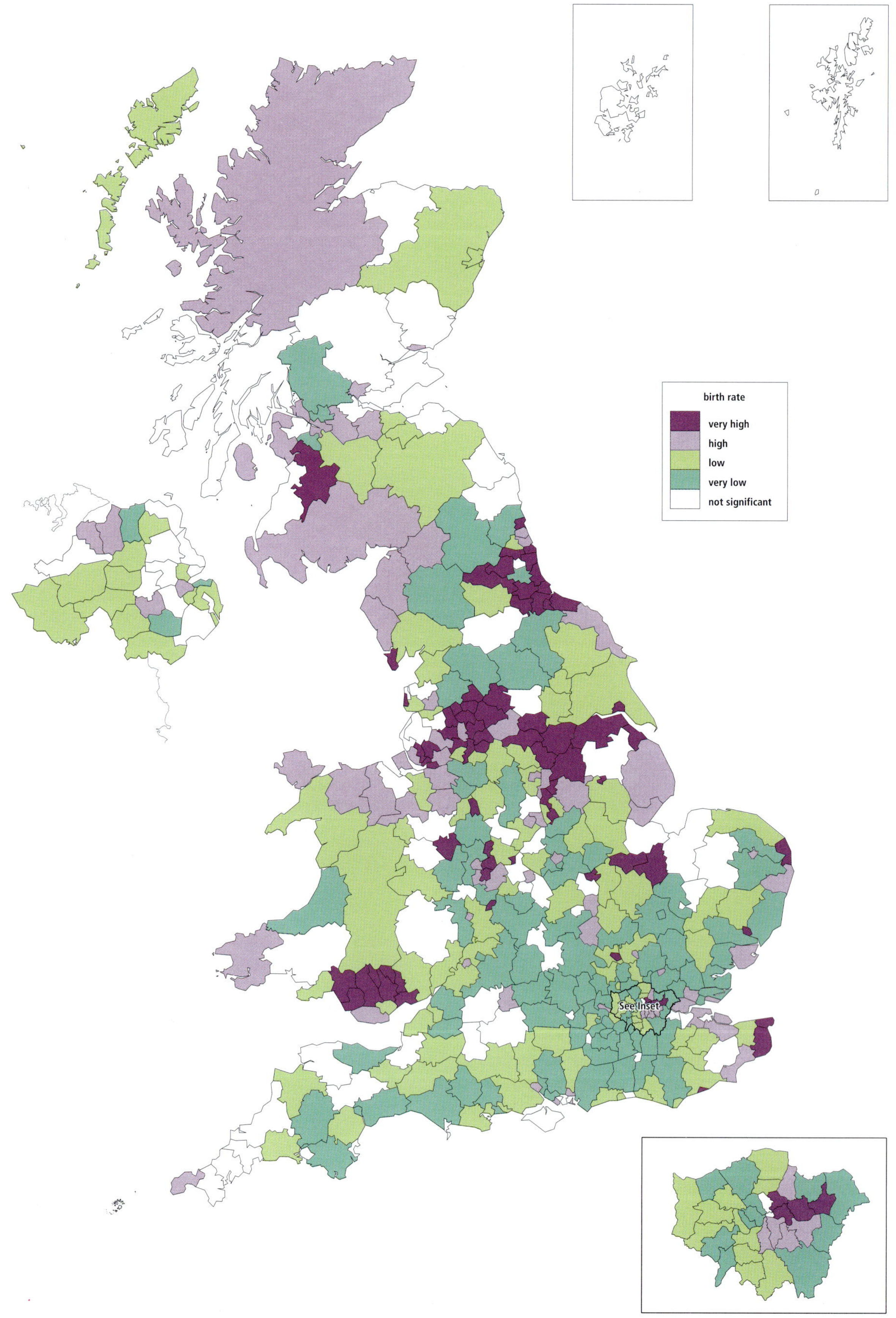

Map 5.30

**Live birth rates by local authority, women aged 20-24
United Kingdom 1991-1997**

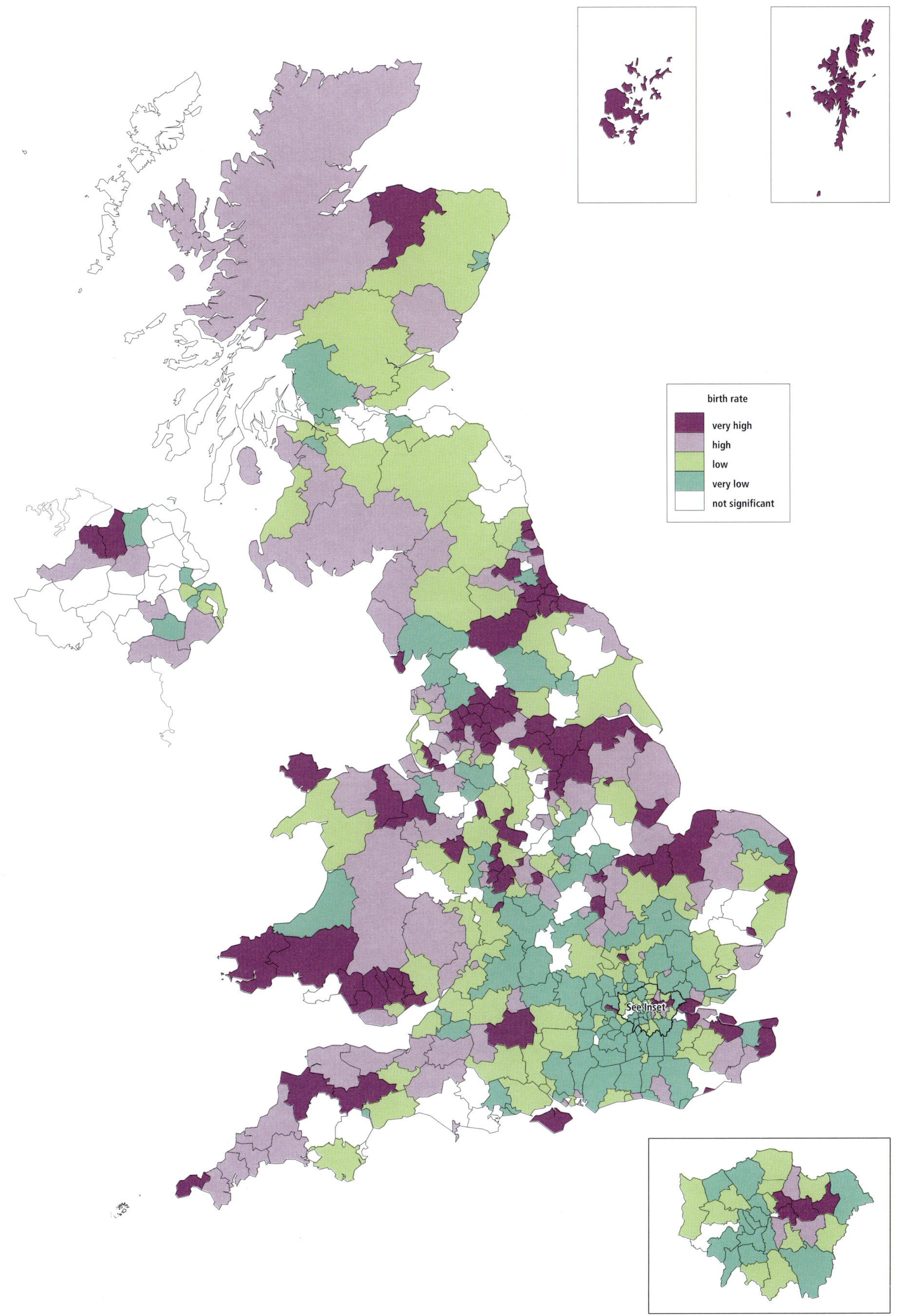

Map 5.31

Live birth rates by local authority, women aged 25-29
United Kingdom 1991-1997

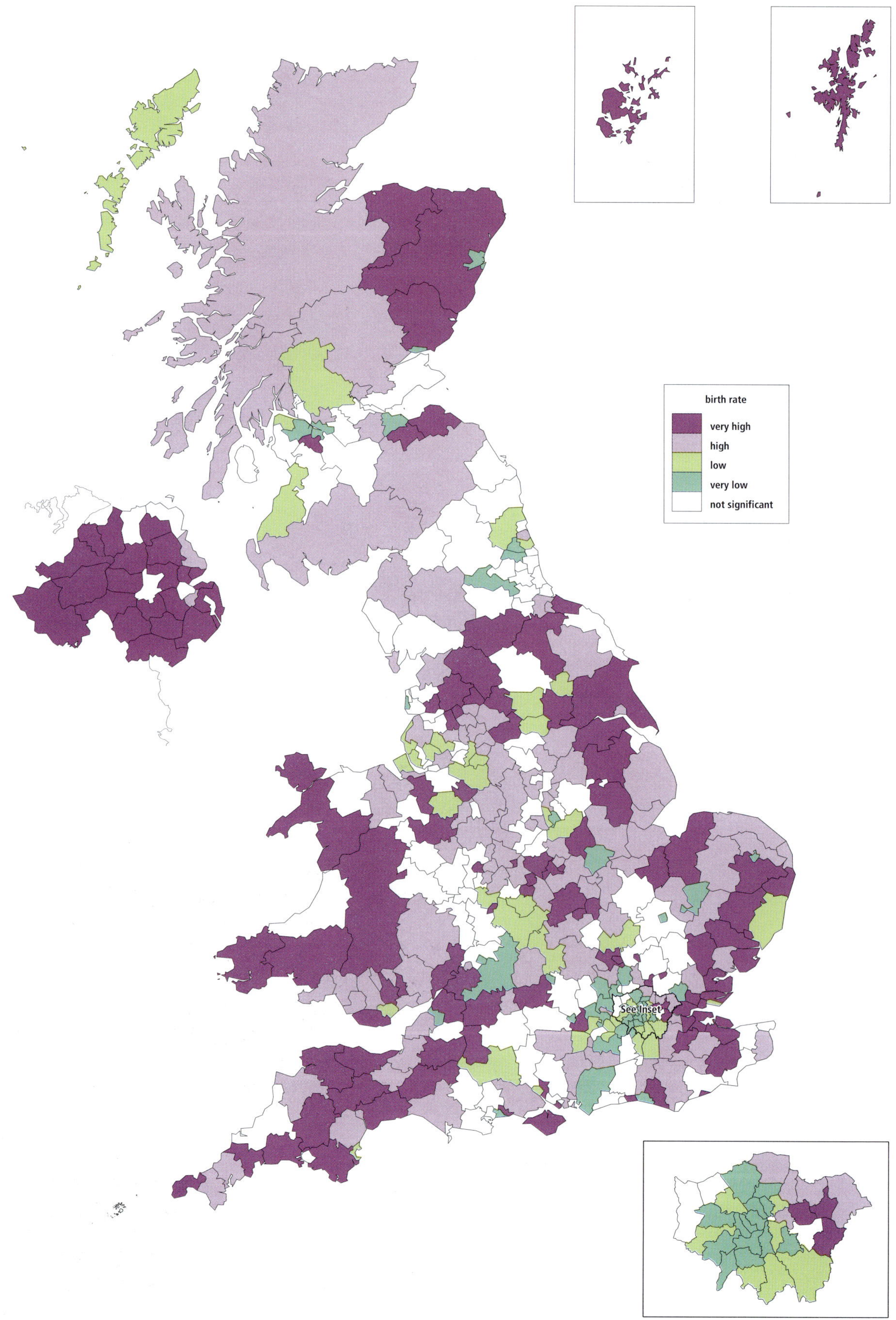

Map 5.32

**Live birth rates by local authority, women aged 30-34
United Kingdom 1991-1997**

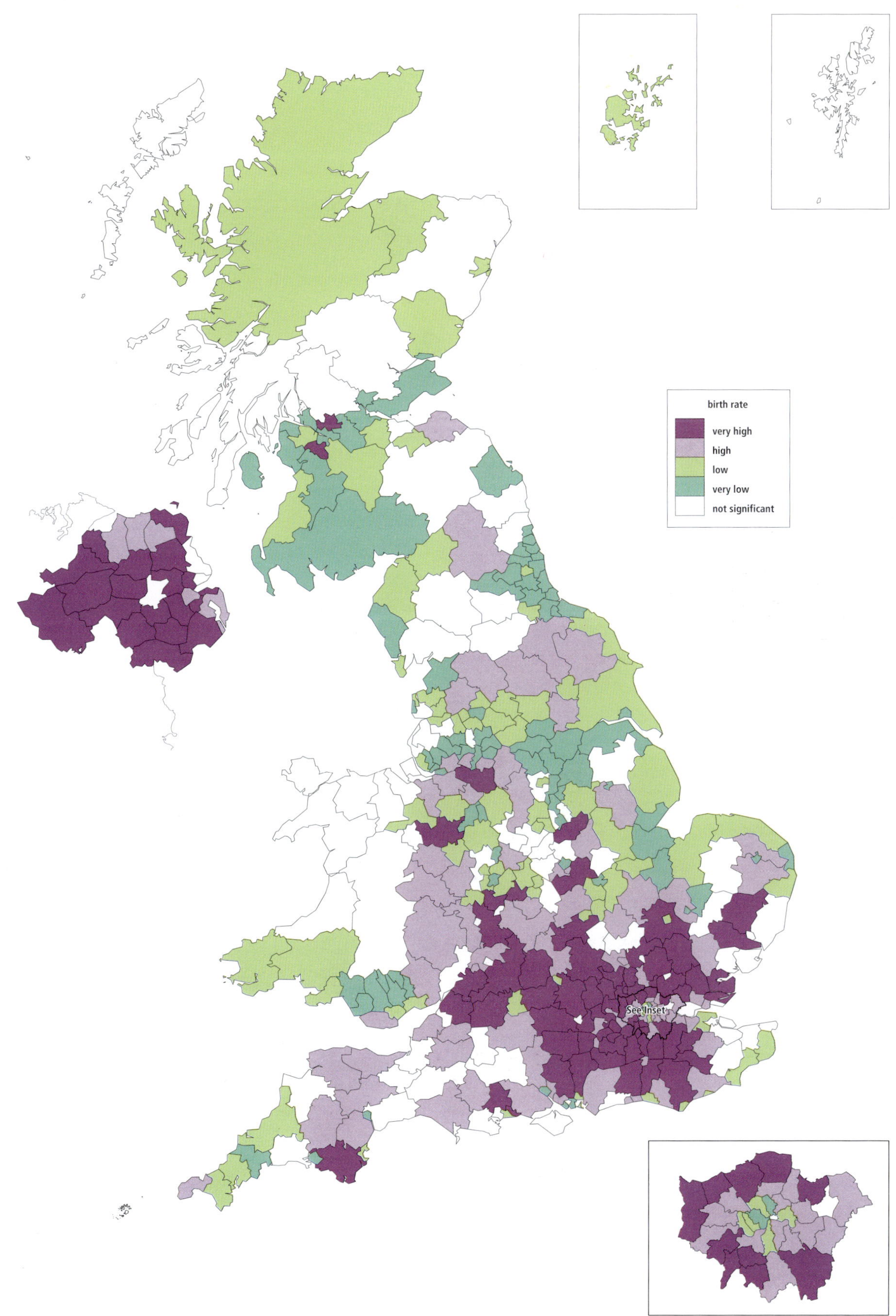

Map 5.33

Live birth rates by local authority, women aged 35-39
United Kingdom 1991-1997

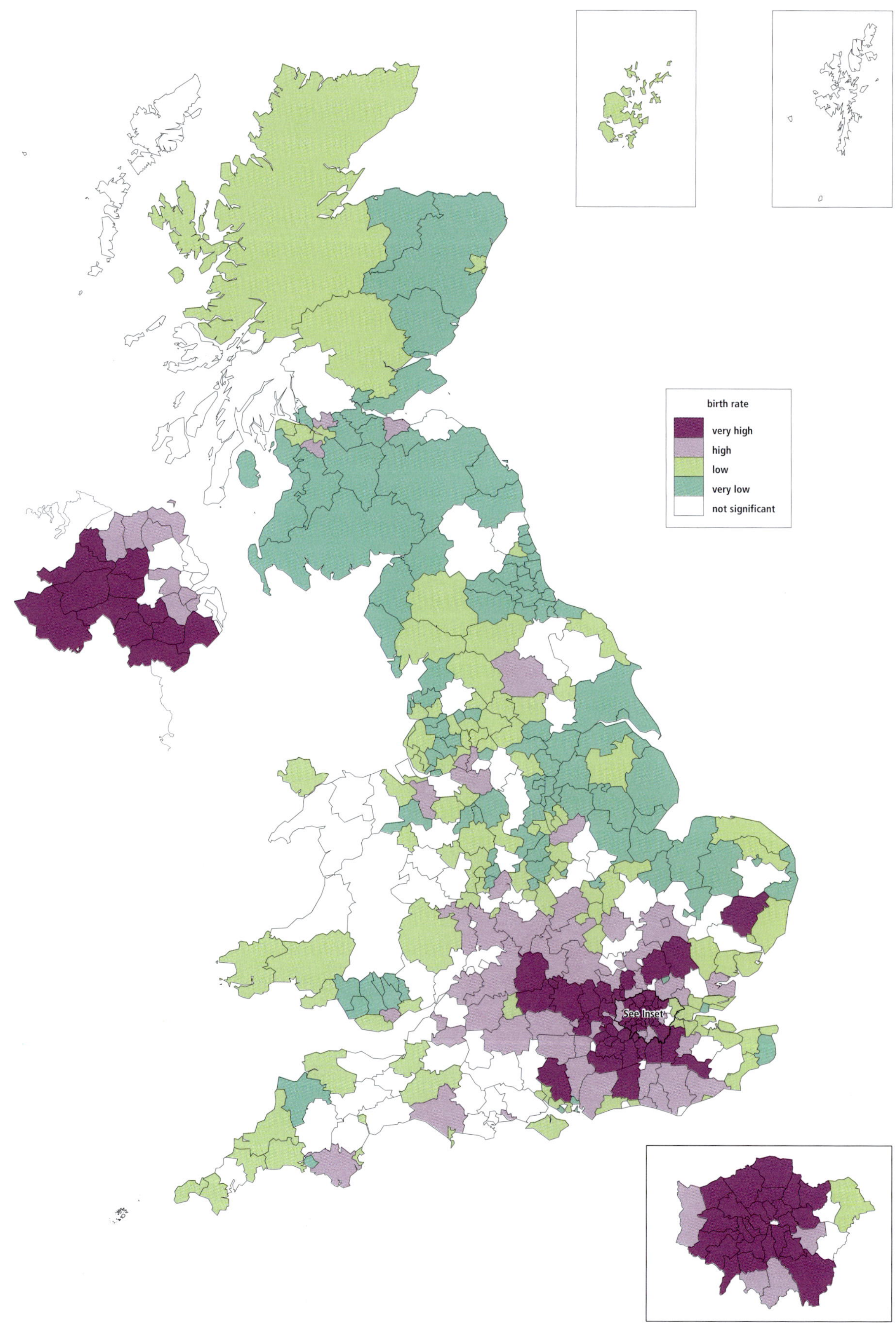

Map 5.34

Live birth rates by local authority, women aged 40 and over
United Kingdom 1991-1997

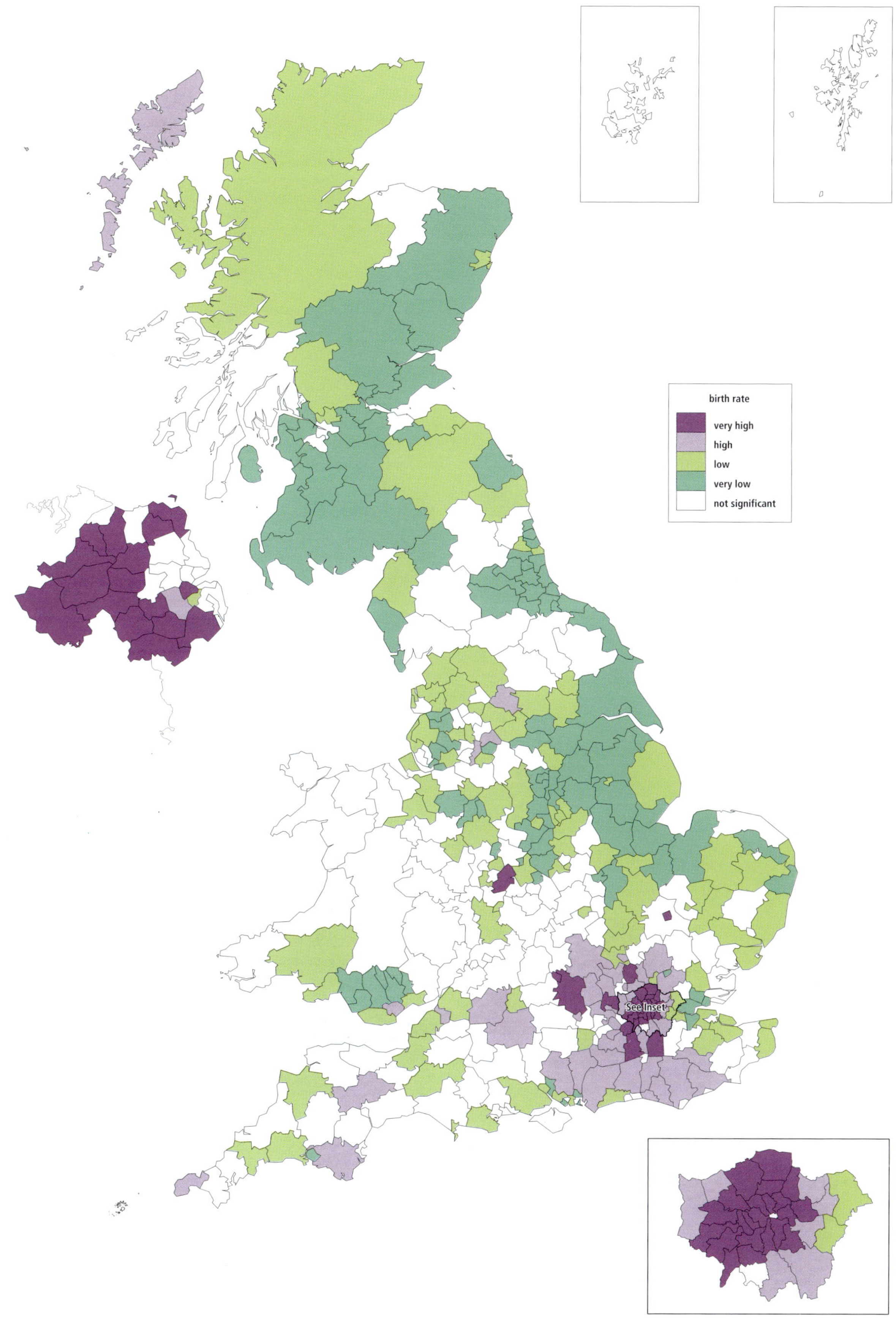

Map 5.35

**Mean age of mother at live birth by local authority
United Kingdom 1991-1997**

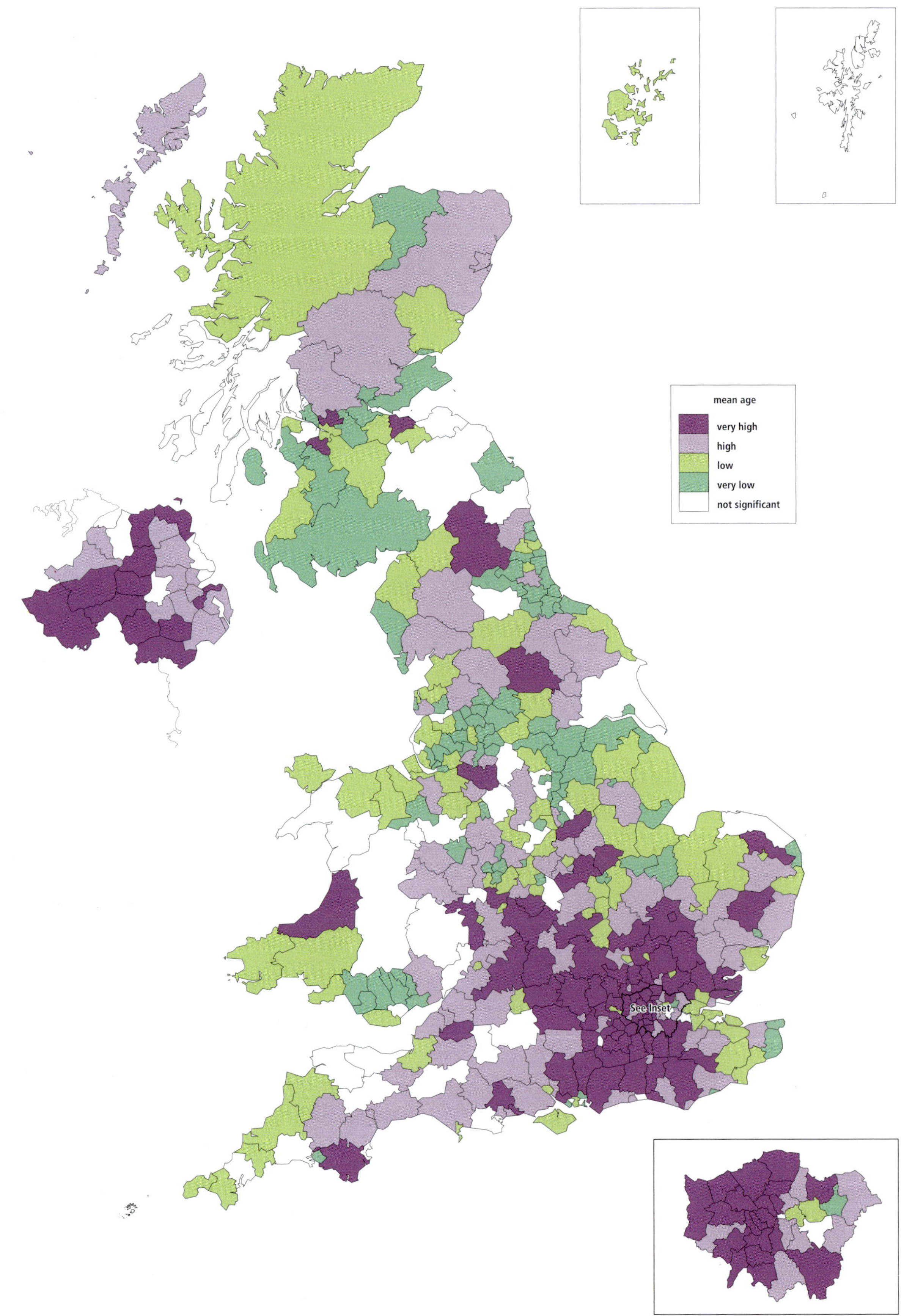

Figure 5.47

**Percentage of live births by type of registration, country and region, women aged under 18
United Kingdom 1991-1997**

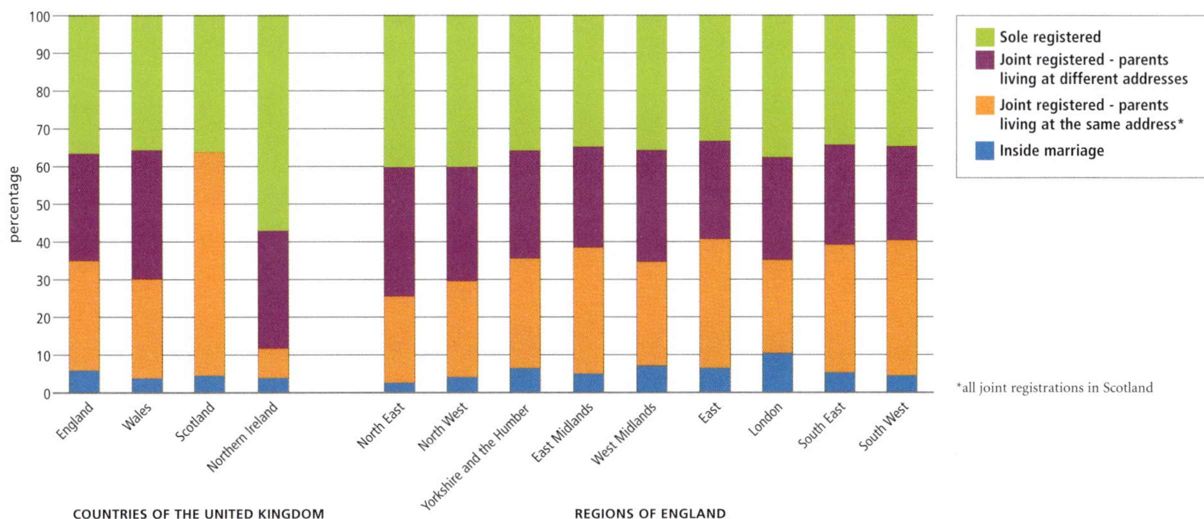

Type of registration

Information on the marital status of the parents is given at
birth registration. Births are generally registered as *inside
marriage* if the parents were married at the date of birth or if
the parents were married when the child was conceived, even if
they later divorced or the father died before the child's birth.
Births occurring outside marriage may be registered either
jointly or solely. A *joint registration* requires both parents to be
present. The addresses of both parents are recorded, so joint
registrations can be either with the parents living at the *same
address* or at *different addresses*. A s*ole registration* records only
the mother's details.[29]

When examining type of registration by country we consider
three types of registration: *inside marriage, sole registered* and
joint registered. This is because in Scotland there was no
distinction recorded between the two types of joint registration
until 1996. This means we cannot make this distinction for
Scotland or the United Kingdom in our analyses. At regional
level, within England, we have briefly considered all the types of
registration. At local authority level we have looked only at sole
registrations for ease of presentation.

The proportion of births outside marriage has been increasing
over the last 20 years. However, not all of these births are to lone
mothers. With an increase in the number of cohabiting couples
and decrease in marriage rates, there has been an increase in
births jointly registered by both parents.[33] Analysing births by
type of registration allows us to look at how the pattern is
changing towards more children being born to cohabiting
couples instead of married couples, whilst the proportion of sole
registrations remains relatively stable. The children of lone
mothers are at increased risk of dying within the first year of
life; this is examined and discussed in more detail in chapter 7.

In this analysis, we have not looked at all-age patterns in the type
of registration, as these would be affected by the differing age
structures of the areas being examined. There are more births
outside marriage at younger ages, so areas with high proportions
of women in these age groups would show higher proportions of
births outside marriage overall. We have considered the age
groups under 18, 18 to 19, 20 to 24 and 25 and over. We have not
discussed 5-year age groups over 25 because the geographic
patterns seen are identical in each of them.

Country and regional level variation
The main differences at the country level were between
Northern Ireland and the other countries. For all the age
groups, England, Wales and Scotland had similar patterns of
registration. At ages under 18 and 18-19, Northern Ireland had
a substantially higher percentage of sole registrations than the
other countries (Figures 5.47, 5.48). For women aged 20-24 and
25 and over, Northern Ireland had a higher proportion inside
marriage than the other countries (Figures 5.49, 5.50).

A comparatively lower percentage of registrations are jointly
registered by parents living at the same address in Northern
Ireland. This pattern has been changing during the 1990s. The
proportion of births that are sole registrations in the under 18 age
group has declined in Northern Ireland, mirrored by an increase
in joint registrations. In the other three age groups the main
trend has been a continuing decline in the percentage of births
registered inside marriage, with a corresponding increase in
births that are joint registrations. This is true for all the countries
of the United Kingdom. Variations at the regional level are
much less marked than at the country level.

Figure 5.48

Percentage of live births by type of registration, country and region, women aged 18-19 United Kingdom 1991-1997

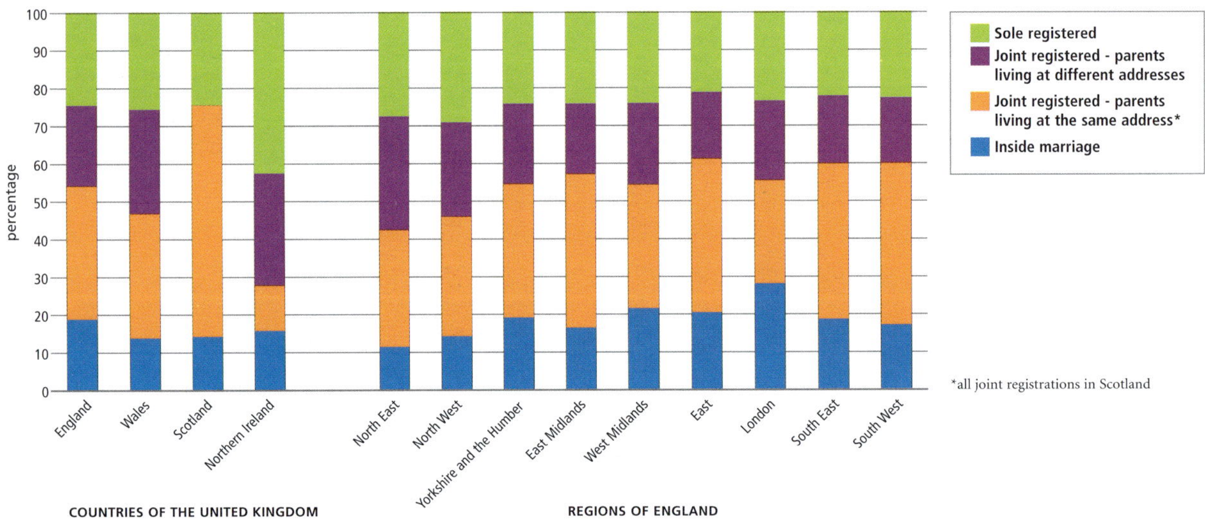

Figure 5.49

Percentage of live births by type of registration, country and region, women aged 20-24 United Kingdom 1991-1997

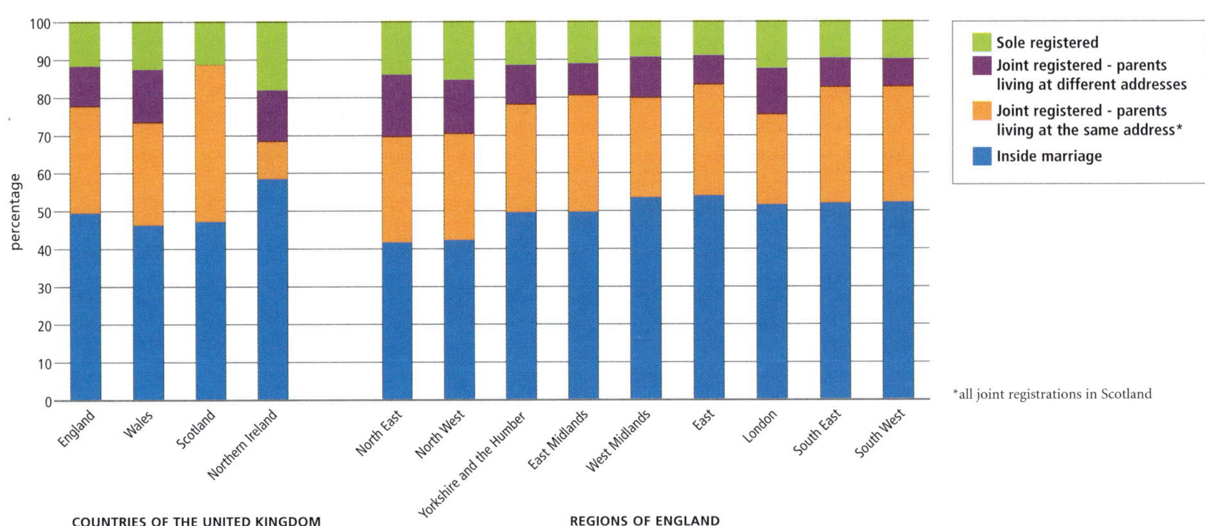

Local authority level variation

The pattern of sole registration described above is clear from the maps at local authority level. For under 18s and 18-19s the percentage of sole registrations was very high in all local authorities in Northern Ireland, and also high in scattered, mostly urban, authorities throughout the rest of Great Britain, particularly in the Liverpool and Manchester areas and south central London (Maps 5.36, 5.37).

For women aged 20-24 the picture was similar, but with more authorities in urban areas showing very high and high percentages, and low percentages being found throughout the rest of Great Britain (Map 5.38). For women aged 25 and over the pattern was different. Very few local authorities in

Northern Ireland had a high proportion of sole registrations (Map 5.39). In this age group authorities with a high proportion of sole registrations tended to be concentrated in inner London and other major centres of population, with the authorities in the rest of the country having a low proportion, particularly in rural areas.

When we examine the figures for women aged 25 and over using ONS classification Groups, the lowest percentages of births registered outside marriage were found in the *Growth Areas* and *Most Prosperous* Groups and the highest percentage of births outside marriage was found in *East Inner London* (Figure 5.51).

Figure 5.50

Percentage of live births by type of registration, country and region, women aged 25 and over United Kingdom 1991-1997

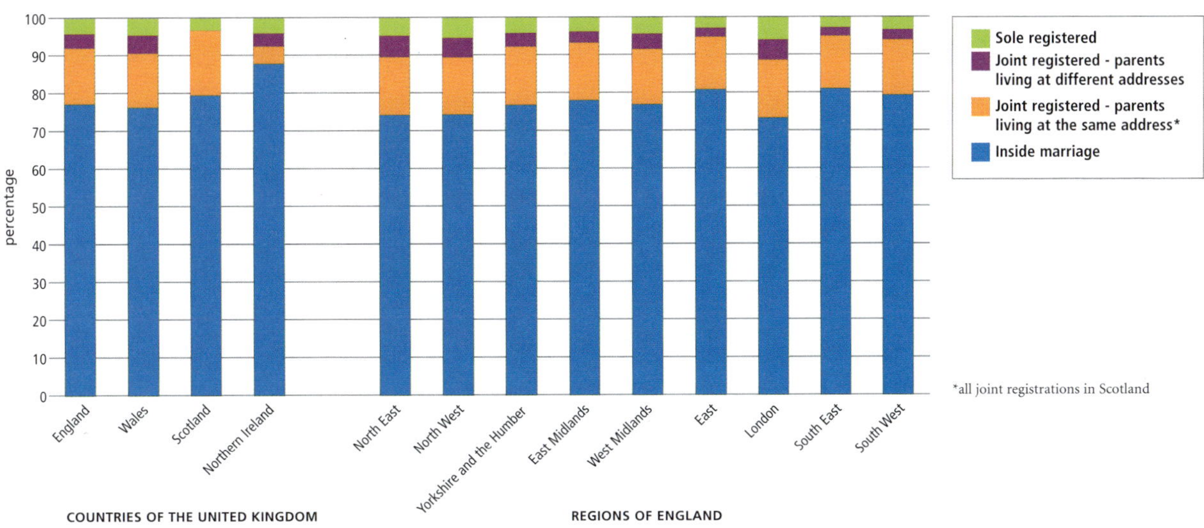

Figure 5.51

Percentage of live births outside marriage by ONS classification Group, women aged 25 and over Great Britain 1991-1997

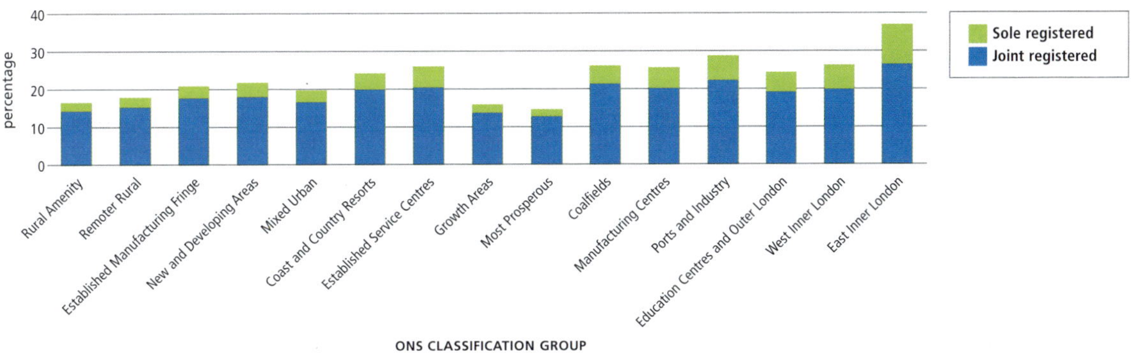

Map 5.36

Percentage of live births that are sole registered by local authority, women aged under 18
United Kingdom 1991-1997

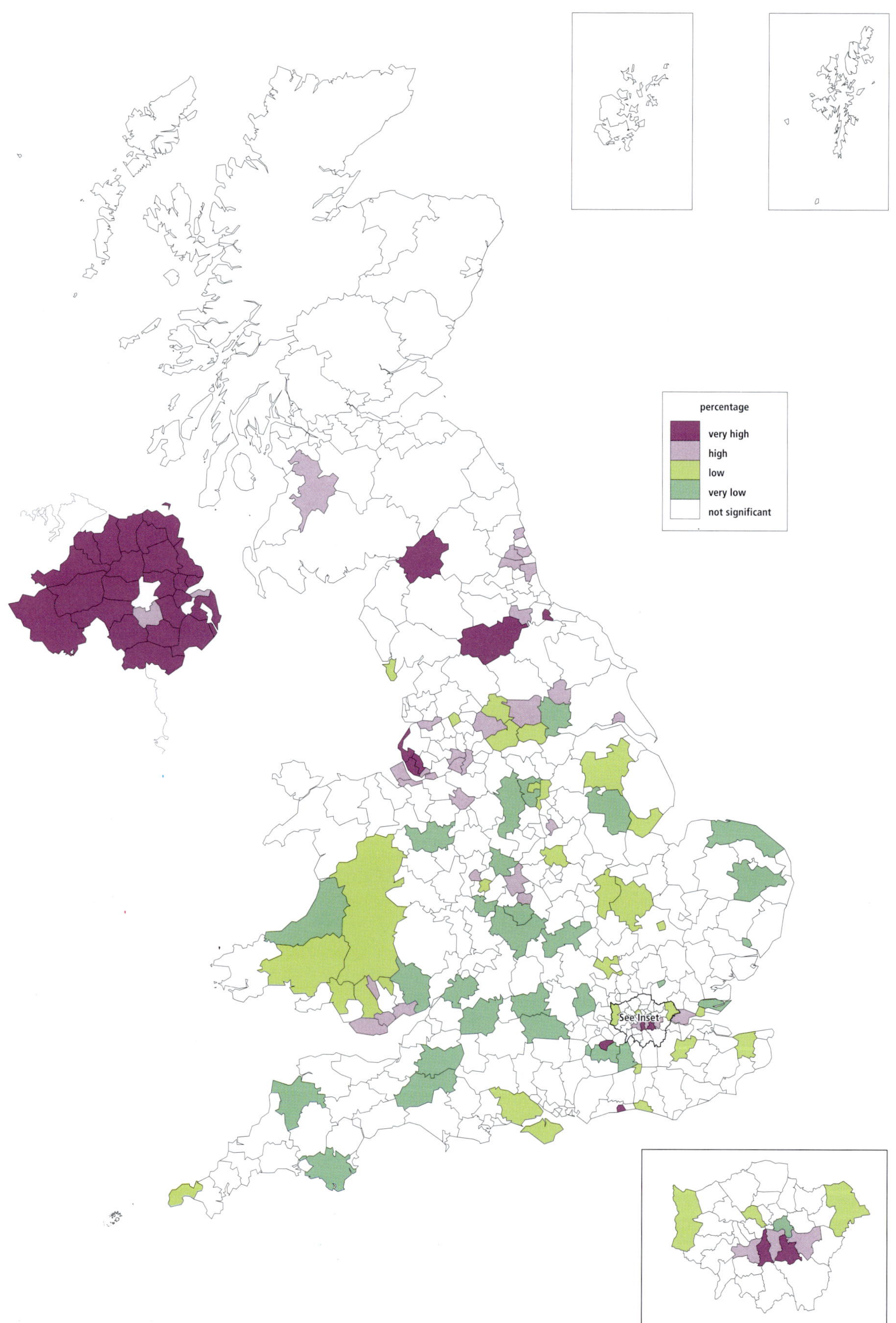

Map 5.37

**Percentage of live births that are sole registered by local authority, women aged 18-19
United Kingdom 1991-1997**

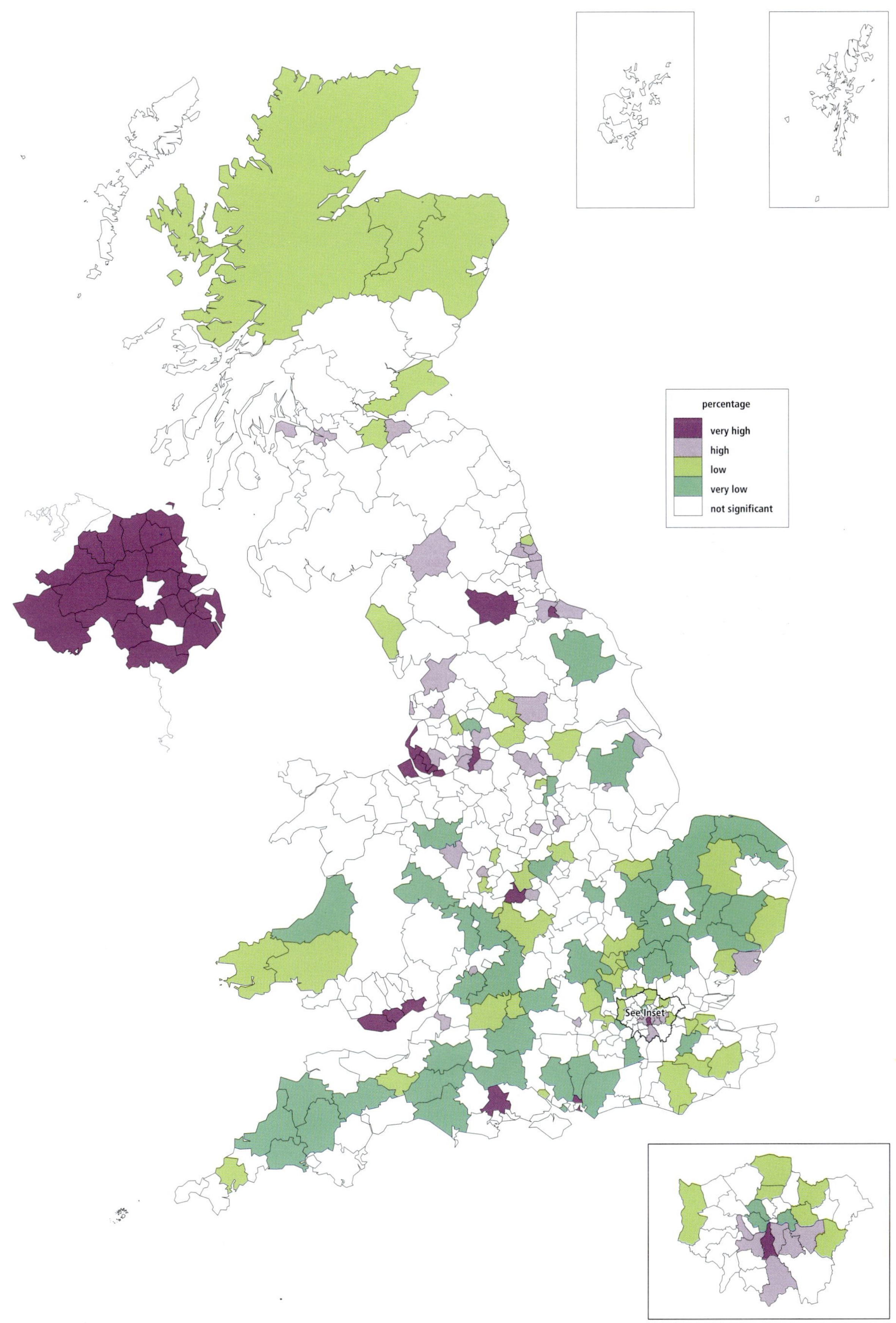

Map 5.38

**Percentage of live births that are sole registered by local authority, women aged 20-24
United Kingdom 1991-1997**

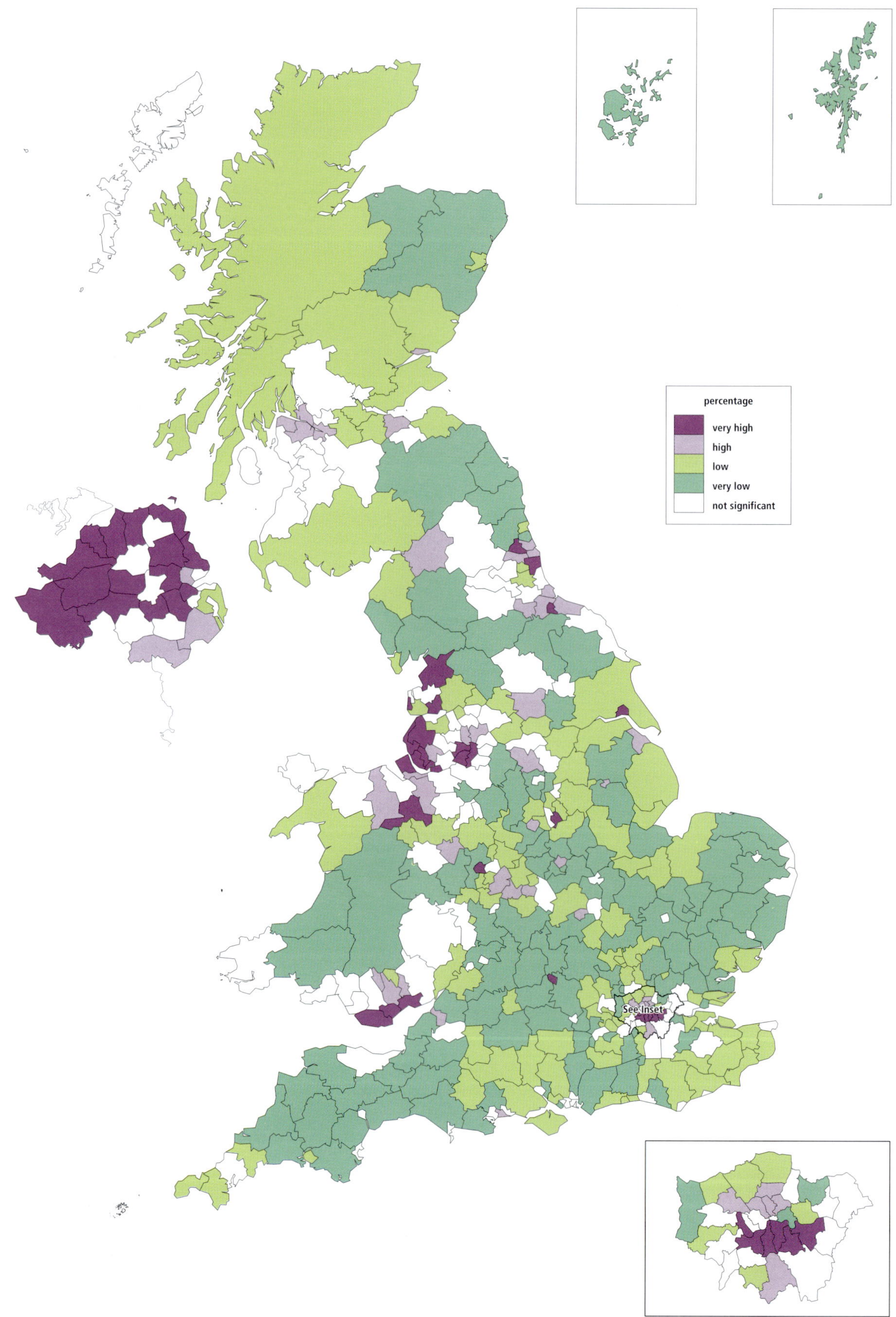

Map 5.39

**Percentage of live births that are sole registered by local authority, women aged 25 and over
United Kingdom 1991-1997**

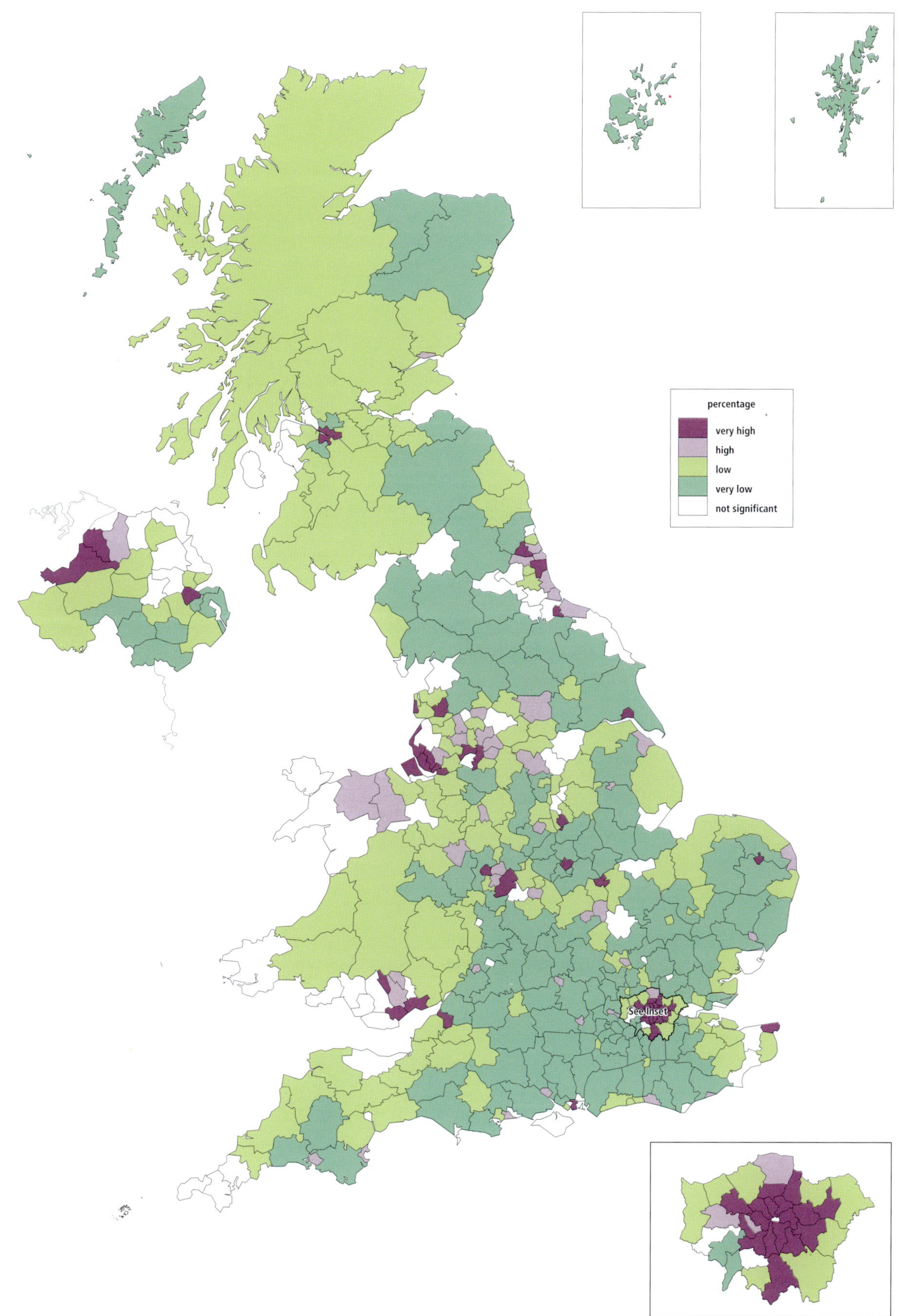

5.5 Variations by deprivation

This section examines the relationship between deprivation and fertility, firstly looking at the relationship for all women, then teenagers and older women. Much of the previously published work on deprivation and fertility has concentrated on the relationship with teenage pregnancies. In this analysis, we examine the relationship between fertility and deprivation within countries and regions to see if there are differences in the relationship within different areas. For all women we have looked at the TFR and mean age of mother at live birth. We have examined type of registration for women aged over 25. For women aged under 18 and 35-39 we have looked at conception, birth and abortion rates and the percentage of conceptions leading to abortion.

There are various ways of measuring the level of deprivation within an area. In this volume we have used the Carstairs and Morris index of deprivation which is described in chapter 4. The method used to allocate wards in England and Wales and postcode sectors in Scotland to a deprivation twentieth and quintile is also described in chapter 4. For the national level we used deprivation twentieths. At the sub-national level we used quintiles.

Data for Great Britain have been used for births and England and Wales for conceptions and abortions, due to the availability of suitable data to which to allocate the deprivation index.

All ages

The TFR showed an increase with deprivation in all countries and regions, although the gradient was less steep in Scotland than elsewhere, which could account for Scotland's lower overall TFR (Figure 5.52). In Great Britain as a whole the TFR ranged from about 1.6 in the lowest deprivation twentieth to just under 3 in the highest deprivation twentieth. London showed the widest difference between quintile 1 and quintile 5, with the TFR in the most deprived areas being 1.8 times higher than the TFR in the least deprived areas, due to the very low TFR in quintile 1, about 1.25.

The mean age of mother at live birth showed a substantial decline with increasing deprivation in all of the countries and regions (Figure 5.53). In Great Britain the mean age at live birth ranged from just under 25 years in twentieth 20 to just under 30 in twentieth 1.

There was an increase in the proportion of births registered outside marriage with increasing deprivation, with all of the countries and regions showing a similar pattern (Figure 5.54). There was an increase in all of the registration types that are outside marriage with increasing deprivation. Large proportions of births registered solely by the mother or jointly by both parents living at different addresses were seen in quintiles 4 and 5.

Women aged under 18

In under 18s there was a very marked gradient of increasing conception and birth rates with increasing deprivation in all of the countries and regions (Figures 5.55, 5.56). In England and Wales as a whole the conception rate in the most deprived areas was over 4 times that of the least deprived areas, and the birth rate in Great Britain was over 7 times higher. The gradient for the birth rate was less steep in Scotland. The majority of the variation in conception and birth rates was found in quintile 5, with a clear north-south divide in birth and conception rates in this quintile. In quintile 1, however, there was not a north-south divide in rates (Figures 5.57, 5.58). Scotland had rates equivalent to those in the south of England.

The percentage of conceptions leading to abortion showed a marked decline with increasing deprivation in all countries and regions (Figure 5.59). In England and Wales as a whole just under 70 per cent of conceptions in under 18s led to an abortion in the least deprived areas, compared to just under 30 per cent in the most deprived areas. The pattern for the abortion rate was less clear (Figure 5.60). There was a gradient with increasing abortion rates with increasing deprivation in England and also in Wales, although the gradient was not as steep in Wales. Within the regions the pattern is less clear, although there was a marked gradient in London. Although the gradient is not clear, the

Figure 5.57

Differences in conception rates by country and region between deprivation quintile 1 and 5, women aged under 18 England and Wales 1992-1994

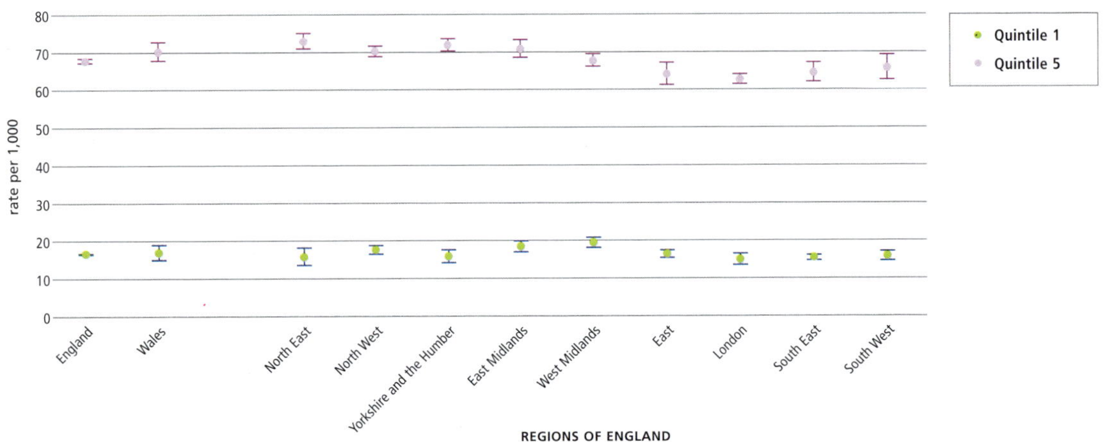

Figure 5.52

Total Fertility Rates by country, region and deprivation
Great Britain 1991-1993

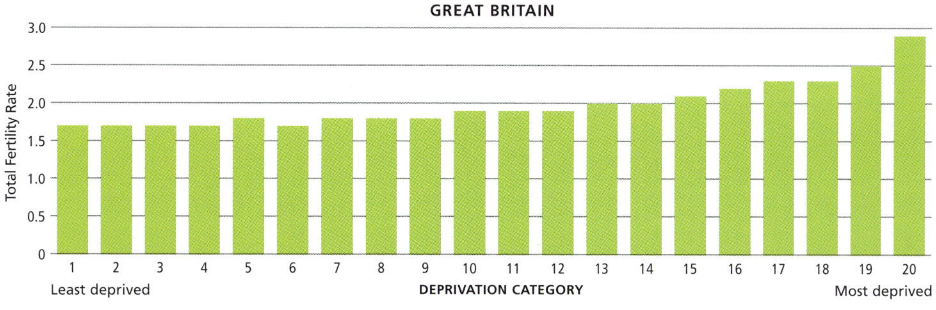

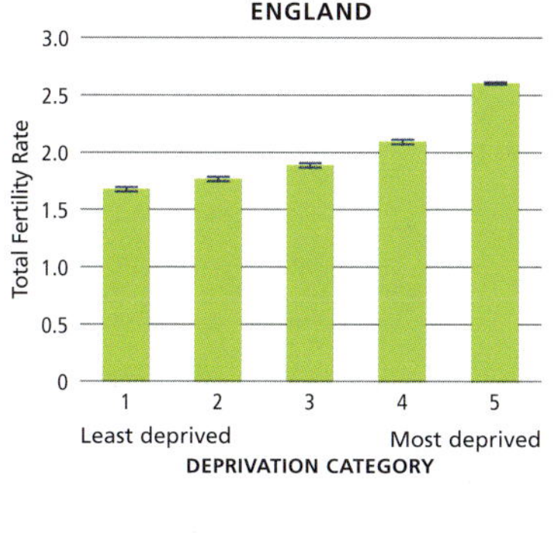

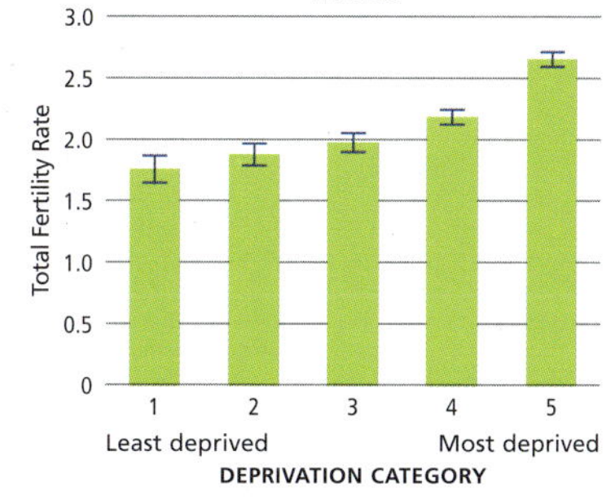

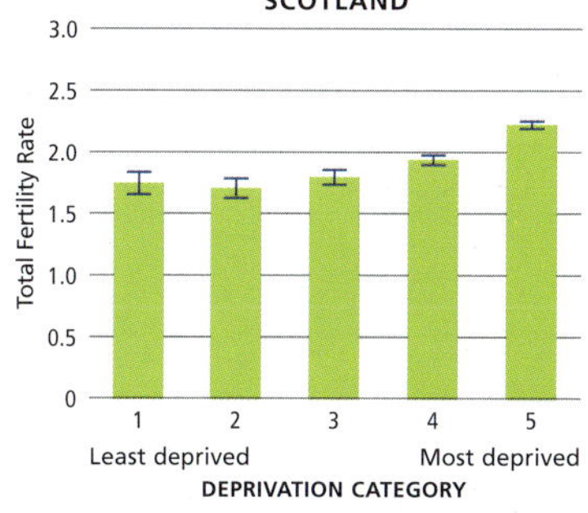

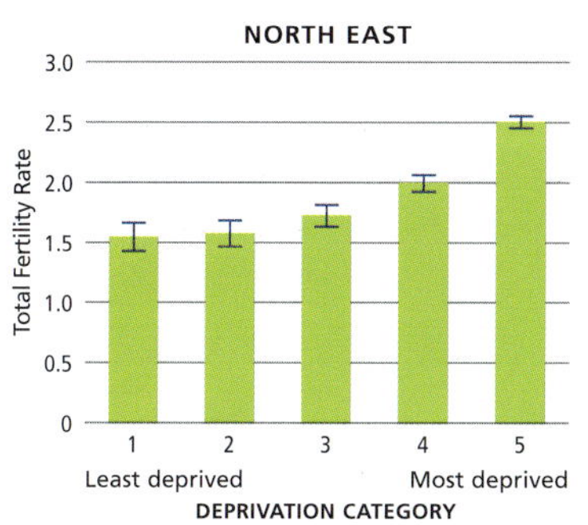

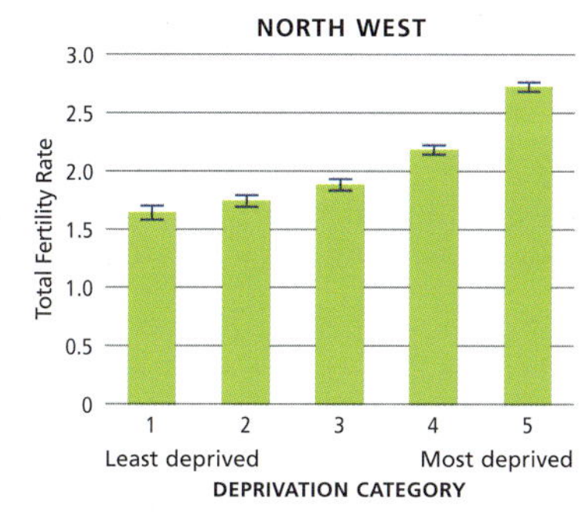

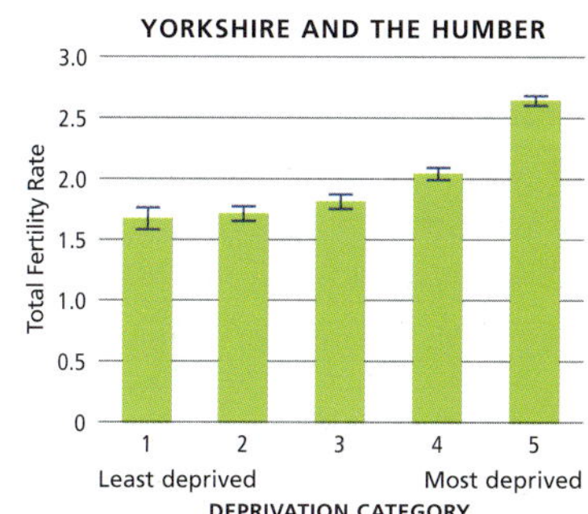

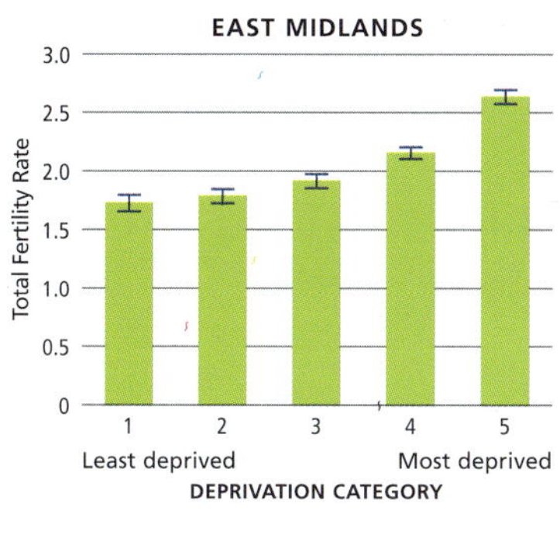

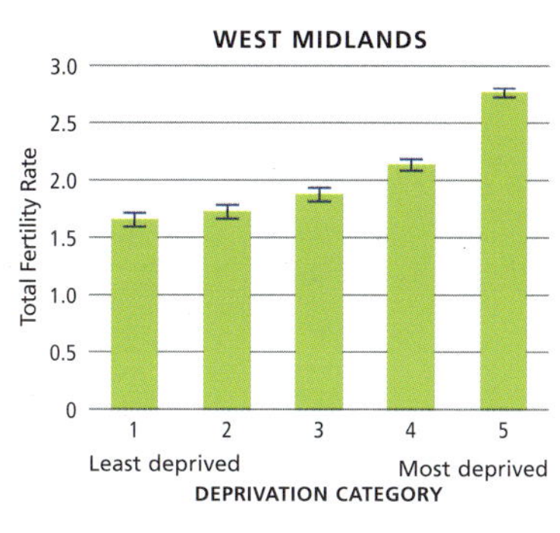

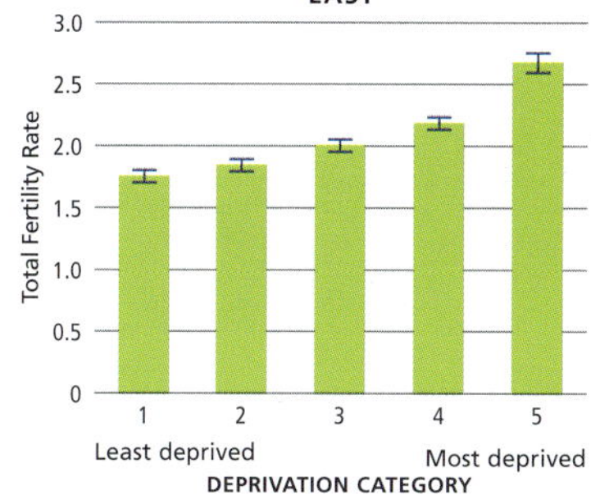

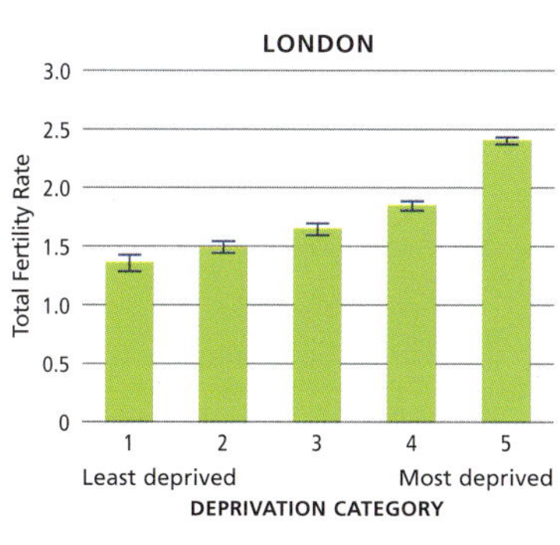

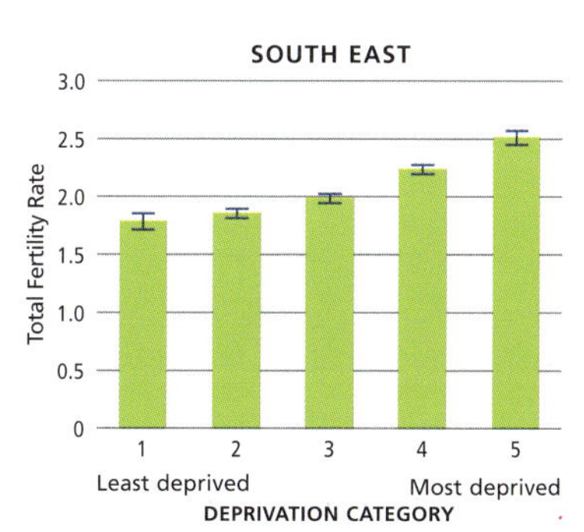

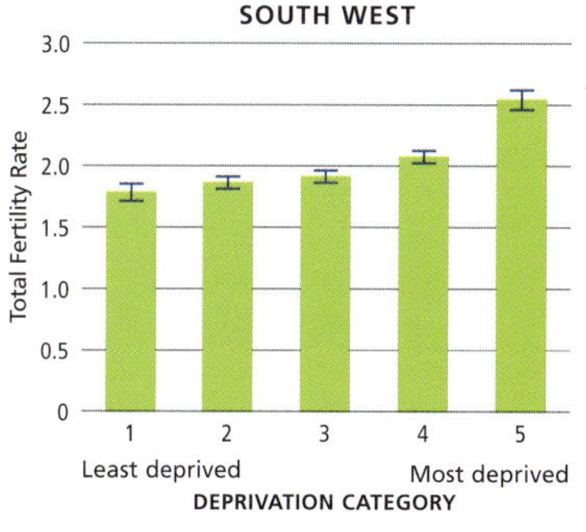

Figure 5.53

Mean age of mother at live birth by country, region and deprivation
Great Britain 1991-1993

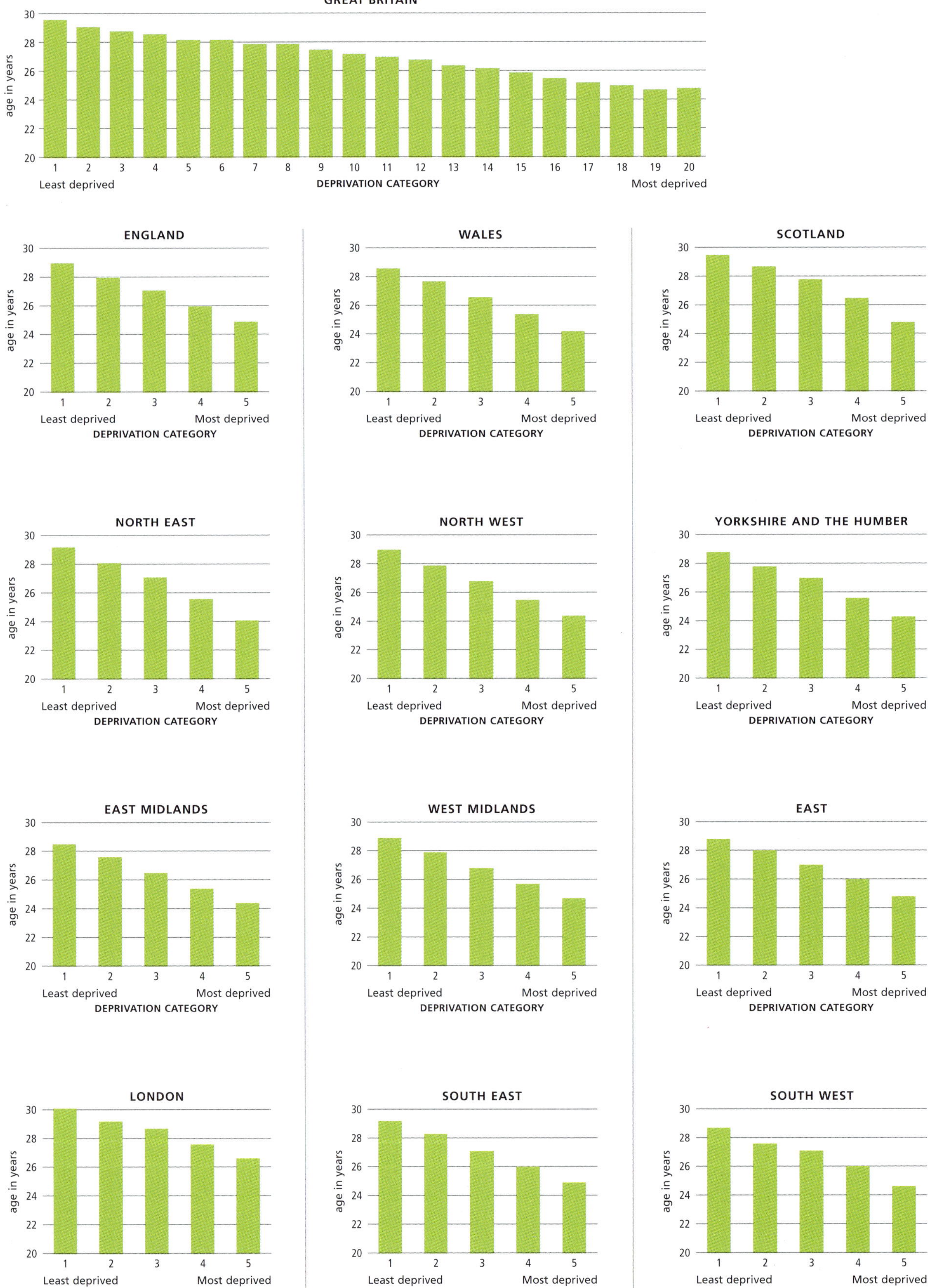

Figure 5.54

**Percentage of live births outside marriage by country, region and deprivation, women aged 25 and over
Great Britain 1991-1993**

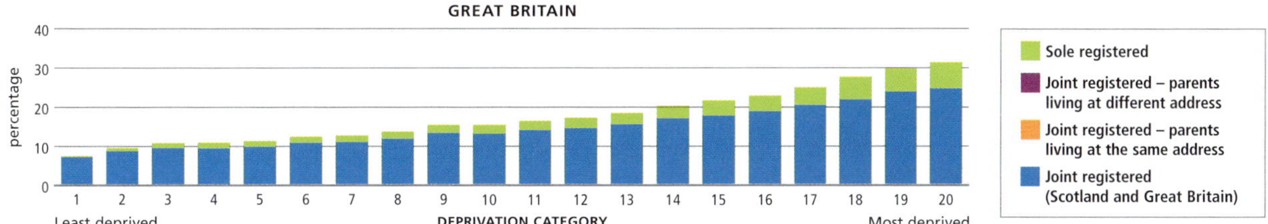

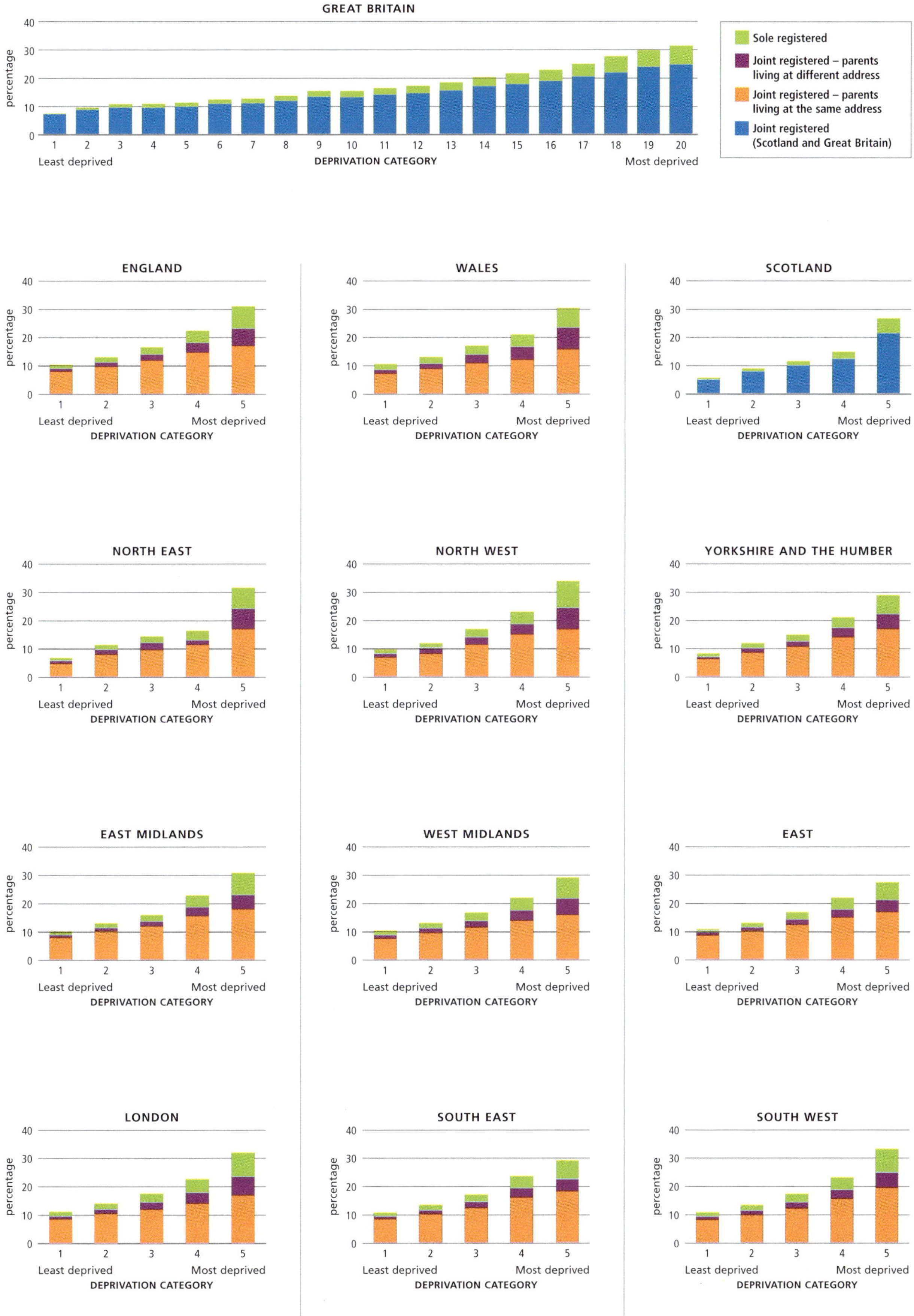

abortion rate in quintile 5 was higher than the rate in quintile 1 in each region (Figure 5.61).

Women in their late thirties

For women aged 35-39 the relationship between deprivation and births, conceptions and abortions is less clear cut than for teenagers, and there is no consistent pattern. In England and Wales as a whole the conception rate in the most deprived twentieth was markedly higher than in the other twentieths, with not much variation outside of this. In Wales the conception rate appeared to decline with increasing deprivation, but in London it was increasing with increasing deprivation, and the rates were higher in London than elsewhere within each deprivation quintile. In some other regions the pattern appeared to be u-shaped, with high rates in the least and the most deprived and lower rates in the centre of the distribution (Figure 5.62).

The pattern for birth rates in these women is also unclear. Scotland, and to a lesser extent Wales, showed decreasing birth rates with increasing deprivation, but in England the pattern was not clear. In London the birth rate increased with increasing deprivation, but in the South West it declined with increasing deprivation. England as a whole showed a u-shaped pattern (Figure 5.63).

In England and Wales as a whole the percentage of conceptions leading to abortion increased with increasing deprivation in women in their late thirties. This pattern was also seen in England, but it was less marked in Wales. In the South East and East of England there was a very clear pattern of an increasing percentage of conceptions leading to abortion with increasing deprivation (Figure 5.64).

The abortion rate in women aged 35-39 increased with increasing deprivation in England and Wales as a whole; this increase was confined to the later twentieths, with no real increase seen before twentieth 17 (Figure 5.65). At country and regional level the patterns are not clear. London showed a marked increase in abortion rates in the most deprived areas compared to the least, but in other regions and Wales no gradient was seen.

Figure 5.58

Differences in live birth rates by country and region between deprivation quintile 1 and 5, women aged under 18 Great Britain 1991-1993

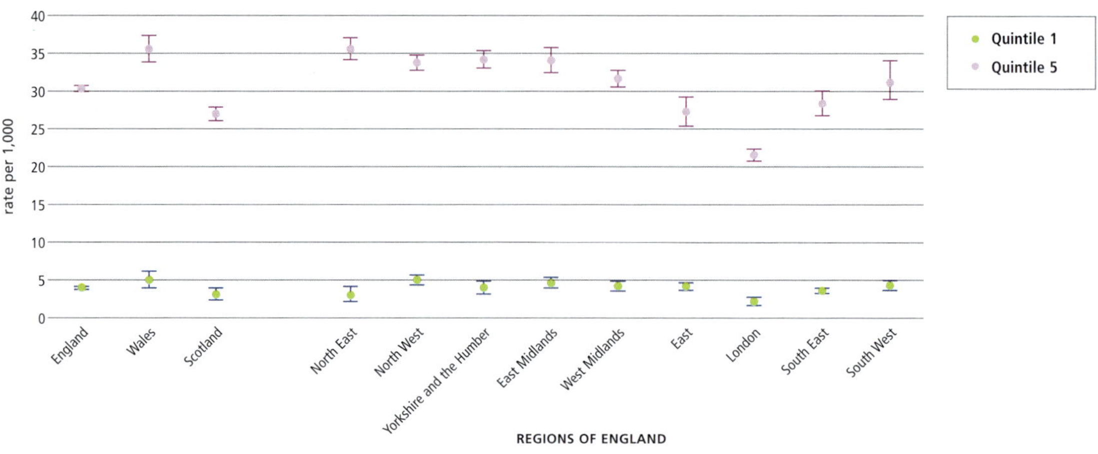

Figure 5.61

Differences in abortion rates by country and region between deprivation quintile 1 and 5, women aged under 18. England and Wales 1992-1994

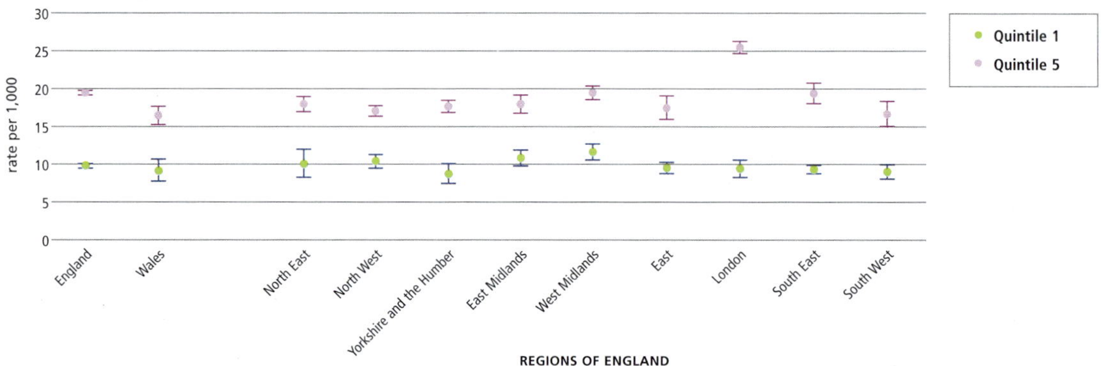

Figure 5.55

Conception rates by country, region and deprivation, women aged under 18
England and Wales 1992-1994

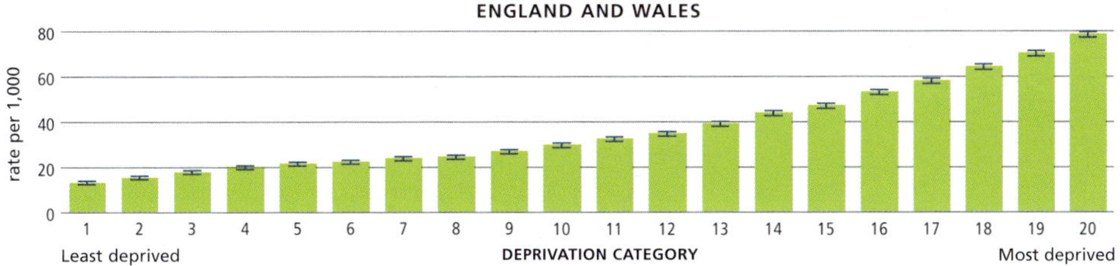

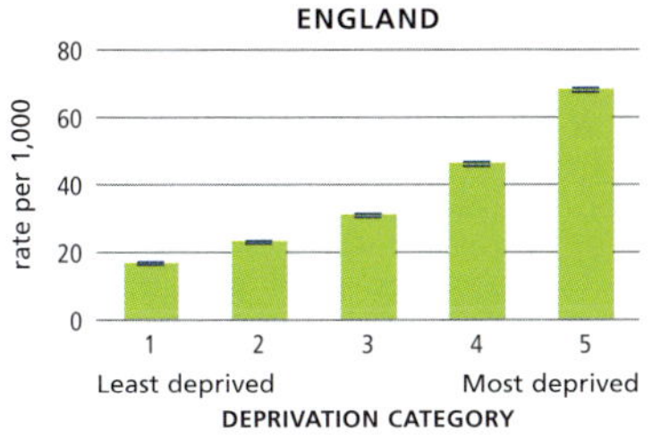

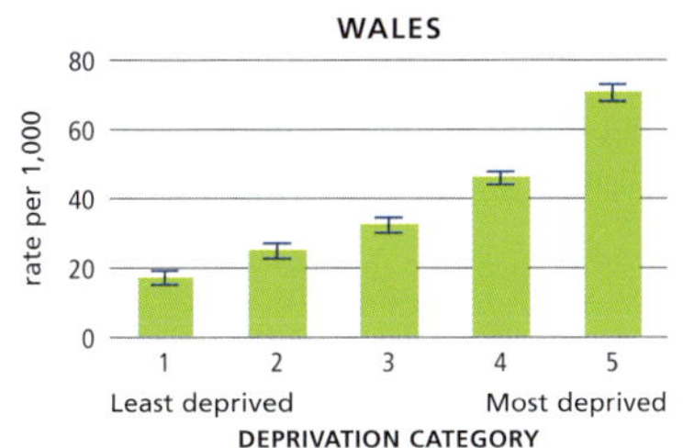

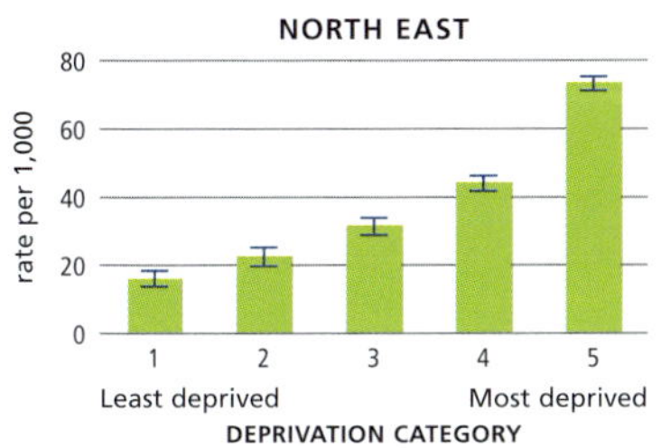

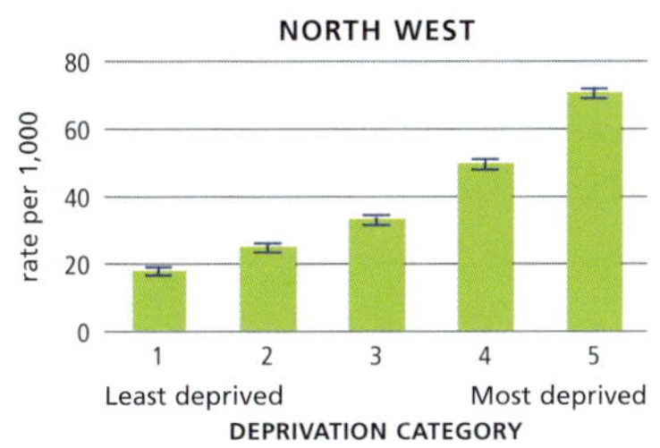

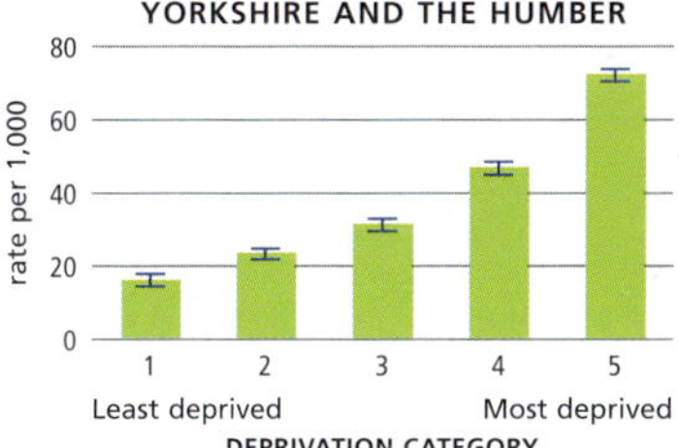

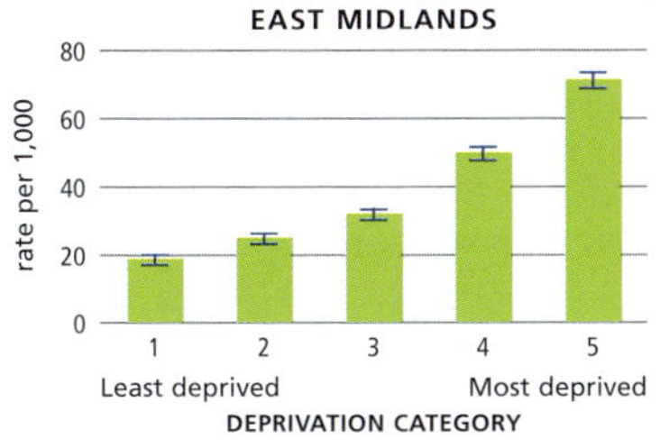

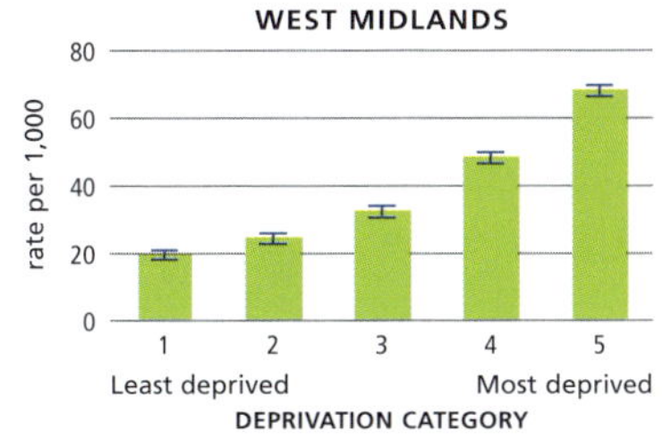

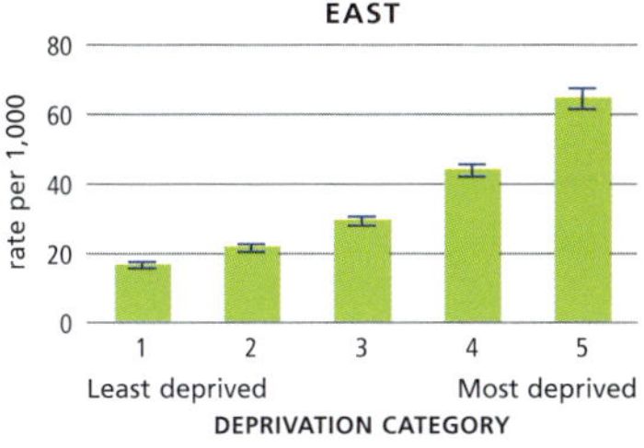

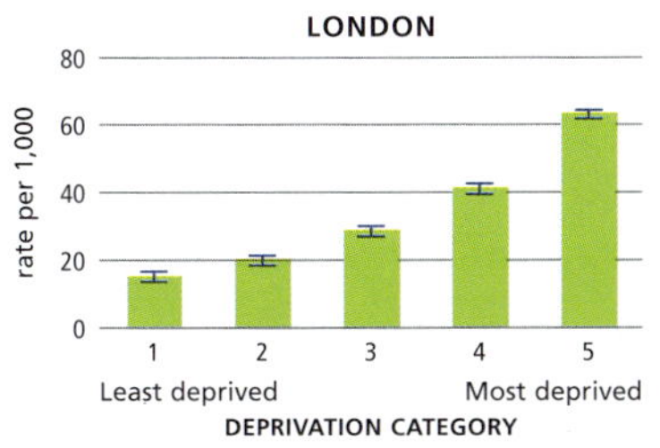

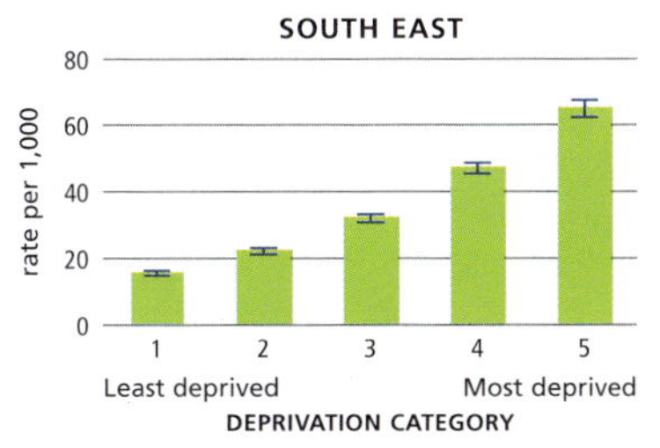

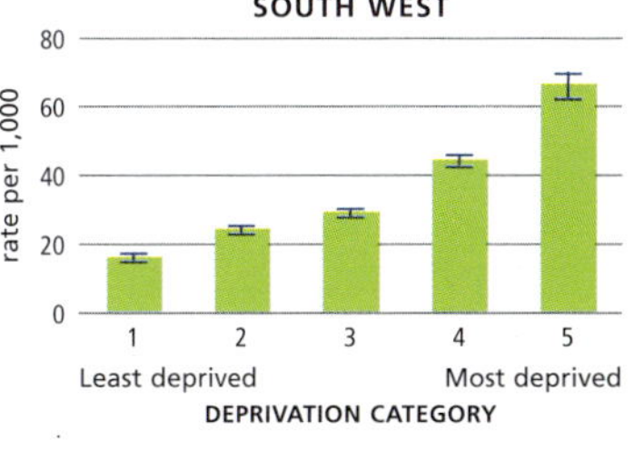

Figure 5.56

Live birth rates by country, region and deprivation, women aged under 18
Great Britain 1991-1993

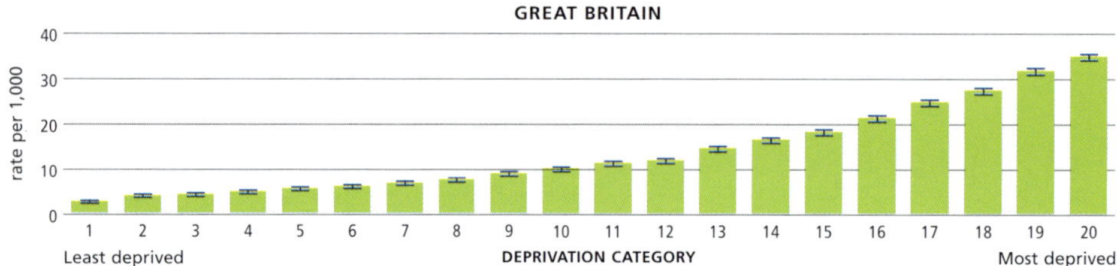

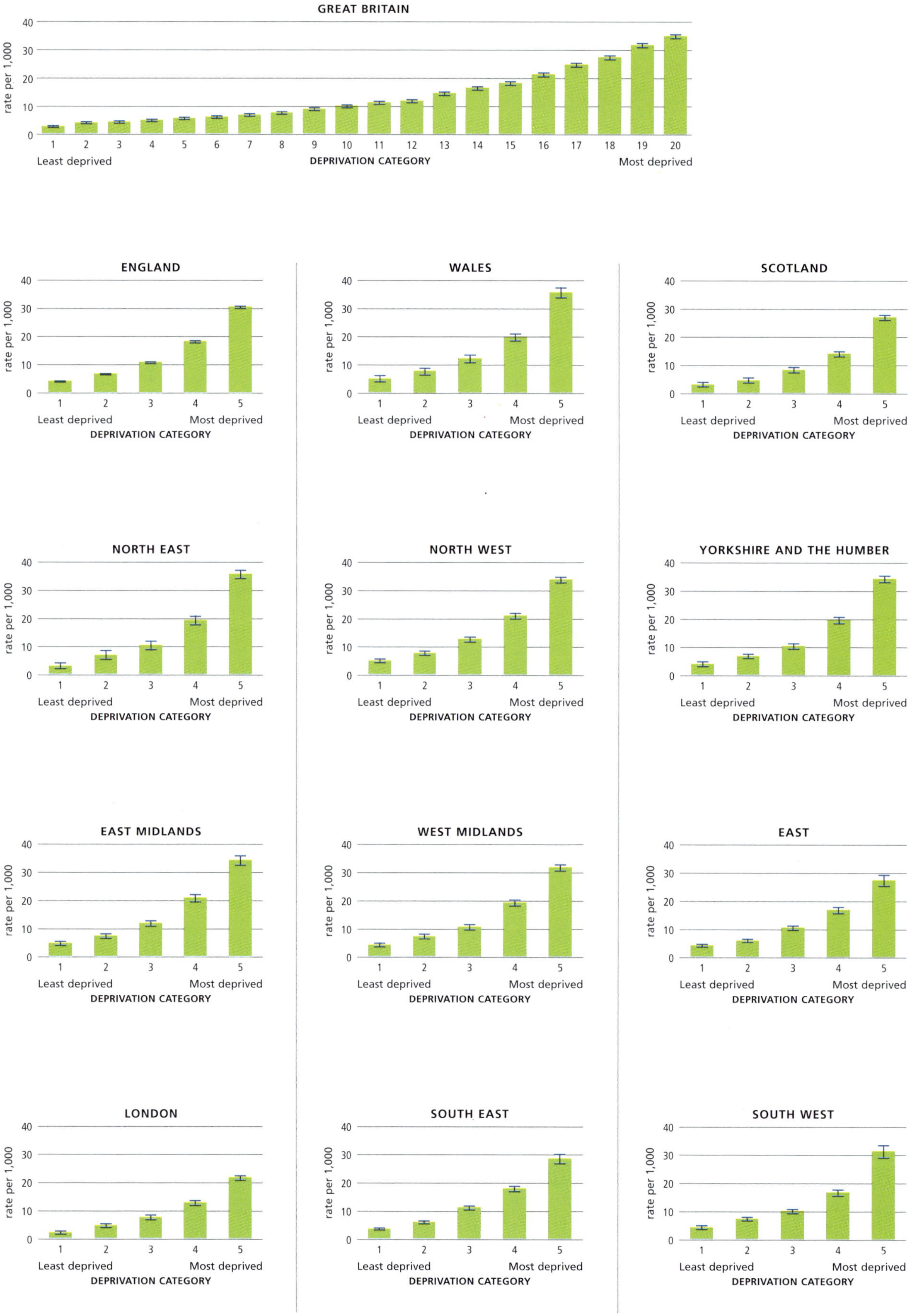

Figure 5.59

Percentage of conceptions leading to abortion by country, region and deprivation, women aged under 18 England and Wales 1992-1994

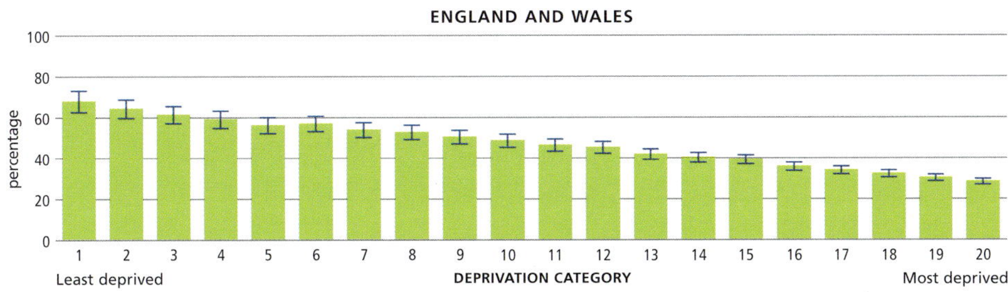

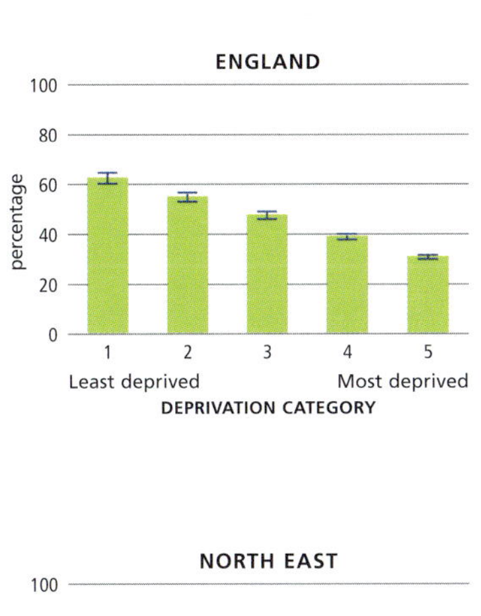

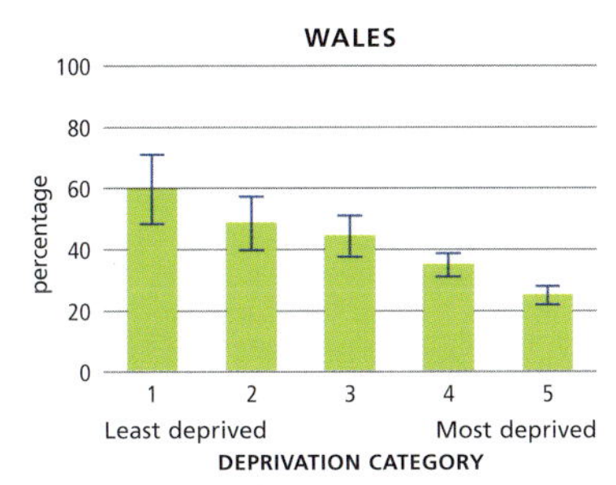

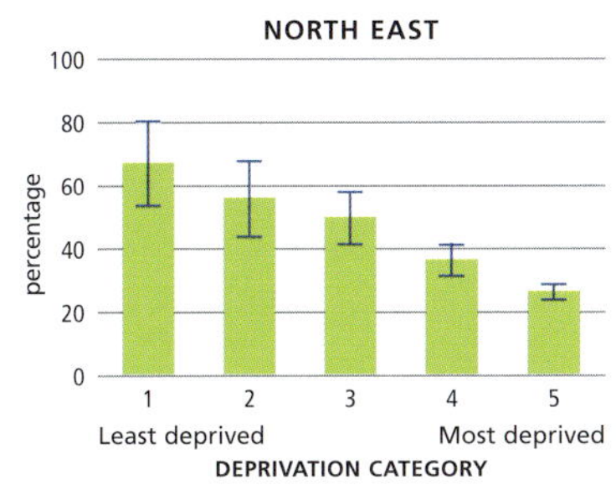

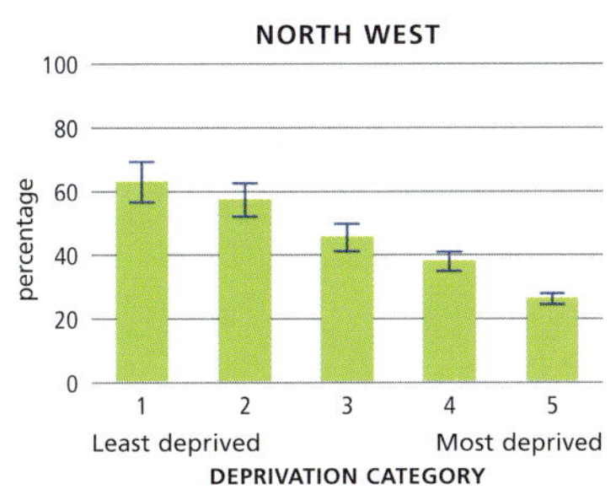

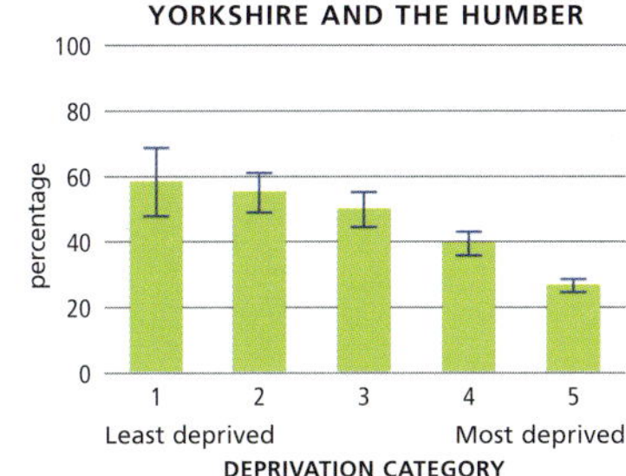

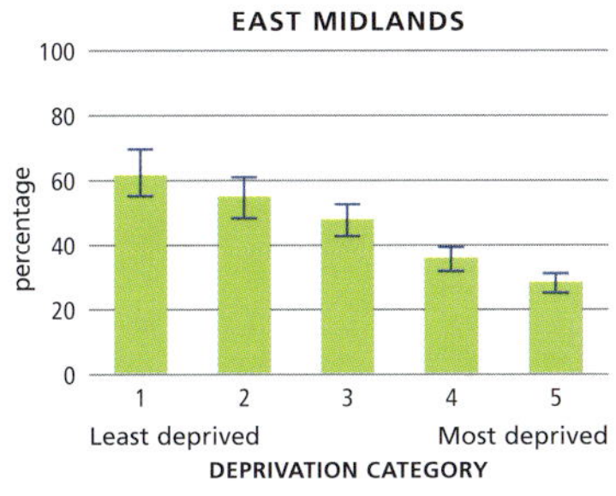

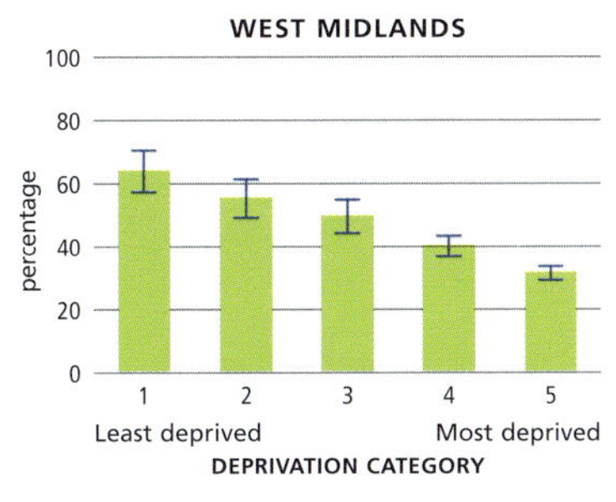

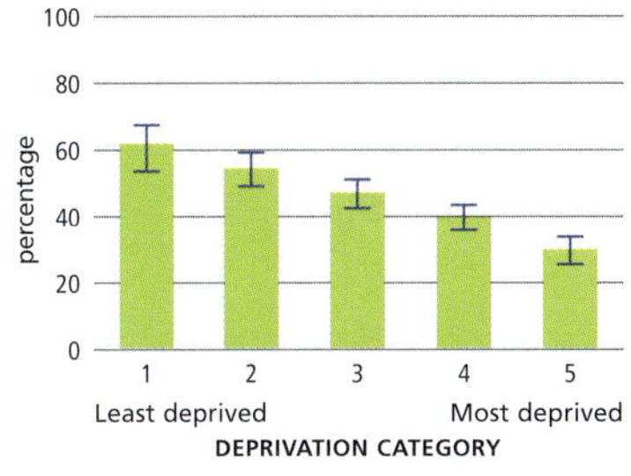

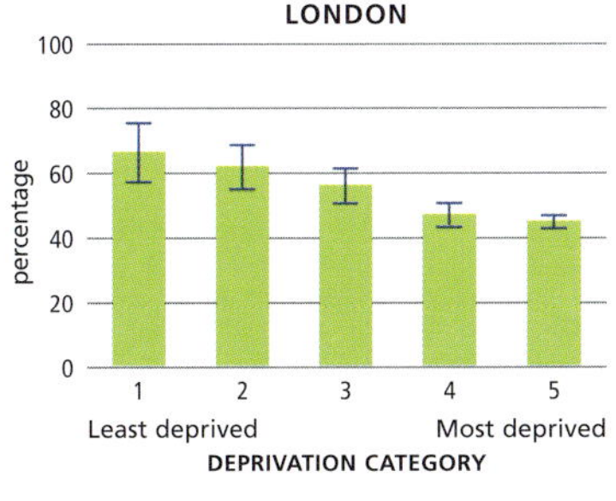

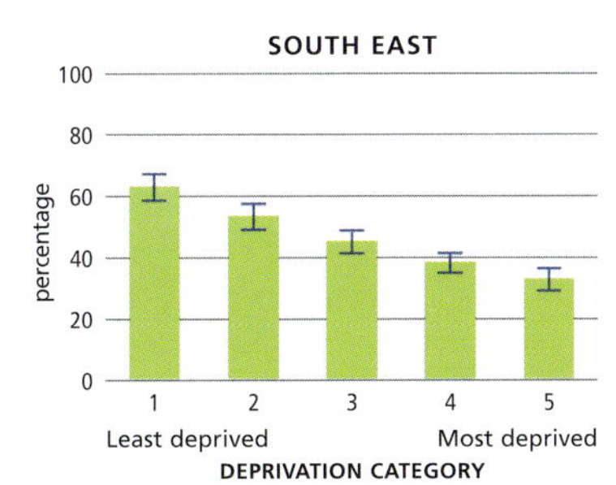

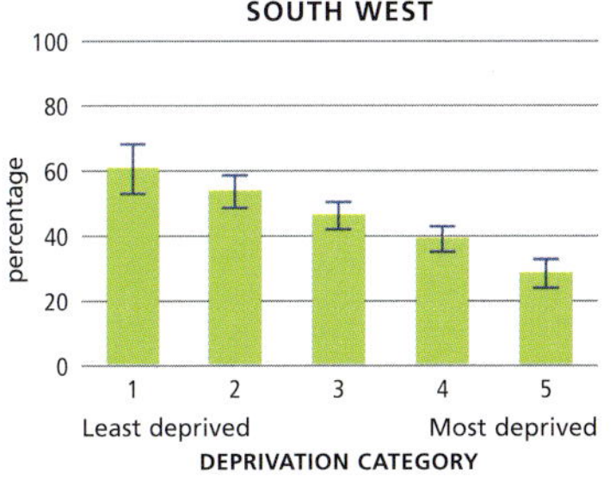

Figure 5.60

Abortion rates by country, region and deprivation, women aged under 18
England and Wales 1992-1994

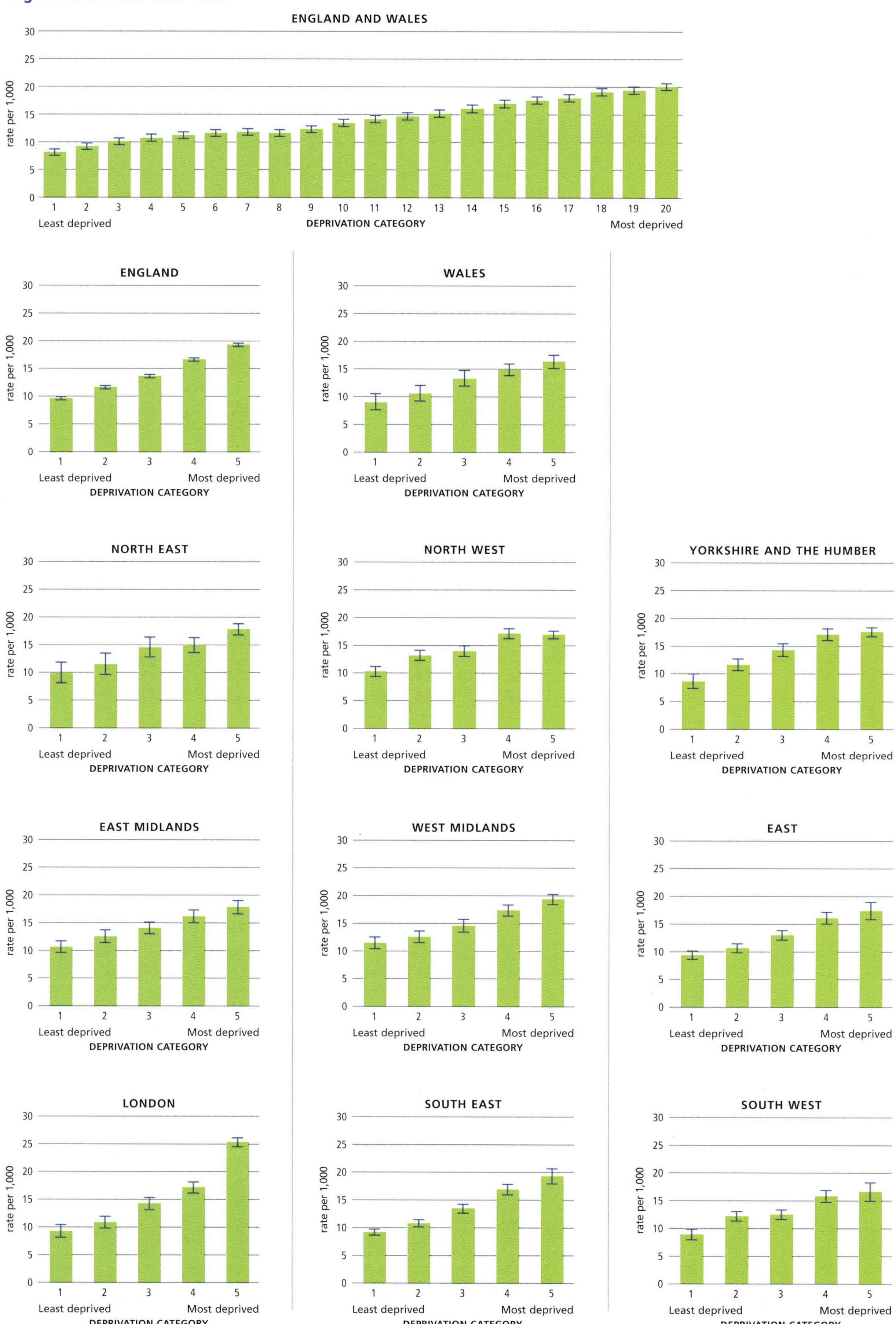

Figure 5.62

Conception rates by country, region and deprivation, women aged 35-39
England and Wales 1992-1994

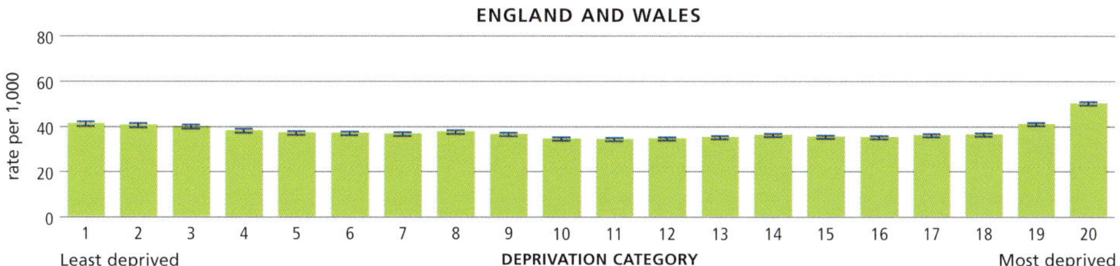

ENGLAND AND WALES

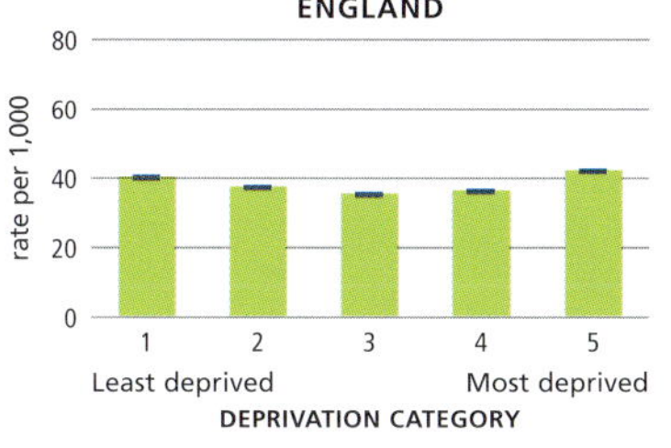

ENGLAND

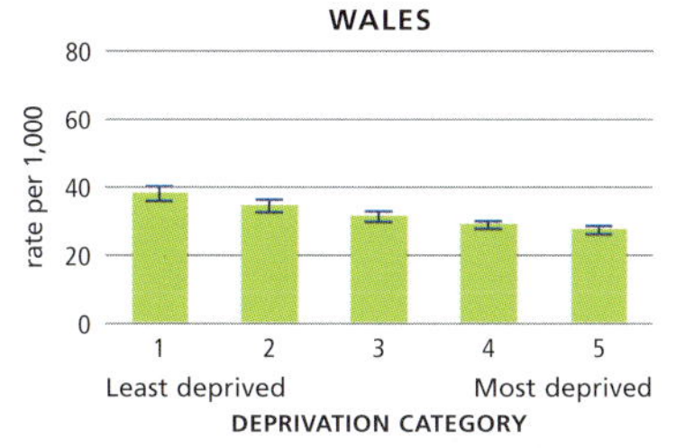

WALES

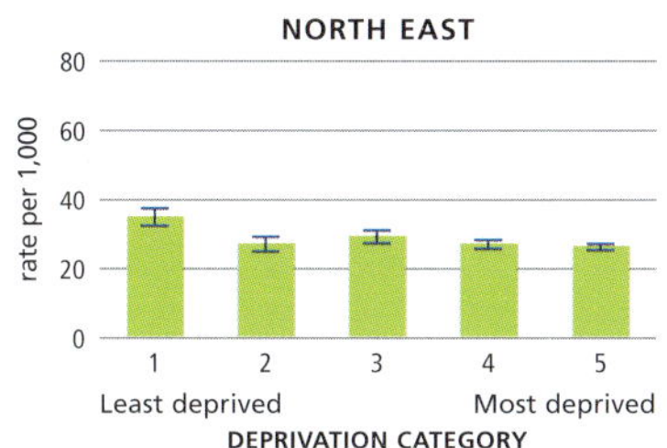

NORTH EAST

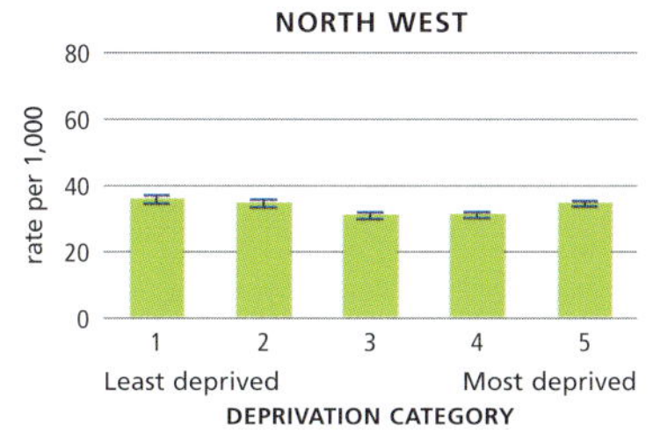

NORTH WEST

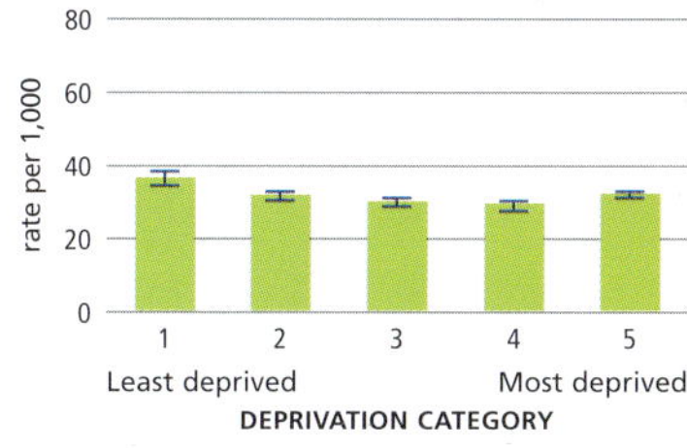

YORKSHIRE AND THE HUMBER

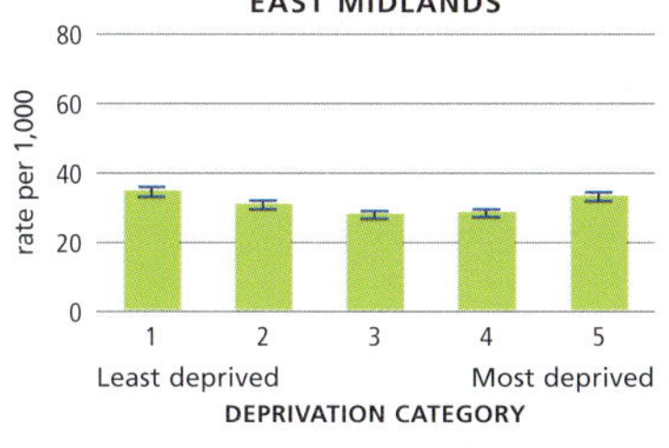

EAST MIDLANDS

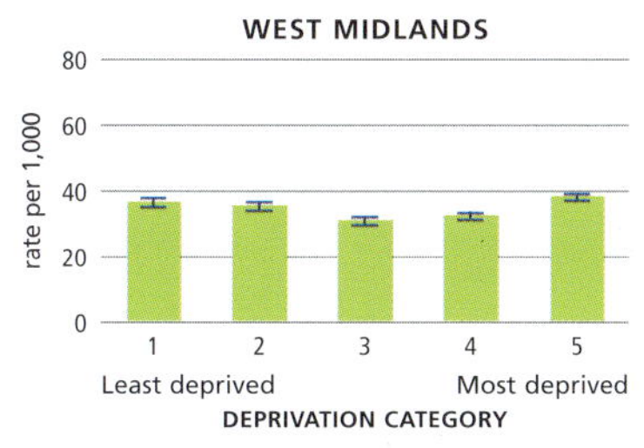

WEST MIDLANDS

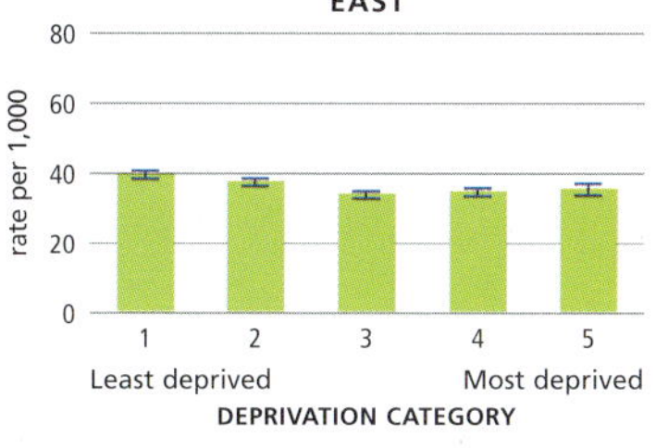

EAST

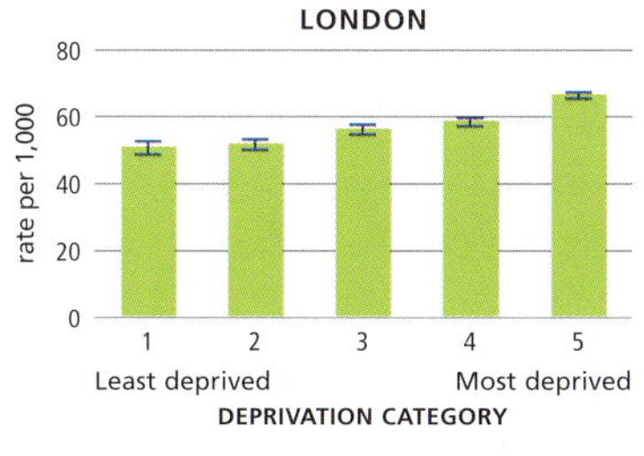

LONDON

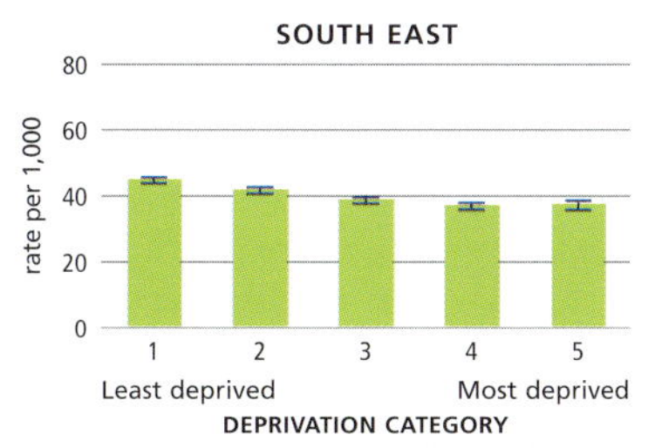

SOUTH EAST

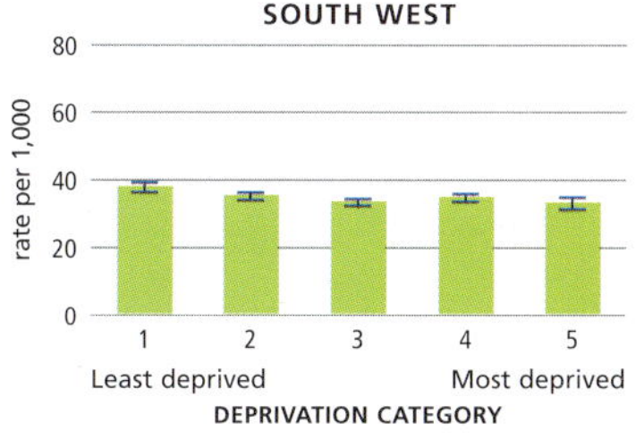

SOUTH WEST

Figure 5.63

**Live birth rates by country, region and deprivation, women aged 35-39
Great Britain 1991-1993**

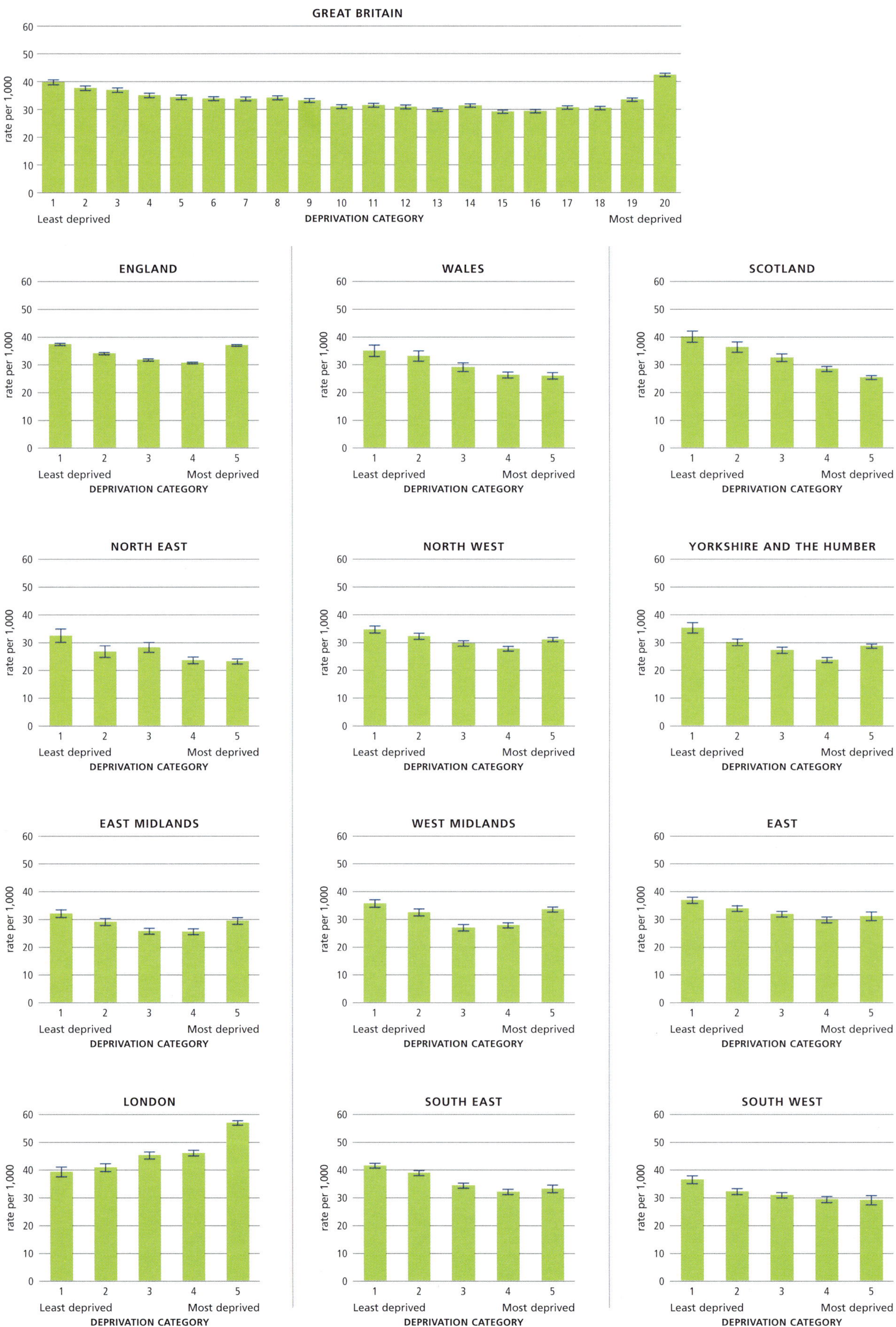

Figure 5.64

Percentage of conceptions leading to abortion by country, region and deprivation, women aged 35-39 England and Wales 1992-1994

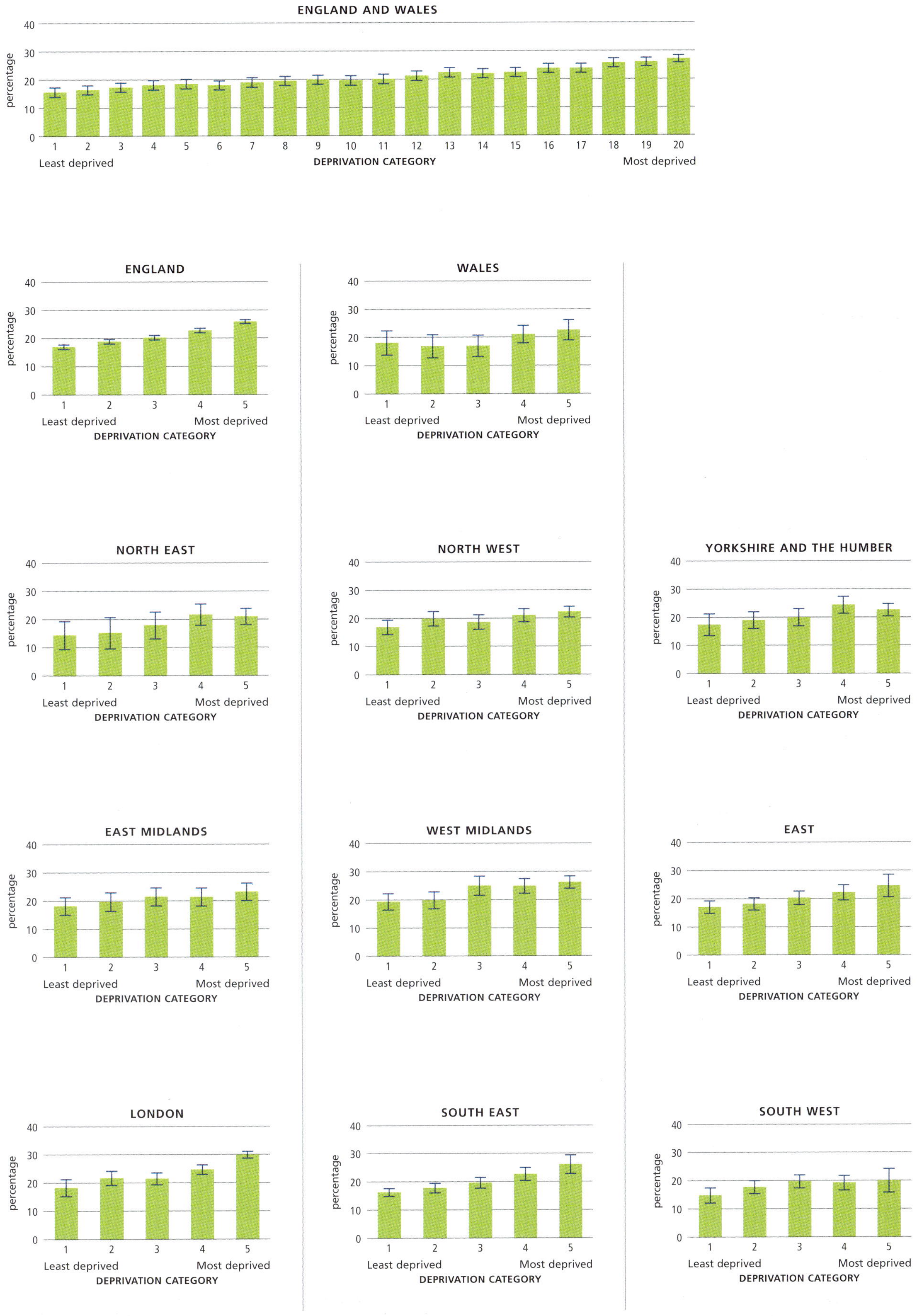

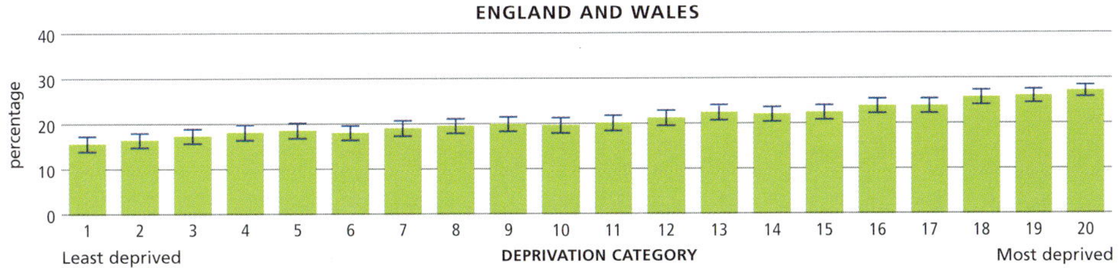

Figure 5.65

**Abortion rates by country, region and deprivation, women aged 35-39
England and Wales 1992-1994**

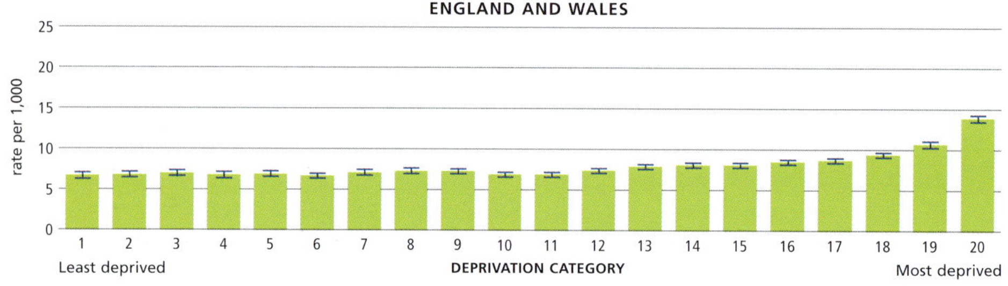

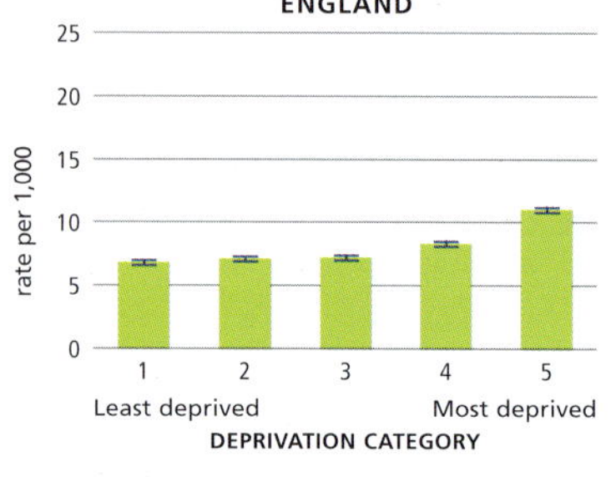

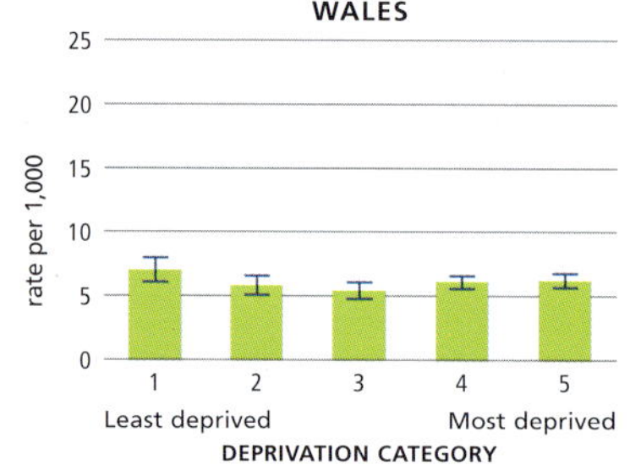

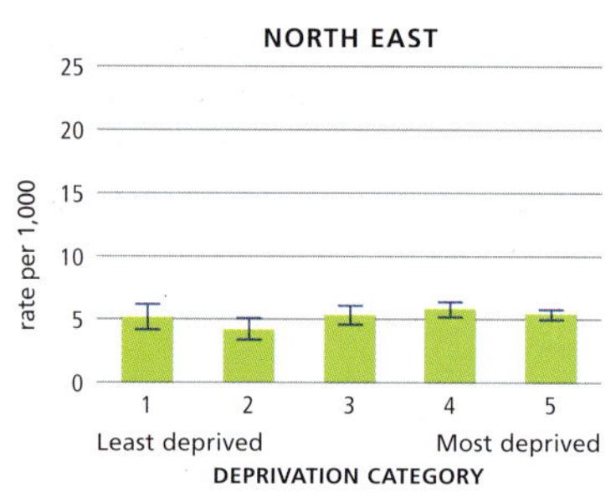

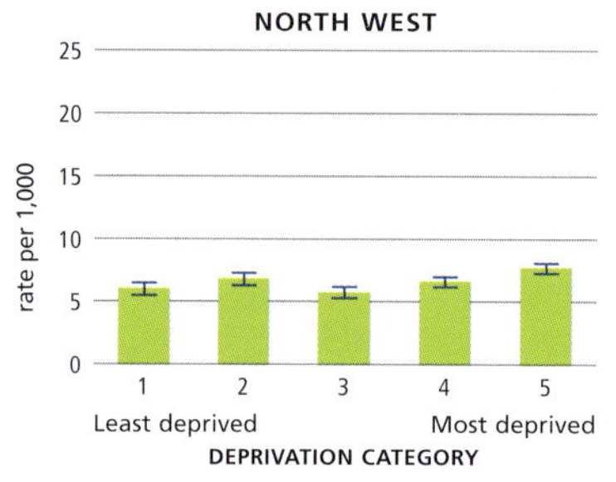

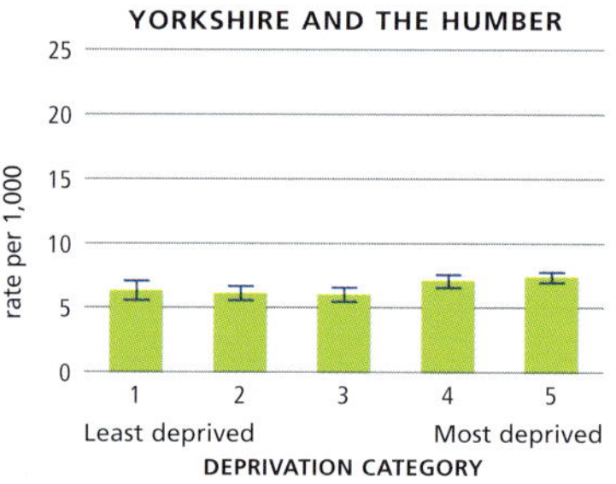

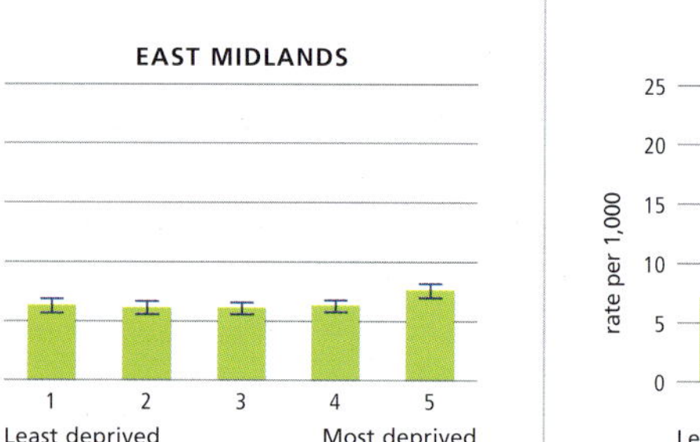

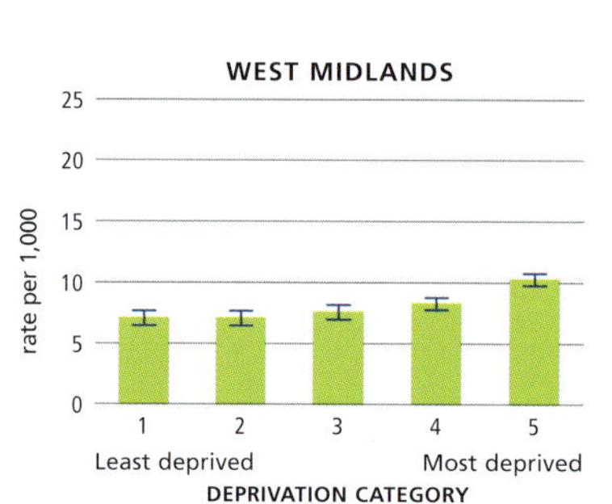

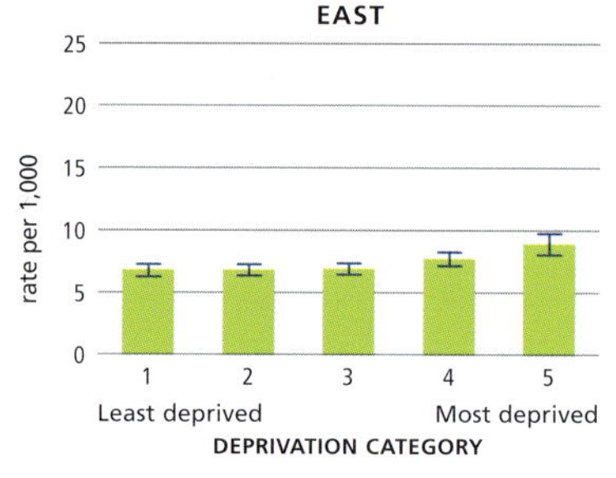

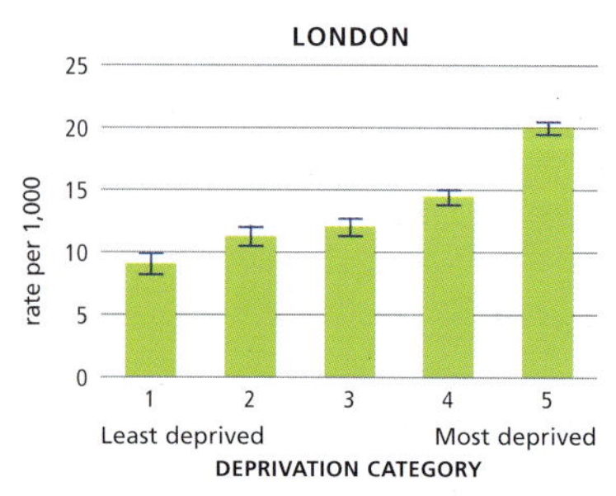

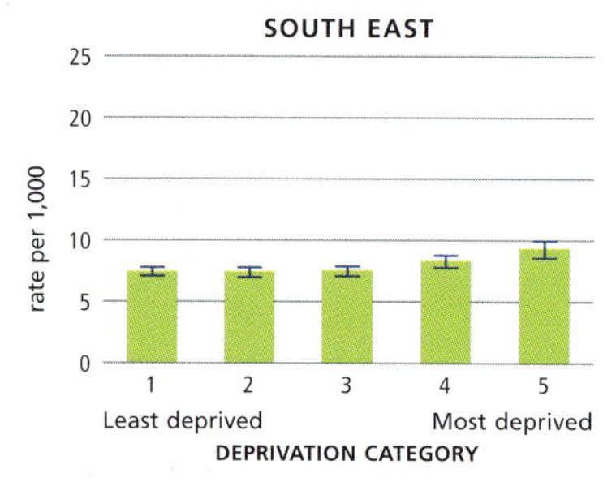

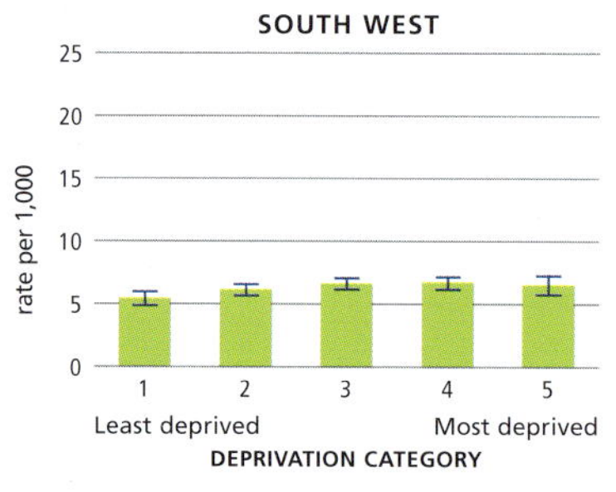

5.6 Discussion

In this discussion we illustrate how the findings from this chapter confirm those of previous studies. We also discuss possible explanations for some of the patterns observed, focusing on the differences in the proportion of births registered inside and outside marriage and on age-specific patterns of fertility.

Northern Ireland as a whole tended to have higher proportions of births registered inside marriage than the rest of the United Kingdom at older ages, but higher proportions registered solely by the mother at younger ages. At local authority level, at older ages, authorities within major centres of population tended to be the ones with a high proportion of births registered solely by the mother. At younger ages, however, there was a concentration of local authorities with high proportions in Northern Ireland and the other local authorities with high proportions were scattered throughout the rest of the United Kingdom.

Those local authorities with high proportions of sole registrations showed some link with those that had larger proportions of single people, with similar distributions seen in Map 3.2 in chapter 3. However, links were also seen with unemployment in younger people (Map 3.7 in chapter 3), and with the proportion of the population living in social housing, in England only (Map 3.15 in chapter 3). This suggests that other factors may be at work, especially as sole registrations increased consistently with increasing deprivation.

Birth rates have been declining in those aged in their twenties and increasing in those in their thirties in all areas. Fertility in women aged 35-39 has increased substantially over the 1990s - the conception rate increasing but the percentage leading to abortion remaining stable or declining, leading to substantial increases in the birth rate. This was particularly apparent in London and the South East - especially in those areas bordering London. High fertility in these women was also seen in prosperous areas. Low fertility in this age group was found in urban and industrial areas outside of London, confirming the findings of earlier work.[20, 21]

Those in Social Classes I and II are known to have higher fertility at older ages, thus we might expect areas with high proportions of the population in Social Classes I and II to have high fertility at older ages. This does appear to be the case when comparing the distribution of fertility at older ages with the distribution of these two Social Classes (shown in Map 3.5 of chapter 3), with high proportions in Social Classes I and II and high fertility in the older age groups in the Home Counties for example.

However, high fertility in London at older ages may also be due to women delaying childbearing in order to follow their career. London is well known to be a destination for young men and women to seek a career, before moving elsewhere to have a family.[34] London also has higher proportions of the population in minority ethnic groups (shown in Table 3.1 in chapter 3) than other areas, and women in these groups are known to have higher fertility.[29] It is unclear as to whether there is any relationship between fertility and deprivation for older women.

London also had high conception rates in all age groups over 20, as well as high percentages leading to abortion, confirming findings of previous work.[20] London also had the highest abortion rates in every age group. This high level of conceptions and abortions compared to other regions may well be as a result of women going to London for an abortion and stating a temporary residence. A substantial number of women from Northern Ireland and the Republic of Ireland travel to England and Wales to seek a termination each year. Although they may state their usual residence in these countries (6,912 women in 1997), they may also state a temporary residence within England and Wales.

High teenage fertility was found in urban and industrial areas, and low teenage fertility in rural and prosperous areas, confirming earlier findings.[20, 21] The results on deprivation and teenage fertility from this chapter also confirm those of earlier work[22, 23, 24] on deprivation with teenage birth rates in the most deprived areas of Great Britain being over 7 times those found in the least deprived and conception rates being 4 times greater in the most deprived areas of England and Wales than in the least.

Those in Social Classes IV and V are known to have higher teenage fertility than those in higher Social Classes, so we might expect areas that have a high proportion of the population in Social Classes IV and V to also be those areas that have high conception and birth rates in under 18s. When we compare the distribution of under 18 fertility rates with the distribution of Social Classes IV and V (Map 3.6 in chapter 3) we see some similarities, with high proportions in Social Classes IV and V and high under 18 fertility in industrial areas of the north and Midlands of England and south Wales.

Migration may also have an impact on the fertility patterns seen in this chapter as migration occurs more in the childbearing years.[35] Migration appears to be associated with childbearing itself, with the desire to move to more spacious accommodation around the birth of a child. The ability to move depends on housing tenure, income and resources, with those living in shared accommodation before the birth of a child being more likely to move. In Figure 3.17 and 3.18 in chapter 3 we saw that the population of London is more affected by migration than other areas of England and Wales, with people most likely to move to the Home Counties from London, seen in Figure 3.15 of chapter 3. This may affect fertility rates in London and in the areas around it, in that if a woman has one child in London and then moves to the Home Counties immediately after the birth, this will have the effect of depressing birth rates in the Home Counties until she has another baby and also increasing rates in London, as it artificially alters the population denominator. Figure 2.4 in chapter 2 suggests that families may migrate from London after having a baby, as it shows higher proportions of those aged under 5 than other regions, but lower proportions aged between 5 and 20. Rates in under 18s and 18-19s may also be altered by the movements of students to university towns and cities. It is difficult to quantify the exact effect this has on rates, however, but it is important to note that it is not simply socio-economic differences between people in the population that affect fertility rates in that population.

References

1 Office for National Statistics. Report: Infant and perinatal mortality by biological and social factors, 1999. *Health Statistics Quarterly* 8 (2000), 76-80.

2 Dattani N, Cooper N, Rodrigues N, Campbell O and Rooney C. Analysis of risk factors for neonatal mortality in England and Wales, 1993-97: based on singleton babies weighing 2500-5499 grams. *Health Statistics Quarterly* 8 (2000), 29-35.

3 Makinson C. The health consequences of teenage fertility. *Family Planning Perspectives* 17 (1985), 132-9.

4 Office for National Statistics. Report: Sudden infant deaths 1999. *Health Statistics Quarterly* 7 (2000), 66-70.

5 Peckham S. Preventing unplanned teenage pregnancies. *Public Health* 107 (1993), 125-133.

6 Wilson J. Maternity Policy. Caroline: a case of a pregnant teenager. *Professional Care of Mother and Child* 5(5) (1995), 139-142.

7 Clarke L, Joshi H, Di Salvo P and Wright J. Stability and instability in children's family lives: longitudinal evidence from two British sources. *Centre for Population Studies Research Paper 97-1*. City University (London: 1997).

8 Di Salvo P. Intergenerational patterns of teenage fertility in England and Wales. *Dissertation submitted in partial fulfilment of the requirements of the MSc in Medical Demography*. London School of Hygiene and Tropical Medicine (1992).

9 Social Exclusion Unit. *Teenage Pregnancy*. The Stationery Office (London: 1999).

10 Coleman D and Salt J. Fertility Trends. in *The British Population: Patterns, Trends, and Processes*. Oxford University Press (Oxford: 1992), 113-174

11 Mutton D, Alberman E and Hook EB. Cytogenetic and epidemiological findings in Down syndrome, England and Wales 1989 to 1993. *Journal of Medical Genetics* 33 (1996), 387-394.

12 Patterson CC, Carson DJ, Hadden DR, Waugh NR and Cole SK. A case-control investigation of perinatal risk factors for childhood IDDM in Northern Ireland and Scotland. *Diabetes Care* 17 (1994), 376-381.

13 McKinney PA, Parslow R, Gurney KA, Law GR, Bodansky HJ and Williams R. Perinatal and neonatal determinants of childhood type 1 diabetes. A case-control study in Yorkshire, UK. *Diabetes Care* 22 (1999), 928-932.

14 Jones ME, Swerdlow AJ, Gill LE and Goldacre MJ. Pre-natal and early life risk factors for childhood onset diabetes mellitus: a record linkage study. *International Journal of Epidemiology* 27 (1998), 444-449.

15 Bingley PJ, Douek IF, Rogers CA and Gale EAM. Influence of maternal age at delivery and birth order on risk of type 1 diabetes in childhood: prospective population based family study. *British Medical Journal* 321 (2000), 420-424.

16 Wood R, Botting B and Dunnell K. Trends in conceptions before and after the 1995 pill scare. *Population Trends* 89 (1997), 5-12.

17 Child TJ, Rees M and Mackenzie IZ. Pregnancy terminations after oral contraception scare. *Lancet* 347 (1996), 1260-1.

18 Flett G, Gurney E, McKessock L, Reid J. Impact of the October 1995 pill scare in Grampian. B*ritish Journal of Family Planning* 24 (1998), 18-20.

19 Office for National Statistics. Annual Update: Births and Conceptions 1998. *Population Trends* 98 (1999), 83-86.

20 Wood R. Subnational variations in conceptions. *Population Trends* 84 (1996), 21-27.

21 Armitage R. Variation in fertility between different types of local area. *Population Trends* 87 (1997), 20-28.

22 Smith T. Influence of socio-economic factors on attaining targets for reducing teenage pregnancies. *British Medical Journal* 306 (1993), 1232-1235.

23 Clements S, Stone N, Diamond I and Ingham R. Modelling the spatial distribution of teenage conception rates within Wessex. *British Journal of Family Planning* 24 (1998), 61-71.

24 Sloggett A and Joshi H. Deprivation indicators as predictors of life events, 1981-1992 based on the ONS Longitudinal Study. *Journal of Epidemiology and Community Health* 52 (1998), 228-233.

25 Office for National Statistics. *The ONS Classification of Local and Health Authorities of Great Britain, Revised in 1999*. SMPS No. 63. Office for National Statistics (London: 2000).

26 Office for National Statistics. Series AB. *Abortion Statistics, England and Wales*. The Stationery Office (London: 1997).

27 Filakti H. Trends in abortion 1990-95. *Population Trends* 87 (1997), 11-19.

28 Breslow NE and Day NE. *Statistical Methods in Cancer Research, Volume II: The Design and Analysis of Cohort Studies*. International Agency for Research on Cancer, World Health Organisation (Lyon: 1987).

29 Office for National Statistics. Series FM1. *Birth Statistics, England and Wales*. The Stationery Office (London: 1997).

30 Calot G. Statement on fertility at the Round Table organised in Wiesbaden on the 25th anniversary of the Bundesinstitut für Bevölkerungsforschung.

31 Ruddock V, Wood R and Quinn M. Birth statistics: recent trends in England and Wales. *Population Trends* 94 (1998), 12-18.

32 Shyrock HS, Siegel JS and Stockwell EG. *The Methods and Materials of Demography. Condensed Edition*. Academic Press (London: 1976), 279.

33 Office for National Statistics. *Social Trends* 31. The Stationery Office (London: 2001).

34 Coleman D and Salt J. Internal Migration. in *The British Population: Patterns, Trends, and Processes*. Oxford University Press (Oxford: 1992), 113-174.

35 Grundy E. Migration and fertility behaviour in England and Wales: a record linkage study. *Journal of Biosocial Science* 18 (1986), 403-423.

Patterns and trends in stillbirths and infant mortality

Justine Fitzpatrick and Nicola Cooper

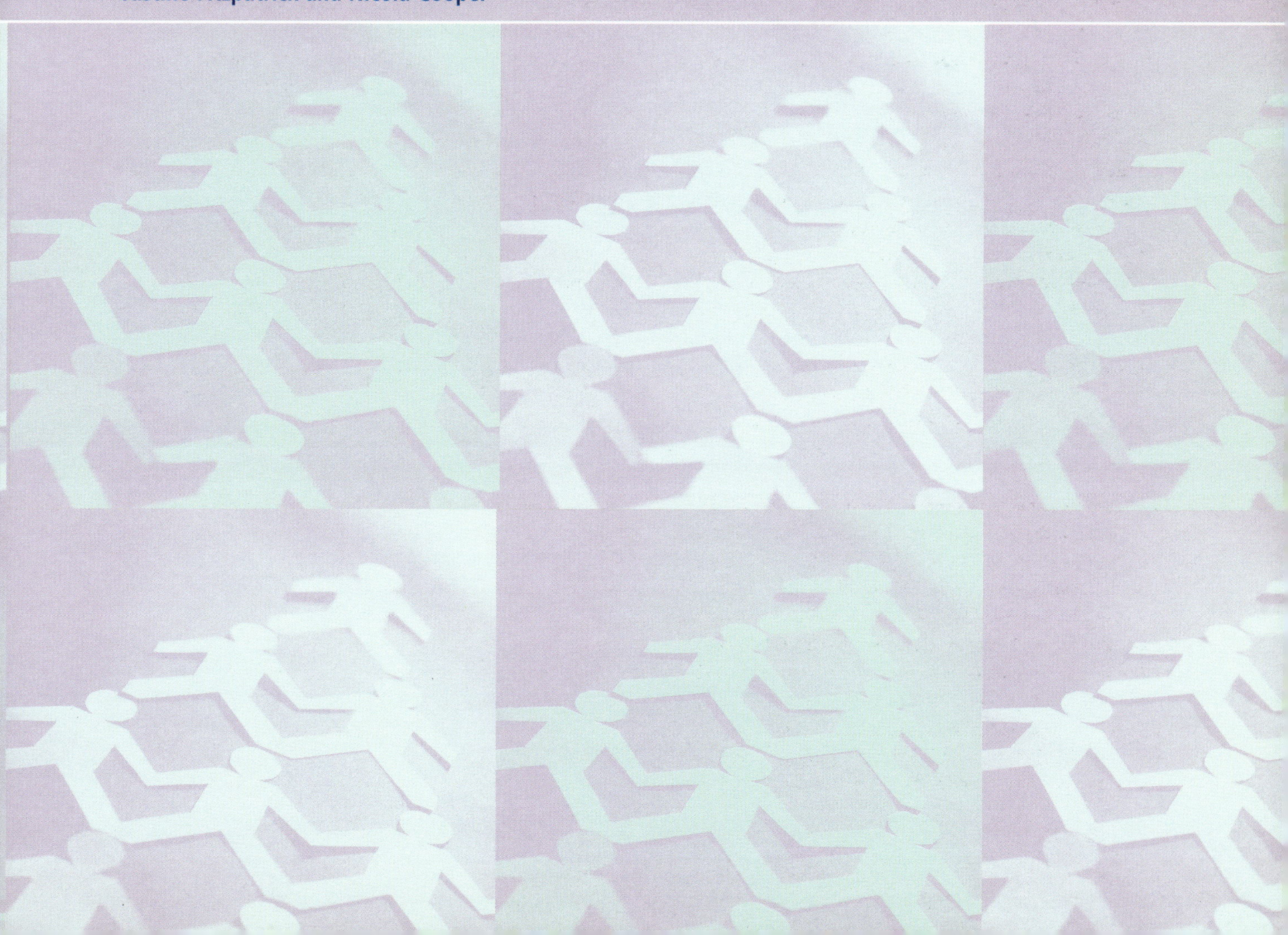

Chapter 6
Patterns and trends in stillbirths and infant mortality

Summary

- There was little variation in stillbirth and infant mortality rates between countries of the United Kingdom. However, Scotland's stillbirth rate was significantly higher than that for the United Kingdom as a whole and Northern Ireland's perinatal mortality rate was significantly higher than that for the United Kingdom.

- The difference between infant mortality rates in the United Kingdom reduced between 1992 and 1996.

- At regional level within England, a north-south divide in stillbirths and infant mortality was apparent; regions in the north and the Midlands had higher stillbirths and infant mortality than regions in the south. The exception to this was London which also had high rates.

- Within countries and regions, authorities with high rates of infant death and stillbirths tended to be found in urban areas. Authorities classified as *East Inner London, Manufacturing Centres* and *Ports and Industry* had the highest rates.

- The most deprived areas within the countries of the United Kingdom and the regions of England had the highest stillbirth and infant mortality rates and the least deprived areas the lowest.

6.1 Introduction

Infant mortality is a widely used indicator of the health of the population and its living conditions, since as the standard of living rises infant mortality falls. *'As mortality in general declines, it concentrates at the two extremes of life'.*[1] The first year of life is a time of great vulnerability, with infancy remaining the most perilous period of childhood in terms of mortality risk. Factors such as ethnicity, socio-economic circumstances, the environment, parental behaviour and sub-standard health care are potential risk factors for infant death.[2,3] This may result in a variation of stillbirth and infant mortality rates between countries, regions and local authority areas.

Geographic variations in infant mortality and stillbirths have been discussed in many previous decennial supplements along with variations by Social Class. Previous decennial supplements have concluded that although Social Class differences in infant mortality do explain some of the difference in mortality between regions, marked differences between regions remain unaccounted for.[4,5]

This chapter describes stillbirths and infant mortality rates in the countries of the United Kingdom in the 1990s, with England studied in further detail at regional level. It also examines variations in rates by local authority within countries of the United Kingdom and within regions of England.

Box 6.1 Definitions of stillbirth and infant mortality rates

Stillbirth rate	=	stillbirths x 1,000
		live births + stillbirths
Perinatal mortality rate	=	(stillbirths + deaths within the first 7 days of life) x 1,000
		live births + stillbirths
Early neonatal mortality rate	=	deaths within the first 7 days of life x 1,000
		live births
Late neonatal mortality rate	=	deaths between 7-27 days of life x 1,000
		live births
Neonatal mortality rate	=	deaths within the first 28 days of life x 1,000
		live births
Postneonatal mortality rate	=	deaths at ages 28 days and over but under one year of life x 1,000
		live births
Infant mortality rate	=	deaths within the first year of life x 1,000
		live births

Inequalities in stillbirth and infant mortality rates are then examined using the ONS classification of local authorities[6] and the Carstairs and Morris index of deprivation.[7] Further details of these classifications are provided in chapter 4 of this volume.

Infant mortality includes all deaths in the first year of life. It is, however, useful to distinguish deaths around the time of birth from those occurring later in the first year. For this purpose a number of definitions are used, covering stillbirths as well as infant death (Box 6.1).

6.2 Geographic patterns in stillbirths and infant mortality

Throughout this chapter, infant mortality rates comprising neonatal mortality (deaths in the first 28 days of life) and postneonatal mortality (deaths in the remainder of the first year of life), are analysed using data for 1991 to 1997. Stillbirth and perinatal mortality rates (stillbirths plus early neonatal deaths) are analysed using data for 1993 to 1997. The Births and Deaths Registration Act 1953 defined a stillbirth as '*a child which has issued forth from its mother after the twenty-eighth week of pregnancy, and which did not at any time after becoming expelled from its mother breathe or show other signs of life*'. New legislation that came into force on 1 October 1992 lowered the gestation age limit for stillbirths from 28 to 24 completed weeks. Figures for stillbirths from 1993 onwards are thus not fully comparable with those for previous years. For this reason, stillbirth and perinatal

mortality are both analysed (using the new stillbirth definition) for 1993 to 1997 only.

Variations by country and region

Table 6.1 shows infant mortality rates by country and region. Figure 6.1 shows the stillbirth and early neonatal mortality components of perinatal mortality rates and Figure 6.2 the neonatal and postneonatal mortality components of infant mortality rates. Scotland had the highest stillbirth, postneonatal and infant mortality rate and the stillbirth rate for Scotland of 6.2 per 1,000 live and stillbirths was significantly higher than the United Kingdom rate of 5.6. Northern Ireland had the same infant mortality rate as Scotland and had the highest perinatal and neonatal mortality rate, but only the perinatal mortality rate (9.4) was significantly higher than the United Kingdom (8.7). Wales was the only country within the United Kingdom that had perinatal (8.2) and neonatal mortality (3.8) rates that were significantly lower than the United Kingdom rates (8.7 and 4.1 respectively). None of the four countries had a postneonatal or infant mortality rate significantly higher or lower than the United Kingdom as a whole.

Analysis of the regions in England showed that as expected there was more variation between regions than between countries. There was a clear north-south divide in infant mortality rates. The North East, North West, Yorkshire and the Humber and West Midlands all had overall infant mortality rates significantly above the United Kingdom rate. The East of England, South East and South West regions had significantly lower rates for

Table 6.1

Infant mortality and stillbirth rates[1] by country and region
United Kingdom 1991-1997

	Stillbirth rate[+]	Perinatal mortality rate[+]	Neonatal mortality rate	Post neonatal mortality rate	Infant mortality rate
United Kingdom	5.6	8.7	4.1	2.2	6.3
England	5.5	8.7	4.2	2.2	6.3
North East	* 6.1	9.2	* 4.5	2.4	* 6.9
North West	5.7	8.8	4.1	* 2.6	* 6.7
Yorkshire and the Humber	5.4	8.9	* 4.6	* 2.6	* 7.2
East Midlands	5.3	8.5	4.3	2.3	6.5
West Midlands	5.9	* 10.1	* 5.3	2.1	* 7.5
East	~ 5.0	~ 7.7	~ 3.4	~ 1.8	~ 5.2
London	* 6.3	* 9.5	4.3	2.3	6.5
South East	~ 5.0	~ 7.7	~ 3.5	~ 1.8	~ 5.3
South West	~ 5.0	~ 7.9	~ 3.7	~ 2.0	~ 5.7
Wales	5.4	~ 8.2	~ 3.8	2.1	6.0
Scotland	* 6.2	9.1	4.0	2.3	6.4
Northern Ireland	5.9	* 9.4	4.5	2.0	6.4

[+]1993-1997 only
*significantly higher than the UK rate
~significantly lower than the UK rate
[1]rates per 1,000

Figure 6.1

**Stillbirth and early neonatal components of perinatal mortality rates by country and region
United Kingdom 1993-1997**

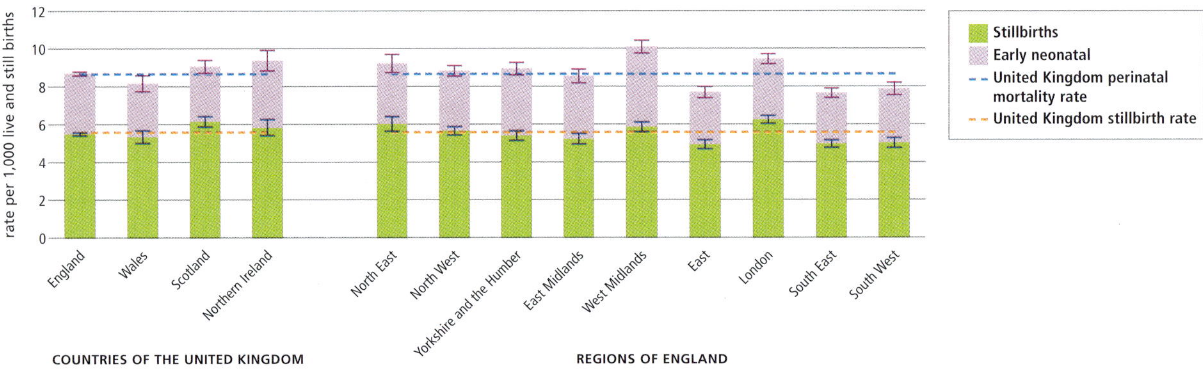

Figure 6.2

**Neonatal and postneonatal components of infant mortality rates by country and region
United Kingdom 1991-1997**

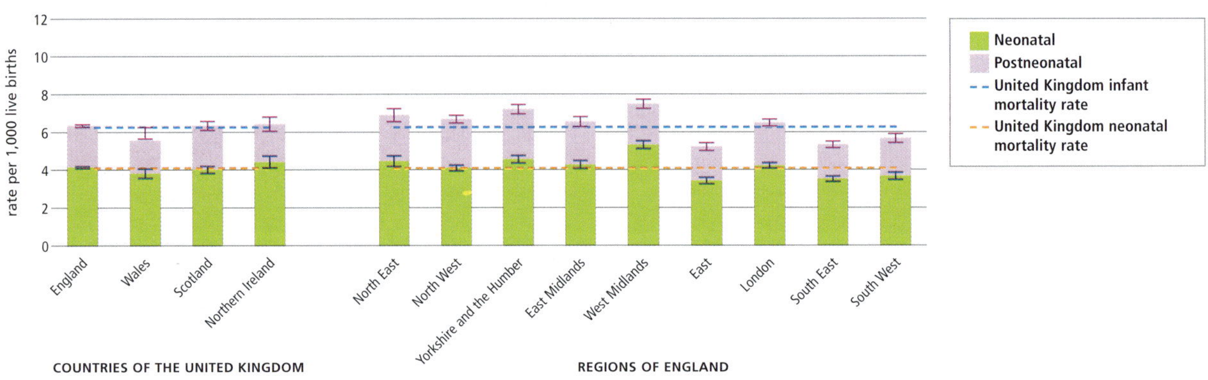

stillbirths and all measures of infant mortality than the United Kingdom as a whole. Stillbirth rates in the North East and London were significantly higher than the rate for the United Kingdom as a whole. There were also significantly higher perinatal mortality rates in the West Midlands and London than in the United Kingdom as a whole. The neonatal mortality rate in the North East, Yorkshire and the Humber and West Midlands was significantly higher than for the United Kingdom. Analysis of postneonatal mortality rates by region showed that rates for the North West and Yorkshire and the Humber were significantly higher than the United Kingdom postneonatal rates.

Trends in infant mortality by country and region

This section looks at trends in infant mortality rates over the period studied. To smooth out the peaks and troughs that occur when dealing with small numbers of deaths, a three-year moving average is presented. We have not presented trends in stillbirths and perinatal mortality rates as comparable data are available only for the period 1993-1997 (see introduction). Where relevant we have indicated whether the differences

between countries and regions have increased over time by looking at the ratio of the rate in the country or region with the highest mortality to the rate in the country or region with the lowest mortality.

Neonatal mortality trends
Northern Ireland had the highest neonatal mortality rate throughout the period 1991-1997 (Figure 6.3). There was a steady fall in the neonatal mortality rate in Scotland, less so for England. The rate for Scotland fell by 14 per cent from 4.3 in 1991-1993 to 3.7 per 1,000 live births in 1995-1997 and this was the lowest rate in the United Kingdom. The neonatal mortality rate for Wales remained relatively stable during the study period and was lower than the rest of the countries in the United Kingdom until 1995-1997. The difference between the countries with the highest and lowest rate in 1995-1997 was similar to the difference in 1991-1993.

Trends in neonatal mortality rates within England by region (Figure 6.4) showed that the West Midlands had the highest rate throughout the period studied, despite a fall of 9 per cent. With

Figure 6.3

**Trends in neonatal mortality rates by country
United Kingdom 1992-1996***

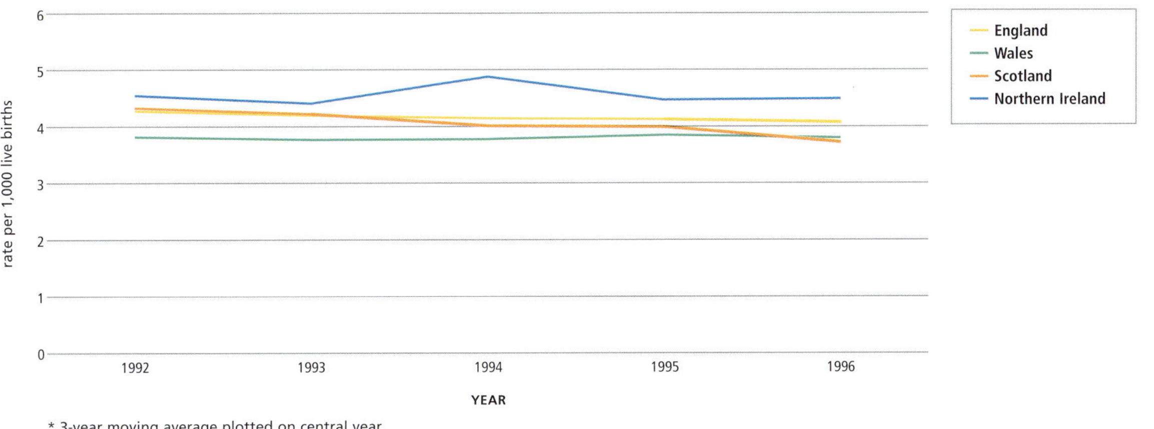

* 3-year moving average plotted on central year

Figure 6.4

**Trends in neonatal mortality rates by region
England 1992-1996***

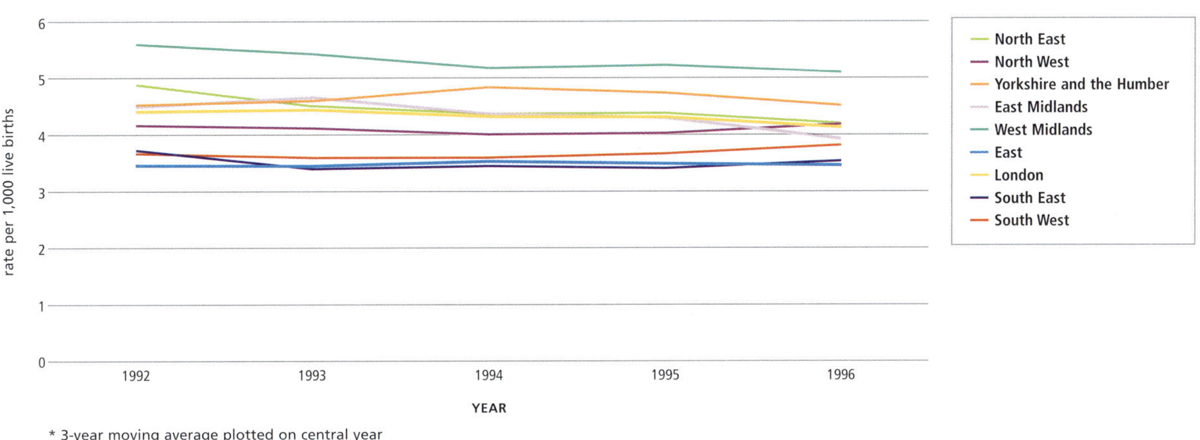

* 3-year moving average plotted on central year

the exception of the North West and the South West all regions saw a decrease in their neonatal mortality over the period studied. The North East and East Midlands regions saw the largest fall in neonatal mortality rates, between 12-14 per cent. The ratio in the rates between the regions with the highest and lowest neonatal mortality rates decreased slightly from 1.6 to 1.5 over the period.

Postneonatal mortality trends
The postneonatal mortality rate fell in all countries over the period studied (Figure 6.5). Northern Ireland consistently had the lowest rate throughout this period. In 1991-1993, Wales and Northern Ireland had the lowest postneonatal mortality rates (2.3 per 1,000 live births), but Wales and Scotland both experienced a more gradual downward trend in postneonatal mortality rates than England and Northern Ireland. This led to a rise in the rate

ratio between the countries in the United Kingdom with the highest and lowest postneonatal mortality rates, from 1.1 in 1991-1993 to 1.3 in 1995-1997.

All regions saw a downward trend in postneonatal mortality rates (Figure 6.6). Yorkshire and the Humber experienced the largest fall in postneonatal mortality rates, of 29 per cent. This was the region with the highest postneonatal mortality rate in the earlier part of the 1990s, before it fell below the rate for the North West in 1995-1997. The region that experienced the smallest fall (10 per cent) in postneonatal mortality rates was the East of England, but this region had the lowest rates at the start of the period studied. Over the study period the ratio of postneonatal mortality rates between the regions in England with the highest and lowest rates narrowed from 1.6 to 1.5.

Figure 6.5

**Trends in postneonatal mortality rates by country
United Kingdom 1992-1996***

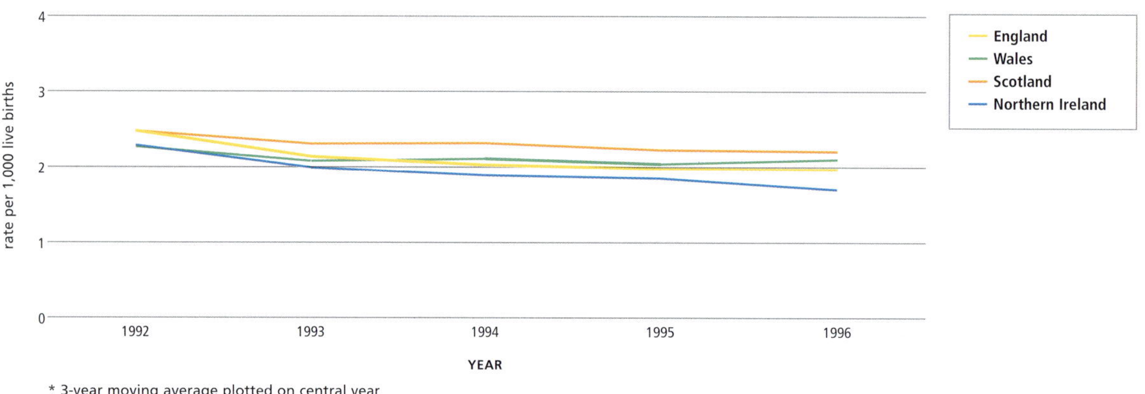

* 3-year moving average plotted on central year

Figure 6.6

**Trends in postneonatal mortality rates by region
England 1992-1996***

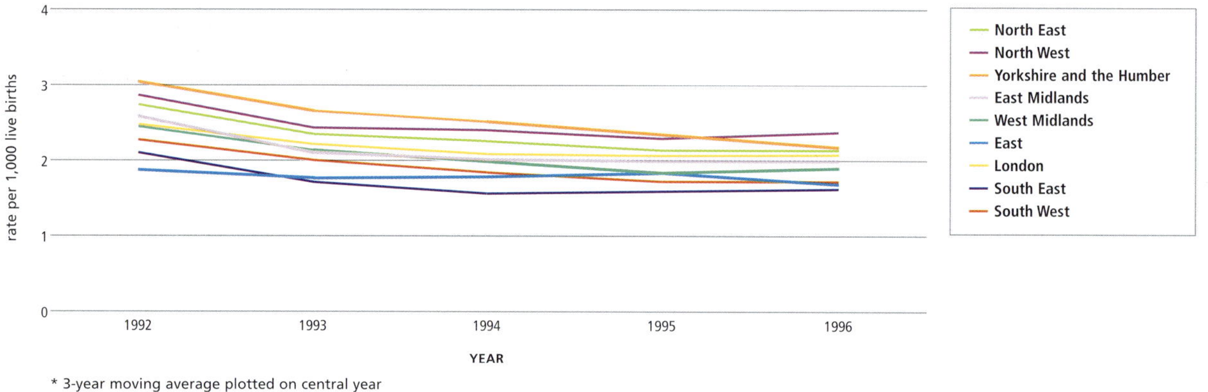

* 3-year moving average plotted on central year

Infant mortality trends

The infant mortality rate fell in all countries, with the largest fall (13 per cent) seen in Scotland (Figure 6.7). As neonatal mortality rates are twice as high as postneonatal rates, trends in infant mortality will largely reflect the trends in neonatal mortality. Northern Ireland had the highest infant mortality rate for much of this period. Wales had the lowest infant mortality rate for the entire period and showed the smallest fall (3 per cent). The ratio of the rate between the countries with the highest and lowest infant mortality rate narrowed from 1.1 to 1.0 between 1991-1993 to 1995-1997.

Infant mortality also fell in all regions. Infant mortality rates for the regions in England ranged from 5.3 to 8.0 in 1991-1993, the south of England regions (East of England, South East and South West) had the lowest rates. The clear north-south divide continued over the period to 1995-1997 (Figure 6.8), but the range in infant mortality rates narrowed to 5.1 to 7.0 in 1995-1997. The West Midlands and Yorkshire and the Humber had the highest infant mortality rates throughout this period. The greatest fall in infant mortality rates occurred in the North East (17 per cent) and the East Midlands (16 per cent). The East of England had the smallest fall in infant mortality, but had the lowest rate at both the beginning and the end of the period studied. The rate ratio between the regions with the highest and lowest infant mortality rate narrowed from 1.5 in 1992 to 1.4 in 1996.

Variations by local authority

Maps 6.1-6.5 show stillbirth and infant mortality rates by local authority in the United Kingdom during the 1990s. The guide to the maps in Appendix A describes the principles used in constructing these maps. Authorities with high stillbirth rates and high rates for all measures of infant death appeared to be concentrated within the major urban areas, in particular London, Manchester, Birmingham and Glasgow. Authorities in other parts of the United Kingdom, for example Devon, Cornwall and Dumfries and Galloway, also had significantly high rates for one or more measure of infant death. Authorities with low rates tended to be located away from

Figure 6.7

**Trends in infant mortality rates by country
United Kingdom 1992-1996***

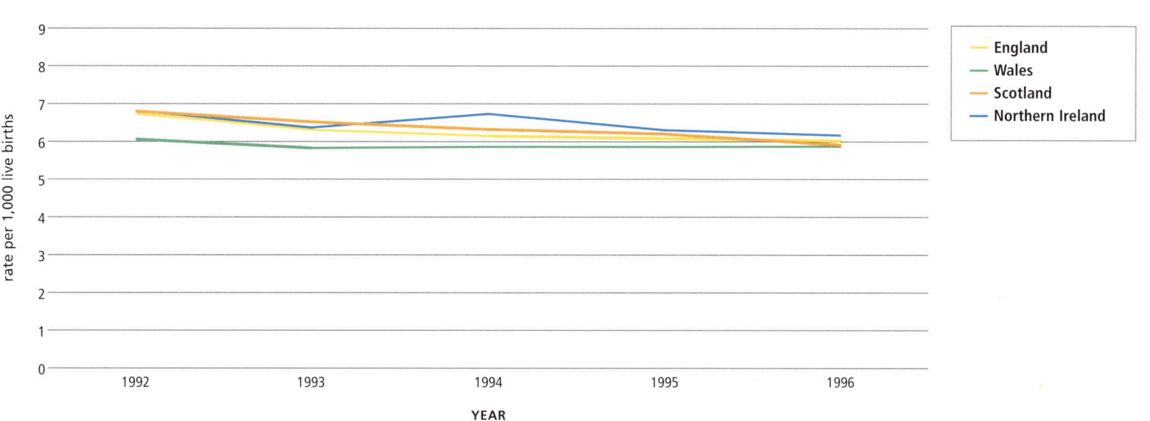

* 3-year moving average plotted on central year

Figure 6.8

**Trends in infant mortality rates by region
England 1992-1996***

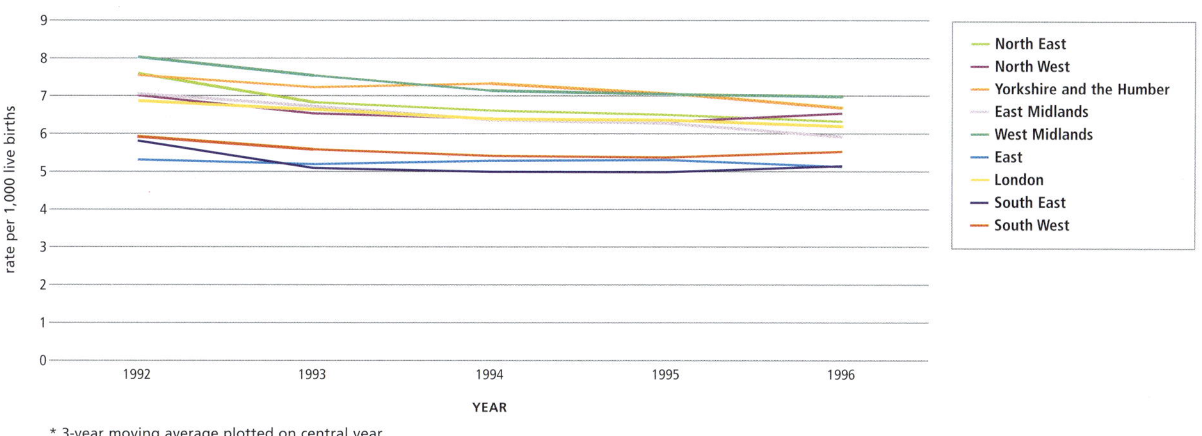

* 3-year moving average plotted on central year

major urban areas. For all measures of infant mortality there was a belt of authorities with low rates across the south of England, reflecting the low mortality for the South East region as a whole.

The overall pattern was similar for all the maps presented here. The maps for perinatal mortality and stillbirths were similar as stillbirths make up a large proportion of perinatal deaths. The maps for neonatal and overall infant mortality were also similar as neonatal deaths make up a large proportion of infant deaths. Many areas had high rates for more than one measure of infant mortality or for stillbirths, for example Birmingham, Glasgow City, Newham and Dumfries and Galloway. Some areas had low rates for more than one measure of infant mortality or stillbirths, for example East Hampshire, Maidstone and the Vale of White Horse.

As the number of infant deaths in any single authority is small, grouping authorities that share similar characteristics may help to draw out geographic patterns in mortality rates. Figure 6.9

shows the stillbirth and neonatal mortality components of perinatal mortality by ONS classification Group. Figure 6.10 shows the neonatal and postneonatal components of infant mortality by ONS classification Group. For stillbirths and perinatal mortality the *East Inner London* Group had the highest rates. Characteristics associated with this group include a large minority ethnic population, large families, high unemployment and high lone parent households. High rates were also found in the *Manufacturing Centres* and *Ports and Industry* Groups. The characteristics of these areas include high unemployment, a large proportion of the population in Social Class IV and V, a high proportion of terraced housing and local authority rented accommodation and a large proportion of the population with a limiting long term illness.

For other measures of infant mortality it was the three Groups mentioned above that had the highest rates, however the highest was found in the *Manufacturing Centres* Group. This Group includes a large proportion of the authorities with very high rates. For infant mortality, eight of the 24 authorities with

Map 6.1

Stillbirth rates by local authority
United Kingdom 1993-1997

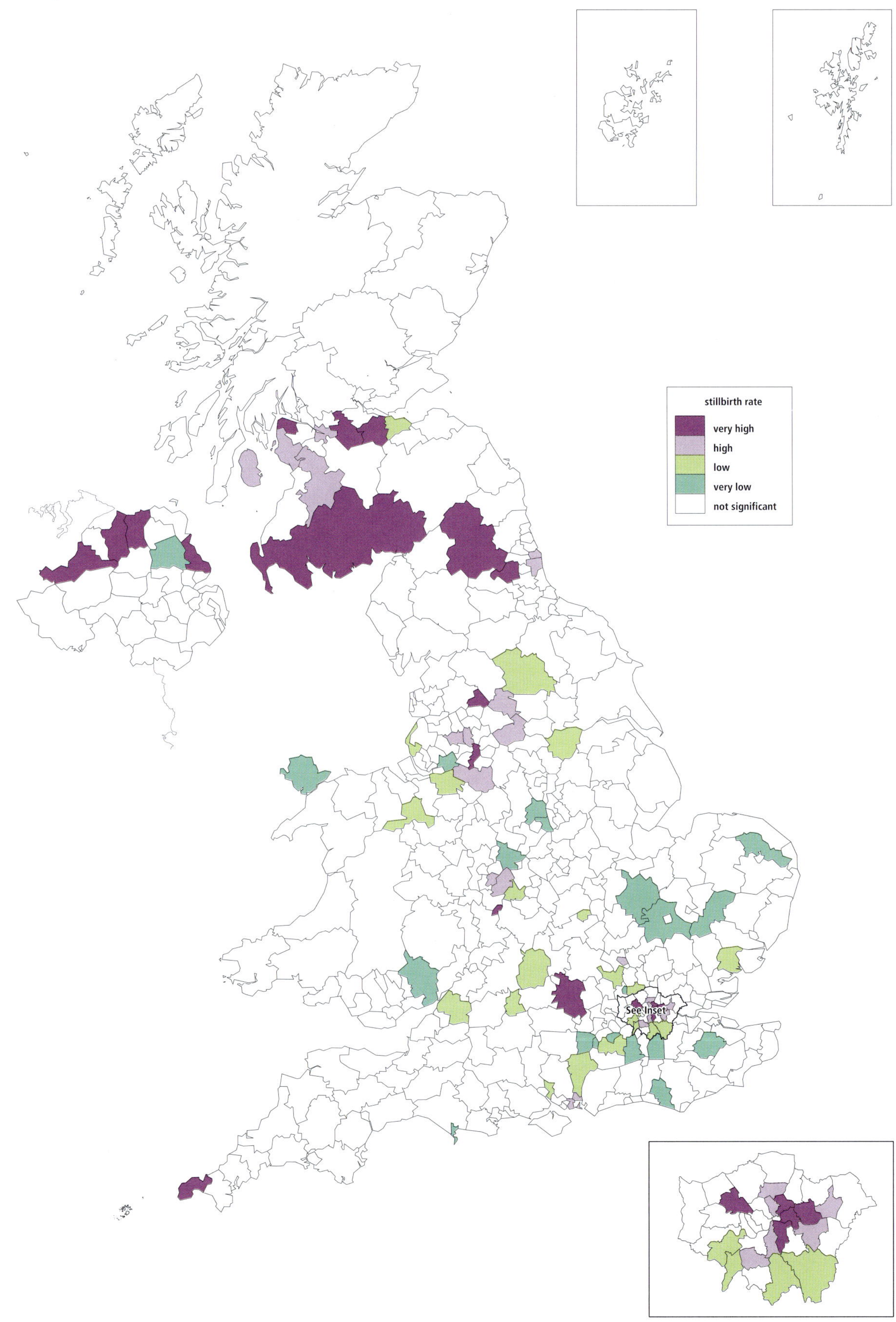

Map 6.2

Perinatal mortality rates by local authority
United Kingdom 1993-1997

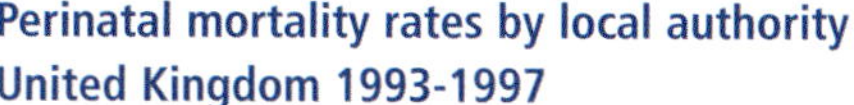

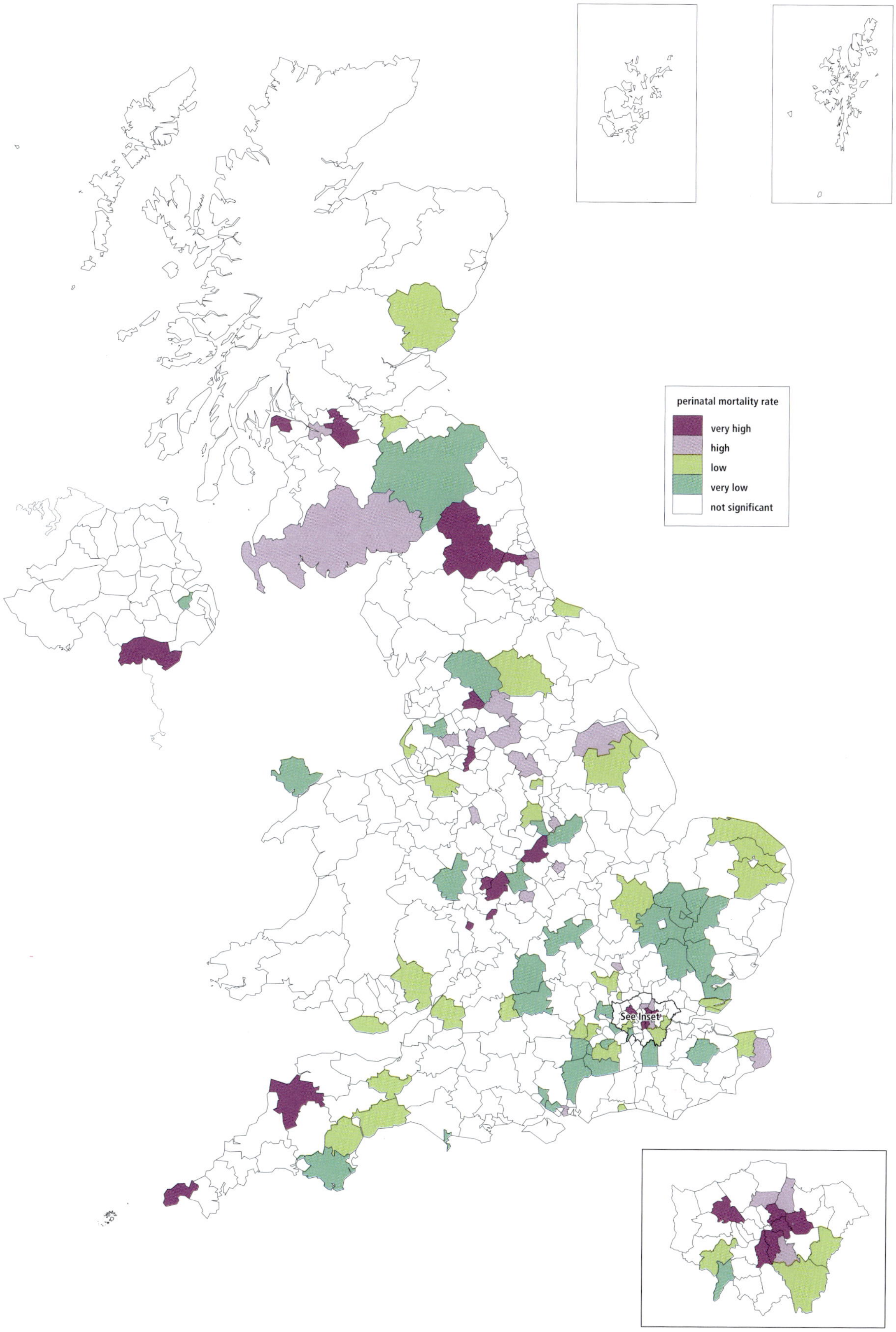

Map 6.3

Neonatal mortality rates by local authority
United Kingdom 1991-1997

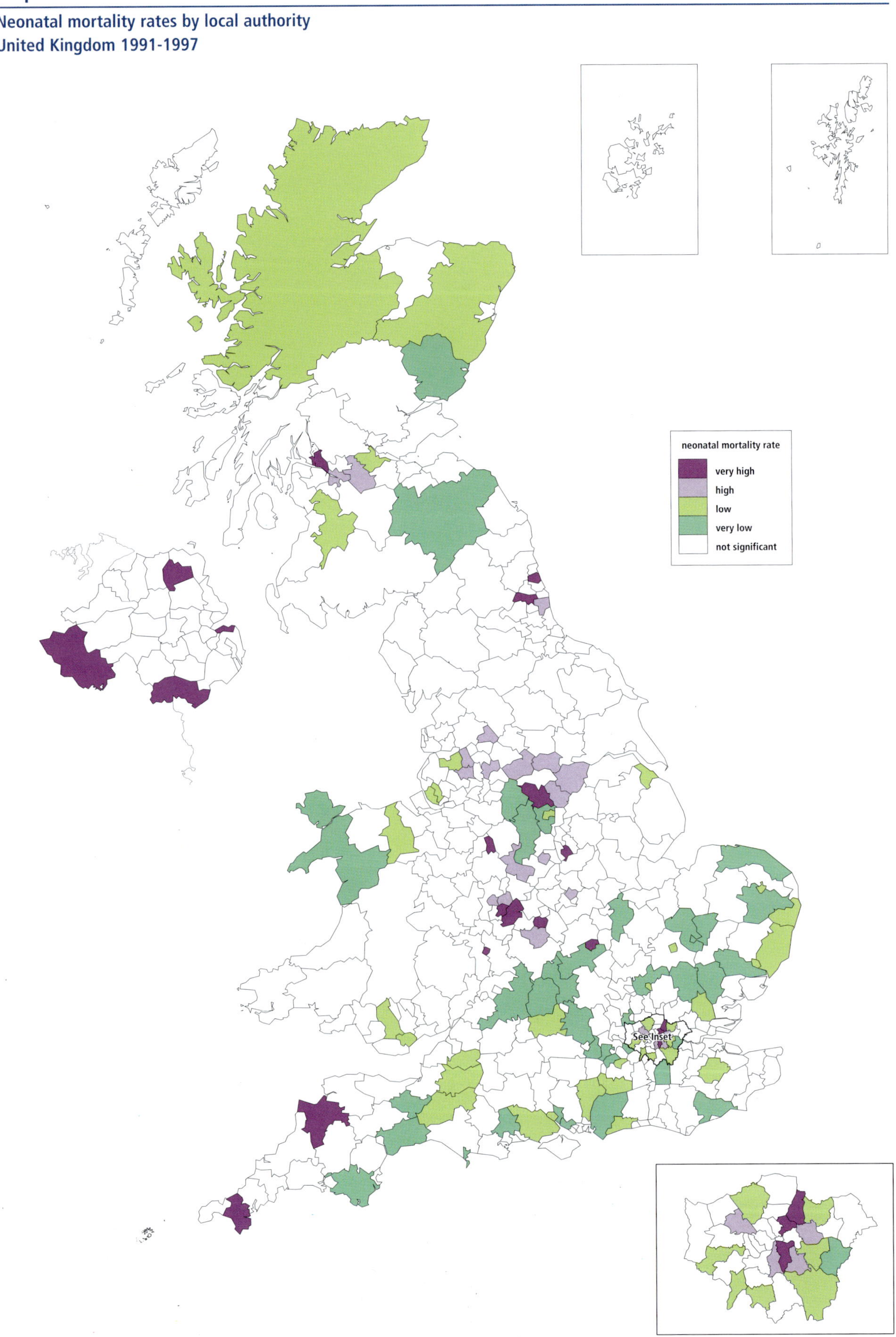

Map 6.4

Postneonatal mortality rates by local authority
United Kingdom 1991-1997

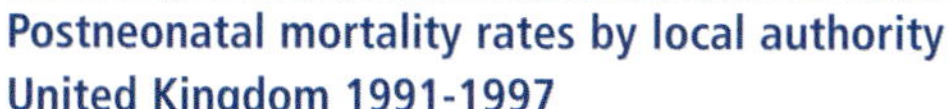

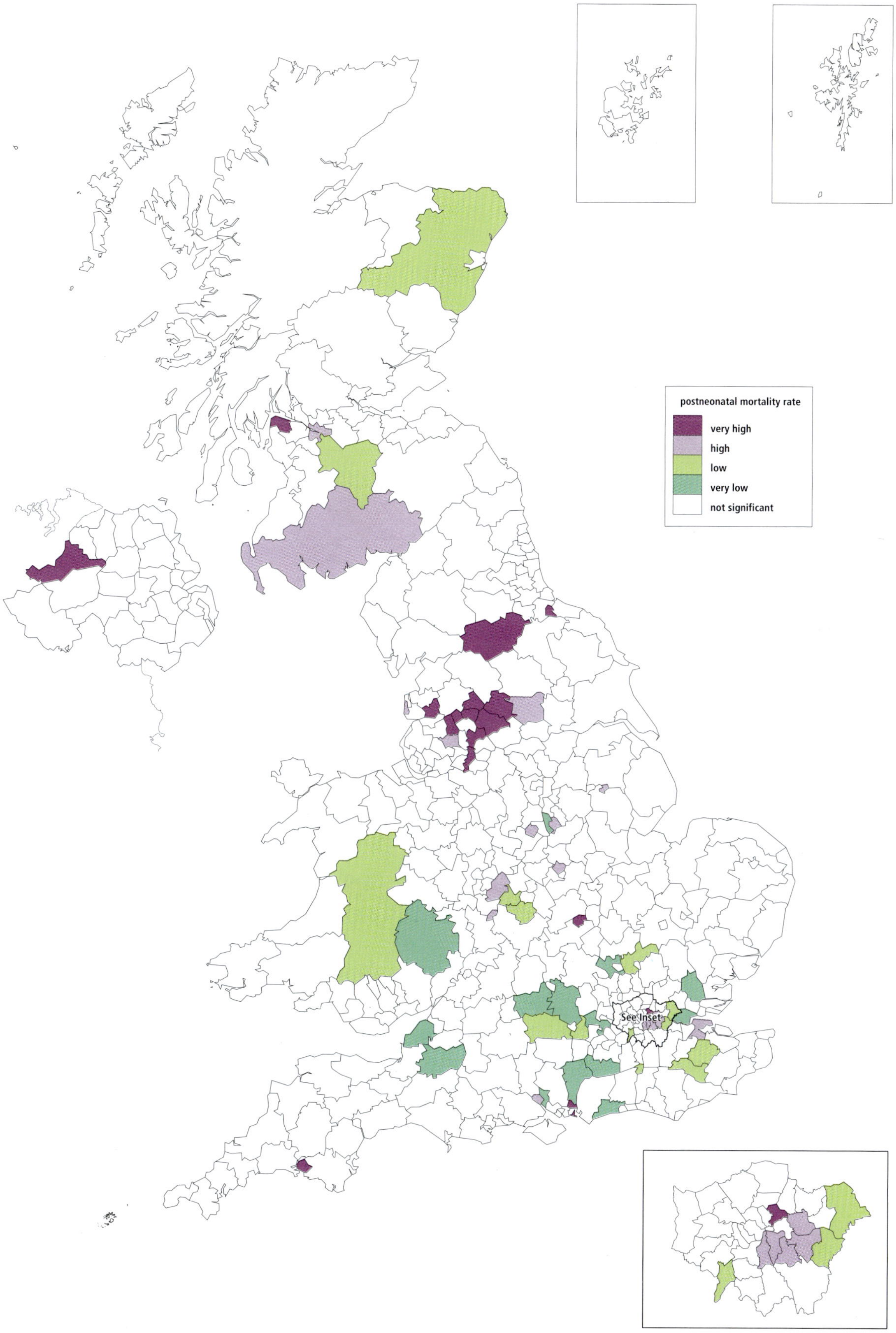

Map 6.5

Infant mortality rates by local authority
United Kingdom 1991-1997

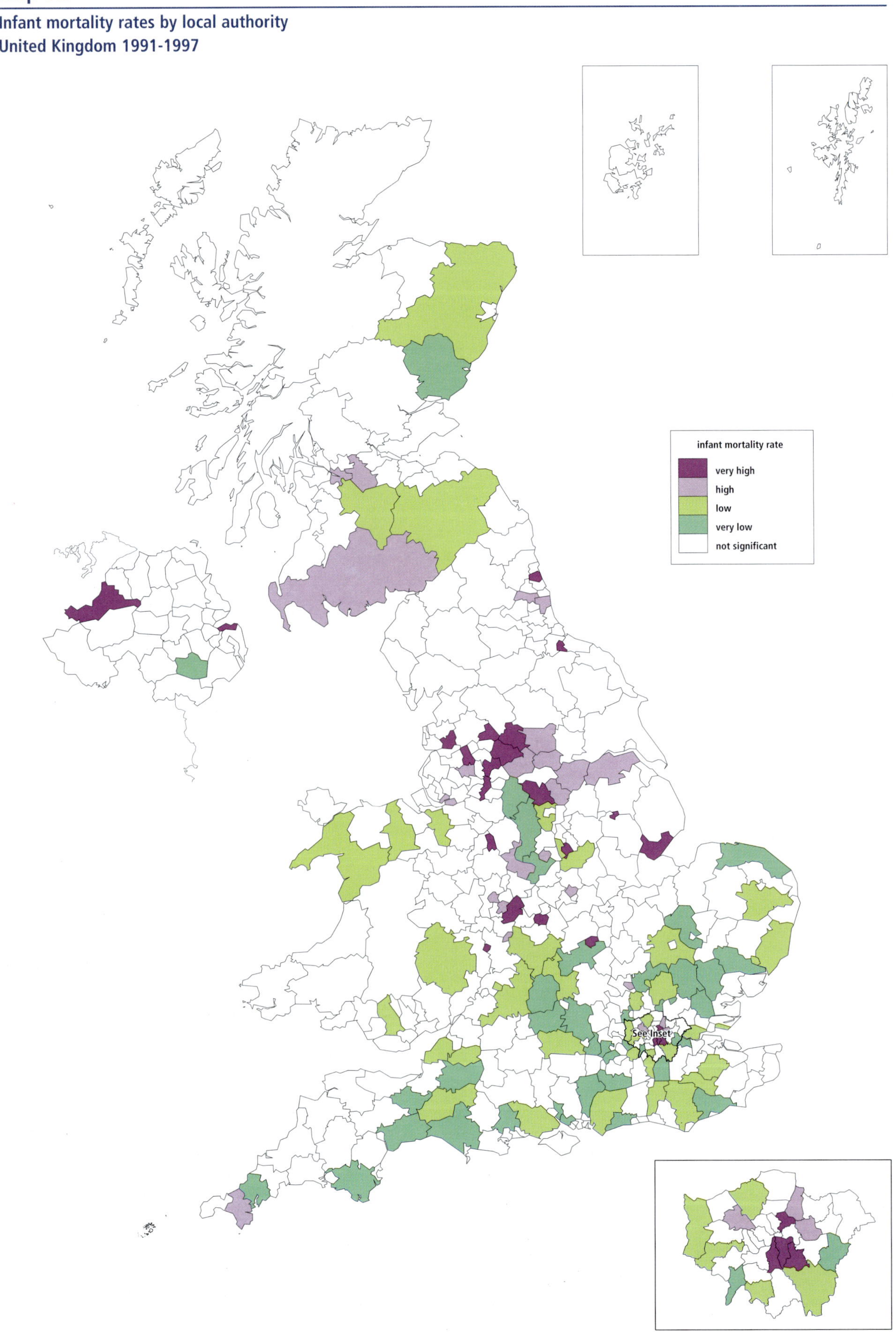

Figure 6.9

**Stillbirth and early neonatal components of perinatal mortality rates by ONS classification Group
Great Britain 1993-1997**

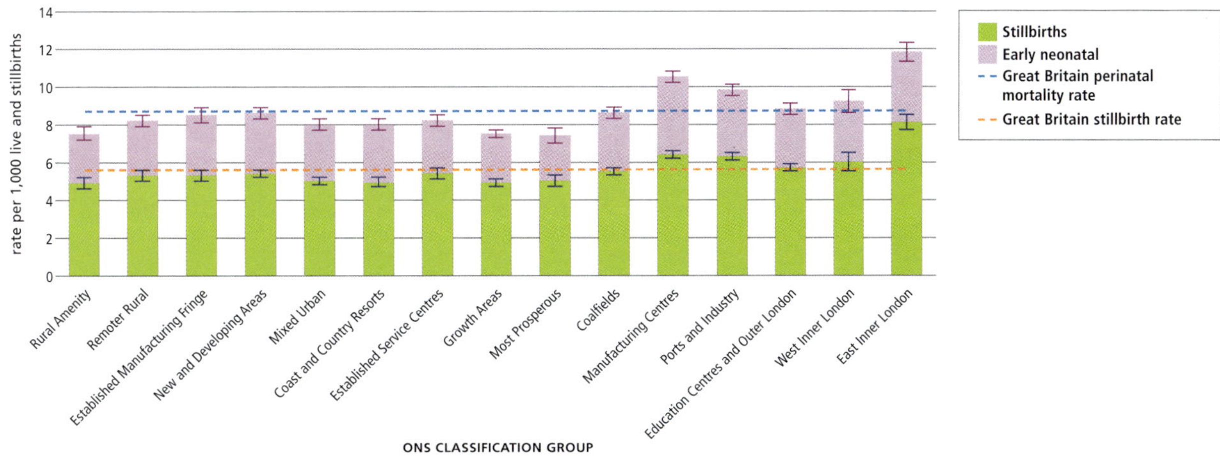

Figure 6.10

**Neonatal and postneonatal components of infant mortality rates by ONS classification Group
Great Britain 1991-1997**

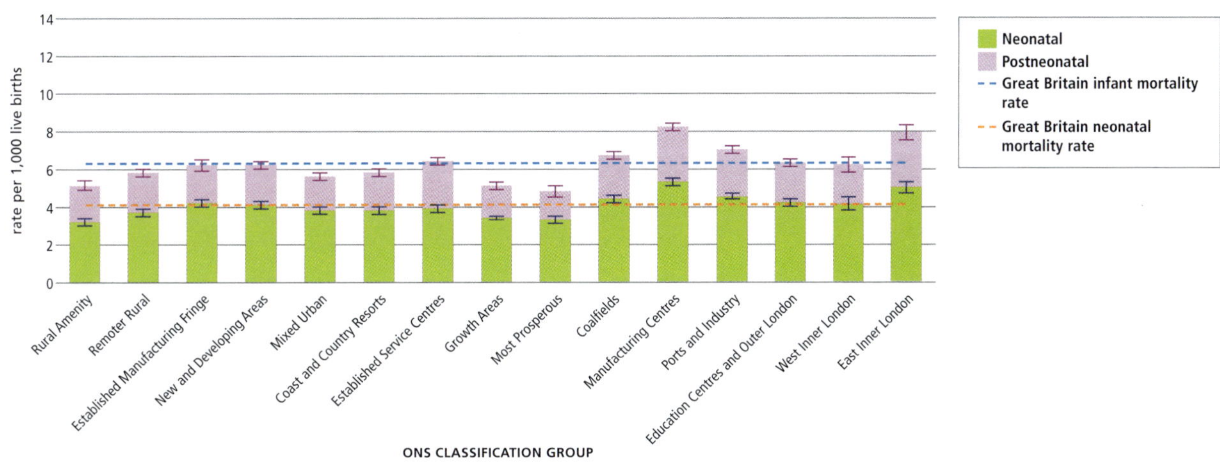

very high mortality were in this Group, compared to eight of the 17 authorities with very high postneonatal mortality.

The *Most Prosperous, Growth Areas* and *Rural Amenity* Groups tended to have low rates for most measures of infant death. Between 35 and 40 per cent of authorities with low mortality were in the *Most Prosperous* Group alone. The characteristics of these areas include low unemployment, high employment in finance and service occupations, a high proportion of the population in Social Class I or II and a high proportion of owner occupied housing.

6.3 Geographic variations in stillbirths and infant mortality by deprivation

The association between stillbirth and infant death rates and deprivation is very complex. Many previous studies have found a positive association between stillbirth rates and deprivation

scores.[8] However, this pattern has been shown to vary throughout England and Wales[8] and other studies, for example using the ONS Longitudinal Study, have found that stillbirth rates were not associated with deprivation.[9] A previous study examining perinatal deaths in the North West Thames Health Region showed that babies born in the most deprived areas had a 16 per cent greater rate of perinatal death than the average for that region and those born in the least deprived areas had an 11 per cent lower rate than the average for that region.[10] This study also suggested that between 1.3 per cent and 14.2 per cent of perinatal deaths would not have occurred if perinatal death rates in the most deprived areas were the same as those areas with average levels of deprivation.

This section examines the pattern of stillbirth and infant mortality rates by the Carstairs and Morris index of deprivation within Great Britain and within the countries of Great Britain and the regions of England. Data for Northern Ireland are not

Figure 6.11

Stillbirth rates by deprivation, country and region
Great Britain 1993-1997

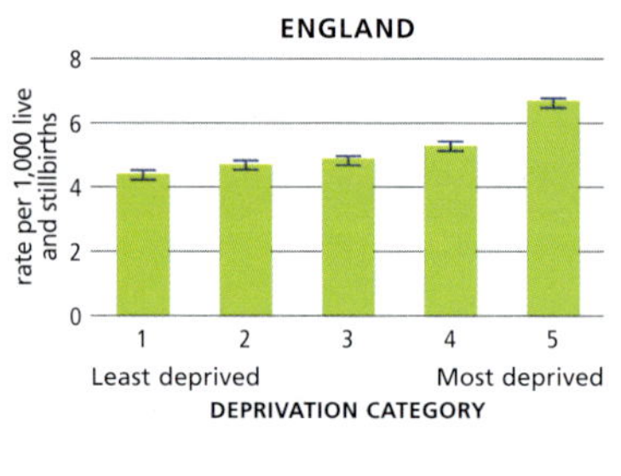

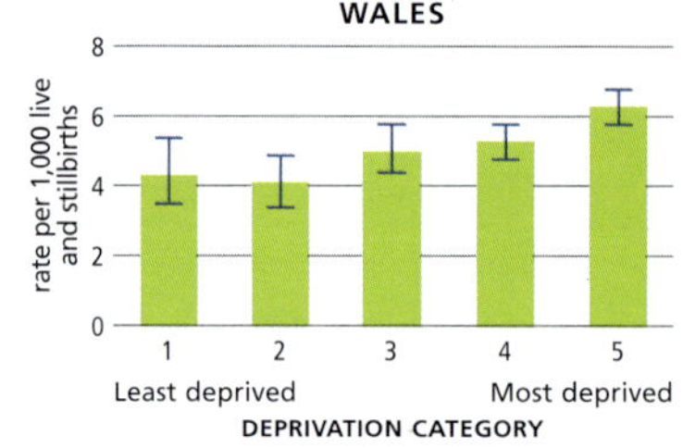

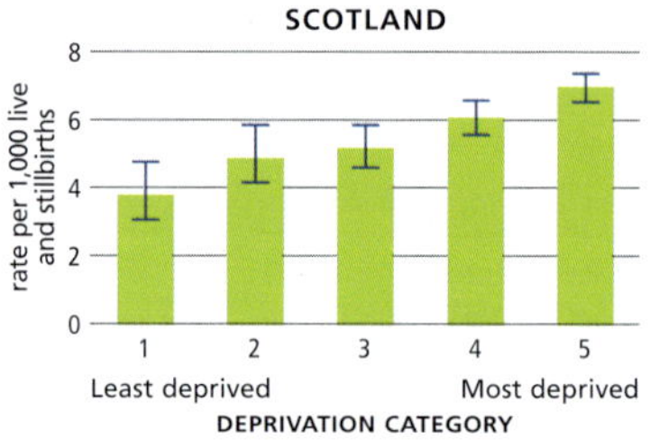

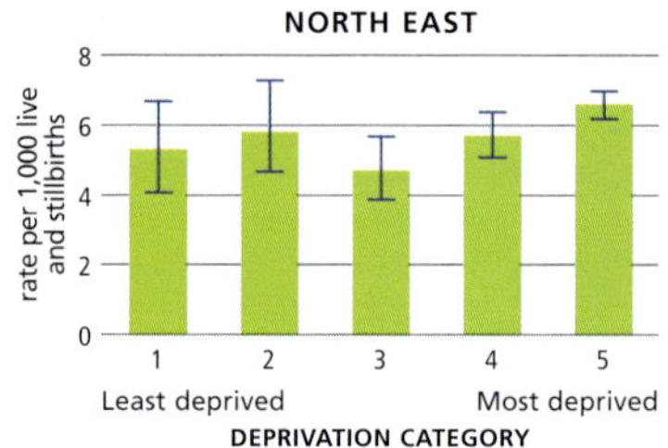

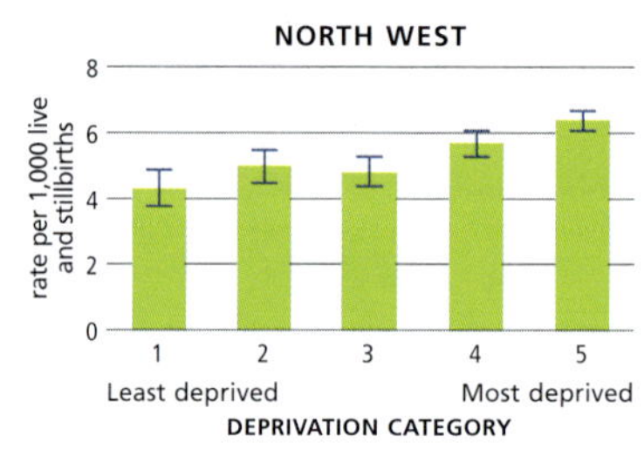

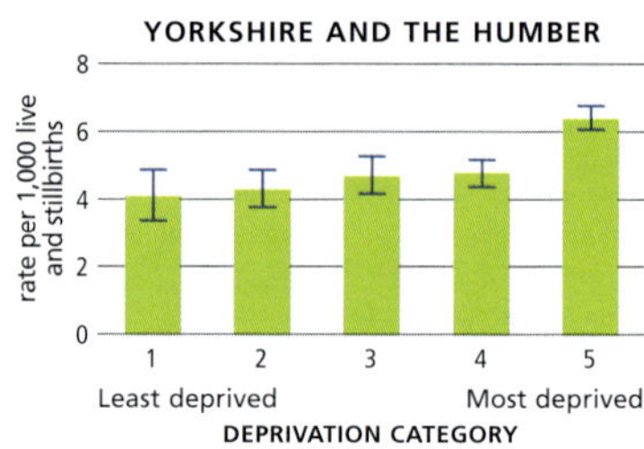

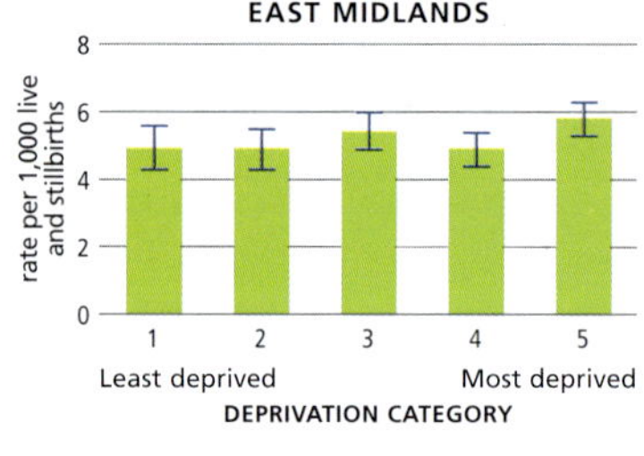

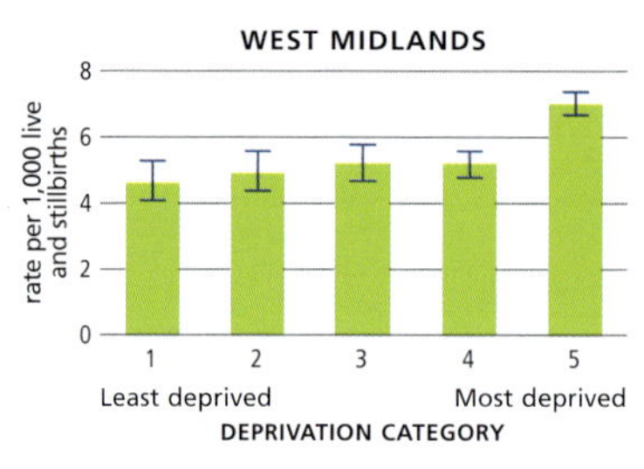

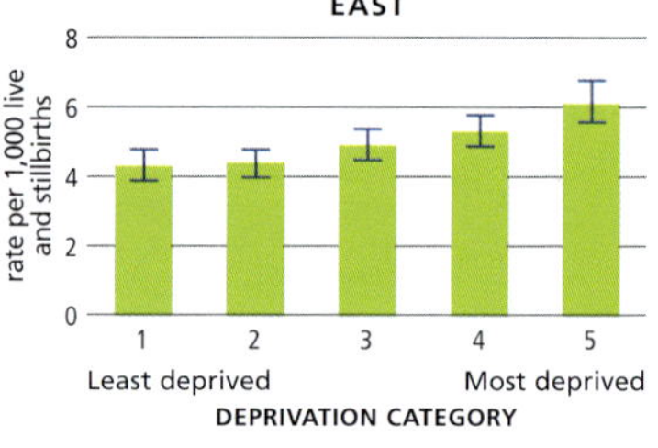

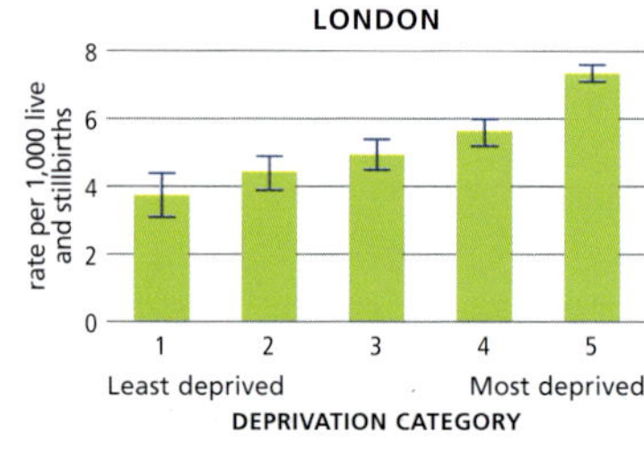

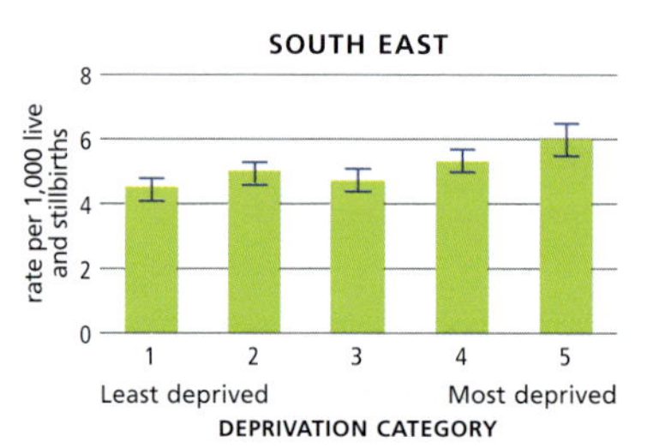

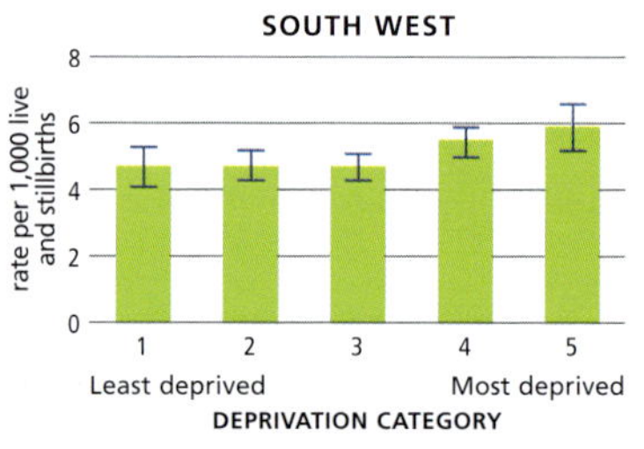

Figure 6.12

Perinatal mortality rates by deprivation, country and region
Great Britain 1993-1997

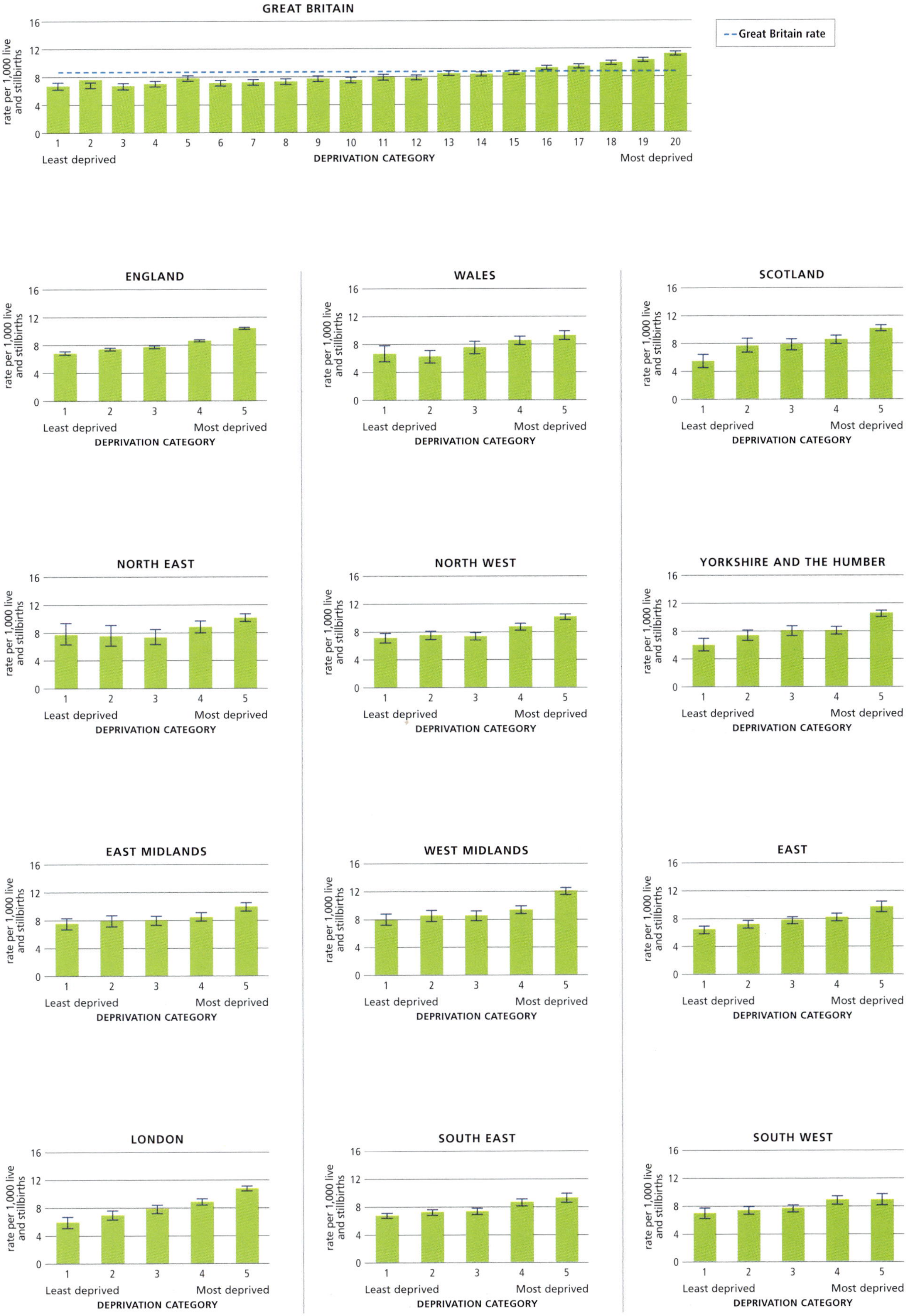

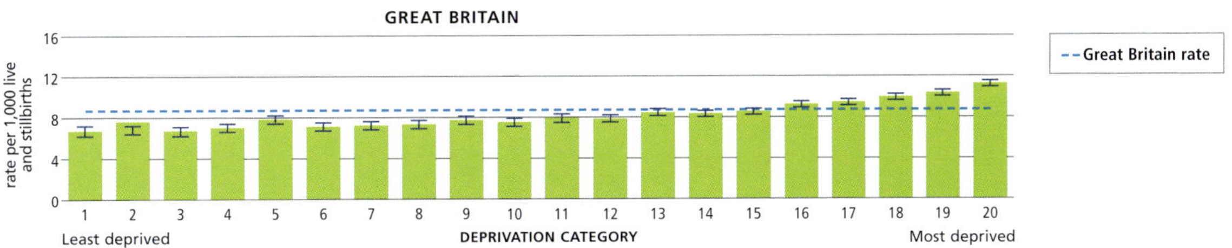

Figure 6.13

Neonatal mortality rates by deprivation, country and region
Great Britain 1991-1997

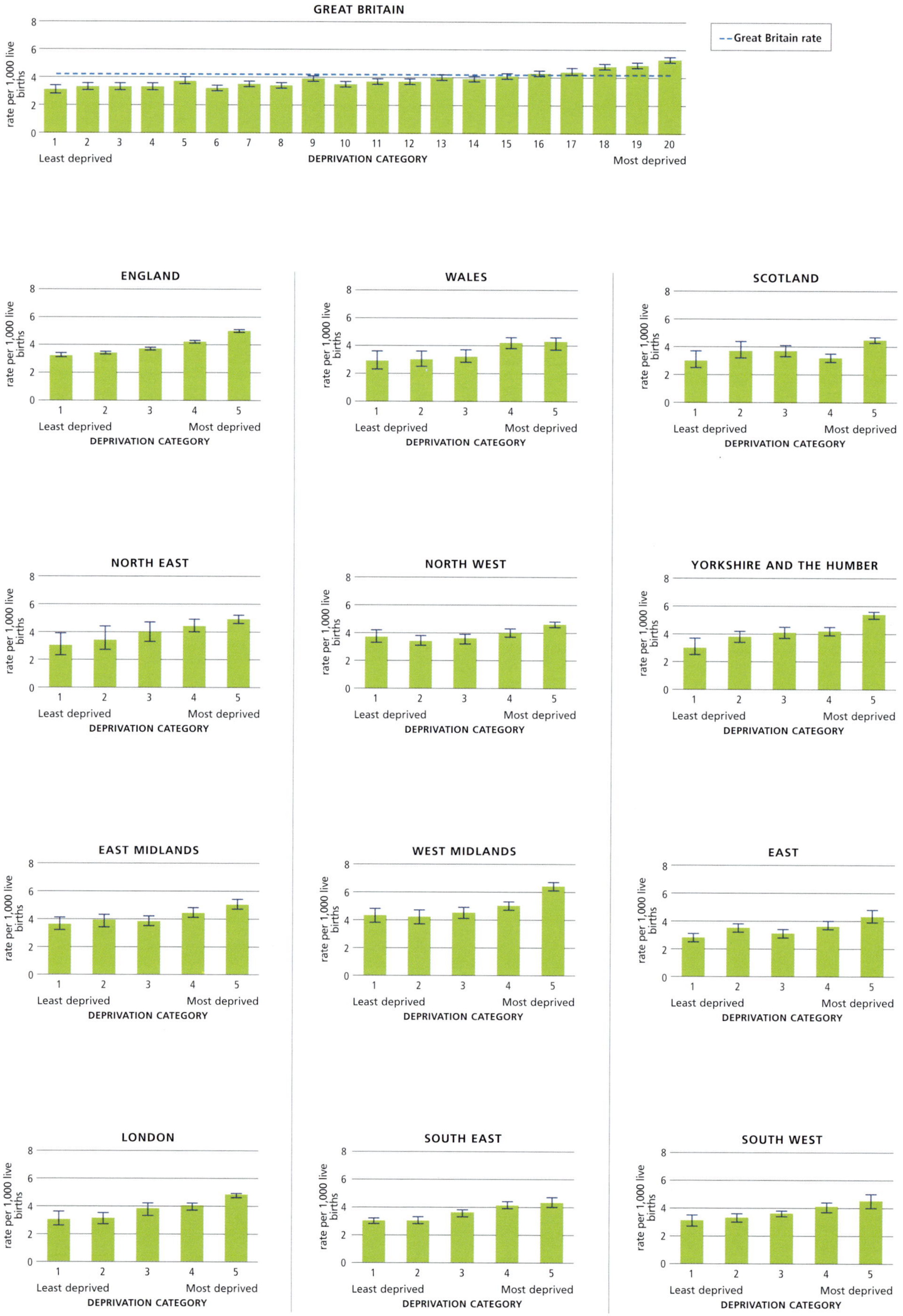

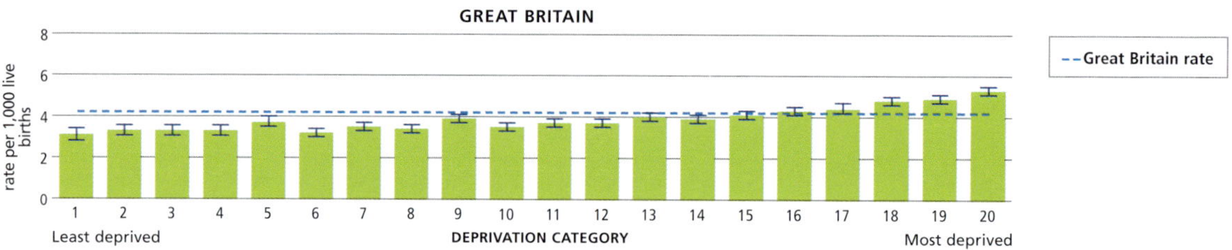

Figure 6.14

Postneonatal mortality rates by deprivation, country and region
Great Britain 1991-1997

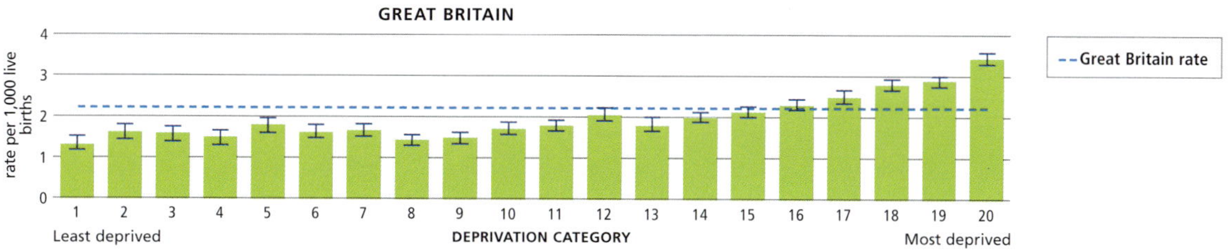

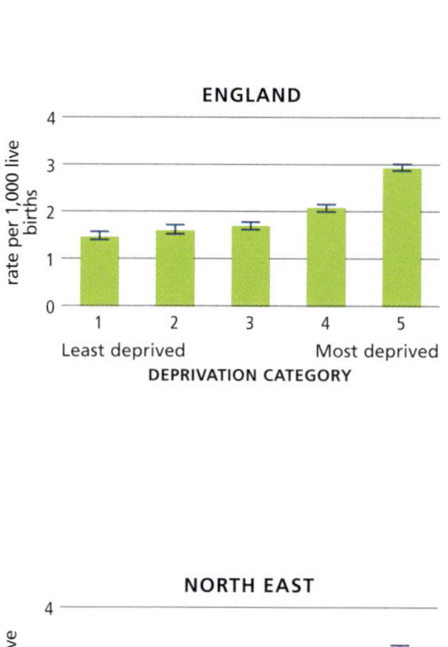

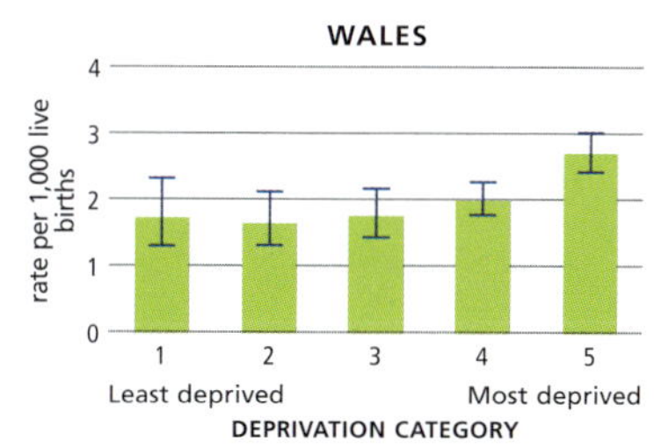

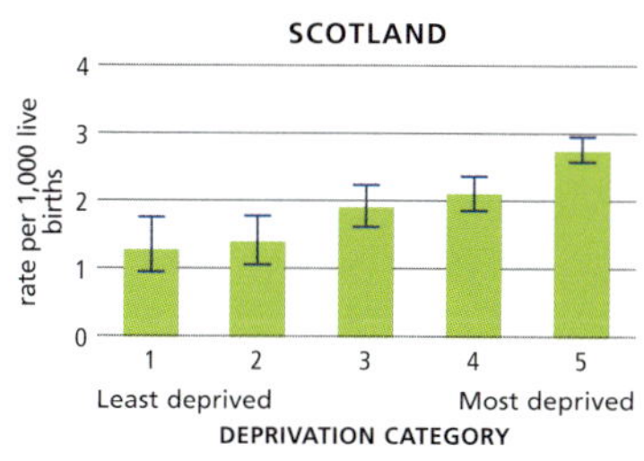

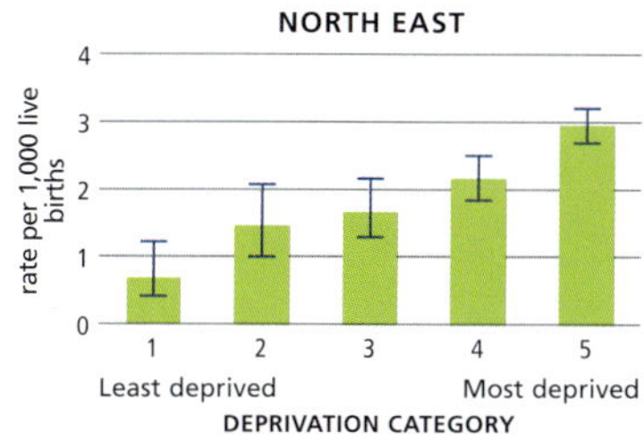

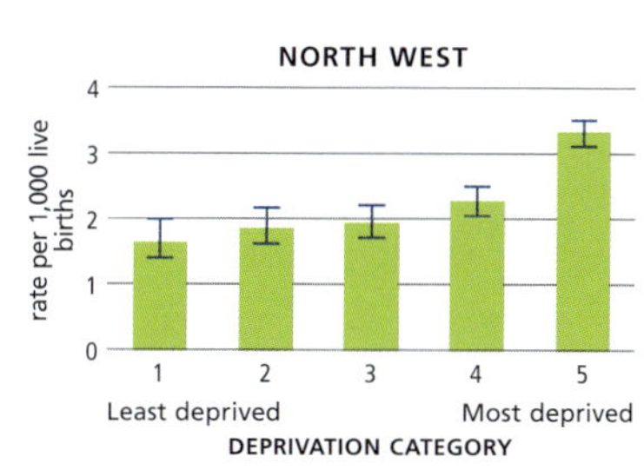

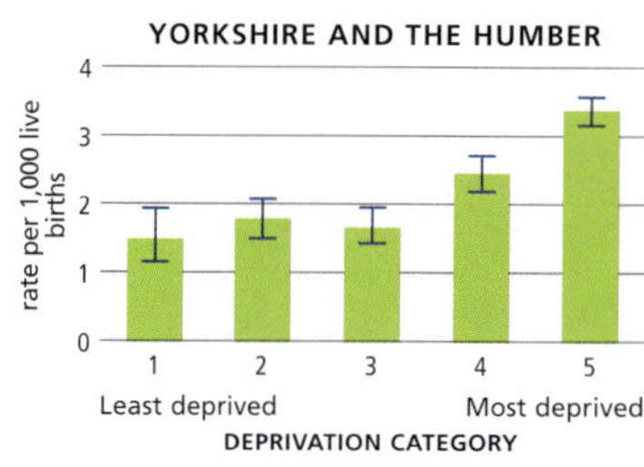

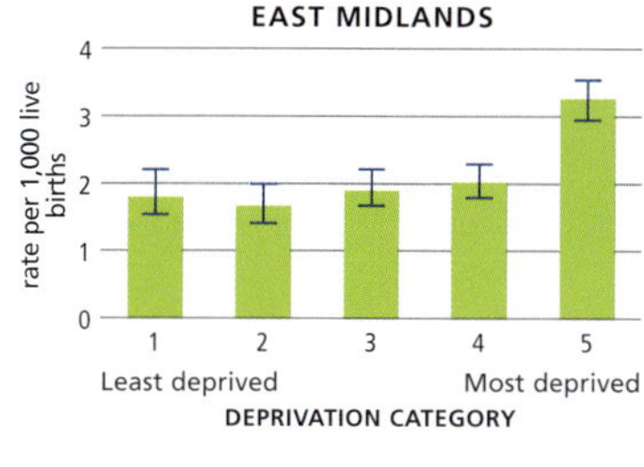

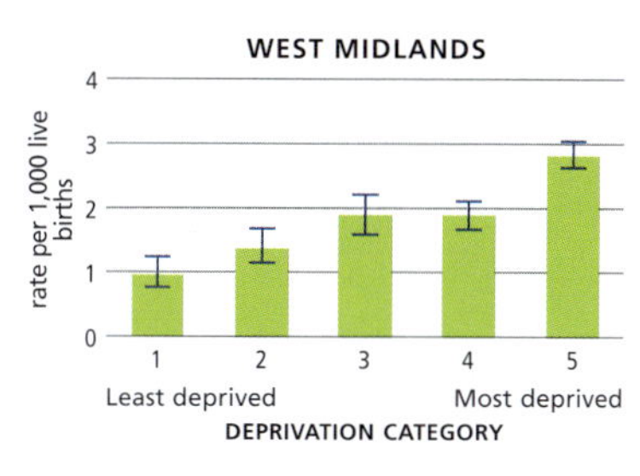

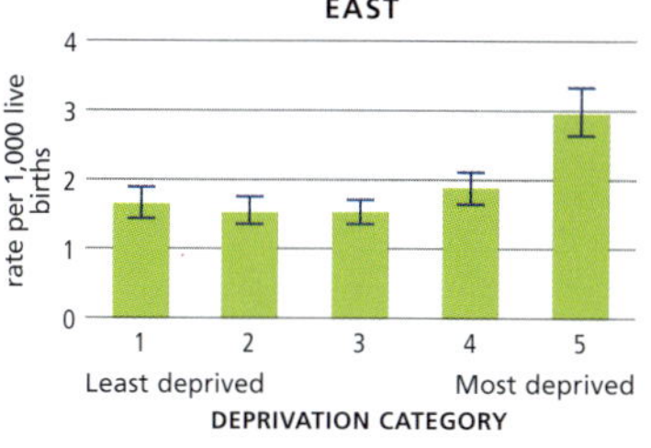

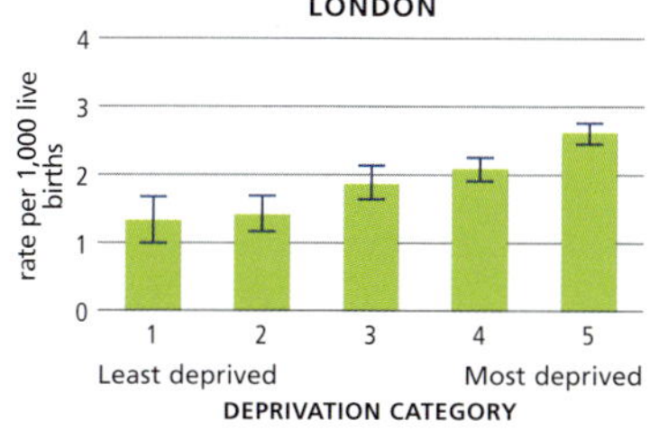

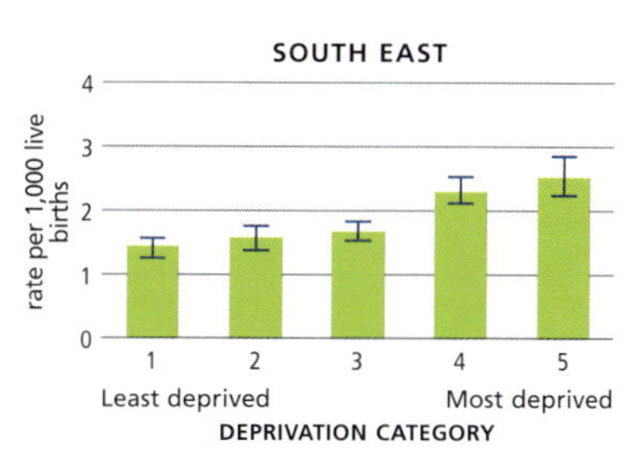

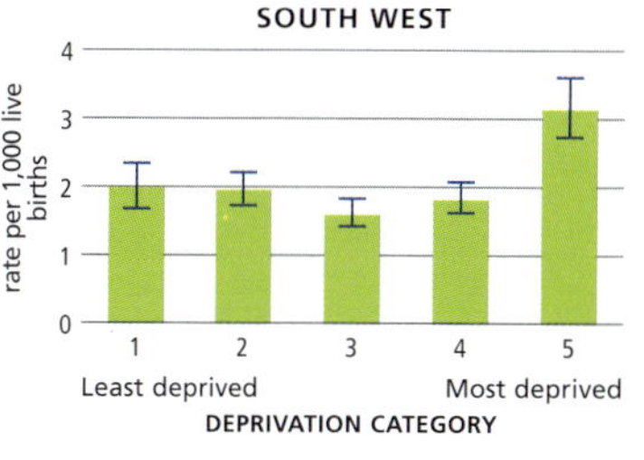

Figure 6.15

Infant mortality rates by deprivation, country and region
Great Britain 1991-1997

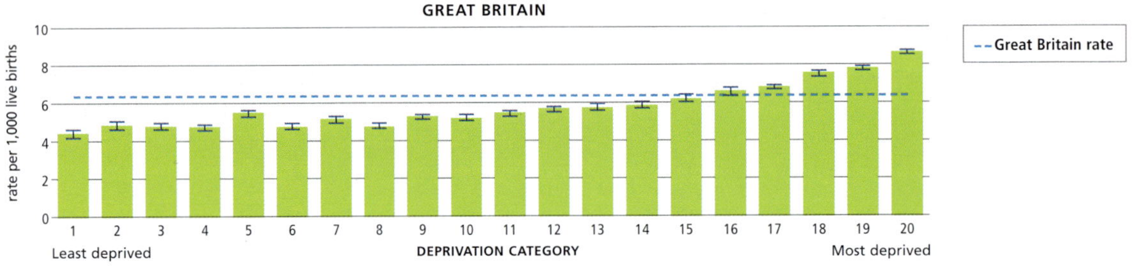

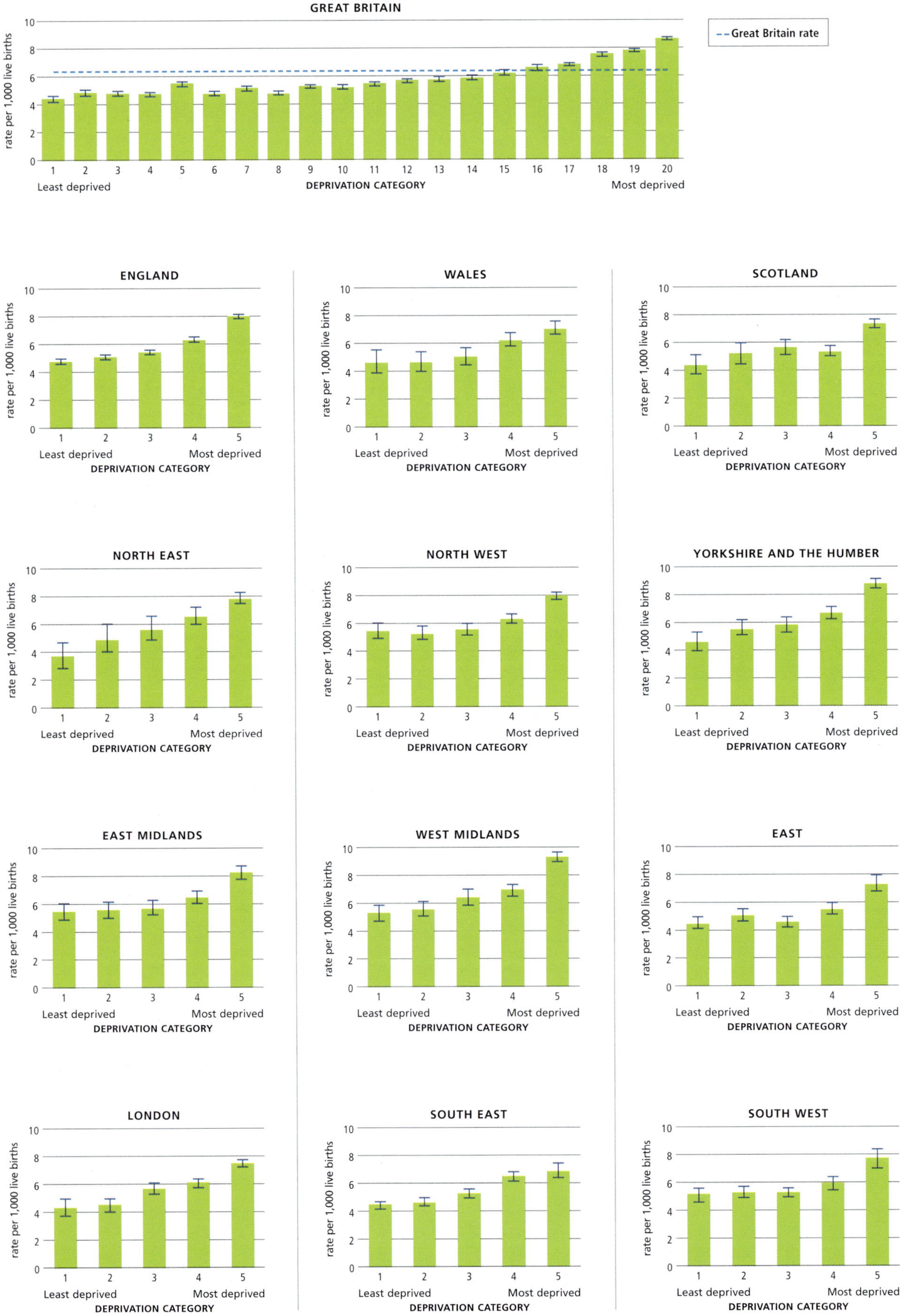

included in this section as a comparable deprivation index for Northern Ireland is not available. Figures 6.11-6.15 show stillbirth and infant mortality rates by this deprivation index. They show rates by deprivation twentieth within Great Britain and rates by deprivation quintile within countries of Great Britain and within regions of England. Chapter 4 describes the deprivation index and the method of allocating a deprivation score to stillbirths and infant deaths.

The analysis of stillbirths and infant mortality by deprivation twentieth in Great Britain shows that for stillbirths and every measure of infant mortality there was a gradual increase in rates with increasing deprivation. Between the first 15 categories the gradient was much flatter, particularly for neonatal, postneonatal and infant mortality. The greatest differences in rates by deprivation were seen in the last five deprivation twentieths.

This relationship between deprivation and stillbirths and infant mortality was apparent in the analysis by deprivation quintile for England. For England, the figures show that stillbirth and infant mortality rates increased with increasing deprivation. Generally, the increase in rates between the first four quintiles was gradual and those within the most deprived quintile had much higher rates than all other quintiles. With the exception of postneonatal mortality, this was not the case for Scotland and Wales. In Scotland and Wales some measures such as stillbirths showed a gradual increase in rates between deprivation quintiles, while for other measures of infant death such as neonatal mortality there was little difference in rates by deprivation quintile.

Within the regions of England a mixed pattern emerged. The population of each region was not evenly divided between each quintile as the quintiles were determined at the Great Britain level (see chapter 4 for further explanation) therefore it is important to take note of the confidence interval around all rates presented in this section. A number of regions showed a similar pattern to that for the country as a whole; particularly the North West, Yorkshire and the Humber, the West Midlands, the East of England and the East Midlands. Flatter gradients were seen in other regions; the South West and the South East. The pattern in the North East varied between the different measures of infant mortality and for stillbirths, largely as a result of the large confidence intervals attached to rates in the first 4 quintiles. Nearly 50 per cent of the population of the North East lived in areas classified to the most deprived quintile, therefore rates for other quintiles tended to be less reliable. London, however, showed the most striking pattern. The gradient of increasing stillbirths, perinatal deaths and infant deaths with increasing deprivation was very clear.

6.4 Discussion

This chapter shows that within England, regions in the north and the Midlands had higher stillbirth and infant mortality rates than regions in the south, but there was little variation between countries of the United Kingdom. There is widespread

concern that improvements in health have been a result of declining mortality and health improvement confined to the most affluent parts of society. Previous studies have found no evidence of a change in inequality over time within England and Wales as a whole, but in some parts of the country inequality has declined.[8] We have studied trends in neonatal, postneonatal and infant mortality throughout the 1990s by country and region. Rates of all three measures by region converged over this time period with the differential between the highest and lowest region being smaller in 1995-1997 than 1991-1993 and at country level, the gap in overall infant mortality fell over the period studied in this chapter.

It is also clear from this chapter that patterns by country and region mask wide variations in stillbirths and infant mortality between local authorities. Within countries and regions, the highest rates tended to be found in urban areas. The ONS classification of local authorities has been used to describe the characteristics of local authorities within Great Britain with higher than average rates of stillbirth or infant death. Areas with high unemployment, a high proportion of the population in Social Class IV or V, a high proportion of terraced and social housing and a high proportion of the population with a limiting long standing illness tended to have the highest rates of stillbirth and infant mortality. In addition, areas with large minority ethnic populations, large families and a high proportion of lone parent households also had high rates of stillbirth and perinatal mortality. Many of these characteristics have been shown to be related to infant mortality.[11]

We have shown that when areas were classified using the Carstairs and Morris index of deprivation there was an association between this and rates of stillbirth and infant mortality. This pattern was visible within most countries of the United Kingdom and regions of England. Within deprivation categories there was little difference in risk of stillbirth or infant death between countries and regions which suggests that differences in the proportion living in deprived areas alone accounts for the differences in rates between countries and regions.

The increased risk of stillbirth and infant death in more deprived communities could be a result of many different factors. The risk of infant death has been shown to be much greater in babies with a birthweight of less than 2,500 grams.[5] Chapter 7 looks at the variation in the percentage of babies born with a low birthweight by region of England and its contribution to variations in infant mortality rates. Research in the West Midlands region has found an association between perinatal death and deprivation for those with birthweight under 2,500 grams, but not for those with birthweight under 1,500 grams.[12]

Chapter 5 in this volume examines teenage births by deprivation and shows clearly that deprived areas had much higher teenage birth rates than non-deprived areas. Other analysis using a wide range of data on teenage pregnancy showed that, compared with all births, babies born to teenagers had higher rates of infant mortality and a higher percentage of babies are born with a low birthweight.[13] Analysis of the known risk factors of infant mortality in chapter 7 helps to explain some of the variations in infant mortality. It confirms findings from earlier studies and shows that babies born to teenage mothers had high rates of infant death. It also confirms that rates of infant death were clearly related to father's Social Class. The proportion of the population in Social Classes IV or V is a variable included in the deprivation index, the most deprived areas have a larger proportion of the population in Social Class IV or V. Chapter 5 also demonstrates that babies born in deprived areas were more likely to be born outside marriage and chapter 7 shows that babies born outside marriage had an increased risk of infant death. However, many other factors, not easily measured or not collected, could have influenced the patterns presented in this chapter, such as household income, infant feeding, the environment, quality of treatment, ethnicity and parity.

References

1 World Health Organisation. *A WHO report on social and biological effects on perinatal mortality*. Volume 1. Statistical Publishing House (Budapest: 1978).

2 West R. Perinatal and infant mortality in Wales; inter-district variations and associations with socio-environmental characteristics. *International Journal of Epidemiology* 17 (1988), 382-396.

3 Dattani N and Cooper N. Trends in cot deaths. *Health Statistics Quarterly* 5 (2000), 10-16.

4 Office for Population Censuses and Surveys. *Occupational mortality. The Registrar General Decennial Supplement for England and Wales 1970-1972*. Series DS no. 1. HMSO (London: 1978), 182.

5 Botting B and Macfarlane A. Geographic variation in infant mortality in relation to birthweight 1983-85 in Britton M. (ed.) *Mortality and Geography* Series DS no. 9. HMSO (London: 1990).

6 Office for National Statistics. *The ONS classification of local and health authorities: revised for authorities in 1999*. Series SMPS no. 63. The Stationery Office (London: 1999).

7 Carstairs V and Morris R. *Deprivation and health in Scotland*. Aberdeen University Press (Aberdeen: 1991).

8 Dummer T, Dickinson H, Pearce M, Charlton M and Parker L. Stillbirth risk with Social Class and deprivation: no evidence for increasing inequality. *Journal of Clinical Epidemiology* 53 (2000), 147-155.

9 Sloggett A and Joshi H. Deprivation indicators as predictors of life events 1981-1992 based on United Kingdom longitudinal study. *Journal of Epidemiology and Community Health* 52 (1998), 228-233.

10 Martuzzi M. Perinatal mortality in an English health region; geographic distribution and association with socio-economic factors. *Paediatric and Perinatal Epidemiology* 12 (1998), 263-276.

11 Macfarlane A and Mugford M. *Birth counts: statistics of pregnancy and childbirth*. The Stationery Office (London: 2000).

12 Bambang S, Spencer N, Logan S and Gill L. Cause-specific perinatal death rates, birth weight and deprivation in the West Midlands, 1991-93. *Child: Care, Health and Development* 26 (2000), 73-82.

13 Botting B, Rosato M and Wood R. Teenage mothers and the health of their children. *Population Trends* 93 (1998), 19-28.

Analysis of infant mortality rates by risk factors and by cause of death in England and Wales

Nicola Cooper

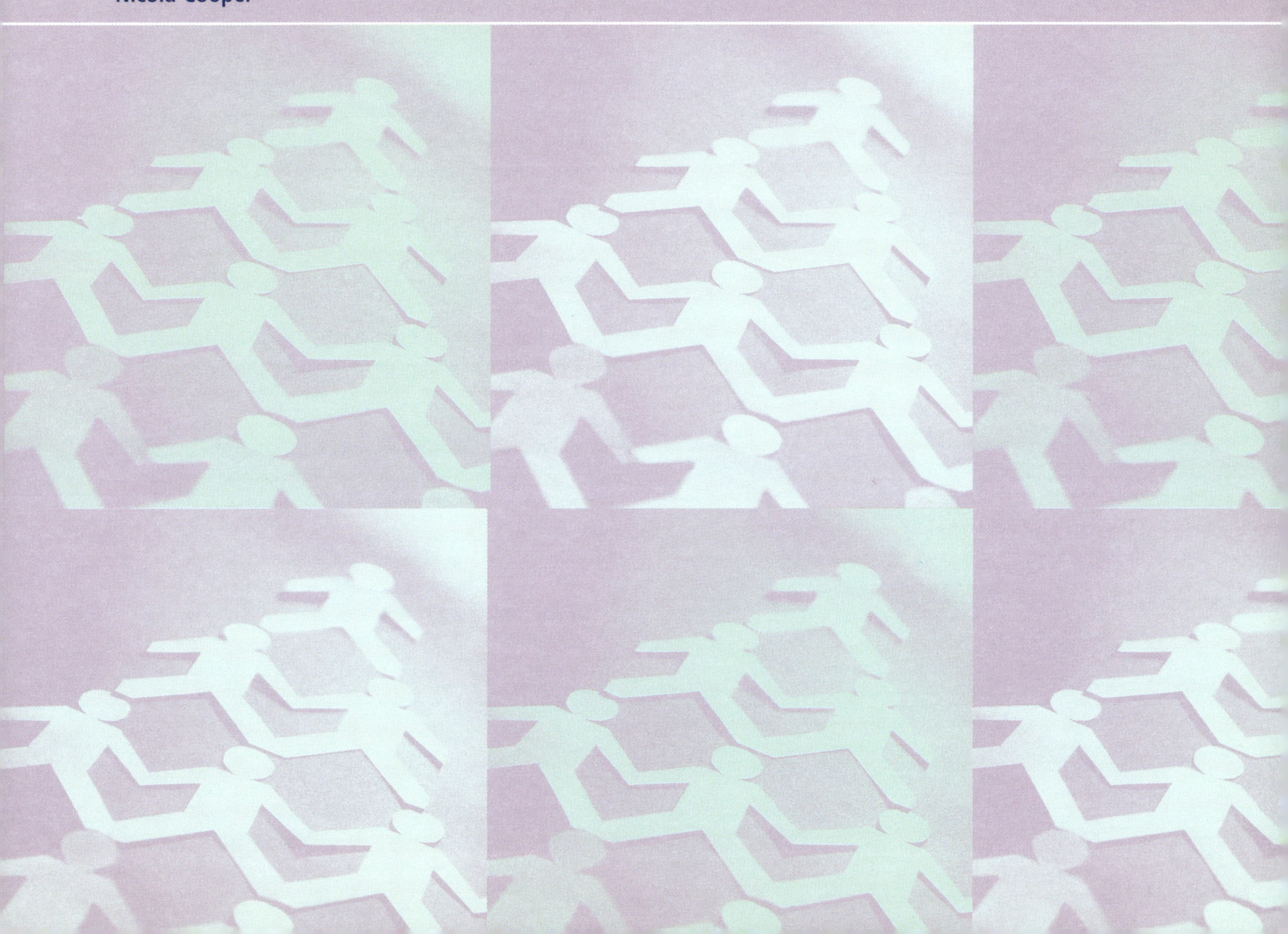

Chapter 7

Analysis of infant mortality rates by risk factors and by cause of death in England and Wales

Summary

- After accounting for very low birthweight (<1,500 grams), the West Midlands still had a high infant mortality rate; with London and the South East having low rates.

- The North West and Yorkshire and the Humber both had high infant mortality rates for babies weighing 2,500 grams or more, the East of England and South East had low rates.

- Geographic differences in infant mortality persisted for mothers aged 20-29 and 30-39, with Yorkshire and the Humber and the West Midlands having higher rates and regions of the south having lower rates.

- Geographic differences in infant mortality still existed for babies born inside marriage. However, for babies born outside marriage and registered by both parents, only the East Midlands had a high infant mortality rate.

- London had a higher infant mortality rate for babies born outside marriage and registered by the mother alone. Equivalent analysis of ONS classification Groups found that *East Inner London* and *West Inner London* both had higher rates.

- When Social Class was accounted for, excess infant mortality for regions was removed from Social Class I, II and V. The geographic differences persisted in Social Classes IIIN, IIIM and IV, with higher rates in the West Midlands and lower rates in the South East. Wales had a significantly lower infant mortality rate for Social Class IIIM.

- Regional differences remained in the infant mortality rates after accounting for mothers born outside England and Wales, with higher rates in Yorkshire and the Humber and the West Midlands and a lower rate in the East of England.

- Babies of mothers born in Scotland and resident in the North East had a higher infant mortality rate. The East Midlands had a higher infant mortality rate for babies born to resident mothers from an 'Other European Union' country. Babies of mothers born in Pakistan and resident in London had a lower infant mortality rate.

- Regional differences persisted for infant deaths from congenital anomalies and immaturity-related conditions, with a higher rate for Yorkshire and the Humber and the West Midlands, and lower rates in the East of England and the South East.

- The North East and North West had higher infant mortality rates from sudden infant death, and the East of England and South East had lower rates.

7.1 Introduction

This chapter looks at geographic variations in overall infant mortality rates by known risk factors[1] for the period 1993-1997 within England and Wales only. The risk factors that were available for analysis were birthweight, mother's age, marital status, Social Class and mother's country of birth. Chapter 6 has already shown that Wales had lower infant mortality than England between 1991 and 1997, and that there was a north-south divide in infant mortality rates within England. In particular, Yorkshire and the Humber and the West Midlands had the highest infant mortality and the East of England, South East and the South West the lowest infant mortality. This section aims to determine whether regional differences in infant mortality persist after controlling for available risk factors. The chapter also analyses infant mortality by cause of death.

7.2 Methods and data

Apart from details about the child's sex, area of residence and occupation of his or her parents, death records do not include the fuller range of information recorded at birth registration. Information on birthweight, mother's age, marital status and mother's country of birth are all collected at birth registration only. For this reason, ONS has linked the death records of infants registered in England and Wales to their corresponding birth records since 1975. In Scotland, there is no routine linkage of birth and infant death registration data, even though extensive facilities for record linkage have been developed.[2] There is no routine linkage of data from birth and infant death registration in Northern Ireland. This chapter, therefore, analyses data for England and Wales only. It also presents data for regions within England and by ONS classification Group.

All babies born between 1st January 1993 and 31st December 1997 (where the mother's residence is known) are included in this analysis. Details of all deaths to babies born in this time period have been obtained and linked to their corresponding birth record. For the individual years 1993-1997, between 1 and 2.3 per cent of infant deaths were not linked to their respective birth records and are therefore excluded from this analysis.

Deaths in the first year of life are becoming increasingly rare. Therefore, to analyse data for Government Office Regions, it was necessary to aggregate data over several years. To examine the geographic variations in infant mortality by known risk factors, data for the years 1993-1997 have been combined.

Table 7.1

Live births and infant mortality rates[+] by birthweight, country and region England and Wales 1993-1997

	Percentage of live births with birthweight stated	Percentage of live births[++]			Number of infant deaths					Infant mortality rate[+]			
		<1,500	<2,500	2,500+	with birthweight stated	<1,500	<2,500	2,500+		with birthweight stated	<1,500	<2,500	2,500+
England and Wales	98.7	1.2	7.2	92.8	19,304	8,494	11,509	7,795		6.0	227.9	49.7	2.6
England	98.7	1.2	7.2	92.8	18,311	8,075	10,933	7,378		6.0	228.0	49.7	2.6
Wales	98.7	1.1	6.7	93.3	993	419	576	417		5.7	226.4	49.2	2.6
North East	99.5	1.1	7.3	92.7	973	396	562	411		6.3	231.0	49.8	2.9
North West	98.3	1.1	7.4	92.6	2,679	1,107	1,541	1,138		* 6.3	229.4	49.4	* 2.9
Yorkshire and the Humber	99.2	1.2	7.5	92.5	2,167	924	1,243	924		* 7.0	246.9	52.8	* 3.2
East Midlands	98.9	1.2	7.2	92.8	1,496	667	913	583		6.0	234.2	50.9	2.5
West Midlands	99.1	1.3	7.9	92.1	2,327	1,077	1,462	865		* 6.9	* 251.9	* 55.1	2.8
East	99.2	1.0	6.5	93.5	1,724	772	1,040	684		~ 5.3	229.9	49.3	~ 2.2
London	97.0	1.3	7.8	92.2	3,056	1,445	1,907	1,149		6.0	~ 211.5	48.4	2.5
South East	98.9	1.0	6.5	93.5	2,347	997	1,349	998		~ 4.9	~ 209.1	~ 43.8	~ 2.2
South West	99.3	1.1	6.6	93.4	1,542	690	916	626		5.6	225.5	50.4	2.4

[+] rate per 1,000 live births

[++] number of live births of stated birthweight (eg <1,500 grams) as a percentage of all live births for which birthweight is known.

* significantly higher than the England and Wales rate

~ signifcantly lower than the England and Wales rate

7.3 Birthweight

A number of studies have found birthweight to be the single most important risk factor for infant mortality.[3,4] The birthweight of a baby may be influenced by social and economic factors prior to the birth. These factors can result in preterm delivery or poor fetal growth with low birthweight. Preterm delivery is also an important risk factor for infant death, but gestation length is not recorded at birth registration in England and Wales.

Previous analysis of singleton live births by birthweight between 1982-1996, shows that the proportion of babies at the upper end of the distribution rose over the period. This suggests that overall, the average birthweight of a singleton has increased.[5,6] In addition, the percentage of low birthweight babies continued to rise in the late 1980s and 1990s.[7] This can be attributed to a rise in the registration of babies weighing under 1,000 grams and to a rise in multiple births. This is thought to be largely due to the increasing survival rate of very preterm babies as a result of improvements in the intensive care received.

The World Health Organisation definitions of birthweight are shown in Box 7.1.

Between 1989 and 1993 ONS's predecessor stopped investigating cases where the birth information was not recorded at birth registration. Subsequently, the number of live birth records with birthweight missing was 3.3 per cent in 1993. During 1994, these investigations were re-introduced, so that by 1997 birthweight was not stated for only 0.17 per cent of all live births.[9] Therefore, any mention of the percentage of live births by birthweight refers to the percentage of stated birthweight, where the birthweight was stated at birth registration.

> **Box 7.1**
>
> **WHO definitions of birthweight**
>
> **Birthweight:** The first weight of the fetus or newborn obtained after birth.
> **Extremely low birthweight:** Less than 1,000g (up to and including 999g).
> **Very low birthweight:** Less than 1,500g (up to and including 1,499g).
> **Low birthweight:** Less than 2,500g (up to and including 2,499g).
>
> Source: *International statistical classification of diseases and related health problems, tenth revision* (1992).[8]

Table 7.2

Live births and infant mortality rates[+] by birthweight and ONS classification Group England and Wales 1993-1997

	Percentage of live births with birthweight stated	Percentage of live births[++]			Number of infant deaths					Infant mortality rate[+]			
		<1,500	<2,500	2,500+	with birthweight stated	<1,500	<2,500	2,500+		with birthweight stated	<1,500	<2,500	2,500+
England and Wales	98.7	1.2	7.2	92.8	19,304	8,494	11,509	7,795		6.0	227.9	49.7	2.6
Rural Amenity	99.3	1.0	6.1	93.9	757	341	458	299		~ 4.8	218.2	48.3	~ 2.0
Remoter Rural	99.1	1.0	6.3	93.7	663	265	372	291		5.8	228.1	52.3	2.7
Established Manufacturing Fringe	98.7	1.1	6.9	93.1	1,001	435	604	397		5.9	231.5	51.7	2.5
New and Developing Areas	99.0	1.2	7.2	92.8	1,523	681	890	633		6.1	228.8	49.3	2.7
Mixed Urban	99.0	1.0	6.5	93.5	1,375	650	857	518		~ 5.3	240.1	50.9	~ 2.1
Coast and Country Resorts	98.8	1.1	6.6	93.4	1,215	519	695	520		5.7	224.8	49.4	2.6
Established Service Centres	99.2	1.2	7.4	92.6	1,207	508	706	501		6.1	215.8	48.2	2.7
Growth Areas	99.0	1.0	6.2	93.8	1,903	854	1,137	766		~ 4.8	219.3	46.2	~ 2.1
Most Prosperous	99.2	0.9	6.0	94.0	543	236	325	218		~ 4.5	216.7	44.8	~ 1.9
Coalfields	99.3	1.2	7.2	92.8	2,130	952	1,263	867		6.4	245.4	52.4	2.8
Manufacturing Centres	99.3	1.3	8.7	91.3	2,812	1,176	1,647	1,165		* 7.7	* 247.5	51.5	* 3.5
Ports and Industry	98.0	1.3	8.1	91.9	1,395	584	834	561		* 7.0	229.6	51.3	* 3.0
Education Centres and Outer London	97.7	1.3	7.7	92.3	1,619	732	992	627		5.8	~ 201.7	46.7	2.4
West Inner London	94.7	1.3	7.4	92.6	360	172	218	142		5.7	206.2	47.0	2.4
East Inner London	95.2	1.6	8.9	91.1	801	389	511	290		* 7.4	228.7	53.0	2.9

[+] rate per 1,000 live births

[++] number of live births of stated birthweight (eg <1,500 grams) as a percentage of all live births for which birthweight is known.

* sigificantly higher than the England and Wales rate

~ significantly lower than the England and Wales rate

England, Wales and Government Office Regions

Table 7.1 confirms findings from chapter 6 and shows that Wales had lower infant mortality than England between 1993 and 1997 and that within England, Yorkshire and the Humber and the West Midlands had the highest rates and the East of England, the South East and the South West the lowest.

Birthweight-specific infant mortality rates show that infant mortality decreases dramatically with increasing birthweight. In England, 1.2 per cent of all live births weigh less than 1,500 grams. In Wales this figure was 1.1 per cent. The infant mortality rate for England for babies born weighing less than 1,500 grams, was 228 per 1,000 live births; whilst the rate for Wales was 226. This was 38 times the overall infant mortality rate in England and 40 times the rate in Wales. This means that 1 in 5 of the around 1 per cent of live births weighing less than 1,500 grams, will die before completing one year of life.

Therefore, it is likely that areas with a large percentage of very low birthweight babies had higher infant mortality rates. However, within England, the West Midlands and London had the highest percentage of live births weighing less than 1,500 grams (1.3 per cent). Table 7.1 does show that the West

Midlands had the highest infant mortality rate of all regions of England for babies weighing less than 1,500 grams, but London had significantly lower infant mortality rates compared to England and Wales within this birthweight category. The rate ratio between the regions in England with the highest and lowest infant mortality rates, for babies weighing less than 1,500 grams was 1.2. This was less than the differential presented for the overall infant mortality rates in this table and in chapter 6 (Table 6.1).

In England, 7.2 per cent of live births had a birthweight less than 2,500 grams, compared to 6.7 per cent in Wales. Babies born weighing less than 2,500 grams in England had an infant mortality rate of 49.7 per 1,000 live births; in comparison, Wales had a rate of 49.2. West Midlands had the highest percentage (7.9 per cent) of babies born weighing less than 2,500 grams and the East of England and the South East the lowest (6.5 per cent). The West Midlands had a significantly higher infant mortality rate for babies born weighing less than 2,500 grams and the South East had a significantly lower rate.

The infant mortality rate for babies weighing 2,500 grams or more in both England and Wales, was 2.6 per 1,000 live births.

Table 7.3

Live births and infant mortality rates[+] by mother's age, country and region
England and Wales 1993-1997

	Percentage of live births				Number of infant deaths				Infant mortality rate[+]			
	<20	20-29	30-39	40+	<20	20-29	30-39	40+	<20	20-29	30-39	40+
England and Wales	6.7	53.8	37.7	1.8	2,135	10,828	6,939	462	9.7	6.2	5.6	8.0
England	6.6	53.6	38.0	1.8	2,019	10,236	6,616	443	9.9	6.2	5.6	8.1
Wales	8.8	57.1	32.7	1.5	116	592	323	19	~ 7.5	5.9	5.6	7.4
North East	10.0	56.4	32.5	1.2	155	548	278	13	10.1	6.3	5.6	7.0
North West	8.4	55.7	34.4	1.5	354	1,538	884	56	9.9	6.4	6.0	8.8
Yorkshire and the Humber	8.4	57.7	32.5	1.4	278	1,293	635	41	10.5	* 7.1	* 6.2	9.4
East Midlands	7.2	56.3	35.1	1.4	172	935	442	37	9.6	6.6	5.0	10.3
West Midlands	7.7	56.8	33.8	1.6	264	1,332	784	64	10.1	* 6.9	* 6.8	* 11.9
East	5.2	53.4	39.7	1.7	160	964	637	28	9.4	~ 5.5	~ 4.9	~ 5.0
London	4.9	48.5	44.2	2.5	266	1,585	1,396	96	10.4	6.2	6.0	7.3
South East	5.0	50.1	42.9	2.0	214	1,253	971	67	8.9	~ 5.2	~ 4.7	7.0
South West	5.7	53.7	38.8	1.8	156	788	589	41	9.9	~ 5.3	5.5	8.2

[+] rate per 1,000 live births

* significantly higher than the England and Wales rate

~ significantly lower than the England and Wales rate

The East of England and the South East had the highest percentage (93.5 per cent) of babies born weighing 2,500 grams or more and West Midlands the lowest (92.1 per cent). The North West and Yorkshire and the Humber both had significantly higher infant mortality rates for babies born weighing 2,500 grams or more compared to England and Wales. The East of England and the South East had significantly lower infant mortality rates for babies weighing 2,500 grams or more compared to England and Wales as a whole, a rate of 2.2 per 1,000 live births. The rate ratio for the regions with the highest and lowest infant mortality rate was 1.4, for babies weighing 2,500 grams or more. Therefore, even within this birthweight category large geographic variations in infant mortality exist.

ONS classification Groups

Table 7.2 shows that *East Inner London* had the highest percentage (1.6 per cent) of live births weighing less than 1,500 grams and *Most Prosperous* the lowest. Chapter 6 has already demonstrated that *East Inner London* and *Manufacturing Centres* had the highest infant mortality rate between 1991 and 1997 and *Growth Areas* and *Most Prosperous* the lowest. Table 7.2 confirms these findings. However, when birthweight was controlled for we can see that the excess infant mortality was much reduced. For babies with birthweight less than 1,500 grams, only *Manufacturing Centres* had a significantly higher infant mortality rate than England and Wales as a whole.

The percentage of babies weighing less than 2,500 grams ranged from 6 per cent in *Most Prosperous* areas to 8.9 (over 47 per cent higher) in *East Inner London*. No ONS classification Group had significantly higher or lower infant mortality than England and Wales for babies born weighing less than 2,500 grams.

Babies weighing 2,500 grams or more accounted for between 91.1 per cent (*East Inner London*) to 94 per cent (*Most Prosperous*) of all live births. *Manufacturing Centres* and *Ports and Industry* both had significantly higher infant mortality rates than England and Wales for babies weighing 2,500 grams or more. *Rural Amenity, Mixed Urban, Growth Areas* and *Most Prosperous* were the areas with significantly lower rates for babies weighing 2,500 grams or more at birth compared to England and Wales.

7.4 Mother's age

Previous analysis of infant mortality rates by mother's age shows that infant mortality is high for mothers aged under 20, is relatively low for mothers in their twenties and thirties; and then rises with age for mothers aged 35 and over. The age at which women have children is influenced by their socio-economic status, including job opportunities, access to further and higher education and training in their employment. In addition, women with high levels of education and training in their employment are more likely to have partners in professional jobs. Thus, relatively few women with partners in

Table 7.4

Live births and infant mortality rates[+] by mother's age and ONS classification Group England and Wales 1993-1997

	Percentage of live births				Number of infant deaths				Infant mortality rate[+]			
	<20	20-29	30-39	40+	<20	20-29	30-39	40+	<20	20-29	30-39	40+
England and Wales	6.7	53.8	37.7	1.8	2,135	10,828	6,939	462	9.7	6.2	5.6	8.0
Rural Amenity	4.5	50.2	43.2	2.1	77	365	313	24	10.9	~ 4.6	~ 4.6	7.4
Remoter Rural	5.9	55.9	36.4	1.8	61	371	233	16	9.0	5.8	5.6	7.8
Established Manufacturing Fringe	7.3	57.0	34.3	1.4	107	593	333	18	8.5	6.0	5.6	7.3
New and Developing Areas	6.6	57.0	35.0	1.4	185	900	491	17	11.0	6.2	5.5	4.9
Mixed Urban	5.2	51.5	41.6	1.7	128	746	542	32	9.5	~ 5.5	~ 5.0	7.1
Coast and Country Resorts	7.2	55.3	35.7	1.8	127	701	437	32	8.1	5.8	5.6	8.4
Established Service Centres	8.2	55.5	34.7	1.5	153	665	402	28	9.3	6.0	5.8	9.2
Growth Areas	4.1	50.1	43.9	1.9	140	980	820	61	8.5	~ 4.9	~ 4.7	8.2
Most Prosperous	3.2	40.9	53.2	2.7	35	240	265	25	9.2	~ 4.8	~ 4.1	7.6
Coalfields	10.1	59.7	29.1	1.1	304	1,254	620	45	8.9	6.2	* 6.3	* 12.2
Manufacturing Centres	9.0	59.6	30.0	1.4	363	1,735	789	51	10.9	* 7.9	* 7.1	9.9
Ports and Industry	9.9	56.2	32.5	1.4	205	838	422	22	10.1	* 7.3	* 6.3	7.6
Education Centres and Outer London	4.5	47.9	45.1	2.5	134	846	730	47	10.4	6.2	5.7	6.7
West Inner London	4.0	41.7	50.8	3.5	24	167	195	18	9.1	6.0	5.8	7.7
East Inner London	6.6	51.7	39.1	2.6	92	427	347	26	12.2	* 7.3	* 7.8	8.8

[+] rate per 1,000 live births

* significantly higher than the England and Wales rate

~ significantly lower than the England and Wales rate

Social Classes I or II have babies before they reach the age of 20. Concern about teenage pregnancy has increased the extent to which data on this subject are compiled and published. Analysis on a wide range of data on teenage pregnancy shows that, compared with all births, babies born to teenagers have high rates of infant mortality and a high percentage of babies are born with a low birthweight.[10] In comparison there are a number of factors affecting a woman's decision to have a child in her late thirties. Some may have long histories of miscarriage or perinatal deaths, others may have remarried or started a new partnership, while others may have only recently decided to start a family. Some births to older women may be to women with a large number of children already, whereas others will be to women who have decided to delay childbearing for some reason. As parity (the number of previous live and stillborn children) is only collected for births inside marriage it is not possible to take these factors into consideration in this chapter.

This section looks at variations in infant mortality rates by mother's age at the time of the child's birth, grouped in four categories (under 20, 20-29, 30-39 and 40 and over).

England, Wales and Government Office Regions

Table 7.3 shows that babies born to mothers aged under 20 had the highest infant mortality rates, a rate of 9.9 per 1,000 live births for England. Wales had a significantly lower infant mortality rate for babies born to mothers aged under 20 compared to England and Wales as a whole, a rate of 7.5 per 1,000 live births. This agrees with other findings that babies born to teenage mothers have around a 60 per cent higher than average infant mortality rate.[11] Seven per cent of all live births in England and 9 per cent of all live births in Wales were to mothers aged under 20. In the North East, mothers aged under 20 accounted for 10 per cent of all live births. In comparison, less than 5 per cent of all live births in London were to mothers aged under 20. Both these regions along with Yorkshire and the Humber and the West Midlands, had infant mortality rates above 10 per 1,000 live births for babies born to mothers aged under 20, although these differences were not significant.

More than half of all live births (54 per cent) in England and (57 per cent) in Wales were to mothers aged 20-29. The infant mortality rate for babies born to mothers aged 20-29 was 6.2 per 1,000 live births in England, and 5.9 in Wales. Yorkshire and the Humber and the West Midlands had significantly higher rates for babies born to mothers aged 20-29 compared to England and Wales. The East of England, South East and South West all had significantly lower infant mortality rates than England and Wales for babies born to mothers aged 20-29. Therefore, large geographic differences in infant mortality can be seen even within specific mother's age groupings. The same regions with high and low overall infant mortality rates had high or low rates for those mothers aged 20-29. A similar pattern was seen for women aged 30-39.

Table 7.5

Live births and infant mortality rates[+] by marital status, country and region
England and Wales 1993-1997

	Percentage of live births			Number of infant deaths			Infant mortality rate[+]		
	Inside marriage	Outside marriage joint registration	Outside marriage sole registration	Inside marriage	Outside marriage joint registration	Outside marriage sole registration	Inside marriage	Outside marriage joint registration	Outside marriage sole registration
England and Wales	65.7	26.7	7.6	11,832	6,477	2,055	5.5	7.4	8.3
England	66.0	26.5	7.5	11,278	6,093	1,943	5.5	7.4	8.3
Wales	61.4	29.8	8.8	554	384	112	5.1	7.3	7.3
North East	57.9	32.2	9.9	486	387	121	5.4	7.8	8.0
North West	60.0	29.7	10.3	1,515	979	338	5.9	7.7	7.6
Yorkshire and the Humber	63.5	28.5	8.0	1,308	706	233	* 6.6	7.9	9.3
East Midlands	65.5	27.3	7.2	887	564	135	5.4	* 8.3	7.4
West Midlands	65.0	26.9	8.0	1,471	735	238	* 6.7	8.0	8.7
East	70.8	23.9	5.2	1,137	522	130	~ 4.9	~ 6.6	7.5
London	66.4	25.2	8.4	1,921	976	446	5.5	7.4	* 10.1
South East	71.3	23.5	5.2	1,576	760	169	~ 4.6	~ 6.7	~ 6.7
South West	68.5	25.4	6.1	977	464	133	5.2	6.6	7.9

[+] rate per 1,000 live births

*significantly higher than the England and Wales rate

~ significantly lower than the England and Wales rate

England had an infant mortality rate of 8.1 per 1,000 live births, for babies born to mothers aged 40 and over. The equivalent rate for Wales was 7.4 per 1,000 live births. In England and Wales, only 1.8 and 1.5 per cent respectively of all live births were born to mothers aged 40 and over. The West Midlands had a significantly higher infant mortality rate for babies born to mothers aged 40 and over than England and Wales and the East of England had a significantly lower rate.

ONS classification Groups

Table 7.4 shows that no ONS classification Group had significantly higher or lower infant mortality rates than England and Wales as a whole for mothers aged under 20.

Manufacturing Centres, Ports and Industry and *East Inner London* all had significantly higher infant mortality rates for women aged 20-29 and 30-39 compared to England and Wales. In comparison, *Rural Amenity, Mixed Urban, Growth Areas* and *Most Prosperous* all had significantly lower infant mortality rates for women aged 20-29 and 30-39 compared to England and Wales. This was a similar pattern to that presented for overall infant mortality. Authorities classified as *Coalfields* had significantly higher infant mortality rates for mothers aged 30-39 and 40 and over; it was the only Group which had a significantly higher rate for women aged 40 and over.

7.5 Marital status

Infant mortality is known to be strongly associated with the parents' marital status.[12] In England and Wales, the proportion of births inside marriage has fallen from 91 per cent in 1976 to 62 per cent in 1998, whilst the proportion registered outside marriage has quadrupled over the period from 9 per cent to 38 per cent.[13]

For details of both parents to be recorded at birth registration for births outside marriage, both parents have to be present at the registration. However, if the father completes a statutory declaration form prior to the registration then his name can be recorded on the birth certificate and the birth is classed as a joint registration outside marriage. If the father does not attend the registration or does not complete a statutory declaration form, then the birth is registered as a sole registration. For sole registration, no details on the father are collected.

In interpreting births by marital status it also has to be borne in mind that marriage patterns vary from culture to culture. In 1997 in England and Wales, only 0.9 per cent of births to women born in Bangladesh were outside marriage, compared with 48.6 per cent of births to women born in the Caribbean Commonwealth.[14]

Table 7.6

Live births and infant mortality rates[+] by marital status and ONS classification Group England and Wales 1993-1997

	Percentage of live births			Number of infant deaths			Infant mortality rate[+]		
	Inside marriage	Outside marriage joint registration	Outside marriage sole registration	Inside marriage	Outside marriage joint registration	Outside marriage sole registration	Inside marriage	Outside marriage joint registration	Outside marriage sole registration
England and Wales	65.7	26.7	7.6	11,832	6,477	2,055	5.5	7.4	8.3
Rural Amenity	73.9	21.5	4.6	502	225	52	~ 4.3	6.7	7.2
Remoter Rural	70.1	24.6	5.2	443	191	47	5.5	6.8	7.9
Established Manufacturing Fringe	66.0	27.4	6.6	632	338	81	5.5	7.1	7.1
New and Developing Areas	66.8	26.4	6.8	944	515	134	5.6	7.7	7.8
Mixed Urban	68.8	25.3	5.9	903	429	116	~ 5.0	~ 6.4	7.5
Coast and Country Resorts	62.9	29.3	7.8	708	453	136	5.2	7.1	8.0
Established Service Centres	60.4	30.0	9.6	640	462	146	5.3	7.7	7.6
Growth Areas	75.4	20.6	4.1	1,396	502	103	~ 4.7	~ 6.1	~ 6.4
Most Prosperous	78.3	18.2	3.5	404	136	25	~ 4.3	6.1	5.9
Coalfields	57.4	33.1	9.5	1,118	843	262	5.8	7.5	8.2
Manufacturing Centres	62.8	28.0	9.1	1,743	880	315	* 7.5	* 8.5	9.3
Ports and Industry	52.3	34.0	13.7	681	597	209	* 6.4	* 8.6	7.5
Education Centres and Outer London	67.9	24.5	7.6	1,035	521	201	5.4	7.5	9.3
West Inner London	68.7	23.0	8.2	231	111	62	5.1	7.3	* 11.4
East Inner London	59.2	28.6	12.2	452	274	166	* 6.7	8.4	* 12.0

[+] rate per 1,000 live births

*significantly higher than the England and Wales rate

~ significantly lower than the England and Wales rate

England, Wales and Government Office Regions

Table 7.5 shows that the lowest infant mortality rates by marital status occurred inside marriage, a rate of 5.5 per 1,000 live births in England and a rate of 5.1 in Wales. Sixty-six per cent of all live births in England and 61 per cent in Wales occurred inside marriage. In comparison, 58 per cent of all infant deaths in England, and 53 per cent in Wales occur inside marriage. For all regions, the lowest infant mortality rates also occurred inside marriage. Both Yorkshire and the Humber and the West Midlands had significantly higher rates of infant death inside marriage than England and Wales as a whole. The East of England and the South East had significantly lower infant mortality rates inside marriage than England and Wales as a whole. This follows the geographic pattern already identified for overall infant mortality.

The infant mortality rate for births registered by both parents outside marriage was 7.4 per 1,000 live births for England and 7.3 per 1,000 for Wales. Within England, the East Midlands had the highest infant mortality rate for live births registered outside marriage by both parents, with a rate of 8.3 per 1,000 live births. The South East and East of England had a significantly lower infant mortality rate than England and Wales for this registration type.

For England, the highest infant mortality rates by marital status were to babies registered outside marriage by the mother alone, a rate of 8.3 per 1,000 live births. This rate was 51 per cent higher than the rate for babies born inside marriage. In Wales, this was not the case, as the rate of 7.3 per 1,000 live births was identical to the rate for babies born outside marriage registered by both parents. London had the highest infant mortality rate of 10.1 per 1,000 live births, for babies registered outside marriage by the mother alone; this was significantly higher than the rate for England and Wales. The South East had a significantly lower infant mortality rate for babies registered outside marriage as sole registration than England and Wales as a whole.

ONS classification Groups

Table 7.6 shows that the geographic pattern of infant mortality for those babies born inside marriage was the same as overall infant mortality.

Manufacturing Centres and *Ports and Industry* both had significantly higher infant mortality rates both inside marriage and outside marriage registered by both parents than England and Wales. The *East Inner London* Group had significantly higher infant mortality rates inside marriage than England and Wales. *East Inner London* and *West Inner London* had significantly higher infant mortality rates outside marriage registered by the mother alone compared to England and Wales. *Mixed Urban* and *Growth Areas* had significantly lower infant mortality rates inside marriage and outside marriage registered by both parents compared to England and Wales. *Growth Areas* also had significantly lower infant mortality rates than England and Wales outside marriage registered by the mother alone. *Rural Amenity* and *Most Prosperous* had significantly lower infant mortality rates inside marriage compared to England and Wales.

7.6 Social Class

The previous section showed that infant mortality rates differ quite markedly according to the marital status of the parents. To an extent this reflects differences in their Social Class distribution. The percentage of births outside marriage and jointly registered by both parents varies strongly by the Social Class of the baby's father.

Mothers occupation at birth has been collected since 1986, but only on a voluntary basis and therefore the information is poorly recorded. Questions have been raised regarding how a mother's occupation should be recorded and classified.[15, 16] Therefore, analysis by Social Class in this section is based on father's occupation.

For this analysis, infant deaths were allocated to Social Classes on the basis of father's occupation at the death of the child, whereas births were allocated to Social Classes on the basis of father's occupation at the birth of the child. Infant deaths cannot be classified on the basis of father's occupation at birth as currently only 10 per cent of all births are coded by father's Social Class and very few of these babies die before completing the first year of life. Analysis in this section is restricted to Social Class variations in infant deaths within marriage, or if outside marriage, registered by both parents and having the father's occupation recorded.

Analysis of infant mortality for 1983-1985 by Social Class and by district health authority was published in the previous *Mortality and Geography* supplement.[17] This showed that districts with the highest proportion of fathers in partly skilled and unskilled manual occupations tended to have the highest percentage of low birthweight babies and the highest infant mortality rates.

England, Wales and Government Office Regions

Of babies born in England between 1993 and 1997, those whose fathers were in Social Class V (unskilled occupations) had an infant mortality rate of 8.8 per 1,000 live births, nearly double the rate (4.5) for those in Social Class I (professional occupations). The Social Class gradients in infant mortality varied for England, Wales and the regions of England (Figure 7.1), with the largest difference between Social Class I and V occurring in Yorkshire and the Humber.

No region had a significantly higher or lower infant mortality rate for Social Class I than England and Wales. West Midlands had significantly higher infant mortality rates than England and Wales for Social Classes IIIN, IIIM and IV. Yorkshire and the Humber had a significantly higher infant mortality rate for Social Class IIIM compared with the rate for England and Wales. The East of England had significantly lower infant mortality rates for Social Classes IIIN and V compared to the rates for England and Wales. The South East had significantly lower infant mortality rates for Social Classes IIIN and IIIM compared with the rate for England and Wales. Wales had a significantly lower infant mortality rate for Social Class IIIM than England and Wales as a whole.

Therefore, there were large geographic differences in infant mortality even within Social Class groupings. Within Social Classes, the largest ratio of infant mortality rates between the regions with the highest and the lowest infant mortality were observed in Social Classes I and V, both had a ratio of 1.6. This contrasts with the results for adult mortality where there was little variation between the regions in the mortality of those in Social Class I (see chapter 12).

ONS classification Groups

No ONS classification Group had a significantly higher or lower infant mortality rate for Social Class I than the rate in this class for England and Wales. With the exception of Social Class I, *Manufacturing Centres* had significantly higher infant mortality rates for all other Social Classes compared to England and Wales. *Ports and Industry* had significantly higher infant mortality rates for Social Class II, IIIM and IV, and *East Inner London* had significantly higher rates for Social Classes II to IIIM compared to England and Wales. *Education Centres and Outer London* was the ONS classification Group which had the steepest Social Class gradient between Social Class I and V (Figure 7.2).

Growth Areas had significantly lower infant mortality rates for Social Classes II, IIIM, IV, and V compared to England and Wales. *Most Prosperous* had a significantly lower infant mortality rate for Social Classes II and IIIM compared to England and Wales. *Remoter Rural* had the lowest infant mortality for Social Class V. However, this was not significantly lower than the rate for England and Wales because of the small number of deaths involved.

Figure 7.1

Infant mortality rates by Social Class, country and region
England and Wales 1993-1997

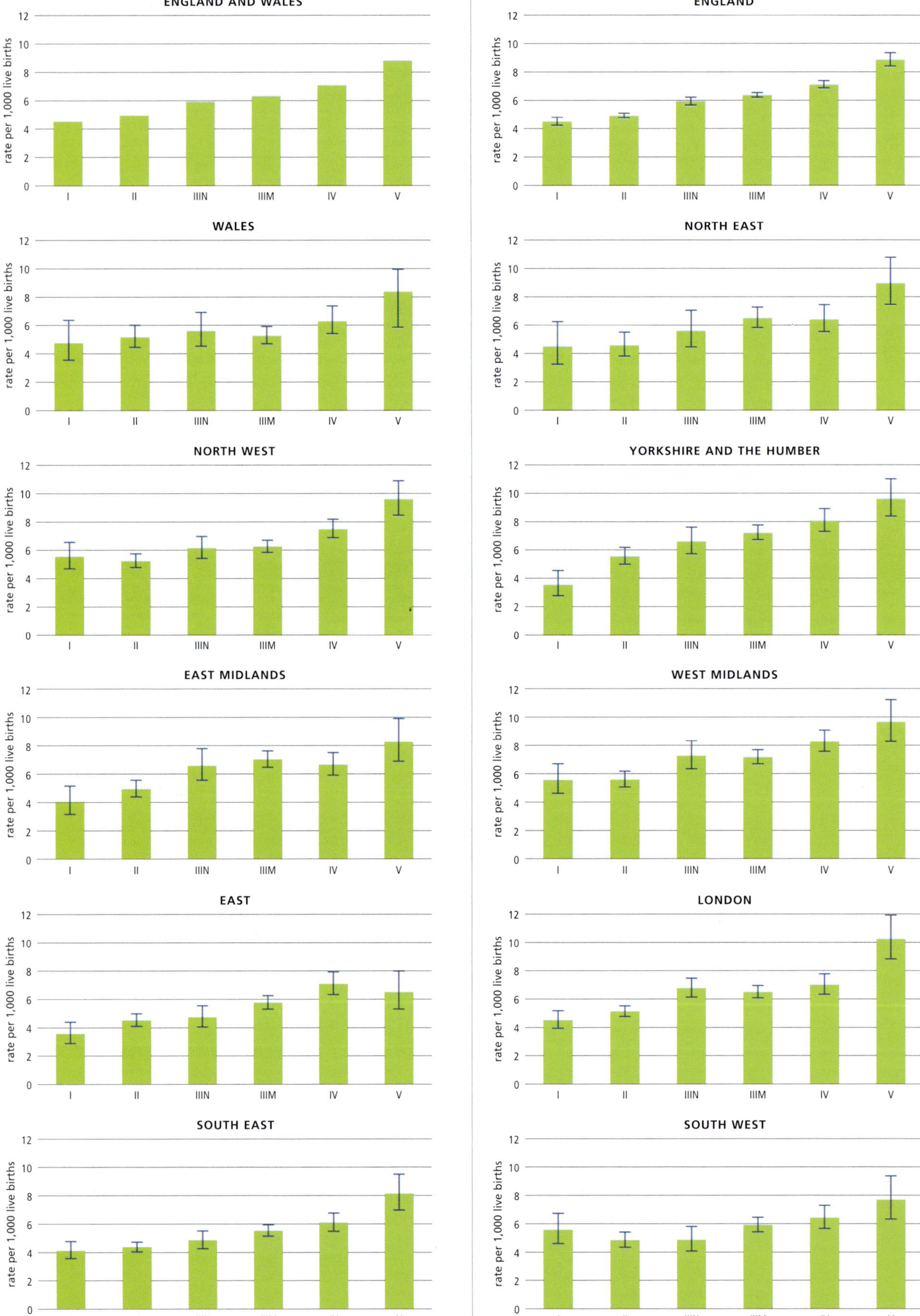

Figure 7.2

Infant mortality rates by Social Class and ONS classification Group
England and Wales 1993-1997

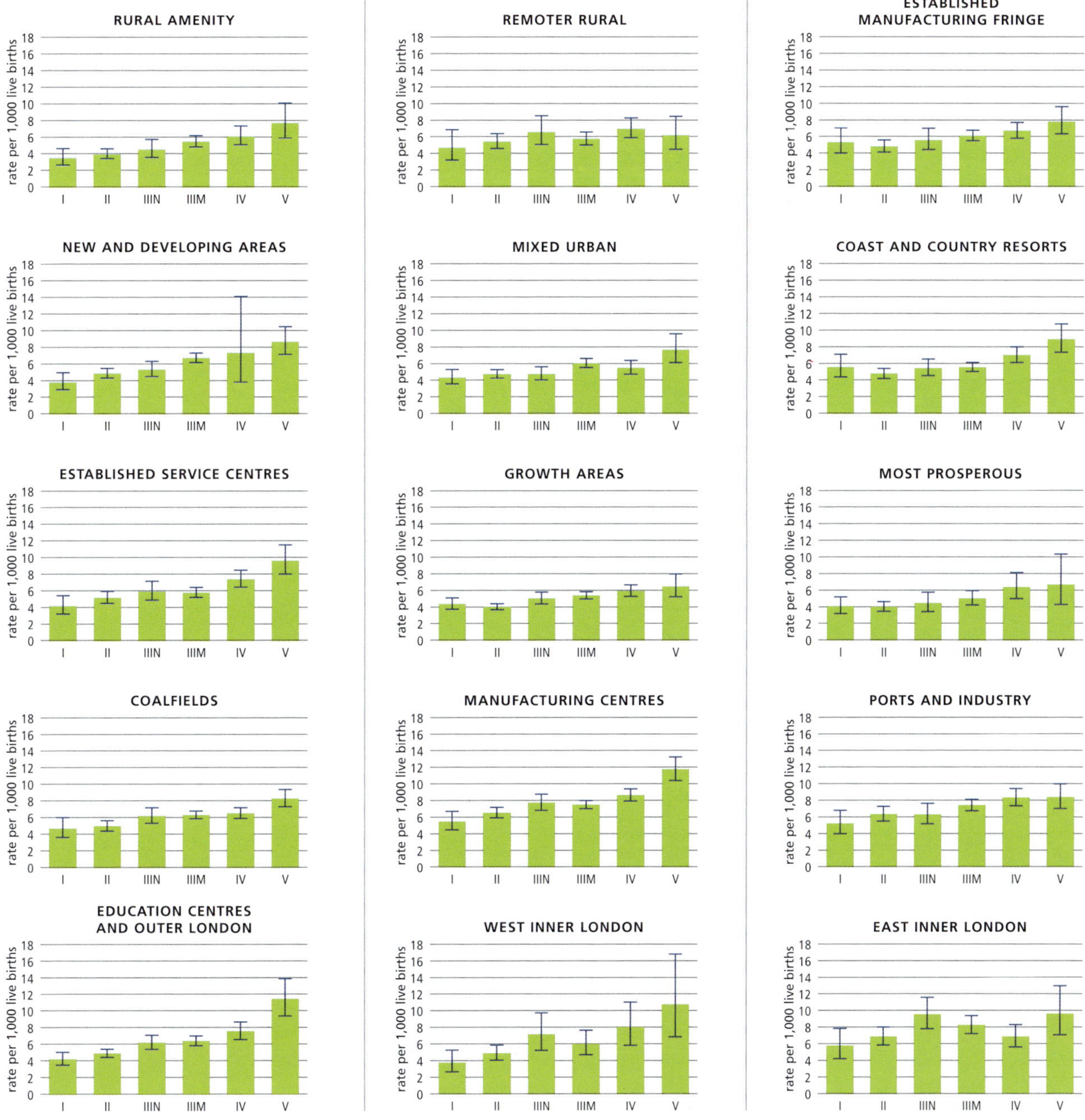

7.7 Mother's country of birth

Mother's country of birth indicates immigrant status but is not a good indicator of ethnic group, with second generation mothers from minority ethnic groups classified as United Kingdom born. The number of women from ethnic minority groups born in the United Kingdom has increased and the number born outside the United Kingdom has decreased. However, mother's country of birth is currently used as a proxy to identify a child's ethnicity, as ethnicity is not recorded at birth or death registration.

Infant mortality data for England and Wales by mother's country of birth for the years 1993-1997 inclusive has been aggregated to provide a large enough data set for analysis. However, the number of infant deaths for the combined years was still only sufficiently large to calculate infant mortality rates at a country or regional level for selected groups of mother's country of birth. The groups studied are mothers born in England or Wales, those born outside England and outside Wales which is further sub-divided into Scotland, other European Union, Bangladesh, India and Pakistan.

Table 7.7

Live births and infant mortality rates[+] by mother's country of birth, country and region England and Wales 1993-1997

Infant deaths by mother's country of birth

Mother's country of birth;	England or Wales	Not born in England or Wales	Scotland	Other European Union	Bangladesh	India	Pakistan
Country							
England and Wales	16,366	3,366	285	246	223	202	736
England	15,403	3,310	277	242	218	200	728
Wales	963	56	8	4	5	2	8
Government Office Region							
North East	896	78	30	10	3	1	16
North West	2,420	311	36	˙26	24	24	112
Yorkshire and the Humber	1,859	320	28	17	17	10	187
East Midlands	1,376	158	19	25	7	20	28
West Midlands	1,977	391	22	9	21	50	181
East	1,522	203	24	21	16	8	47
London	1,873	1,311	48	65	113	72	73
South East	2,073	407	52	50	14	13	73
South West	1,407	131	18	19	3	2	11

Live births by mother's country of birth

Mother's country of birth;	England or Wales	Not born in England or Wales	Scotland	Other European Union	Bangladesh	India	Pakistan
Country							
England and Wales	2,796,830	476,227	48,776	44,725	33,093	34,102	62,916
England	2,630,603	466,805	47,382	43,353	32,341	33,830	62,256
Wales	166,227	9,422	1,394	1,372	752	272	660
Government Office Region							
North East	144,232	10,024	2,824	1,247	951	330	1,061
North West	386,605	42,729	6,645	3,088	3,361	3,233	10,738
Yorkshire and the Humber	279,633	34,392	4,447	2,778	1,658	1,947	13,798
East Midlands	224,696	25,595	4,209	2,630	898	3,903	2,391
West Midlands	296,808	42,529	3,236	2,357	4,030	5,986	14,554
East	291,151	37,303	5,202	4,657	2,273	1,428	3,797
London	330,786	192,814	7,547	13,590	16,926	13,449	10,152
South East	422,531	59,301	9,148	8,957	1,735	2,975	5,228
South West	254,161	22,118	4,124	4,049	509	579	537

Infant mortality rates[+] by mother's country of birth

Mother's country of birth;	England or Wales	Not born in England or Wales	Scotland	Other European Union	Bangladesh	India	Pakistan
Country							
England and Wales	5.9	7.1	5.8	5.5	6.7	5.9	11.7
England	5.9	7.1	5.8	5.6	6.7	5.9	11.7
Wales	5.8	5.9	-	-	-	-	-
Government Office Region							
North East	6.2	7.8	* 10.6	-	-	-	-
North West	* 6.3	7.3	5.4	8.4	7.1	7.4	10.4
Yorkshire and the Humber	* 6.6	* 9.3	6.3	-	-	-	13.6
East Midlands	6.1	6.2	-	* 9.5	-	5.1	11.7
West Midlands	* 6.7	* 9.2	6.8	-	8.4	8.4	12.4
East	~ 5.2	~ 5.4	4.6	4.5	-	-	12.4
London	5.7	6.8	6.4	5.6	6.7	5.4	~ 7.2
South East	~ 4.9	6.9	5.7	5.6	-	-	14.0
South West	5.5	5.9	-	-	-	-	-

[+] rate per 1,000 live births   *significantly higher than the England and Wales rate   ~ significantly lower than the England and Wales rate

- The rates for areas with less than 20 infant deaths for the combined 1993-1997 period have not been calculated because of the small numbers involved

England, Wales and Government Office Regions

The infant mortality rate for babies born to mothers from England or Wales was 5.9 per 1,000 live births for England, compared to a rate of 5.8 for Wales (Table 7.7). Babies born to mothers from outside England or Wales accounted for 18 per cent of all live births in England, and 21 per cent of all infant deaths in England. The infant mortality rate for babies born to mothers from outside England or Wales was 7.1 per 1,000 live births for England. In Wales, babies born to mothers from outside England or Wales accounted for only 6 per cent of both live births and infant deaths. There were only 56 infant deaths in Wales to mothers born outside England or Wales, with a rate of 5.9 per 1,000 live births. The small number of infant deaths in Wales to mothers born outside England or Wales means that further analysis by mother's country of birth is not meaningful.

The infant mortality rate in England was highest for infants of mothers born in Pakistan (11.7 per 1,000 live births), double the rate for babies of mothers born in England or Wales. Previous analysis of infant death by birthweight and mother's country of birth showed that babies of women born in Pakistan had exceptionally high infant mortality rates and a higher incidence of low birthweight babies compared with other groups of babies.[9] The West Midlands, and Yorkshire and the Humber, had the highest number of births to mothers born in Pakistan and also high infant mortality rates for mothers born in Pakistan. The infant mortality rate for England for babies born to mothers from Bangladesh was 15 per cent higher than the rate for babies born to mothers from England or Wales.

Over 41 per cent of all live births in England, to mothers born outside England or Wales, occurred to mothers resident in London. London also accounted for 40 per cent of all the infant deaths in England to babies born to mothers outside England or Wales. For those mothers born in Bangladesh and India, 52 per cent and 40 per cent respectively of all live births in England occurred to women resident in London. However, London had a lower infant mortality rate than England for babies born to mothers from India and a significantly lower infant mortality rate for babies born to mothers from Pakistan than England and Wales as a whole.

The West Midlands and Yorkshire and the Humber had significantly higher infant mortality rates for babies born to mothers outside England or Wales, and the East of England had significantly lower rates. The North East had a significantly higher infant mortality rate for mothers born in Scotland (10.6 per 1,000 live births) compared to England and Wales. The East Midlands had a significantly higher infant mortality rate for mothers from other European Union countries (9.5 per 1,000 live births) compared to England and Wales.

Analysis by mother's country of birth and region shows a wide variation in infant mortality rates by region for specific countries, which may reflect the small numbers involved. These infant mortality rates show only those babies born to first generation immigrant mothers and therefore, is not a complete picture of infant mortality by ethnicity.

7.8 Cause of death

The ONS cause classification is currently used to classify the causes of infant deaths. It is a cause grouping for infant deaths that has been derived to provide the maximum information about preventability and yet meets the national and international responsibilities of ONS.[18] The classification is a hierarchical one. For neonates all conditions mentioned on the death certificate, and for postneonates the underlying cause of death, is used to direct the death to the first appropriate class of the nine mutually exclusive categories, as shown in Box 7.2.

The infant mortality rate for deaths attributed to congenital anomalies for both England and Wales was 1.5 per 1,000 live births. Twenty-six per cent of all infant deaths in England and 27 per cent in Wales had a mention of congenital anomaly on the death certificate. The West Midlands and Yorkshire and the Humber had a significantly higher rate of infant deaths from congenital anomalies than England and Wales (Table 7.8). There were significantly lower rates of infant deaths from congenital anomalies in the East of England and South East. The rate ratio between the regions with the highest and lowest rates was 1.5. For further analysis and explanation of the geographic variations in infant deaths from congenital anomalies see chapter 8 of this volume.

There were 96 infant deaths from antepartum infections in England and 5 in Wales. The West Midlands had a significantly higher rate of infant deaths from antepartum infections, compared with the rate for England and Wales as a whole.

In England and Wales, infant deaths from immaturity-related conditions resulted in the highest infant mortality rate. This was 2.2 per 1,000 live births in England. In comparison, Wales had a significantly lower rate of infant death from immaturity-related conditions than England and Wales, a rate of 1.9 per 1,000 live births. Thirty-seven per cent of infant deaths in England and 33 per cent of infant deaths in Wales, were from immaturity-related conditions. Yorkshire and the Humber, East Midlands and West Midlands all had significantly higher rates of infant death from immaturity-related conditions compared with the rate for England and Wales. The East of England, South East, South West all had significantly lower rates of infant death from immaturity-related conditions. Infant deaths from immaturity-related conditions have a strong correlation to preterm birth reflected by low birthweight babies. The West Midlands had a significantly higher rate of infant death from immaturity-related conditions compared to England and Wales and was one of the regions with the highest percentage of live births weighing less than 1,500 grams. The South East with the lowest proportion of live births weighing under 1,500 grams had the lowest rate of infant deaths from immaturity-related conditions.

There were 1,581 infant deaths attributed to asphyxia, anoxia or trauma in England and 96 in Wales, a rate of 0.5 per 1,000 live births for both England and for Wales. No region had a significantly higher or lower rate for infant deaths from asphyxia, anoxia or trauma compared with the rate for England and Wales.

Box 7.2 ONS classification of infant deaths and associated codes from the International Classification of Diseases, Ninth Revision (ICD9)

Group	Description	ICD9 codes
1	Congenital anomalies	Main or other infant conditions: 270-273, 277, 279.0, 279.2-9, 282, 284.0, 286.0-4, 287.3, 288.1-2, 330, 335.0, 343, 348.0, 359.0-3, 424.0-3, 425.0-1, 425.3-4, 426, 571.4-9, 655.1, 740-743, 745-746, 747.1-9, 748, 749.0-2, 750.1-751.9, 752.4, 752.6-9, 753, 754.3, 754.8, 755.2-757.3, 757.8-9, 758, 759, 774.0, 777.0
2	Antepartum infections	Main or other infant conditions: 090, 279.1, 762.7, 770.0, 771.0-2 Main or other maternal conditions: 655.3
3	Immaturity-related conditions	Main infant conditions: 761.0-1, 761.8, 765.0-1, 769.0, 770.2, 770.4-5, 770.7-8, 772.1, 774.2, 774.7, 776.6, 777.5, 779.6 Main or other maternal conditions: 761.0-1, 761.8, 765.0-1, 769.0, 770.2, 770.4-5, 770.7-8, 772.1, 774.2, 774.7, 776.6, 777.5, 779.6
4	Asphyxia, anoxia, or trauma	Main or other infant conditions: 760.0, 761.6-7, 762.0-2, 762.4-6, 763, 764, 766-768, 770.1, 772.2, 779.0-2 Main or other maternal conditions: 641-642, 760.0, 761.6-7, 762.0-2, 762.4-6, 763, 764, 766-768, 770.1, 772.2, 779.0-2
5	External conditions	Main infant conditions: 260-263, 507.0-8, 778.1-3, 779.3, 800-999
6	Infections	Main or other infant conditions: 001-088.0, 091-139.0, 254.1, 320-326.0, 382, 420-422, 460-466.1, 475-476.1, 480-491, 494.0, 510-511, 513.0-1, 540-542.0, 567, 590, 599.0, 771.3-8
7	Other specific conditions	Main or other infant conditions: 254.1-9, 255, 283, 286.7, 762.8-9, 772.0, 772.3-9, 773.0-5, 774.1, 774.3-6, 775, 776.0-5, 776.7-9, 777.1-4, 777.6-9, 778.0, 778.4-9, 779.4-5 Main or other maternal conditions: 140-253, 254.1-9, 255, 283, 286.7, 331, 423, 427, 441-442, 493, 556-558, 760.2, 760.5-6, 762.3, 762.8-9, 772.0, 772.3-9, 773.0-5, 774.0-1, 774.3-6, 775, 776.0-5, 776.7-9, 777.1-4, 777.6-9, 778.0, 778.4-9, 779.4-5, 785.5
9	Sudden infant death	Main or other infant conditions: 798.0-2, 798.9, 799.1
0	Other conditions	All other codes

Table 7.8

Infant mortality rates[+] by cause of death and region
England and Wales 1993-1997

Number of deaths

	Congenital anomalies	Antepartum infections	Immaturity related conditions	Asphyxia, anoxia or trauma	External conditions	Infections	Other specific conditions	Sudden infant death	Other conditions
	1	2	3	4	5	6	7	9	0
England and Wales	5,058	101	7,168	1,677	360	1,591	354	1,908	1,364
England	4,790	96	6,834	1,581	345	1,503	333	1,795	1,293
Wales	268	5	334	96	15	88	21	113	71
North East	234	3	343	92	19	75	11	130	57
North West	690	9	972	191	64	218	42	325	198
Yorkshire and the Humber	563	13	773	191	57	171	53	185	163
East Midlands	397	2	608	131	19	119	26	126	94
West Midlands	656	27	878	193	42	182	38	193	140
East	442	9	622	144	25	163	32	153	119
London	780	15	1,246	283	49	277	53	287	238
South East	621	10	861	233	44	181	53	234	164
South West	407	8	531	123	26	117	25	162	120

Rates

	Congenital anomalies	Antepartum infections	Immaturity related conditions	Asphyxia, anoxia or trauma	External conditions	Infections	Other specific conditions	Sudden infant death	Other conditions
	1	2	3	4	5	6	7	9	0
England and Wales	1.5	0.0	2.2	0.5	0.1	0.5	0.1	0.6	0.4
England	1.5	0.0	2.2	0.5	0.1	0.5	0.1	0.6	0.4
Wales	1.5	0.0	~ 1.9	0.5	0.1	0.5	0.1	0.6	0.4
North East	1.5	0.0	2.2	0.6	0.1	0.5	0.1	* 0.8	0.4
North West	1.6	0.0	2.3	0.4	0.1	0.5	0.1	* 0.8	0.5
Yorkshire and the Humber	* 1.8	0.0	* 2.5	0.6	* 0.2	0.5	* 0.2	0.6	* 0.5
East Midlands	1.6	0.0	* 2.4	0.5	0.1	0.5	0.1	0.5	0.4
West Midlands	* 1.9	* 0.1	* 2.6	0.6	0.1	0.5	0.1	0.6	0.4
East	~ 1.3	0.0	~ 1.9	0.4	0.1	0.5	0.1	~ 0.5	0.4
London	1.5	0.0	2.4	0.5	0.1	0.5	0.1	0.5	0.5
South East	~ 1.3	0.0	~ 1.8	0.5	0.1	~ 0.4	0.1	~ 0.5	0.3
South West	1.5	0.0	~ 1.9	0.4	0.1	0.4	0.1	0.6	0.4

[+] rate per 1,000 live births

* significantly higher than the England and Wales rate

~ significantly lower than the England and Wales rate

There were 345 infant deaths from external conditions in England and 15 in Wales, both with a rate of 0.1 per 1,000 live births. Yorkshire and the Humber had a significantly higher rate of infant deaths from external conditions compared to the rate for England and Wales.

Infections accounted for 8 per cent of all infant deaths in England and 9 per cent in Wales. The infant mortality rate for infant deaths from infections for both England and for Wales was 0.5 per 1,000 live births. The South East had a significantly lower rate (0.4) of infant deaths from infections compared to the rate for England and Wales.

In England there were 333 infant deaths classified as 'other specific conditions' and 21 in Wales, both with a rate of 0.1 per 1,000 live births. The category 'other specific conditions' groups together all other conditions that specifically relate to infants and are not previously mentioned in the ONS cause classification. Yorkshire and the Humber had a significantly higher rate for infant deaths from 'other specific conditions' compared with England and Wales.

Ten per cent of all infant deaths in England and 11 per cent of all infant deaths in Wales were assigned to the category 'sudden infant death', both with a rate of 0.6 per 1,000 live births. These figures were based on the ONS cause classification of infant deaths and do not represent all mentions of Sudden Infant Death Syndrome, as published in other ONS publications.[19, 20] Analysis shows the North East and North West both experienced significantly higher rates for sudden infant death compared with the rate for England and Wales. The East of England and South East both had significantly lower rates of sudden infant death compared with England and Wales.

7.9 Discussion

Analysis of the known risk factors of infant mortality in this chapter helps to explain some of the geographic variations in infant mortality presented in chapter 6 by demonstrating that when some factors were controlled for excess infant mortality was reduced.

Chapter 6 showed that within England, regions in the north and the Midlands had higher infant mortality rates than regions in the south. Further analysis has shown much of the difference in rates can be explained by the percentage of live births that were of low birthweight. However, even when we look at infant mortality rates for babies of a particular birthweight, differences between the countries and the regions still exist. London had a significantly lower infant mortality rate for babies born weighing less than 1,500 grams despite being the region with the highest percentage of live births of this birthweight. This could be considered the result of a range of factors and may be a reflection of the intensive care and the medical facilities available to babies in London.[21, 22] Infant deaths from immaturity-related conditions were seen to be directly related to the percentage of low birthweight live births in any given region. Other studies have clearly shown that both birthweight and gestational age have

independent associations with mortality.[3] Unfortunately, information about gestational age of the baby at birth is not collected at birth registration in England and Wales. Therefore, no analysis by gestational age could be undertaken.

Analysis of mother's age showed that babies born to mothers aged under 20 had the highest infant mortality rate and in addition it is likely that a greater percentage were of low birthweight.[7] However, geographic differences in infant mortality rates still exist when looking at particular mother's age groups alone. Yorkshire and the Humber and the West Midlands both had higher rates for mothers aged 20-29 and 30-39 and the latter also had higher rates for mothers aged 40 and over. For all age groups, lower rates by mother's age occurred in regions in the south of England.

The East of England and South East had low infant mortality rates for births both inside marriage and outside marriage registered by both parents. Yorkshire and the Humber and West Midlands both had high infant mortality rates for births inside marriage. The infant mortality rate for births registered outside marriage by the mother alone was significantly higher in London than elsewhere. The percentage of births inside marriage varies strongly by Social Class of the baby's father and by the mother's country of birth. Analysis of all the Social Classes shows that Yorkshire and the Humber and the West Midlands regions had higher than average infant mortality rates for Social Class IIIN, IIIM and IV. Lower than average infant mortality rates by Social Class occurred in the East of England and South East.

As expected, analysis by mother's country of birth shows that the overall geographic pattern was repeated for babies born to mothers born in England or Wales. The North West, Yorkshire and the Humber and West Midlands all had high rates and East of England and South East had low rates for babies born to mothers from England or Wales. For babies born to mothers outside England or Wales, Yorkshire and the Humber and West Midlands had significantly higher rates whilst the East of England had a significantly lower rate. The rates seen in babies born to mothers from England or Wales will include an increasing number of second generation immigrant mothers and the rates may be a reflection of this.[23] Finally, the lower infant mortality rates for babies to mothers born in Pakistan but resident in London compared to the rate for England could be the result of many factors including good access to facilities and support for these mothers.[24] Statistics examining average birthweight and infant deaths by mothers country of birth show that babies of women born in Pakistan have exceptionally high mortality rates and a higher incidence of low birthweight compared with other groups of babies.[9]

Analysis of infant deaths from congenital anomalies and immaturity-related conditions showed a clear north-south split. For both causes of death, Yorkshire and the Humber and West Midlands had high infant mortality rates compared to England, with the regions in the south having lower rates. The regions in the south also had lower infant mortality rates for sudden infant death and regions of the north had higher infant mortality from sudden infant death. Infant deaths from immaturity related conditions have a strong correlation to preterm birth reflected by low birthweight babies. This was clearly demonstrated in the West Midlands and South East.

It has been clearly demonstrated that the known risk factors for infant mortality are interrelated. Low birthweight is a main factor contributing to immaturity related deaths. Birthweight is affected by mother's age and country of birth as well as factors which are not routinely measured, including mother's nutrition and the availability of social support. Mother's age, mother's country of birth and Social Class all influence the parents' marital status. Birthweight remains the strongest and most important risk factor associated with neonatal mortality.[4] Over 67 per cent of the infant deaths referred to in this chapter occurred in the neonatal period, thus making birthweight a very important risk factor in infant mortality. The differentials in infant mortality rates that exist between regions suggests the potential for improvement in infant mortality rates in the future.

References

1 Office for National Statistics. Report: Infant and perinatal mortality by social and biological factors, 1999. *Health Statistics Quarterly* 8 (2000), 76-80.

2 Heasman MA and Clarke JA. Medical record linkage in Scotland. *Health Bulletin* 37(4) (1979), 97-103.

3 Coory M. Does gestational age in combination with birthweight provide better statistical adjustment of neonatal mortality rates than birthweight alone? *Paediatric and Perinatal Epidemiology* 11 (1997), 385-391.

4 Dattani N, Cooper N, Rooney C, Rodrigues L and Campbell O. Analysis of risk factors for neonatal mortality in England and Wales, 1993-97: based on singleton babies weighing 2,500-5,499 grams. *Health Statistics Quarterly* 8 (2000), 29-35.

5 Power C. National trends in birthweight: implications for future adult disease. *British Medical Journal* 308 (1994), 1270-1271.

6 Alberman E. Are our babies becoming bigger? *Journal of the Royal Society of Medicine* 84 (1991), 257-260.

7 Macfarlane AJ and Mugford M. *Birth Counts: Statistics of pregnancy and childbirth*. Volume 1, text. The Stationery Office (London: 2000).

8 World Health Organisation. *International statistical classification of diseases and related health problems*. Tenth revision. Volume 1. WHO (Geneva: 1992).

9 Office for National Statistics. *Mortality Statistics 1997: Childhood, infant and perinatal*. Series DH3 No. 30. The Stationery Office (London: 1998).

10 Botting B, Rosato M and Wood R. Teenage mothers and the health of their children. *Population Trends* 93 (1998), 19-28.

11 Drever F, Fisher K, Brown J and Clark J. *Social Inequalities 2000*. The Stationery Office (London: 2000).

12 Dattani N. Mortality in children aged under 4. *Health Statistics Quarterly* 2 (1999), 41-49.

13 Botting B and Dunnell K. Trends in fertility and contraception in the last quarter of the 20th century. *Population Trends* 100 (2000), 32-39.

14 Office for National Statistics. *Birth Statistics*. Series FM1 No. 26. The Stationery Office (London: 1998).

15 Cooper J and Botting B. Analysing fertility and infant mortality by mother's Social Class defined by occupation. *Population Trends* 70 (1992), 15-21.

16 Botting B and Cooper J. Analysing fertility and infant mortality by mother's Social Class as defined by occupation - Part II. *Population Trends* 74 (1993), 27-33.

17 Botting B and Macfarlane AJ. Geographic variation in infant mortality in relation to birthweight 1983-85 in Britton M (ed). *Mortality and geography: a review in the mid 1980s, England and Wales*. Series DS No. 9. HMSO (London: 1990), 48-57.

18 Alberman E, Botting B, Blatchley N and Twidell A. A new hierarchical classification of causes of infant deaths in England and Wales. *Archives of Disease in Childhood* 70 (1994), 403-409.

19 Dattani N and Cooper N. Trends in Cot Deaths. *Health Statistics Quarterly* 5 (2000), 10-16.

20 Office for National Statistics. Report: Sudden infant deaths 1999. *Health Statistics Quarterly* 7 (2000), 66-70.

21 NHS Executive. *Paediatric Intensive Care 'A Framework for the Future'*. Report from the National Co-ordinating Group on Paediatric Intensive Care to the Chief Executive of the NHS Executive 1997.

22 Martuzzi M, Grundy C and Elliott P. Perinatal mortality in an English health region: geographical distribution and association with socio-economic factors. *Paediatric and Perinatal Epidemiology* 12 (1998), 263-276.

23 Mason D. *Race and Ethnicity in Modern Britain*. Oxford University Press (Oxford: 1995), 95-106.

24 The Health of Londoners Project. *Child health in London. The health and social characteristics of London's children*. The Health of Londoners Project (London: 1999).

Geographic variation in congenital anomaly notifications in England and Wales

Ruth Yates and Lois Cook

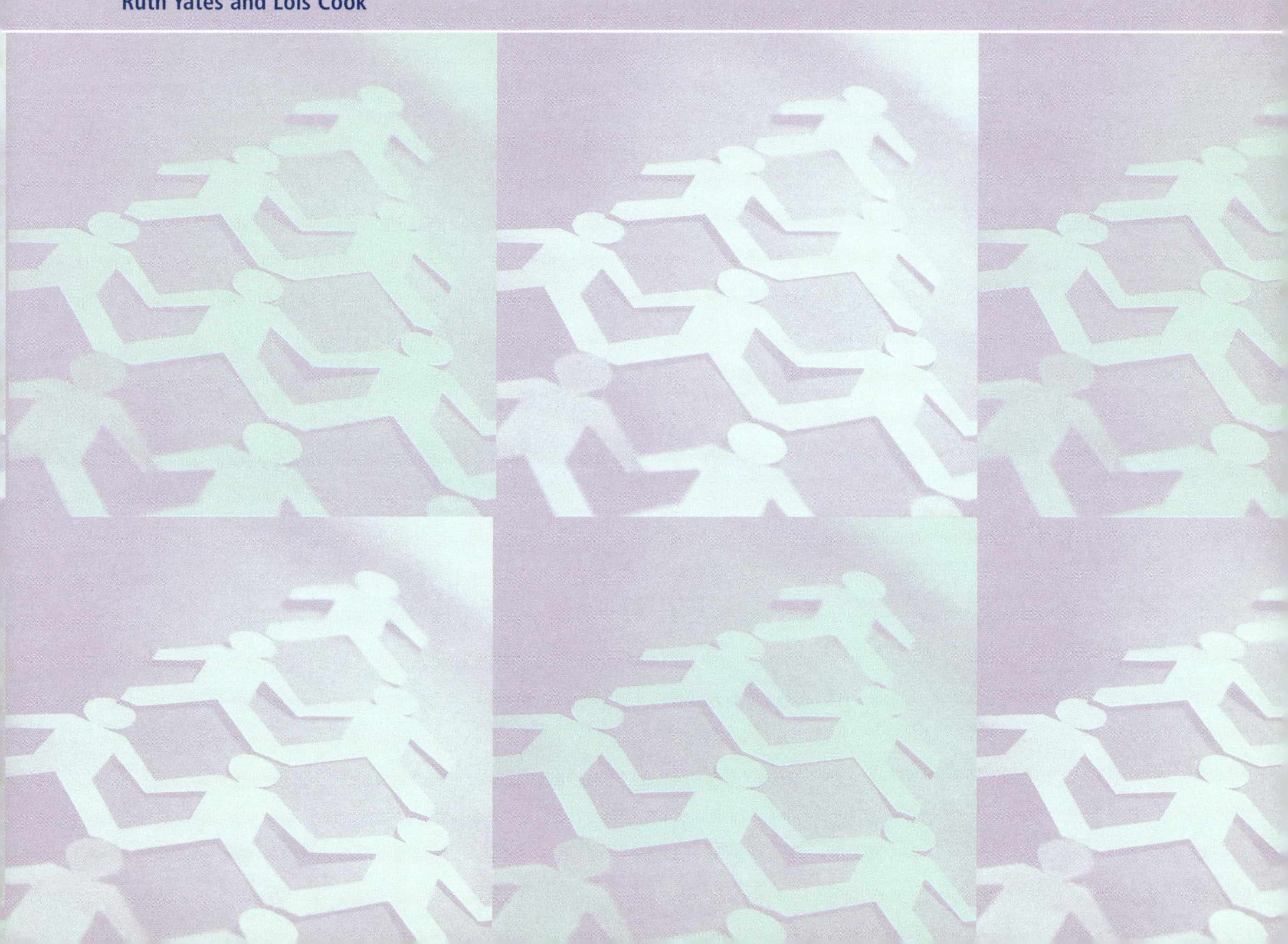

Chapter 8
Geographic variation in congential anomaly notifications in England and Wales

Summary

• There is a degree of under-reporting to the National Congenital Anomaly System (NCAS) as different anomalies have different levels of reporting and community trusts vary in their reporting practices. While this does not invalidate the surveillance function of NCAS, geographical variations in congenital anomalies are often the result of notification procedures.

• Variation in rates of abortions carried out under special grounds E of the 1967 Abortion Act (where there is a substantial risk that if the child were born it would suffer from such physical or mental abnormalities as to be seriously handicapped) between regions may reflect both access and attitudes toward diagnostic tests and abortion services. Notification rates to NCAS may have been low in the south of England because larger proportions of affected fetuses were terminated.

• A relationship between maternal age and Down syndrome is evident in rates reported to NCAS and abortions carried out under grounds E. The highest rates were found in the *Most Prosperous* ONS classification Group, which, along with the London Groups, had high conception rates for women aged 35-39.

• Regional and ONS classification Group analysis of neural tube defects indicated higher combined notification and abortion rates in areas with greater proportions of

conceptions to younger mothers, for example the North East. However, it is likely that socio-economic and genetic variables also contributed to this distribution.

• Abortions with a mention of heart and circulatory anomalies were low, only constituting under a quarter of all known cases. However there were regional differences with high rates in the East of England and low in the West Midlands, probably a reflection of differential access to prenatal diagnosis and abortion services.

• Although high notification rates to NCAS were recorded in Yorkshire and the Humber and low rates in London, limb reductions had little geographic variability.

• A north-south gradient for rates of abdominal wall defects was evident with higher combined notification and abortion rates in the North West and the North East and lower rates in London and the South East. This may be a result of higher rates of gastroschisis among offspring of young mothers, more commonly found in the north of England than the south, but could also reflect higher levels of deprivation in the north.

• Notification rates for polydactyly in London were three times those in the North East, a pattern at odds with regional variations in most other types of anomaly. This is probably due to the fact that it is a condition associated with black minority ethnic groups and London has the largest proportion of these groups in England and Wales.

8.1 Introduction

Congenital anomalies account for many deaths in young children and can also result in serious disability. The cause of many congenital anomalies remains unknown; there is considerable research interest in interactions between genetic and environmental factors. Such research has created a greater understanding of exogenous causes of many anomalies. Furthermore, birth prevalence of congenital anomalies has been affected by more sophisticated and widely available prenatal diagnostic services. Such determinants of the birth prevalence of congenital anomalies are subject to regional variation. An examination of rates may indicate regional risk factors.

For England and Wales, national information on congenital anomalies is available from three sources: notifications to the National Congenital Anomaly System (NCAS), death registration and abortion notifications for fetal anomalies. This chapter explores variations in congenital anomalies between 1992 and 1997 for Wales and the regions of England, using all three sources. Reasons for regional differences in rates for congenital anomalies include different reporting practices,

access to diagnostic and abortion services, demographic characteristics such as the average age at conception and the genetic characteristics of a population. These are discussed throughout this chapter. In addition, variation in the rate of congenital anomalies by ONS classification Group and the Carstairs and Morris index of deprivation are discussed. Chapter 4 provides the details on these classifications.

NCAS covers England and Wales only. The Scottish Congenital Anomaly Register (SCAR) is a separate system which has data from 1988. SCAR data are not comparable to NCAS data as they are collected in different ways; information is obtained from hospital admission and discharge records for children aged under 1 year. From April 1997 the information collected in these records changed, which means that we are unable to compare the data over the time period covered in our analysis. Another consequence of this change in data collection has been a fall in the number of congenital anomalies recorded in Scotland since 1996. For these reasons data from SCAR are not included in our analysis. Our analysis does not cover Northern Ireland as there are no national data available for Northern Ireland for the period covered.

8.2 Information sources

The National Congenital Anomaly System

The National Congenital Anomaly System (NCAS) was established in 1964 in response to the Thalidomide epidemic in order to detect other such hazards more quickly. The system records congenital anomalies for live births and stillbirths. Notification to NCAS is **voluntary** and is reported by local community trusts, which use birth notifications as their main source of information. The main purpose of NCAS is surveillance, while it also provides the best available birth prevalence data for England and Wales. The data from NCAS is passed on to the International Clearinghouse for Birth Defects Monitoring Systems (ICBDMS), for international studies into the prevalence and epidemiology of congenital anomalies. In 1990 NCAS adopted the European Registration of Congenital Anomalies (EUROCAT) exclusion list and a number of minor anomalies were excluded.[1] Some of these minor anomalies continued to be reported meaning the number of notifications to NCAS was higher in the early 1990s than for the following years.

Until 1995 the notification of a congenital anomaly had to take place within 10 days of birth. Consequently anomalies not easily diagnosed within the first few days of life were not always reported (for example heart anomalies). Since 1995 cases have been notified whenever they are identified. However, some systems within community trusts are not set up to report late diagnoses of anomalies to NCAS leading to a continued under reporting for certain conditions. In addition, there is a degree of under reporting to NCAS regardless of when the diagnosis is made. Just as different anomalies have different levels of under reporting, community trusts have different reporting practices. While such problems do not invalidate the surveillance function of NCAS, variations across England and Wales can be due to differences in notification procedures rather than differences in prevalence.

In addition to NCAS there are a number of regional congenital anomaly registers (Map 8.1).[2] The regional registers usually have multi-source ascertainment, which, combined with a working relationship with data suppliers, results in more complete data than NCAS. As Map 8.1 indicates coverage by a regional register varies throughout England and Wales which can have a number of effects on the data supplied to NCAS. Firstly, a number of regional registers now supply data directly to NCAS.[3] For instance, NCAS received data for Wales via the Congenital Anomaly Register and Information Service (CARIS)[4] for 1997 and these data are used in these analyses. Other registers have not supplied data before 1998. When registers pass on data to NCAS, notifications for this region are more complete so rates are usually higher. If a register does not provide data to NCAS, the interest at a local level can stimulate a higher rate of notification to NCAS. Conversely, the existence of a regional register can mean that data providers reporting at the local level are reluctant to fill out additional forms for NCAS and this can result in under-reporting. It is very difficult to predict the impact that regional registers have on the NCAS data.

Notification rates to NCAS (referred to in this chapter as the notification rate) are presented per 10,000 live and stillbirths.

Abortion notifications for fetal anomaly

Some congenital anomalies can be detected prenatally and, in these cases, parents may choose to terminate the pregnancy. Although abortion data are not part of NCAS, ONS processes abortion information on behalf of the Department of Health. Abortions for suspected, potential or confirmed fetal anomaly are recorded under grounds E of the Abortion Act 1967, where: *there is a substantial risk that if the child were born it would suffer from such physical or mental abnormalities as to be seriously handicapped.*

Data used here include abortions carried out under grounds E alone and in combination with any other grounds. The abortion notification form requires practitioners to record information about confirmed or suspected diagnoses in the fetus. As a fetus terminated under grounds E can suffer from more than one congenital anomaly, the abortion rates for individual conditions presented in this chapter include any mention of an anomaly on the abortion notification.

Prior to 1992, the postcode of usual residence was not retained for analysis of abortions once the administrative area information (such as the local authority or health authority applicable at the time) was derived. These data cannot, therefore, be recast to the latest boundaries. Analysis in this volume is based on boundaries in 1999 and has therefore been restricted to 1992 onwards for this chapter.

Rates for abortions carried out under grounds E (referred to as the abortion rate in this chapter) are expressed per 10,000 live and stillbirths. Abortions are not included in the denominator, as most abortions carried out under other grounds are not examined for anomalies. This leads to considerable under-ascertainment of anomalies among abortions. Furthermore most grounds E abortions would result in birth were it not for prenatal diagnosis. Notification of abortions is statutory; however, it should be noted that there are concerns that grounds E abortions are under notified. Technology available for prenatal diagnosis of congenital anomalies has advanced considerably in recent years, with conditions such as neural tube defects, abdominal wall defects and chromosomal anomalies being detected in the early stages of pregnancy.

Combined rates of notification to NCAS and abortions under grounds E for fetal anomaly (referred to as combined rates in this chapter) are also expressed per 10,000 live and stillbirths.

Infant death registration

In this chapter we also present data on infant deaths where a congenital anomaly has been mentioned on the death certificate (ONS cause group congenital anomaly). Box 7.2 in chapter 7 describes the ONS cause classification and presents detailed analysis of infant mortality by cause of death. For chapter 7 it was only possible to use data for 1993 onwards, therefore analysis in this chapter is restricted to 1993 onwards to allow comparison. Rates of infant death with a mention of congenital anomaly are presented per 10,000 live births.

Map 8.1

**Coverage of the regional Congenital Anomaly Registers
England and Wales 1997**

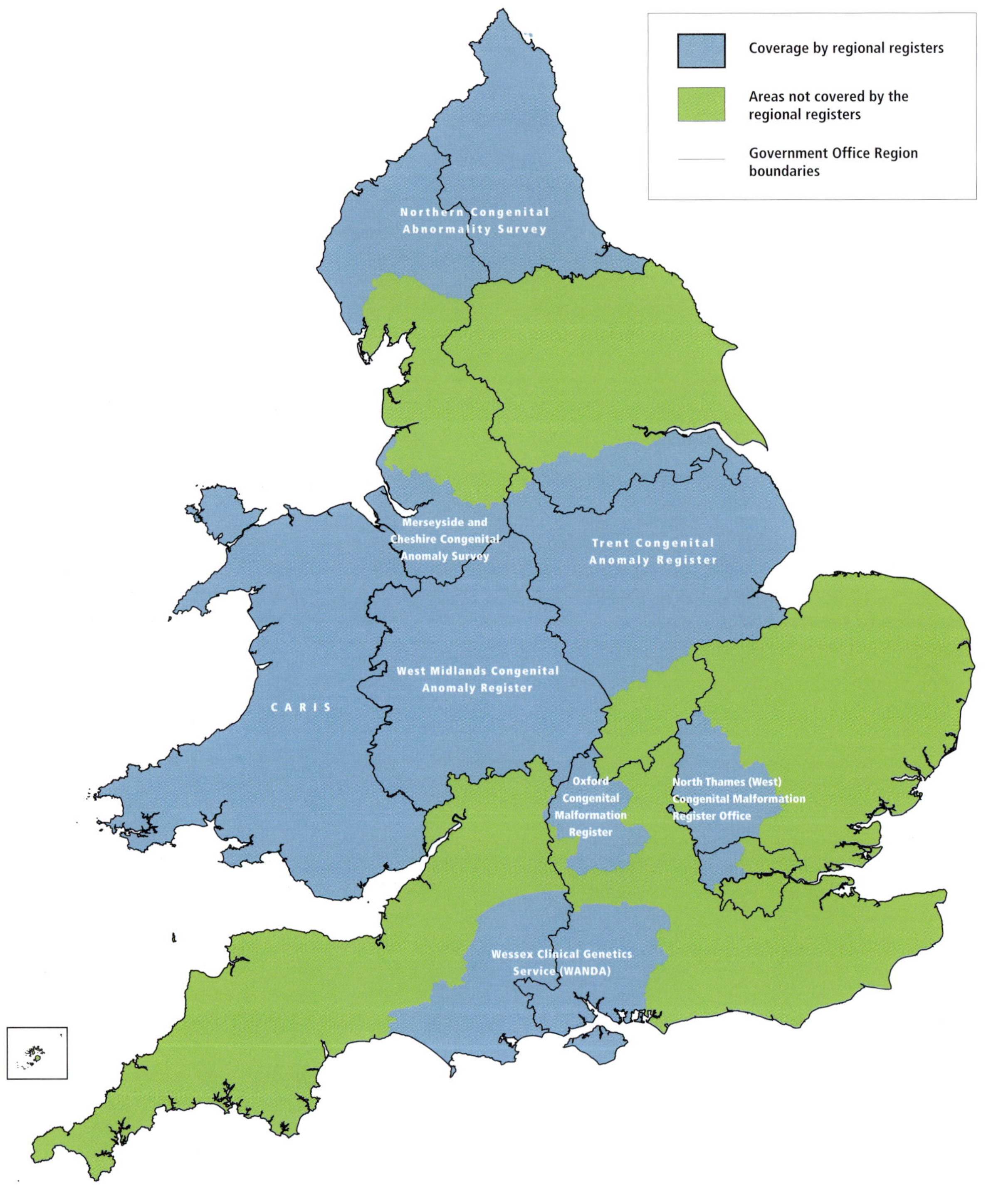

Figure 8.1

All babies notified to NCAS by country and region England and Wales 1992-1997

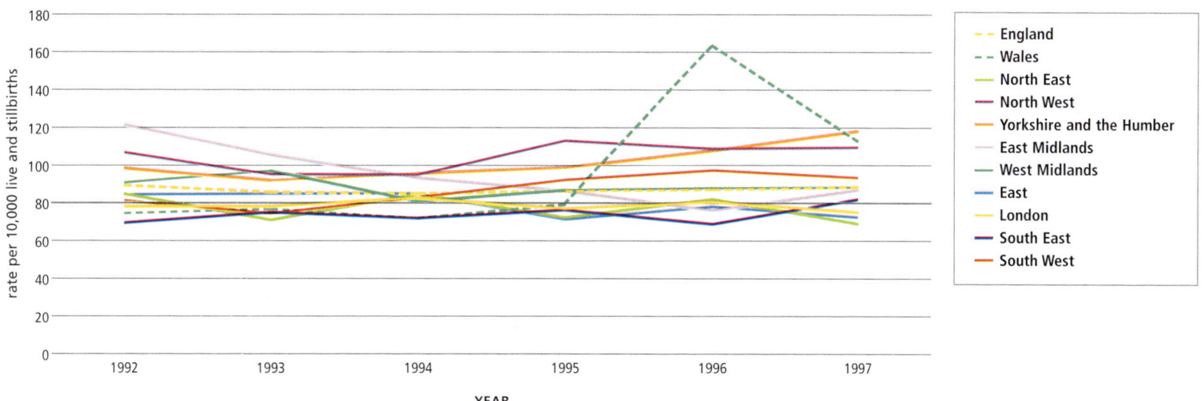

8.3 All anomalies

The overall congenital anomaly notification rate to NCAS in England and Wales for the period 1992-1997 was 87.2 per 10,000 live and stillbirths. There were higher rates in the North West (104.1) and Yorkshire and the Humber (101.1) and lower rates in the South East (73.5) and London (78.3) indicating that rates for all babies notified may reflect broader north-south divides in health (Map 8.2).[5] The existence of a congenital anomaly register in the North East which did not exchange data with NCAS made this region an exception to the north-south divide, with a rate of 77.3. This is because community trusts are unlikely to report to both a national and regional register. NCAS rates for England and Wales as a whole remained consistent for the period 1992-1997 whilst regional trends varied considerably (Figure 8.1). For instance, the rate in the East Midlands fell from 120.9 to 86.4, in comparison the rate in Wales rose from 74.3 to 112.7.

Infant deaths with mention of congenital anomalies had a rate of 15.4 per 10,000 live births for the period 1993-1997 (Figure 8.2). Significantly higher rates occurred in the West Midlands (19.3) and Yorkshire and the Humber (17.9) and lower rates in the South East (12.9) and the East of England (13.4).

Only 0.2 per cent of all abortions were carried out under grounds E. England and Wales had a rate of 28.0 per 10,000 live and stillbirths, remaining consistent for the period. Highest rates were in the East of England (36.6) and the South East (35.2) with lower rates in the West Midlands (21.0) and the South West (21.5). Abortions notified under grounds E combined with notifications to NCAS (Figure 8.3) showed similar combined rates in the South East (108.8), North East (102.8) and the West Midlands (109.6), indicating that NCAS rates may be low in the south of England as larger numbers of affected fetuses were terminated. Variation in rates of abortions carried out under grounds E between regions may reflect both access and attitudes towards diagnostic tests and abortion. As Figures 8.4 and 8.5 indicate, there are substantial variations in rates of abortions and notifications to NCAS between local authorities within

regions. Particularly large variations in rates between local authorities suggest important differences between local areas within regions.

Regional differences highlighted above imply a possible north-south gradient in notification to NCAS. There were considerable variations in notification rates concealed by analysing by the regions and Wales and exceptionally high rates in certain local authorities were likely to impact on the overall rates for the regions. For instance, notifications in 1996 and 1997 were higher in Wales as CARIS provided data to NCAS for these years[4] and generally lower for regions such as the South East, where regional registers did not exist. Small numbers prevent meaningful analysis at local authority level. The ONS classification of local authorities groups similar authorities together and provides simple indicators of local authority characteristics. This is discussed in more detail in chapter 4. The analysis of congenital anomaly rates by ONS classification Group also helps to overcome systematic geographical distortions caused by regional variations in data collection although some Groups are geographically clustered. As discussed geographic variation in abortion notifications carried out under grounds E reflects a number of factors including regional differences in access to diagnostic and termination services. This may be less of a problem when looking at rates by ONS classification Group.

Analysis by ONS classification Group indicated higher rates of congenital anomalies notified to NCAS 1992-1997 in local authorities in England and Wales classified as *Ports and Industry* (122.5) (Figure 8.6). However, geographic factors remain relevant, as authorities in this Group are located entirely in northern England. The combination with abortions data indicated a similar pattern with *Ports and Industry, West Inner London* and *Remoter Rural* areas having the highest combined rates. Geographic factors are also important in Groups with low rates, for instance NCAS rates were lower in *East Inner London* (a Group entirely located in London), a likely reflection of poor notification practices.

Map 8.2

Notifications to the National Congenital Anomaly System and abortions carried out under grounds E by country and region England and Wales 1992-1997

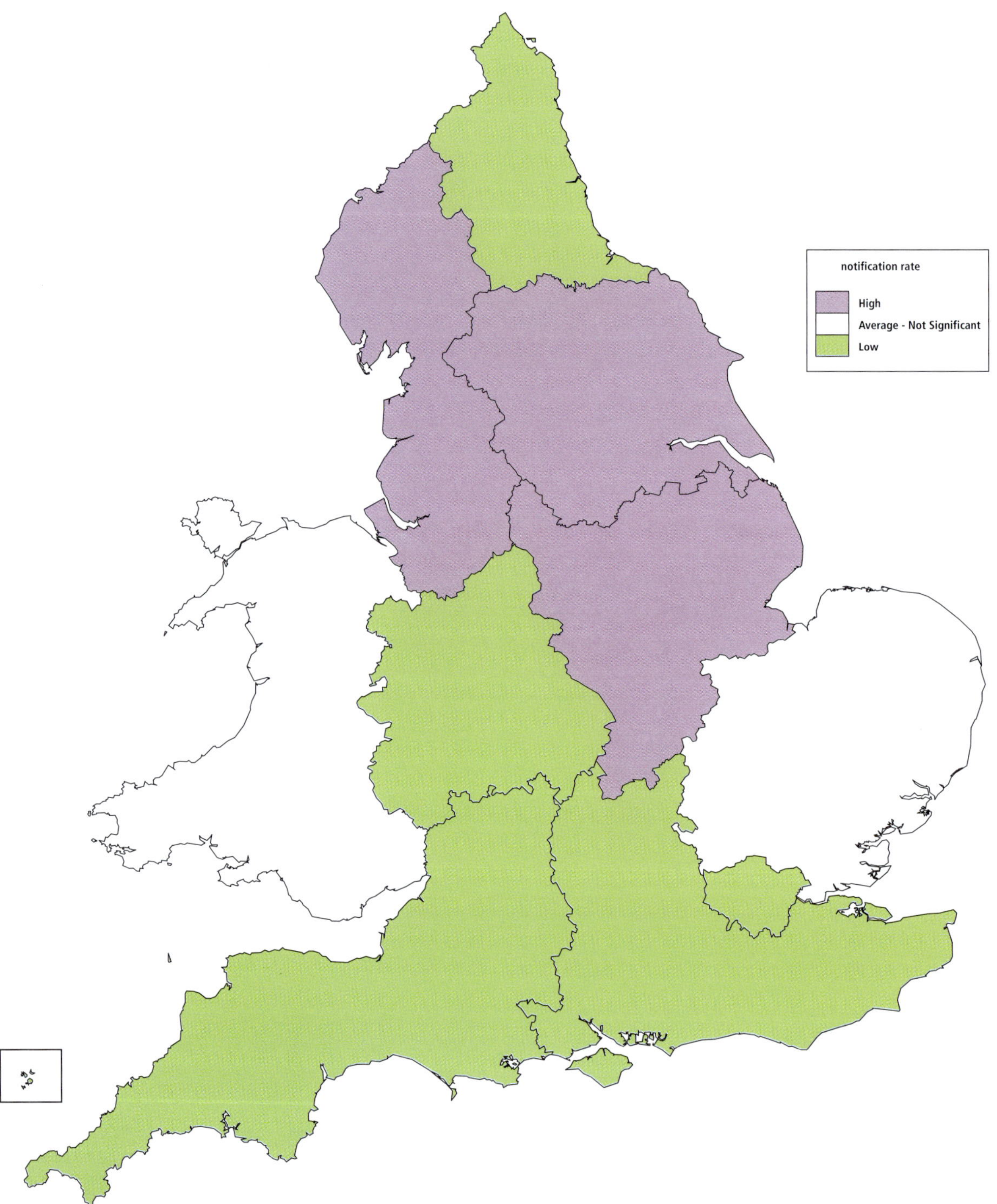

Figure 8.2

**Infant death registrations with mention of a congenital anomaly by country and region
England and Wales 1993-1997**

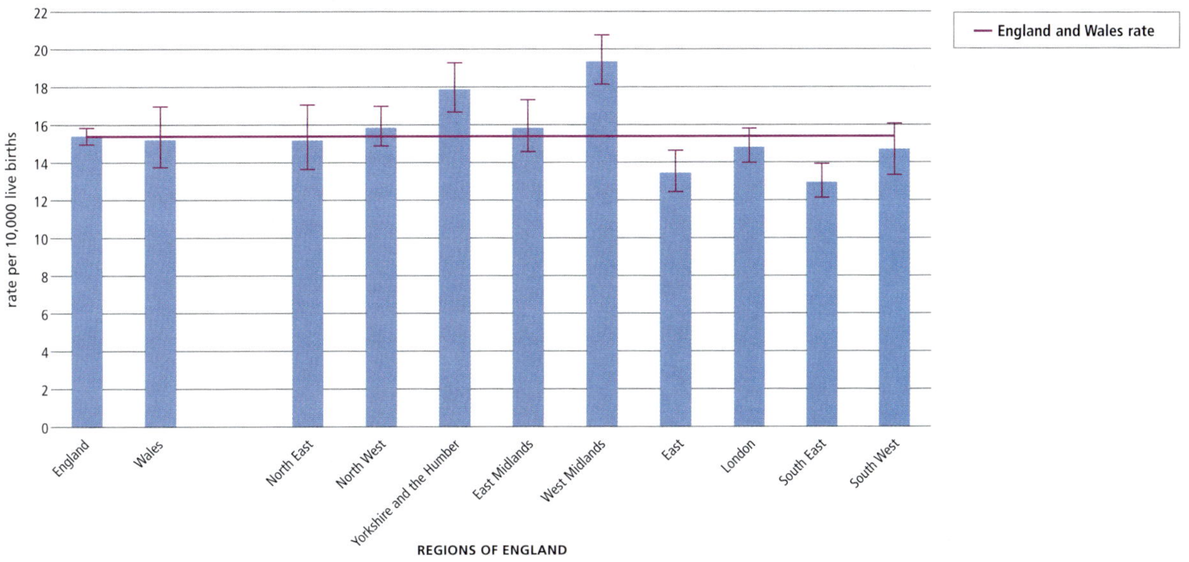

Figure 8.3

**All babies notified to NCAS and notifications of abortions carried out under grounds E by country and region
England and Wales 1992-1997**

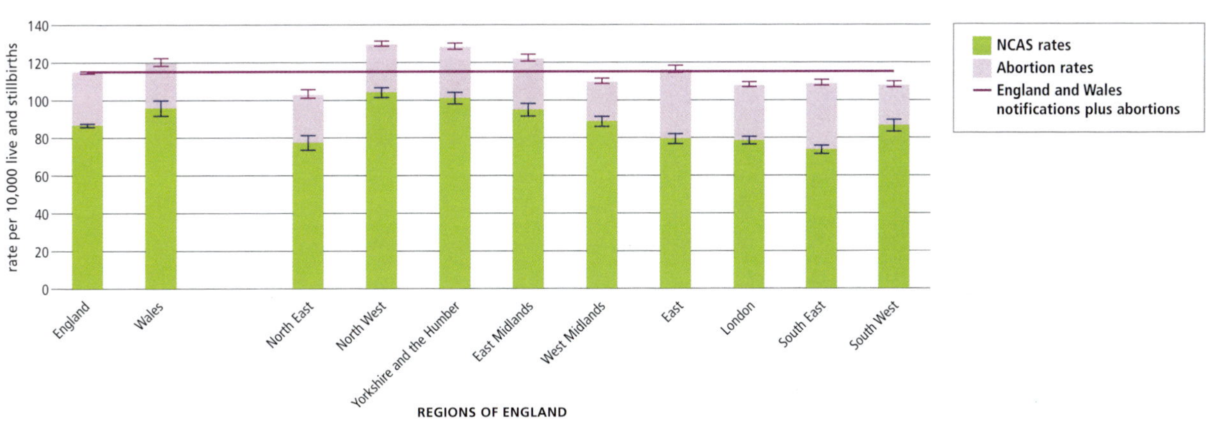

Figure 8.4

**All babies notified to NCAS by local authority within countries and regions
England and Wales 1992-1997**

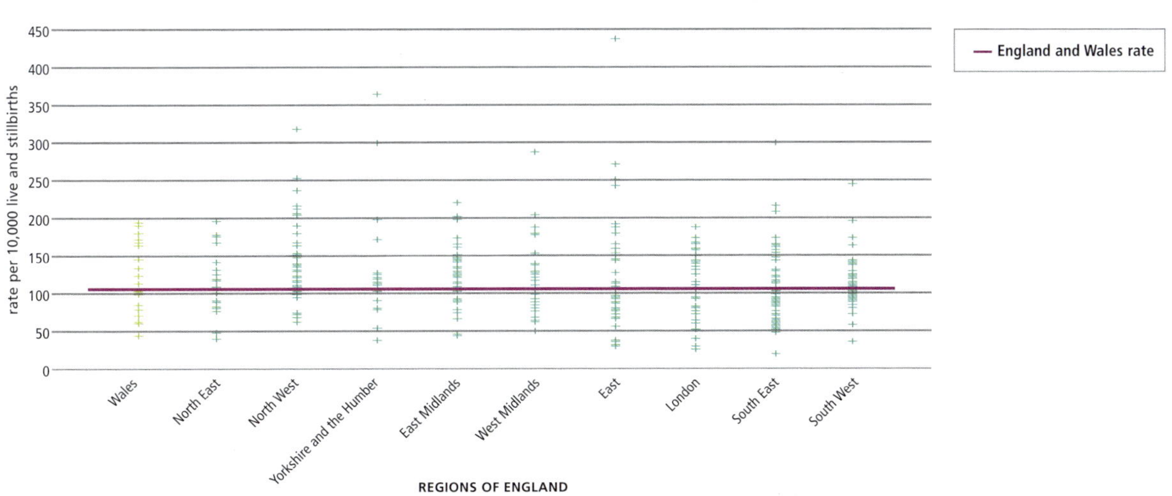

Figure 8.5

All notifications of abortions carried out under grounds E by local authority within countries and regions England and Wales 1992-1997

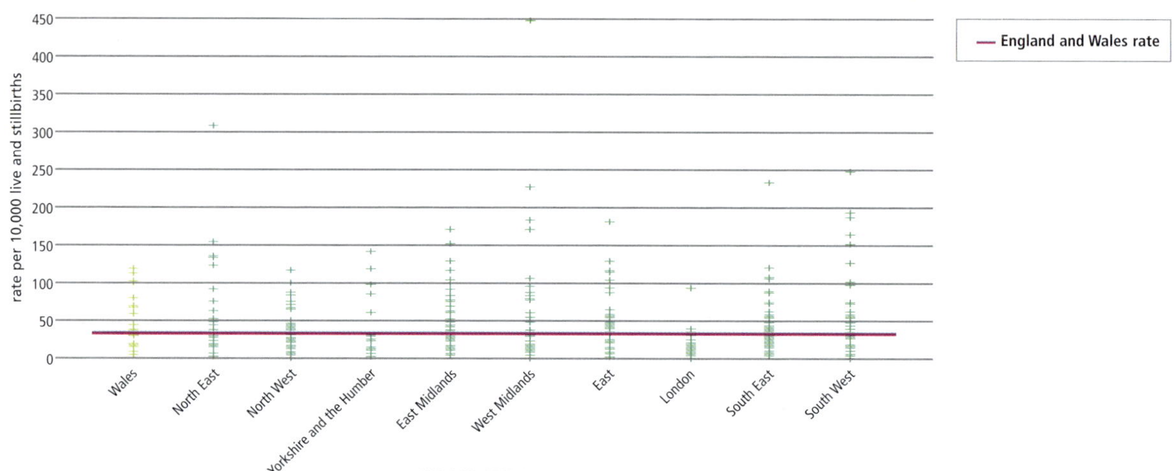

Figure 8.6

All babies notified to NCAS and notifications of abortions carried out under grounds E by ONS classification Group England and Wales 1992-1997

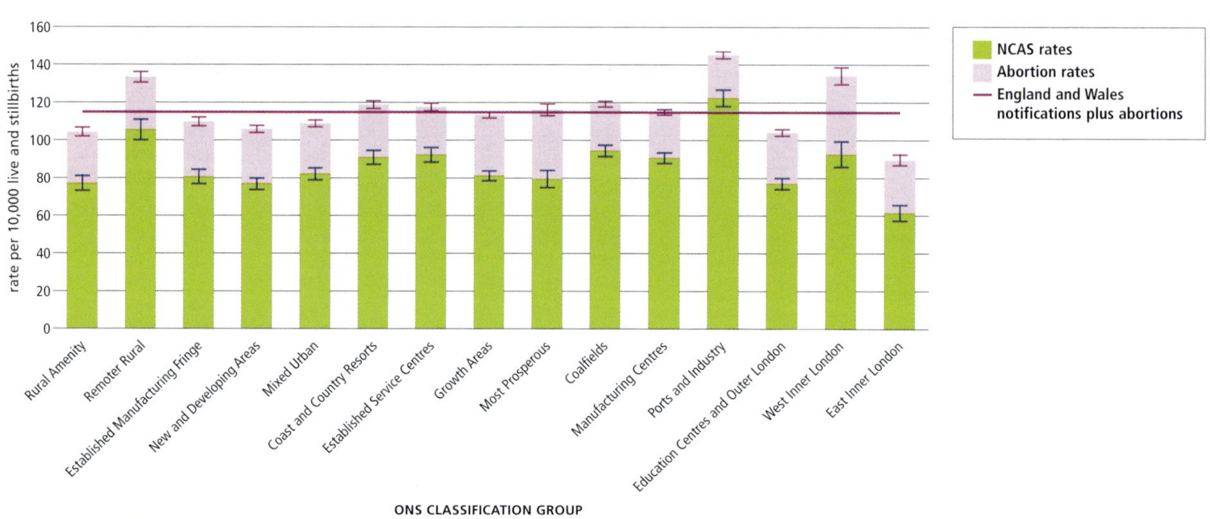

Although overall patterns of notification for babies with congenital anomalies are informative there are important differences between types of anomaly which impact completeness of notification to NCAS. For instance, those anomalies visible at birth are more completely notified than internal and chromosomal defects.[4] Exogenous factors may also vary by anomaly, for instance, certain congenital anomalies, such as Down syndrome, are more likely to be found in offspring of older mothers who are more concentrated in certain regions. The geographic distribution of fertility by mother's age is discussed in chapter 5. In addition when the data in this chapter were analysed by deprivation, no significant differences by deprivation were found. As different anomalies have different causes it makes sense to look at geographic variations in individual anomalies.

8.4 Down syndrome

Down syndrome is a chromosomal anomaly; a group of disorders encompassing a broad range of severity. A chromosome abnormality is the result of either abnormal numbers of chromosomes or rearrangement of chromosomal genetic material and often results in death. Analysis of infant deaths where chromosomal anomalies are mentioned showed marked regional variation with a rate of 1.9 per 10,000 live births for England and Wales, 1993-1997 (Figure 8.7).

Down syndrome is the most common of the more severe types of chromosomal malformations, present in 6 per cent of all children reported to NCAS and over 60 per cent of those with chromosomal anomalies. It is a condition caused by an excess

Figure 8.7

Infant death registrations with mention of chromosomal anomaly by country and region
England and Wales 1993-1997

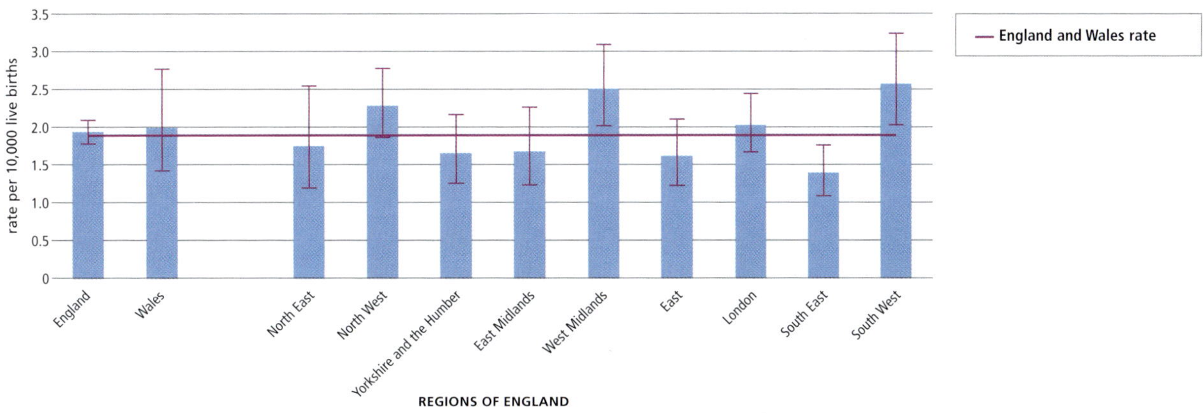

Figure 8.8

Notifications of Down syndrome to NCAS and notifications of abortions carried out under grounds E with mention of Down syndrome by country and region
England and Wales 1992-1997

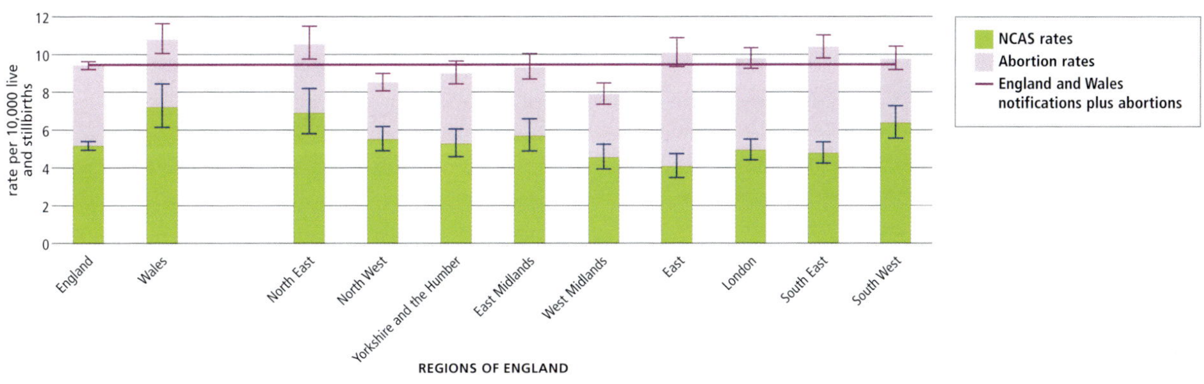

Figure 8.9

Notifications of Down syndrome to NCAS and notifications of abortions carried out under grounds E with mention of Down syndrome by ONS classification Group
England and Wales 1992-1997

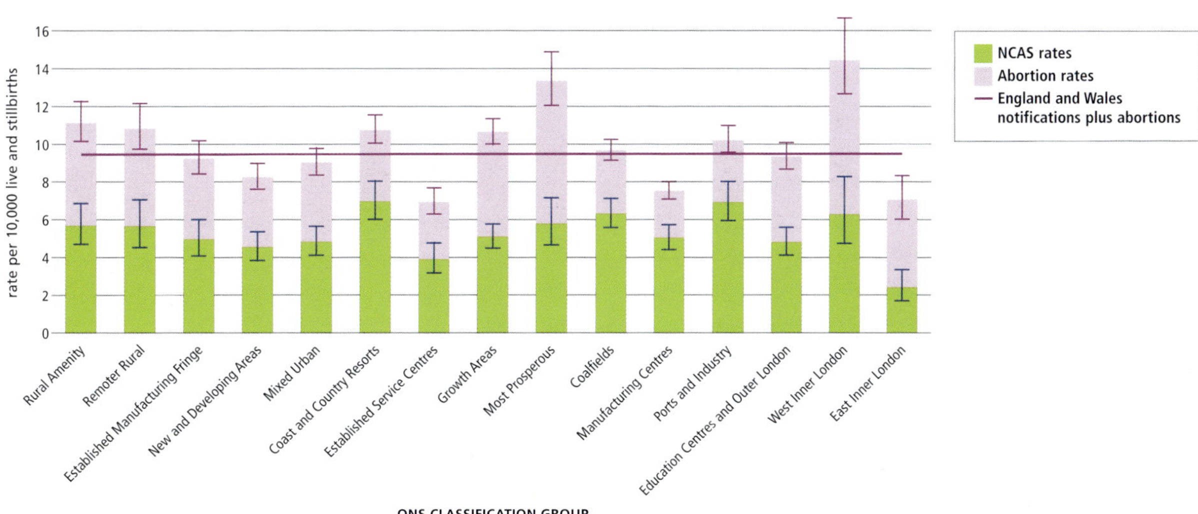

Figure 8.10

Notifications of Down syndrome to NCAS and notifications of abortions carried out under grounds E with mention of Down syndrome by deprivation
England and Wales 1992-1997

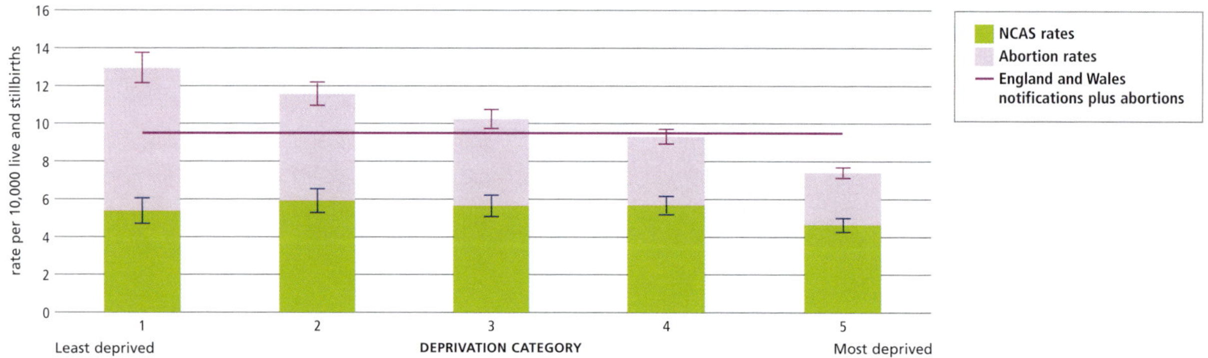

of chromosome 21 material, disturbing development and resulting in a physical appearance allowing straightforward diagnosis at birth. The condition carries increased risk for anomalies, mental retardation, weaker immune systems, premature ageing and death. The condition is permanent although anomalies can be treated surgically and mental development can be increased with adequate care.

Down syndrome notifications to NCAS constituted a rate of 5.3 per 10,000 live and stillbirths for England and Wales, lower than the rates generally recorded on other national registers.[6] Significantly higher rates in Wales (7.2) and the North East (6.9) were probably due to improved data for 1997 when NCAS made a specific request to data suppliers to compare records with NCAS and report missing cases. Information on Down syndrome for 1997 is more complete than for other years.[7] This is reflected in increased rates for England and Wales as a whole and for Wales and the North East in particular in 1997. Consequently the data for this period may not reflect actual trends in Down syndrome rates over time, but rather changes in notification procedures. The National Down Syndrome Cytogenetic Register data suggests that there was actually a decline in the prevalence of the condition over the period.[8] As an anomaly that can be detected prenatally, increases in proportions of Down syndrome cases detected and terminated are likely to account for decreasing notification rates to NCAS.

Down syndrome has greater prevalence among offspring of older mothers,[9] having implications for the increasing numbers of women delaying childbearing.[10] Our analysis confirmed this, with higher notification rates to NCAS for Down syndrome babies born to mothers in older age groups being evident at the England and Wales level; rates of 14.9 for mothers aged 35 and over compared to 4.0 for those aged under 35. As they are most likely to conceive an affected child, older pregnant women are more likely to be offered prenatal diagnosis, consequently there are relatively high rates of detection and subsequent terminations. As Figure 8.8 shows, NCAS data alone may underestimate actual prevalence of Down syndrome in regions identified as having large proportions of older mothers, such as

the East of England where abortion rates are noticeably high (6.0 per 10,000 live and stillbirths).

High combined notification and abortion rates for Down syndrome were evident in the *Most Prosperous* (13.4) and *West Inner London* (14.4) Groups (Figure 8.9). These Groups are known to have higher fertility in older women (Figure 5.45 in chapter 5). *East Inner London* also has high fertility in older women, but low notification rates for Down syndrome. This could be a reflection of under-notification. Deprivation analyses suggest that the least deprived mothers were more likely to have an affected fetus, possibly also a reflection of older maternal age (Figure 8.10). Figure 5.63 in chapter 5 shows fertility among women aged 35-39 by deprivation.

8.5 Central nervous system anomalies

Central nervous system (CNS) anomalies are among the most common birth defects, often resulting in serious disability and infant mortality. Over 4 per cent of children reported to NCAS had such anomalies. The brain and/or spinal cord (and their protecting skull or spinal column) fail to develop properly; the condition develops soon after conception, usually before the mother knows she is pregnant. CNS anomalies include neural tube defects (see below) and congenital hydrocephalus (the accumulation of cerebrospinal fluid, either within the brain ventricles or between the brain and the skull). There is a relationship between maternal age and CNS anomalies with both younger and older mothers more likely to conceive an affected child.[11]

Notifications to NCAS for CNS anomalies in the period had a rate of 3.7 per 10,000 live and stillbirths in England and Wales as a whole. Increases in Welsh rates between 1995 (2.2) and 1996 (3.8) were largely due to improved data from CARIS.[4] Regional and Group analysis indicated higher rates in areas with high rates of conception among young mothers, for instance, the North West (4.8), the West Midlands (4.8), *Ports and Industry* (6.2) and *Manufacturing Centres* (5.3) (Figures 8.11 and 8.12). Areas with lower rates tended to have smaller proportions of conceptions to

Figure 8.11

Notifications of CNS anomalies to NCAS and notifications of abortions carried out under grounds E with mention of CNS anomalies by country and region
England and Wales 1992-1997

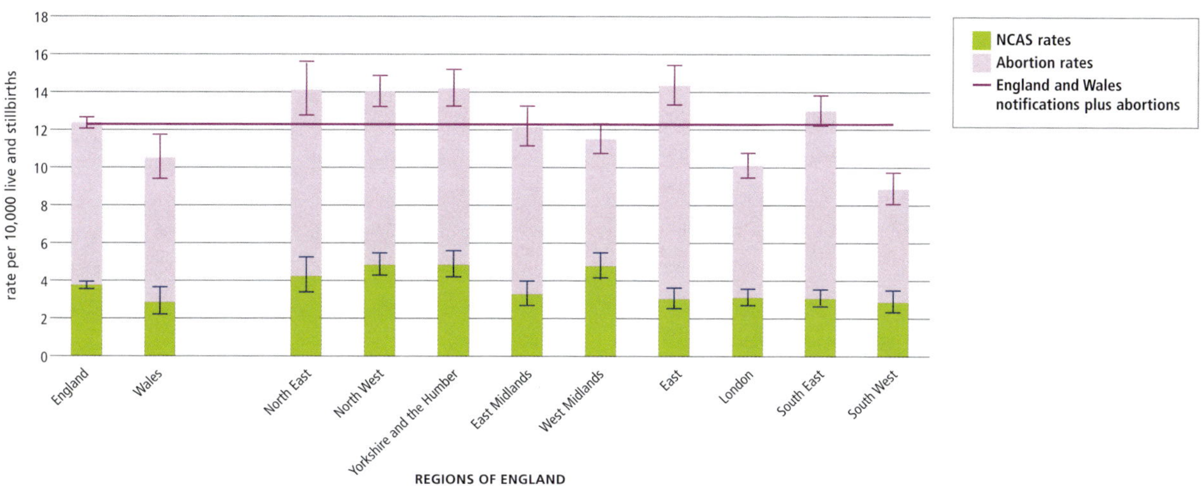

Figure 8.12

Notifications of CNS anomalies to NCAS and notifications of abortions carried out under grounds E with mention of CNS anomalies by ONS classification Group
England and Wales 1992-1997

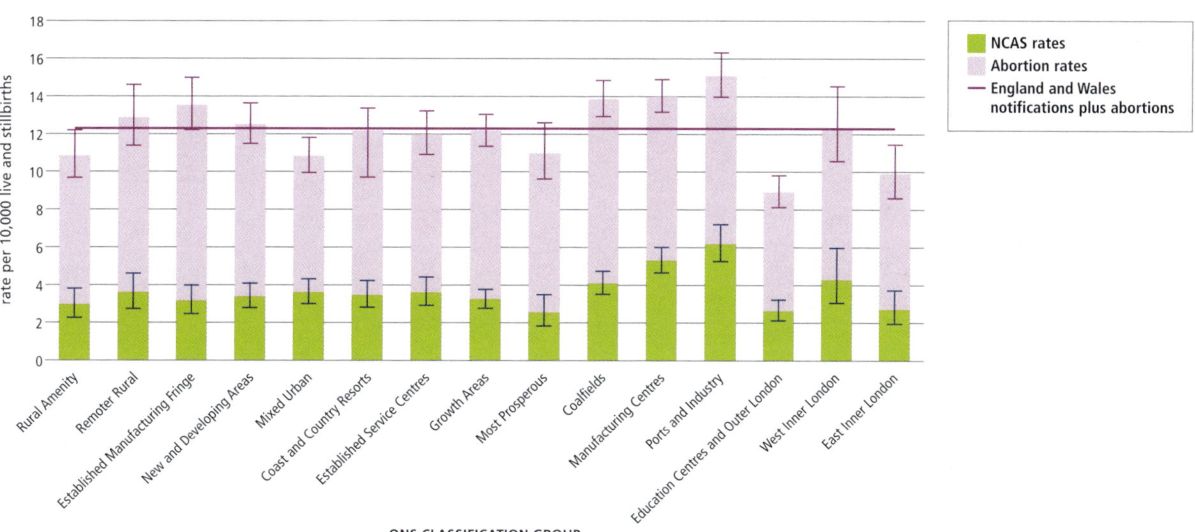

young mothers. Infant death registrations with mention of CNS anomalies reflect this pattern. However, it is likely that socio-economic and genetic variables also contributed to this distribution; generally areas with higher levels of deprivation had higher conception rates for younger mothers. Chapter 5 of this volume demonstrates this. Prenatal screening and diagnosis mean a large proportion of cases result in termination. Although there was little regional variation, rates of abortion under grounds E with CNS mentioned were high in the East of England (11.3) and low in the South West (6.0) (Figure 8.11).

There are three major kinds of neural tube defects (NTDs); anencephaly, a high mortality condition where most of the brain and skull are absent; encephalocele, where the brain protrudes through a gap in the skull; and spina bifida where the

neural tube is split and one or more vertebrae fail to form properly. The majority of pregnancies involving NTDs end in either termination or stillbirth. There is a genetic background to many NTD cases and risk of reoccurrence in subsequent children does exist. However there are also exogenous factors. Folic acid supplements taken around time of conception can reduce the likelihood of NTD occurrence in the fetus. A government-sponsored campaign initiated in the late 1990s to raise awareness among health professionals and women of childbearing age will have had little impact on this analysis which only looks at data for 1992-1997. However, regional differences in diet could explain variations in rates. Results from the 1995 Infant Feeding Survey[12] suggested that only 53 per cent of recent mothers under 20 understood the importance of increasing the intake of folic acid in early

Figure 8.13

Notifications of NTDs to NCAS and notifications of abortions carried out under grounds E with mention of
NTDs by country and region
England and Wales 1992-1997

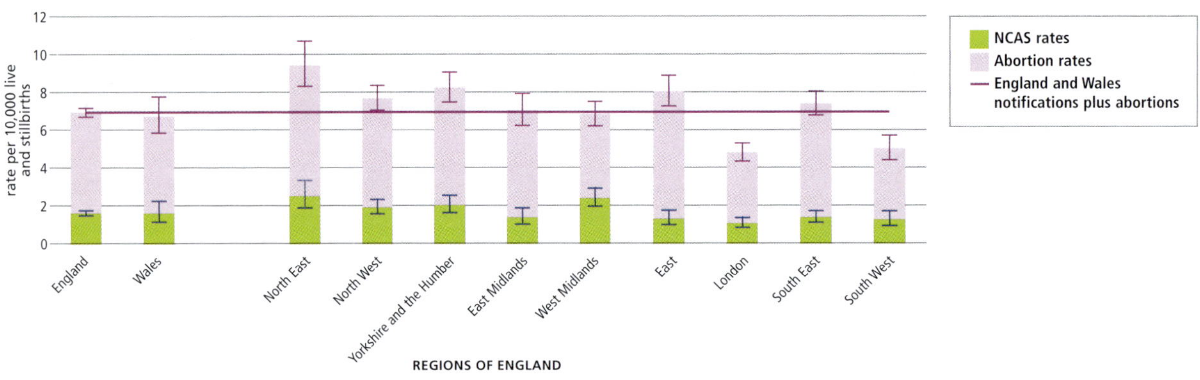

Figure 8.14

Notifications of NTDs to NCAS and notifications of abortions carried out under grounds E with mention of
NTDs by country and region
England and Wales 1993-1996*

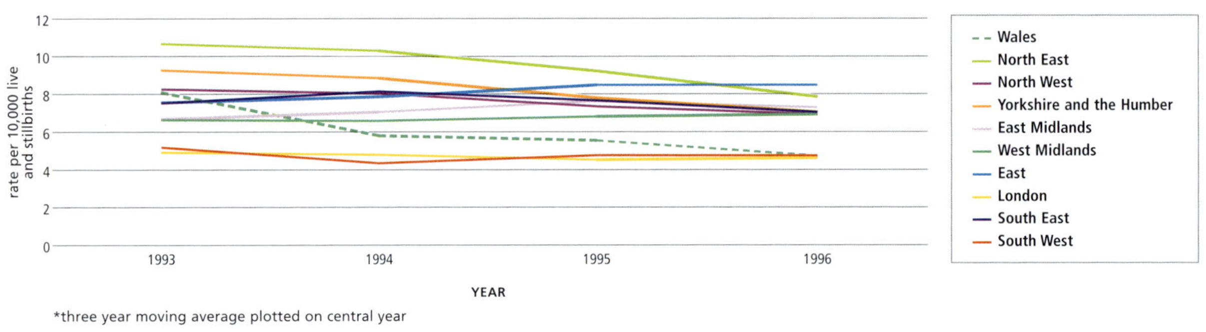

*three year moving average plotted on central year

Figure 8.15

Infant death registrations with mention of heart and circulatory anomalies by country and region
England and Wales 1993-1997

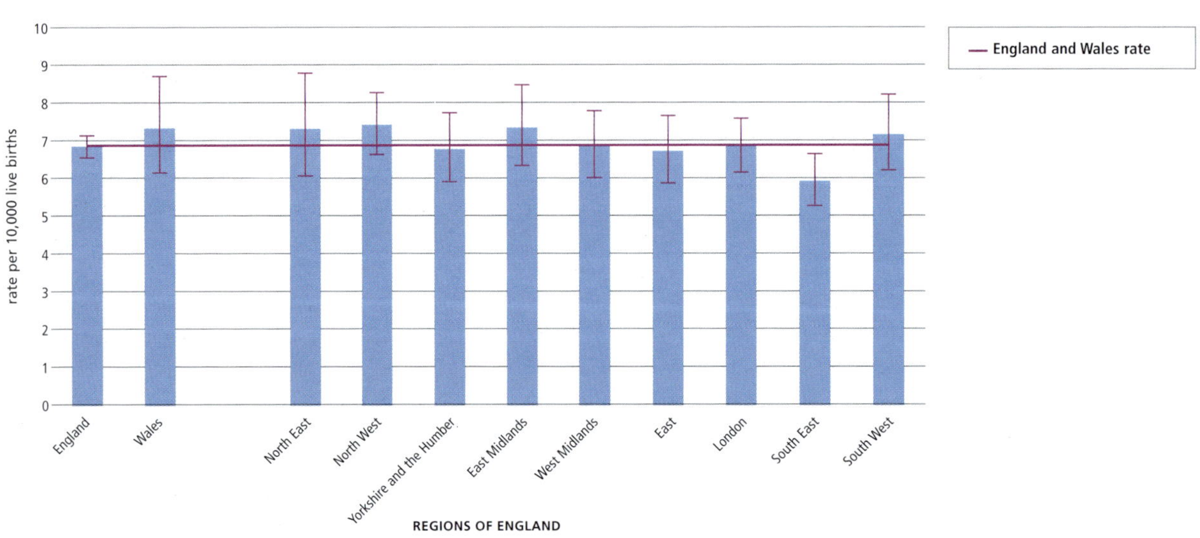

Figure 8.16

Notifications of heart and circulatory anomalies to NCAS and notifications of abortions carried out under grounds E with mention of heart and circulatory anomalies by country and region
England and Wales 1992-1997

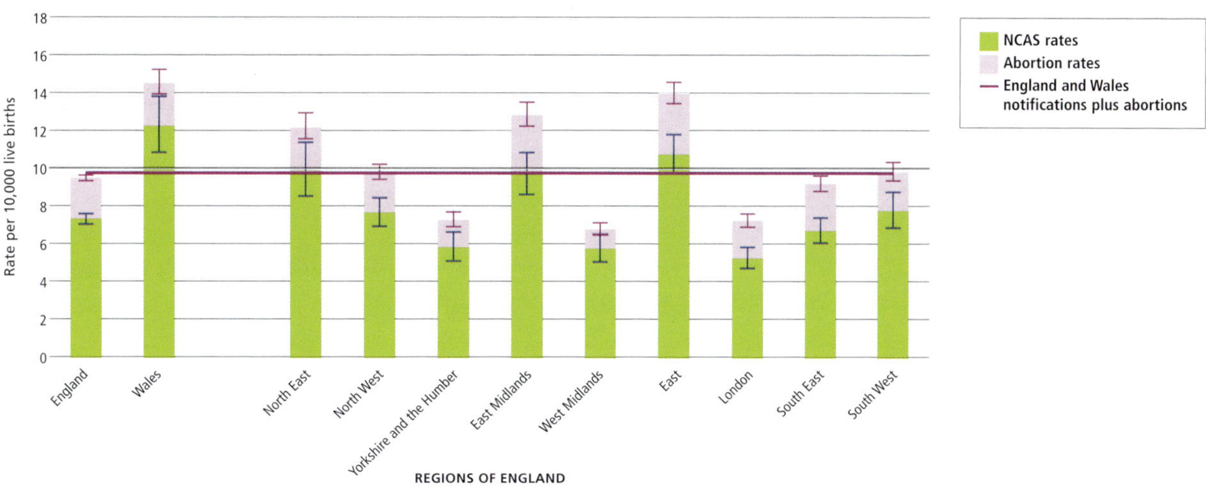

Figure 8.17

Notifications of heart and circulatory anomalies to NCAS and notifications of abortions carried out under grounds E with mention of heart and circulatory anomalies by ONS classification Group
England and Wales 1992-1997

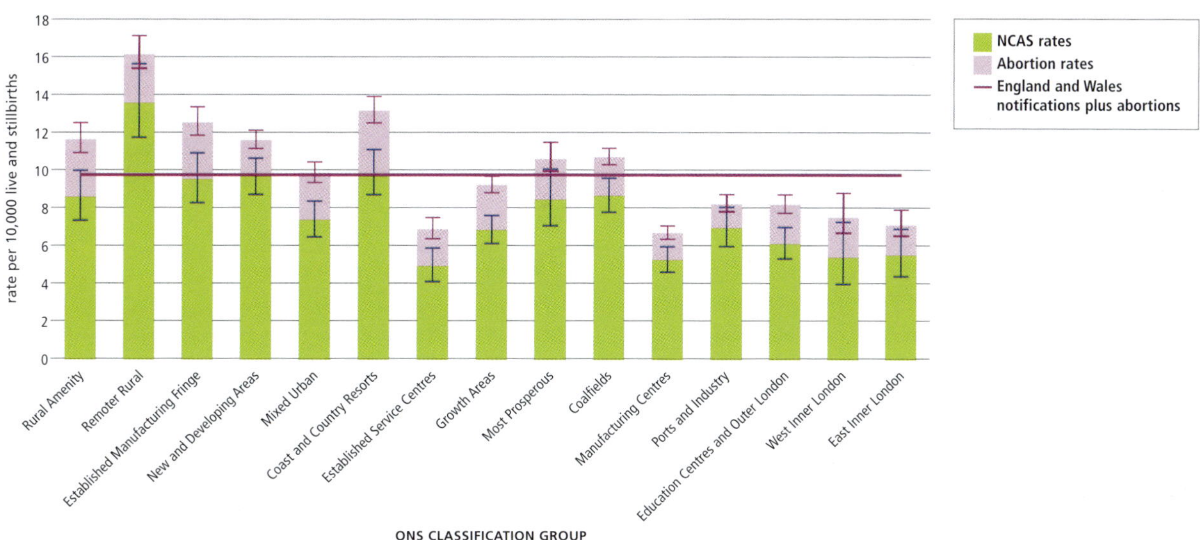

pregnancy (compared to 80 per cent of those mothers over 30). Furthermore, The National Food Survey 1997 indicated that younger households consumed far less fresh vegetables and cereals (foods rich in folates) than older households.[13]

The rate for NTD notifications made to NCAS was 1.6 per 10,000 live and stillbirths for the period, accounting for nearly 2 per cent of babies notified. Regional patterns reflected those for CNS anomalies (Figure 8.13). The National Diet and Nutrition Survey[14] indicates greater consumption of cereals (often fortified with folic acid) in London and the South East where NTD rates were low. Deprivation analysis shows no significant relationship between deprivation and NTD rates. However, genetic as well as environmental factors are important.

The rate to NCAS combined with mentions on abortions carried out under grounds E fell from 7.5 in 1992 to 5.9 in 1997 (Figure 8.14). This downward trend was echoed at the regional level, especially in the North East where rates more than halved from 11.2 to 5.4 with similar decreases in Yorkshire and the Humber. This reflects a long term decrease in rates for NTDs using NCAS data, however, other studies suggest that the rate remained unaltered throughout the 1990s.[15] The rates by ONS classification Group reflected those of CNS anomalies.

8.6 Heart and circulatory anomalies

Of the children born with heart and circulatory anomalies one third die soon after birth and one third require surgery.[16] Infant deaths with mention of such anomalies had a rate of 6.9 per

Figure 8.18

Notifications of cleft anomalies to NCAS and notifications of abortions carried out under grounds E with mention of clefts by country and region
England and Wales 1992-1997

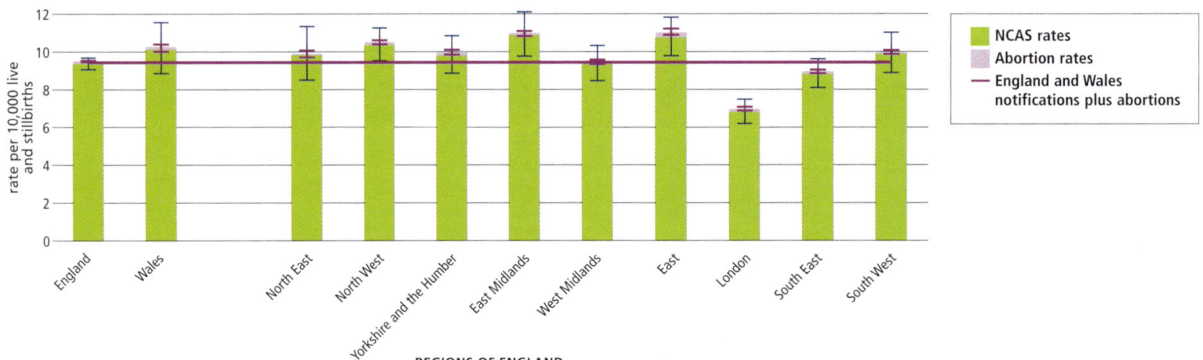

10,000 live births in England and Wales for the period 1993-1997, with no significant regional variation (Figure 8.15). The likelihood of inheritance for heart anomalies depends on the condition; women considered at greatest risk can have prenatal screening.

Heart and circulatory anomalies were reported in over 8 per cent of babies notified to NCAS for the period, with a rate of 7.6 per 10,000 live and stillbirths for England and Wales. Significantly lower rates were recorded in London (5.3) and higher rates in the North West (7.7) and Wales (12.3), the latter rates reflecting improved data from CARIS (rates increased from 9.0 in 1992 to 26.8 in 1997) (Figure 8.16). Similar increases occurred in the North East and Yorkshire and the Humber whilst other regions had reasonably consistent rates. Abortions for heart and circulatory anomalies are low, only constituting under a quarter of all known cases (Figure 8.16). However there were regional differences with rates high in the East of England (3.3) and low in the West Midlands (1.0), probably a reflection of differential access to prenatal diagnosis and abortion services. The Group analysis seemed to suggest that there might have been higher rates of heart anomalies in rural rather than urban areas (Figure 8.17) and deprivation analysis showed no significant variation.

8.7 Cleft palate, cleft lip and cleft lip and palate

These conditions are coded separately but can be analysed together as clefting of the lip or/and palate. Clefts can be repaired surgically with complete cosmetic and functional restoration by school age. Genetic factors can incur familial recurrence risk but environmental factors have also been put forward, such as certain drugs and maternal smoking.[17] Cleft anomalies have high levels of notification, present in 11 per cent of all babies reported to NCAS. Such levels are a likely reflection of straightforward diagnosis at birth. Clefts are not routinely detected prenatally and are relatively simple to correct surgically; rates for abortions carried out under grounds E with mention of clefts are therefore low and too small for regional analysis (Figure 8.18). Similarly death registrations are not analysed here, as it is not a fatal condition.

The overall rate for clefts in the period was 9.5 per 10,000 live and stillbirths for England and Wales, within the range of rates experienced by other national congenital anomaly registers.[6] Regional patterns for cleft anomalies were similar to those for all babies notified (Figure 8.18) with lower rates in London region and London ONS classification Groups. There was no statistically significant relationship between the condition and deprivation. As a condition that can be easily diagnosed at birth, it is well notified and causal factors are debatable, it is therefore difficult to conclude what regional variations in rates mean.

8.8 Hypospadias and epispadias

Hypospadias and epispadias are malformations of the genitals present in around 9 per cent of babies notified to NCAS. They are examined together although hypospadias has greater prevalence. Hypospadias is a malposition of the urethral opening on the underside of the penis. It has an extremely broad range of severity; milder forms (which constitute the majority of cases) were part of the 1991 NCAS exclusion list. Hypospadias arises early in embryonic development and is a process driven by androgens and usually requires correctional surgery. It has been postulated that exogenous hormones may be a causal factor but no definite non-genetic cause has been confirmed. Possibility of environmental causes has raised concerns about whether milder forms should have been excluded from NCAS. Epispadias affects both sexes; in males the urethra opens on the dorsal side of the penis and in females the urethra may open above or into the clitoris. Like hypospadias the severity of the condition varies, there is some evidence of genetic causes and little is known of exogenous factors; milder forms can be repaired surgically. Although they can be detected prenatally their severity is such that terminations are not usual and so will not be considered here. Also they are not fatal conditions so infant deaths will not be analysed.

Figure 8.19

**Notifications of hypospadias and epispadias to NCAS by country and region
England and Wales 1992-1997**

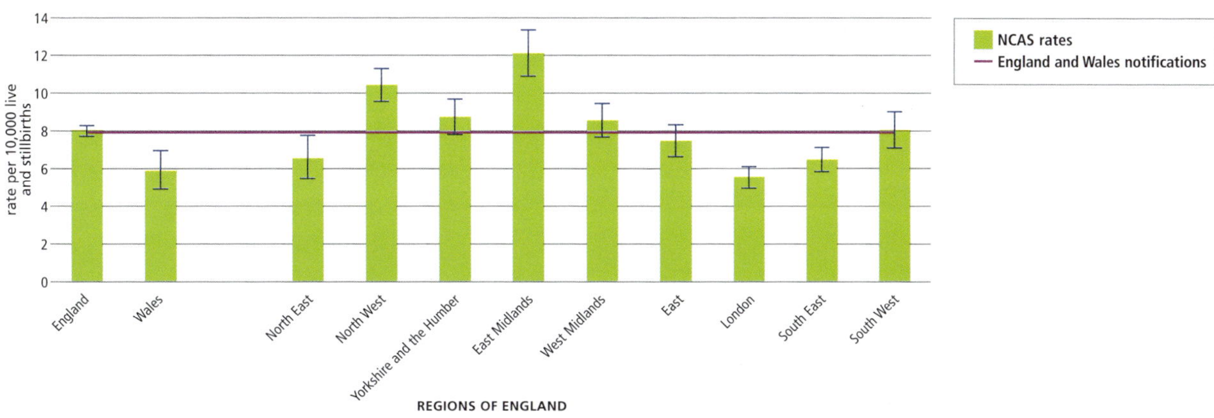

Figure 8.20

**Notifications of limb reduction anomalies to NCAS and notifications of abortions carried out under grounds E with
mention of limb reductions by country and region
England and Wales 1992-1997**

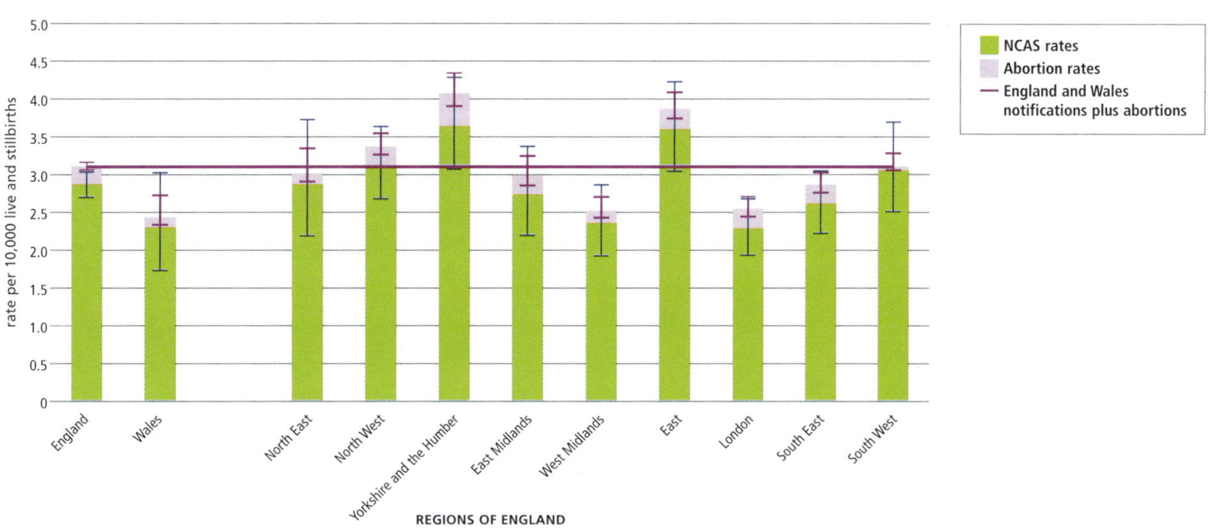

The notification rate for hypospadias and epispadias to NCAS
for the period was 7.9 per 10,000 live and stillbirths in England
and Wales (Figure 8.19). Regional variation reflected the rates
for all babies notified with the exception of significantly higher
rates in the East Midlands (12.1). England and Wales saw an
overall decrease in rates from 7.9 in 1992 to 7.4 in 1997 echoed
in the East Midlands (from 14.0 to 9.1) and London (from 5.3
to 4.2), decreases which are a likely affect of the exclusion list.
Deprivation analysis has been carried out and there was no real
variation. Group analysis reflected the pattern for all anomalies
with high rates in *Ports and Industry* (10.7) and lower rates in
the London areas.

8.9 Limb reductions

Limb reductions show considerable variation in severity, from
the missing end of a finger to the complete absence of a limb or
limbs. Where appropriate prosthesis can be used, surgery is
usually not an option. As isolated anomalies, limb defects are
not hereditary but may be symptoms of other conditions that
are. The drug most associated with this anomaly is thalidomide
(no longer used by pregnant women) and although other
exogenous causes have been investigated there is no other
proven link.

Limb reductions are reported in over 3 per cent of babies
notified to NCAS. The overall rate to NCAS for the period was
2.8 per 10,000 live and stillbirths in England and Wales, a rate

Figure 8.21

**Notifications of limb reduction anomalies to NCAS and notifications of abortions carried out under grounds E with mention of limb reduction anomalies by ONS classification Group
England and Wales 1992-1997**

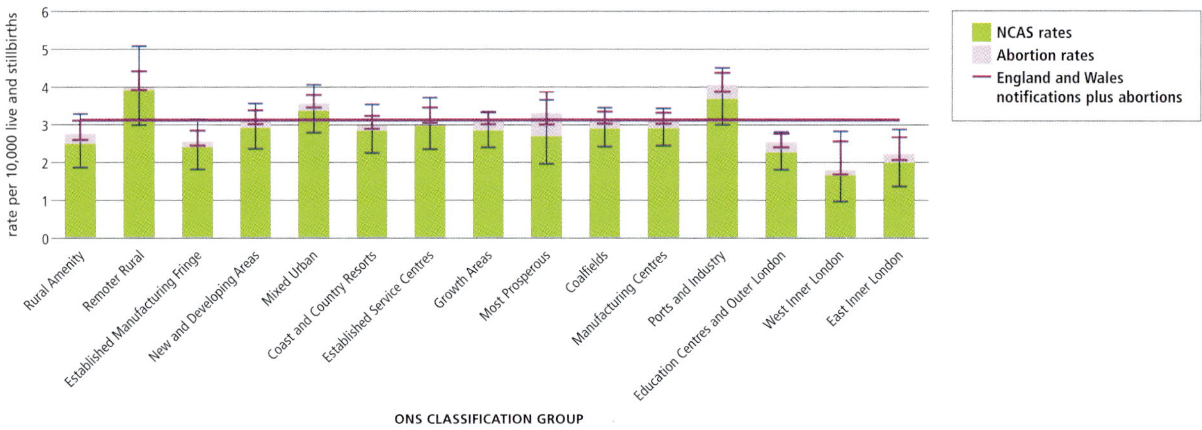

Figure 8.22

**Notifications of eye anomalies to NCAS and notifications of abortions carried out under grounds E with mention of eye anomalies by country and region
England and Wales 1992-1997**

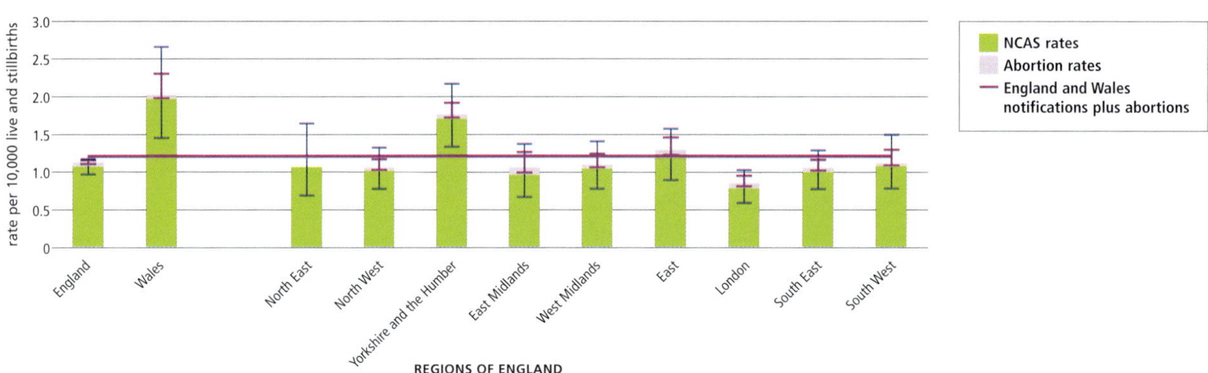

similar to other national registers.[6] Although high rates were recorded in Yorkshire and the Humber (3.6) and low rates in London (2.3), limb reductions had little geographic variability and rates remained consistent for the period (Figure 8.20). Exceptions are the North East and the East Midlands where rates halved over the period. Despite relatively low rates for abortions carried out under grounds E with mention of limb reductions, NCAS rates in the *Remoter Rural* Group were higher (3.9). High rates were also evident in *Ports and Industry* (3.7) with lower rates in the London Groups (Figure 8.21). There was no clear relationship with deprivation. As limb reduction anomalies are not fatal, infant death registrations have not been analysed.

8.10 Eye anomalies

Malformations and inherited disorders of the eyes range in severity from cataracts and defects of the iris, to anophthalmia (absence of both eyes) and are often accompanied by other serious anomalies. Eye anomalies represent only 1 per cent of all notifications to NCAS with an overall rate of 1.1 per 10,000 live and stillbirths in England and Wales (Figure 8.22).

Rates were similar to those for all babies notified, with higher rates in Wales (2.0) (again impacted by notification from CARIS which saw rates in Wales increase from 0.8 in 1992 to 2.9 in 1997)[4] and Yorkshire and the Humber (1.7) and lower rates in London (0.8). The numbers of eye anomalies mentioned on notifications for abortions carried out under grounds E were very small and showed little regional variation (Figure 8.22). Rates remained reasonably consistent over the period. Significantly higher rates were recorded in *Remoter Rural* (2.3) and *Ports and Industry* (2.2), consistent with the rates for all anomalies (Figure 8.23). Analysis revealed no clear relationship with deprivation and infant death registrations have not been analysed, as it is not a fatal condition.

Figure 8.23

Notifications of eye anomalies to NCAS and notifications of abortions carried out under grounds E with mention of eye anomalies by ONS classification Group
England and Wales 1992-1997

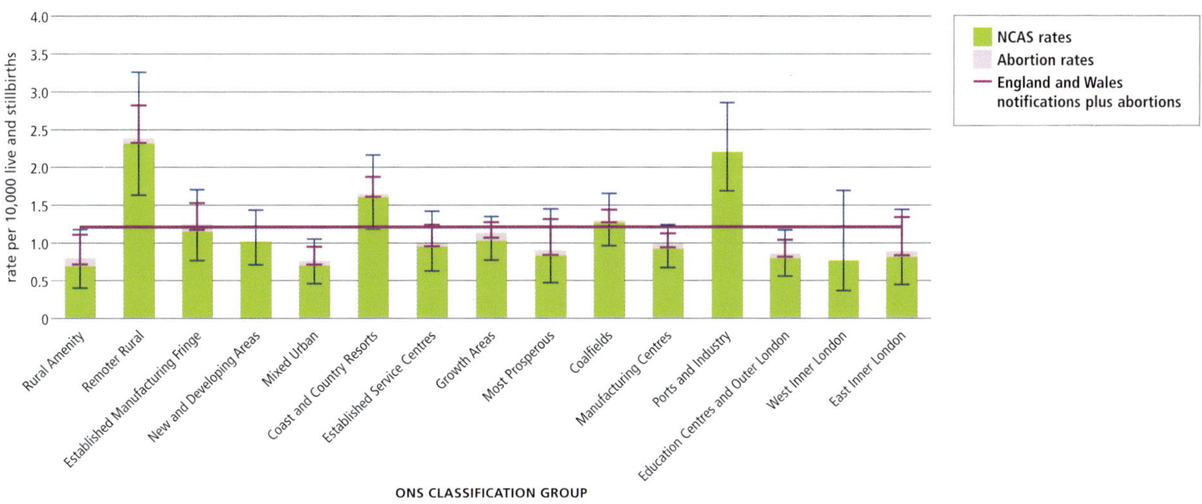

Figure 8.24

Notifications of abdominal wall anomalies to NCAS and notifications of abortions carried out under grounds E with mention of abdominal wall anomalies by country and region
England and Wales 1992-1997

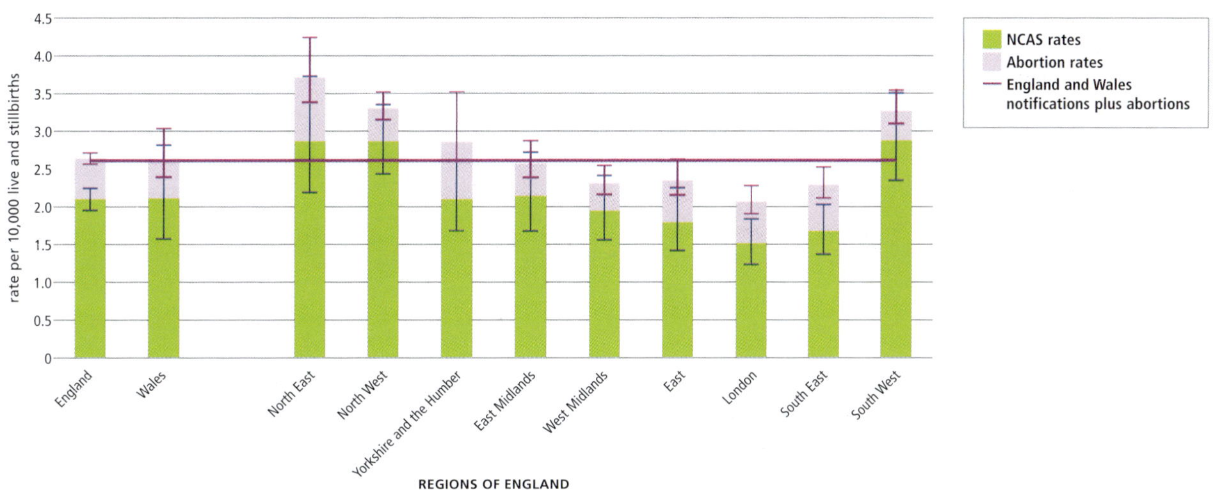

8.11 Abdominal wall anomalies

The two main types of anomaly in this group both originate in early development. Omphalocele, a repairable malformation, is often part of a genetic or chromosomal syndrome and associated malformations result in high mortality; it is characterised by an abnormally large umbilicus. Gastroschisis is a non-hereditary condition where the intestine protrudes from a hole in the abdomen, it can usually be surgically repaired to complete normality and mortality is comparatively low, any exogenous causes remain doubtful. Over 2 per cent of babies reported to NCAS have abdominal wall anomalies. Although they can be detected prenatally, terminations are rare because of the mild severity of the conditions.

Abdominal wall anomalies had a rate of 2.1 per 10,000 live and stillbirths in England and Wales, a rate similar to other national congenital anomaly registers.[6] A north-south gradient was evident with higher rates in the North West (2.9) and the North East (2.9) with lower rates in London (1.5) and the South East (1.7) (Figure 8.24). This might be a result of higher rates of gastroschisis among offspring of young mothers[11] more commonly found in the north of England than the south, but could also reflect higher levels of deprivation in the north. There were also higher levels of abdominal wall anomalies mentioned in notifications of abortions carried out under grounds E in the North East (0.8) and Yorkshire and the Humber (0.8). Relatively consistent rates for England and Wales mask regional fluctuations. Rates almost halved in the East Midlands from 3.7 in 1993 to 1.9 in 1997 and

Figure 8.25

Notifications of abdominal wall anomalies to NCAS and notifications of abortions carried out under grounds E with mention of abdominal wall anomalies by ONS classification Group
England and Wales 1992-1997

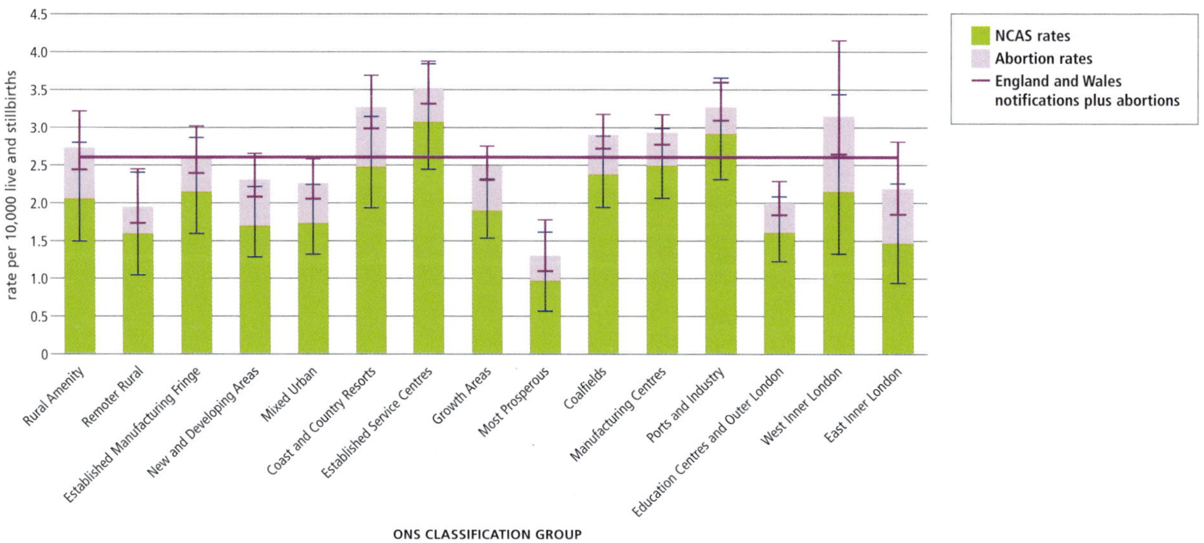

Figure 8.26

Notifications of abdominal wall anomalies to NCAS and notifications of abortions carried out under grounds E with mention of abdominal wall anomalies by deprivation
England and Wales 1992-1997

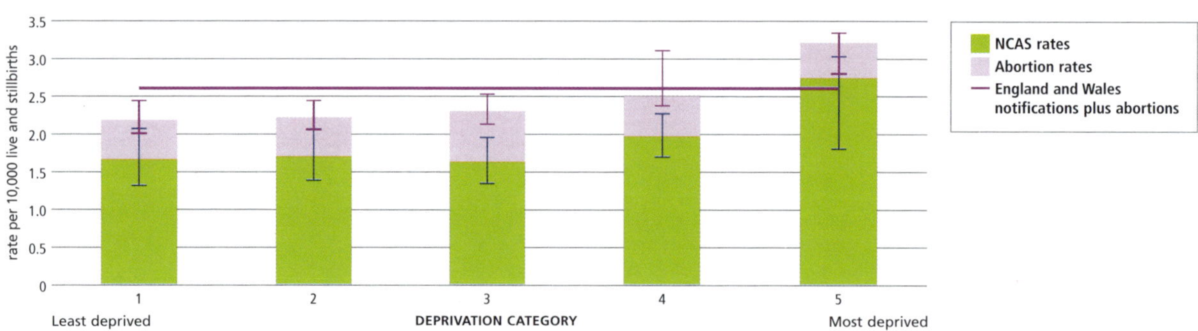

fell from 4.1 in 1994 to 1.0 in 1997 in the North East. Conversely, rates in the South West more than doubled from 1.7 in 1992 to 4.0 in 1997. Infant death registrations with a mention of these anomalies are too small in number to conduct a regional analysis.

As with other conditions significantly higher rates were notified for *Ports and Industry* (2.9) with lower rates of notification in the *Most Prosperous* Group (1.0) (Figure 8.25). Abortions carried out under grounds E where abdominal wall anomalies are mentioned had higher rates in *Coast and Country Resorts* (0.8) and *West Inner London* (1.0).

Deprivation analysis indicated significantly higher rates of notification to NCAS for abdominal wall anomalies in the most deprived areas, which could be associated with higher levels of young motherhood (Figure 8.26). However, this is not apparent for abortion under grounds E with mention of abdominal wall defects.

8.12 Polydactyly

Polydactyly is the occurrence of more than the usual number of fingers or toes. Notifications to NCAS for polydactyly represented a rate of 6.8 per 10,000 live and stillbirths for England and Wales and were present in nearly 8 per cent of babies notified. Polydactyly is a condition associated with black minority ethnic groups.[18] London has the largest proportion of black minority ethnic groups of all the regions and Wales (see Figure 3.8 in chapter 3). The rates for polydactyly in London (12.5) were three times those in the North East (3.8) (Figure 8.27), a pattern at odds with regional patterns for most other types of anomaly. Significantly higher rates were notified in *East Inner London* (13.2) and *West Inner London* (13.2). The areas with especially high rates for the period were almost all in London and authorities with large black minority ethnic populations. As Figure 8.28 demonstrates, there was also a link with areas classified as

Figure 8.27

**Notifications of polydactyly to NCAS by country and region
England and Wales 1992-1997**

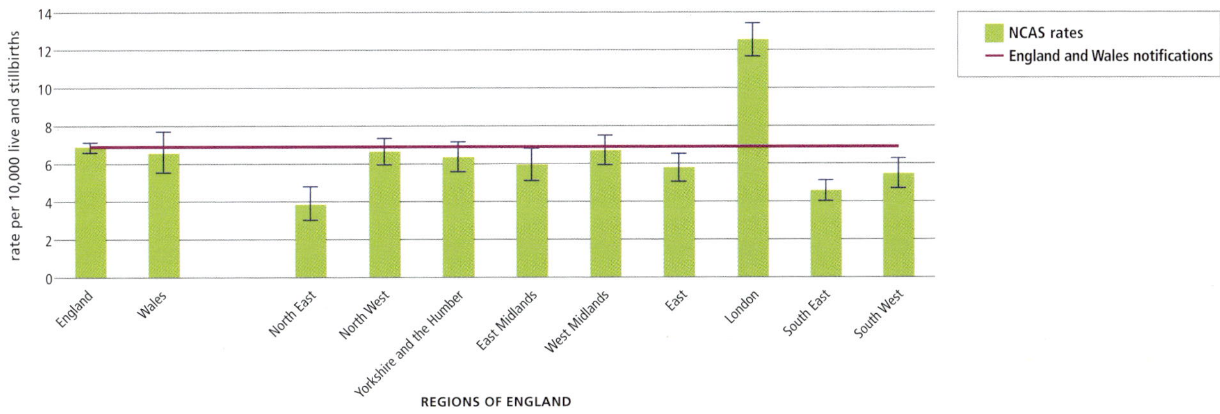

Figure 8.28

**Notifications of polydactyly to NCAS by deprivation
England and Wales 1992-1997**

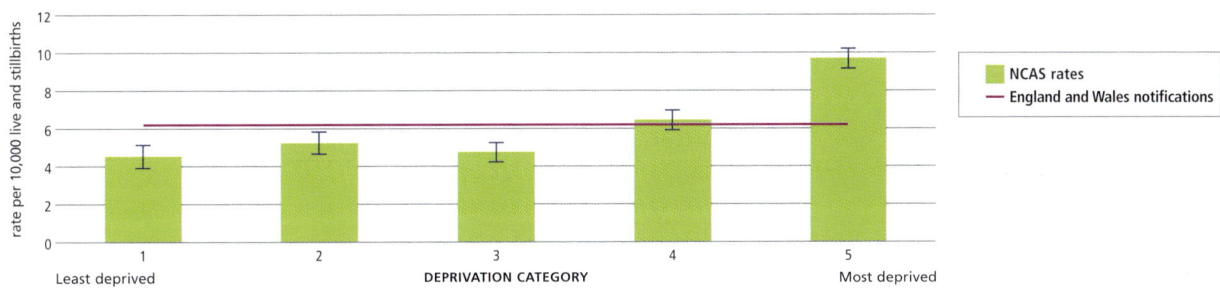

most deprived; this could be a reflection of the location of minority ethnic groups rather than an exogenous association with deprivation. Rates for England and Wales, experienced a small decline from 7.2 in 1992 to 6.6 in 1997, a trend reflected in all regions with the exception of the East Midlands, where rates declined from 7.1 in 1992 to 3.9 in 1997. Although there were abortions carried out under grounds E and infant death registrations with mention of polydactyly, the numbers are too small to be analysed by region.

8.13 Deformities of the feet

Deformities of the feet, a group of anomalies which includes talipes (club foot), account for nearly 12 per cent of babies notified to NCAS and had an overall rate of 10.3 per 10,000 live and stillbirths, ranging from 7.8 in the South East to 13.9 in the East Midlands (Figure 8.29). Numbers of abortions carried out under grounds E and infant death registrations with mention of deformities of the feet are too small for meaningful regional analysis. Rates remained consistent for England and Wales over the period, however, in the East Midlands and the North East rates halved, while in Wales, the North West and the South West they increased. Rates were significantly higher in *Ports and Industry* (16.8) and *Coalfields* (12.3) and lower in *West Inner London* (4.9) and *Most*

Prosperous (7.5) (Figure 8.30). Analysis showed no clear relationship between deformities of the feet and deprivation.

8.14 Discussion

The quality of the data is the main problem encountered in an analysis of regional differences in the occurrence of congenital anomalies using NCAS. As a surveillance system NCAS offers an invaluable service; fluctuations in rates over time are monitored for each health authority. The system is based on the assumption that data supplied to NCAS is collected in a similar way over time for each health authority but not necessarily for England and Wales. NCAS has levels of under-reporting that vary by health authority and to some extent regional variations reflect variations in reporting rather than occurrence.

Regional variations in levels of reporting occur for a number of reasons. For instance, data from Wales is impacted by the existence of a congenital anomaly register. When data exchange with CARIS began the multi-source data collection provided NCAS with more complete information on congenital anomalies in Wales. A consequence of this is that rates in Wales have risen. Most registers have not provided NCAS with data for 1992-1997 but as mentioned earlier, the impact of a regional register on NCAS data is difficult to quantify.

Figure 8.29

Notifications of deformities of the feet to NCAS by country and region
England and Wales 1992-1997

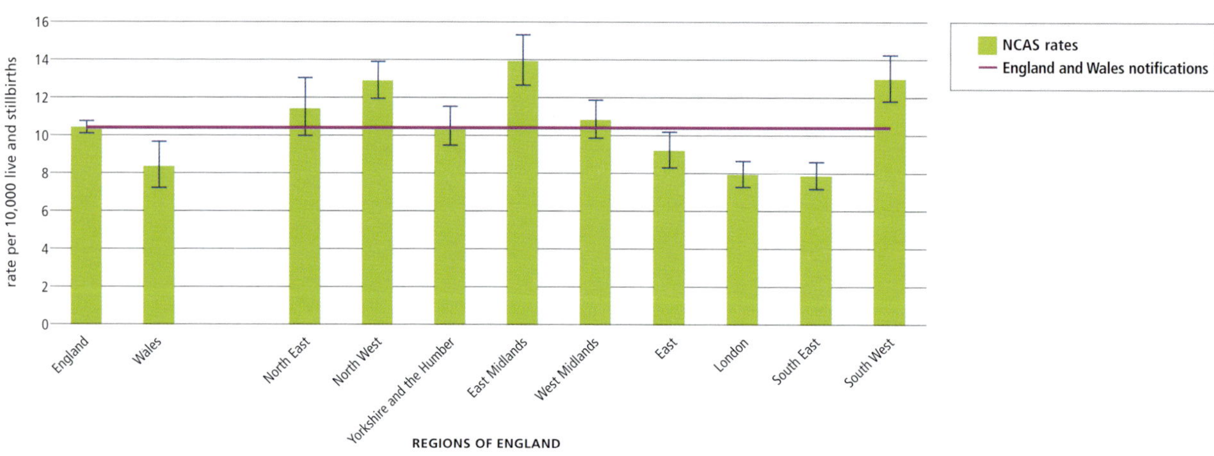

Figure 8.30

Notifications of deformities of the feet to NCAS by ONS classification Group
England and Wales 1992-1997

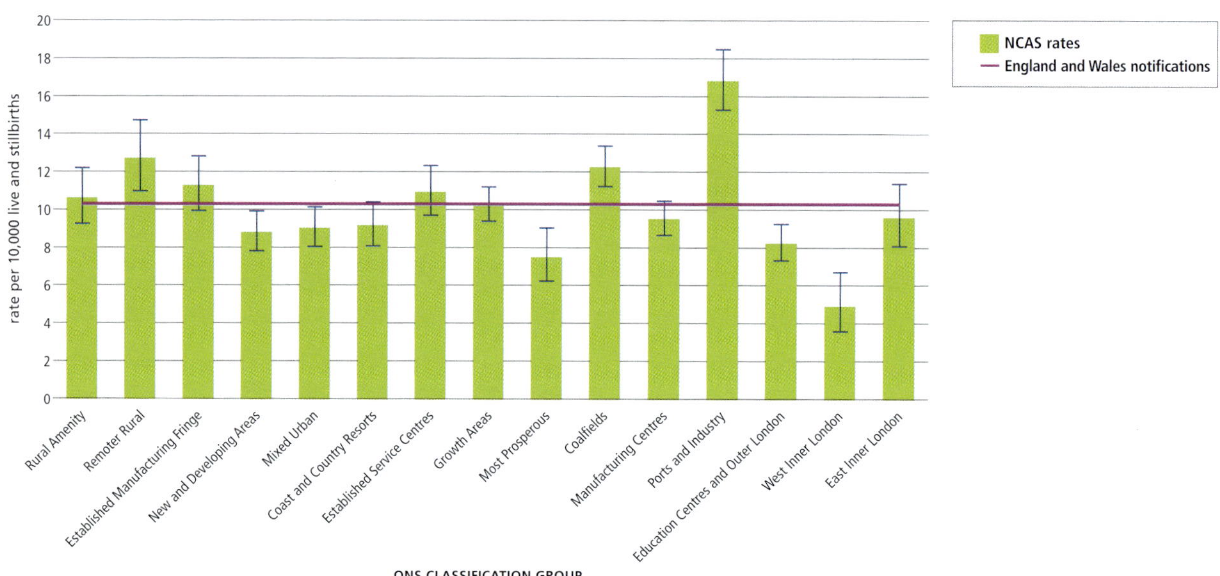

Even when differences in levels of notification are taken into consideration, lack of understanding and certainty about the causes of many anomalies make regional variations difficult to explain. London and its ONS classification Groups demonstrate low rates for most anomalies which is probably a manifestation of under-notification, however rates for polydactyly are high; a reflection of suggested links with black minority ethnic groups rather than notification practices.

Notification of abortions carried out under grounds E is statutory and as such does not have the same problems as notifications to NCAS. However, abortions carried out under grounds other than E are not examined for fetal anomalies and we cannot assume that notifications under grounds E represent all cases of terminations of fetuses affected by congenital anomalies. Higher rates in the East of England and the South East derive partly from older mothers being offered prenatal

diagnosis as routine. As these regions have larger proportions of older mothers, a larger proportion of women will have prenatal screening. Regional variation in access to diagnostic and abortion services is also an issue.

Taking limitations of the data and tentative conclusions about the causes of anomalies into consideration, the characteristics of regions can be related to their rates for specific anomalies. Down syndrome has high rates in regions with larger proportions of older mothers. Conditions such as NTDs and abdominal wall defects have higher rates in regions considered more deprived with larger proportions of younger mothers. Looking at rates across Groups supports such analysis. In the case of Down syndrome combined rates were highest in the *Most Prosperous*, *West Inner London* and *Growth Areas* Groups, all characterised by older mothers.

References

1 Office for National Statistics. *Congenital Anomaly Statistics Notifications, England and Wales.* Series MB3, no.14. The Stationery Office (London: 2000)

2 Office for National Statistics. *BINOCAR Report.* Office for National Statistics (London: 2000)

3 North Thames West Congenital Malformation Register, Merseyside and Cheshire Congenital Anomaly Survey, Congenital Anomaly Register and Information Service (CARIS) in Wales from 1998 and Trent Congenital Anomaly Register.

4 Botting B. The impact of more complete data from Wales on the National Congenital Anomaly System. *Health Statistics Quarterly* 5 (2000), 7-9.

5 Reid A and Harding S. Trends in regional deprivation and mortality using the longitudinal study. *Health Statistics Quarterly* 5 (2000), 17-24.

6 International Centre for Birth Defects. *Annual Report 1999 - International Clearinghouse for Birth Defects Monitoring Systems.* International Centre for Birth Defects (Rome: 1999).

7 Botting B. Improving the completeness of Down syndrome notification. *Health Statistics Quarterly* 6 (2000), 14-17.

8 Huang T, Watt HC, Wald NJ, Morris JK, Mutton D and Alberman E. Reliability of statistics on Down's syndrome notifications. *Journal of Medical Screening* 4 (1997), 95-97.

9 Cuckle H. Maternal age-standardisation of prevalence of Down syndrome. *Lancet* 354 (1999), 529.

10 Office for National Statistics. Annual Update: Births and Conceptions 1998. *Population Trends* 98 (1999), 83-86.

11 Botting B, Rosato M and Wood R. Teenage mothers and the health of their children. *Population Trends* 93 (1998), 19-28.

12 Office for National Statistics. *Infant Feeding Survey 1995.* The Stationery Office (London: 1997).

13 Ministry of Agriculture Fisheries and Food. *National Food Survey 1997.* The Stationery Office (London: 1997).

14 Office for National Statistics. *The National Diet and Nutrition Survey.* HMSO (London: 1990).

15 Abramsky L, Botting B, Chapple J and Stone D. Has advice on periconceptional folate supplementation reduced neural tube defects? *Lancet* 354 (1999), 998.

16 Hindmarch C. *On the Death of a Child.* Radcliffe Medical Press (Oxon: 2000), 24.

17 International Centre for Birth Defects. *Congenital Malformations Worldwide. A report from The International Clearinghouse for Birth Defects Monitoring Systems.* International Centre for Birth Defects (Elsevier: 1991).

18 Buyse M. *Birth Defects Encyclopedia.* Blackwell Scientific Publications (Cambridge, Mass. USA: 1990), 1397-1398.

Geographic patterns in cancer incidence

Penny Babb, Anita Brock, Jenny Jones and Mike Quinn

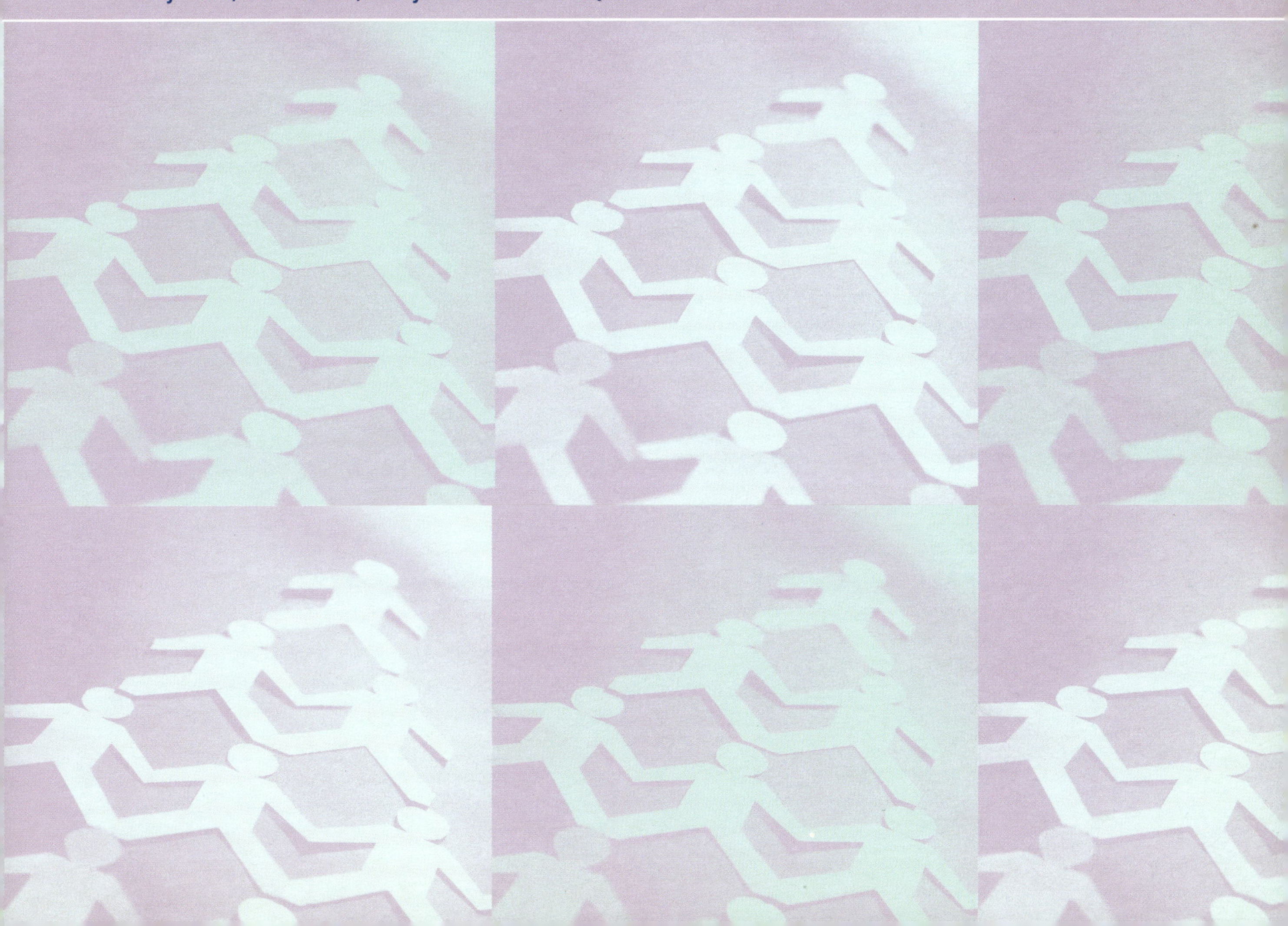

Chapter 9
Geographic patterns in cancer incidence

Summary

- In England, the incidence of lung cancer (compared with the United Kingdom average) was very high in both males and females in the North East (and to a lesser extent the North West) and low in the Midlands and south – apart from London.

- There was far less variability in the incidence of breast cancer, but rates were generally higher in the south of England than in the north.

- Of the countries of the United Kingdom, England had the lowest overall incidence of prostate cancer but there was a substantial band of higher incidence in the southern regions.

- The incidence of colorectal cancer in England was lower than in the other United Kingdom countries.

- Wales had the highest breast cancer incidence and fairly high rates of colorectal cancer.

- Scotland had the highest overall incidence of lung cancer for both sexes, and even higher rates than in England across all the deprivation categories in both males and females. Scotland also had relatively high incidence of colorectal cancer.

- Northern Ireland had the lowest incidence of lung and breast cancers but the highest incidence of prostate and colorectal cancers.

- Lung cancer incidence shows clear socio-economic variations with people living in more deprived areas at greater risk of developing the disease.

- The incidence of breast and prostate cancers show similar inverse associations with socio-economic status, with lower incidence in people living in the most deprived areas of Great Britain.

9.1 Introduction

Local variations in the incidence of different types of cancer are of importance both in aiding our understanding of the epidemiology of the diseases and in assisting local planning of clinical and public health resources. This chapter reviews the incidence of the three most common cancers in men (lung, prostate and colorectal) and in women (breast, colorectal and lung) which account for over 50 per cent of all registrations in each sex. The numbers and rates of newly diagnosed cases (incidence) in 1991-1993 are presented for each country of the United Kingdom (1993-1995 for Northern Ireland) and

Government Office Regions of England. The incidence of each of the cancers is then examined for each local authority in Great Britain – within England, grouped by its region – as well as by the ONS classification of local authorities. The variation in incidence with socio-economic deprivation (measured by the Carstairs and Morris index) is also examined. These classifications are described in chapter 4 of this volume. Analyses of variations in cancer survival by health region were included in the volume *Cancer Survival Trends in England and Wales, 1971-1995: deprivation and NHS Region.*[1]

9.2 Methods and data

Cancer registration in the United Kingdom is carried out by nine regional registries in England and registries in Wales, Scotland and Northern Ireland. ONS compiles national data for England and Wales from the receipt of individual registrations from the English regional registries and the registry in Wales. The United Kingdom cancer registration system is described in detail in the volume *Cancer trends in England and Wales 1950-1999.*[2] Incidence data collected by the registries of Scotland and Northern Ireland (and aggregated into five-year age groups) have been provided to ONS to give the Great Britain or United Kingdom picture where possible. Incidence data for years up to and including 1996 are available from the cancer registry for Scotland (ISD Scotland).[3] Data for Northern Ireland are only available for years 1993-1995[4] (the Northern Ireland Registry recommenced operation in the early 1990s); this should be borne in mind when comparing incidence with other parts of the United Kingdom where there have been long-term downward trends in lung cancer in males and short-term fluctuations in both breast and prostate cancer (resulting from screening). Incidence data for England and Wales were complete for years up to and including 1993 at the time the analyses reported here were prepared, although final data for 1994-1997 are now available.[2,5] For the purposes of the analyses of cancer incidence by local authority, only data for years 1991-1993 have been used. The Northern Ireland data have not been used at the local authority level, as the area of residence of the patient is not specified for a large proportion of records; the local authority analyses are, therefore, for Great Britain only.

Box 9.1 Comparative incidence ratio (CIR):

This is the ratio of the age-standardised rate (ASR) for the country/region/ONS classification Group to the ASR for the United Kingdom (or Great Britain) multiplied by 100 (i.e. it is expressed as a percentage).

It is useful in highlighting the areas with higher or lower incidence compared with the country as a whole.

9.3 Lung cancer

On average 28,100 new cases of lung cancer were diagnosed in males in the United Kingdom each year during 1991-1993 and 14,200 cases in females (Table 9.1). Around 80 per cent of all lung cancer cases occurred in England (22,800 and 11,300 in males and females, respectively). In Scotland there were on average 3,100 new cases of lung cancer diagnosed in males each year and 1,800 new cases in females, accounting for around 12 per cent of such cases in the United Kingdom. Lung cancer cases in Wales and Northern Ireland accounted for around 5 per cent and 2 per cent, respectively, of such cases in the United Kingdom.

Scotland had the highest age-standardised incidence rates of the four countries within the United Kingdom, for both sexes (118 per 100,000 males and 51 per 100,000 females), while the lowest rates occurred in Northern Ireland for males (80) and in England for females (33). Incidence in males was 9 per cent higher in Wales than in England.

Table 9.1

Incidence of lung cancer: average annual number of new cases and rates per 100,000 population United Kingdom 1991-1993

Males

| Country/Region | Average annual number of cases | Rate per 100,000 | | | | | | |
		Crude Rate	ASR[1]	CIR[2]	Age group 15-44[1]	45-64[1]	65-74[1]	75+[1]
United Kingdom[3]	28,060	98.9	90.2	100.0	2.8	109	480	705
England	22,840	96.4	87.3	96.8	2.7	103	466	694
North East	1,640	128.9	117.5	130.3	3.4	143	646	879
North West	3,680	109.7	102.0	113.1	3.5	133	538	737
Yorkshire and the Humber	2,550	103.9	94.9	105.3	3.4	114	517	720
East Midlands	1,900	95.0	84.7	94.0	2.6	96	449	703
West Midlands	2,510	96.6	89.0	98.7	2.6	106	494	669
East	2,160	84.5	74.3	82.4	2.2	80	399	639
London	3,020	89.5	91.3	101.3	2.9	104	468	784
South East	3,310	87.6	76.9	85.3	2.5	86	404	651
South West	2,070	89.7	69.8	77.4	1.7	82	366	577
Wales	1,590	112.8	95.5	105.9	3.2	119	501	733
Scotland	3,050	123.5	118.2	131.1	3.2	153	622	877
Northern Ireland[4]	580	71.7	79.6	88.3	3.6	110	430	514

Females

| Country/Region | Average annual number of cases | Rate per 100,000 | | | | | | |
		Crude Rate	ASR[1]	CIR[2]	Age group 15-44[1]	45-64[1]	65-74[1]	75+[1]
United Kingdom[3]	14,160	47.8	34.9	100.0	1.9	52	191	192
England	11,330	45.9	33.3	95.4	1.9	49	182	187
North East	910	68.1	50.7	145.3	2.2	83	272	248
North West	1,960	55.4	40.6	116.4	2.5	63	223	207
Yorkshire and the Humber	1,250	49.2	36.2	103.9	2.3	55	201	183
East Midlands	820	39.9	29.7	85.3	1.7	45	163	159
West Midlands	1,070	40.2	30.0	86.1	1.6	45	169	158
East	990	37.7	26.8	76.9	1.3	37	146	168
London	1,660	46.9	37.5	107.5	1.9	53	209	223
South East	1,640	41.6	28.3	81.1	1.6	39	152	182
South West	1,020	42.0	26.0	74.6	1.8	36	139	167
Wales	740	49.5	34.2	98.2	2.1	52	193	170
Scotland	1,780	67.5	50.5	144.9	2.5	79	275	263
Northern Ireland[4]	320	37.6	33.5	95.9	2.2	56	181	147

1   Directly age-standardised rate per 100,000 using the European standard population.
2   Comparative incidence ratio: the ratio of the region ASR and the ASR for the United Kingdom multiplied by 100.
3   The United Kingdom figure is an estimate as data for years prior to 1993 are not available for Northern Ireland (see note 4).
4   The data for Northern Ireland are for years 1993-1995.
The age-standardised rate in children aged under 15 is 0.2 per 100,000 or less in all countries and regions.

Figure 9.1

**Lung cancer CIR by country and region (United Kingdom = 100), all ages
United Kingdom 1991-1993**

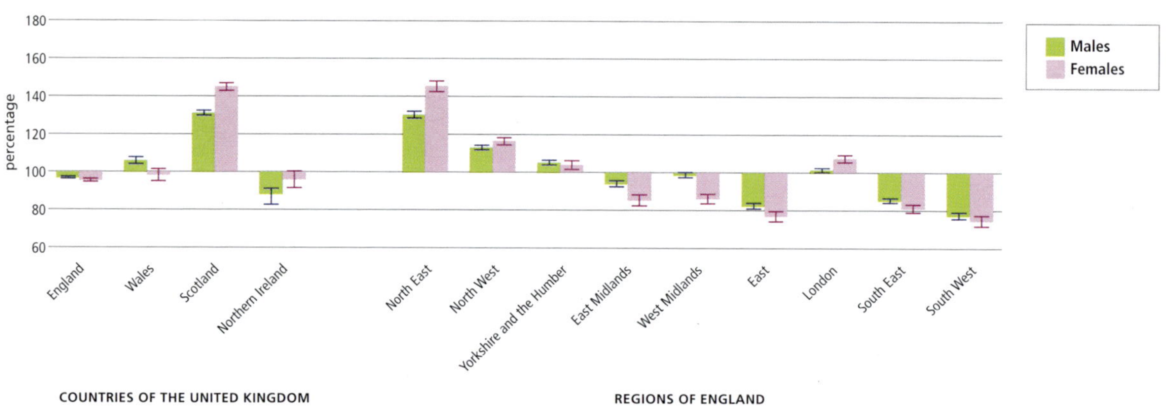

Figure 9.2

**Lung cancer ASR by local authority within countries and regions, males all ages
Great Britain 1991-1993**

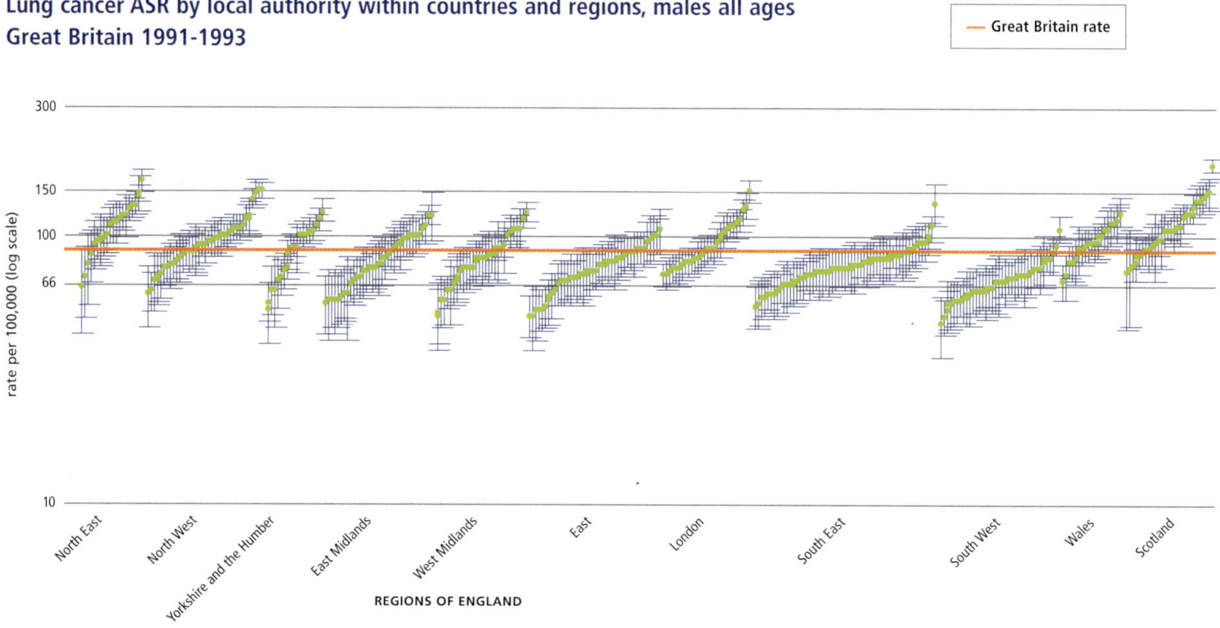

Figure 9.1 shows comparative incidence ratios (CIRs) for lung cancer. For an explanation of CIRs see Box 9.1. Among the regions of England, the North East had the highest incidence of lung cancer in both males and females, with levels similar to those occurring in Scotland. For males the rate was about 30 per cent higher than the average for the United Kingdom; for females it was 45 per cent higher. The East of England, South West and South East had the lowest incidence of lung cancer, with rates about 20 per cent below the United Kingdom average. Overall, the northern regions of England tended to have rates higher than the average for the United Kingdom, while those for the southern parts of England had lower than average incidence. However, the incidence of lung cancer in Yorkshire and the Humber in both males and females was only around 4-5 per cent higher than the average for the United Kingdom, and the incidence in females in London was 7 per cent greater than the average.

Lung cancer incidence rises steeply with age with the highest rates occurring in adults aged 65 or over (Table 9.1). Lung cancer incidence in females was greater in the 65-74 age group than in those aged 75 or over in the Midlands and northern parts of England and in Scotland and Northern Ireland, while for men, incidence was highest in the elderly in all areas of the United Kingdom.

The distribution of the age-standardised incidence rates by local authority in each country and region of England are shown (with their 95 per cent confidence limits) for males and females in Figures 9.2 and 9.3. Within every region or country there is a very wide range between the local authorities with the highest and lowest incidence. The lower overall incidence in the southern regions of England (Figure 9.1) was confirmed by the large number of local authorities below the average for Great Britain, with very few showing significantly higher incidence than the average. In contrast, a substantial number (but by no

Figure 9.3

**Lung cancer ASR by local authority within countries and regions, females all ages
Great Britain 1991-1993**

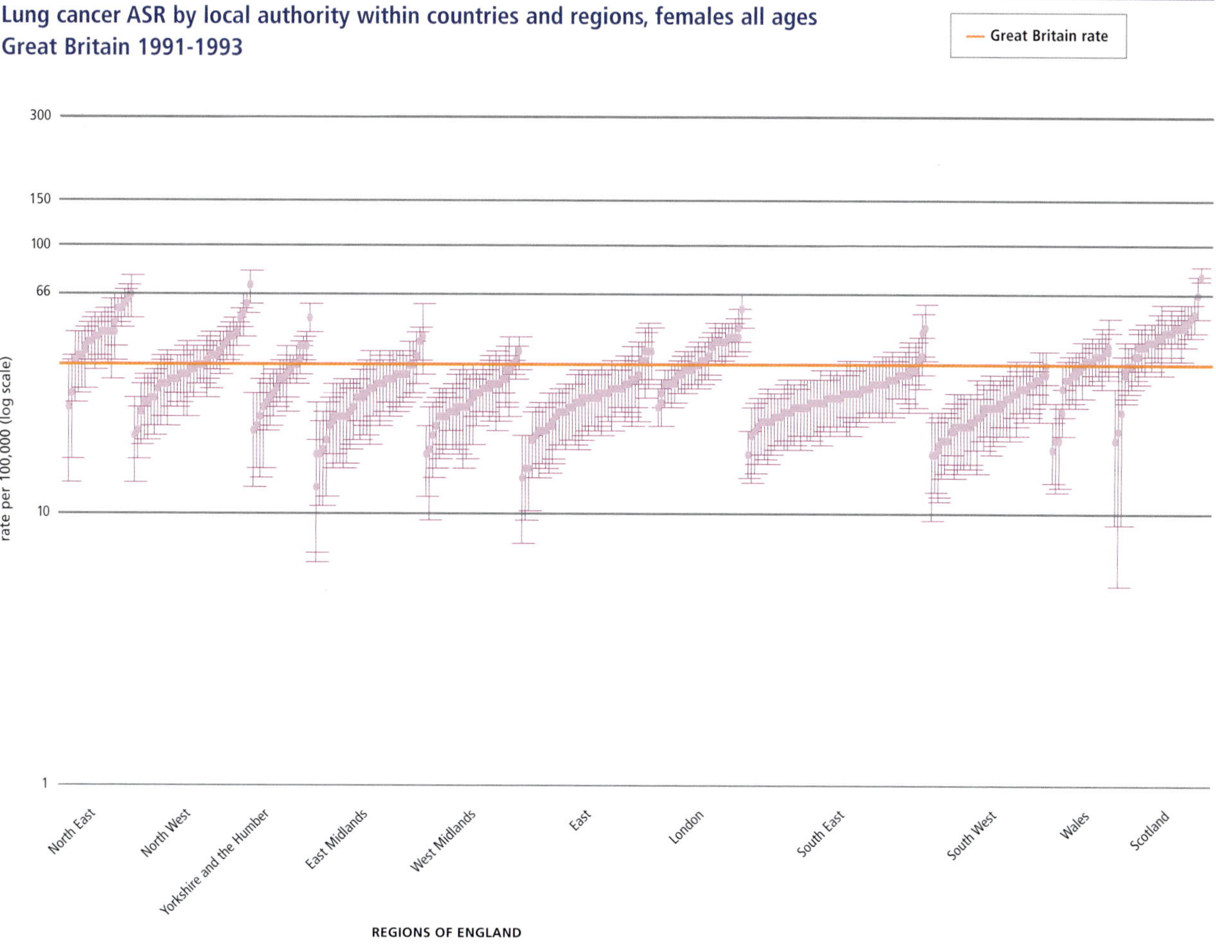

Figure 9.4

**Lung cancer CIR by ONS classification Group (Great Britain = 100), all ages
Great Britain 1991-1993**

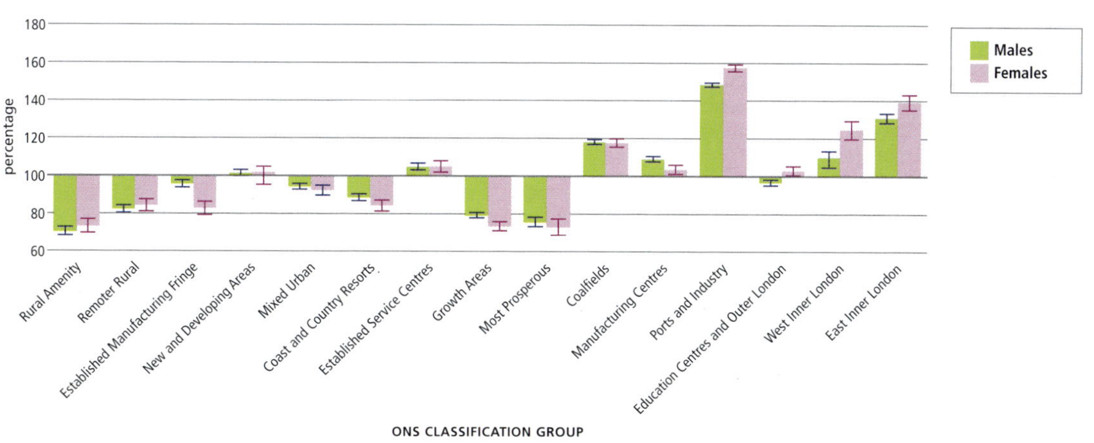

means all) of the local authorities in Scotland and the North East of England were above the average.

The areal variation in the incidence of lung cancer is shown in further detail for local authorities in Great Britain (i.e. excluding Northern Ireland) in Maps 9.1 to 9.4. Maps 9.1 and 9.3 give the quintile distribution of the directly age-standardised incidence rates and clearly show the higher incidence occurring in authorities in Scotland, the northern parts of England (particularly the urban areas of the North West and North East), south Wales and London (shown by the large areas of dark blue). Lower incidence was found in the majority of authorities in the southern parts of England (predominantly white or pale blue areas). Maps 9.2 and 9.4

Figure 9.5

Lung cancer ASR by local authority within ONS classification Groups, males all ages Great Britain 1991-1993

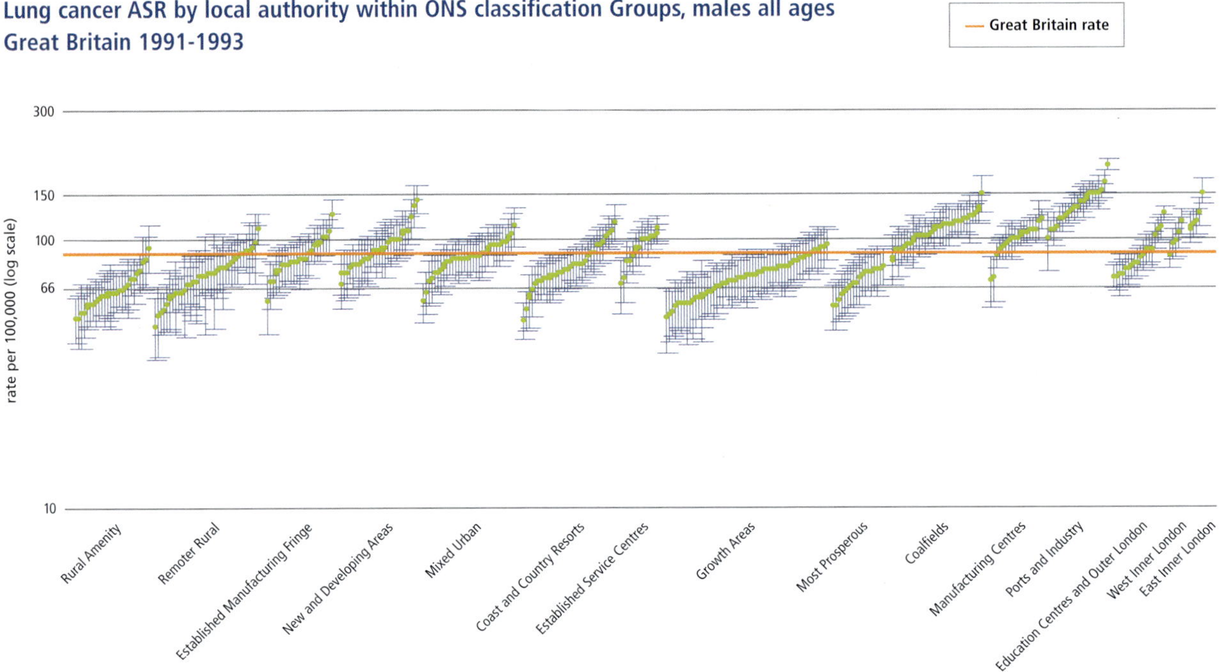

show the areas with statistically significantly higher or lower directly age-standardised incidence rates than for Great Britain as a whole.

The lung cancer CIRs for local authorities within ONS classification Groups are shown in Figure 9.4. Industrial areas showed the highest incidence, with *Ports and Industry* showing an excess of almost 50 per cent in men and over 50 per cent in women. Other high rates occurred in *East Inner London* – 30-40 per cent above the average. Particularly low incidence was seen in rural areas *(Rural Amenity, Remoter Rural)* and *Coast and Country Resorts, Growth Areas* and *Most Prosperous*, with rates around 20 per cent below the average for Great Britain. The distribution of age-standardised incidence rates of lung cancer in males for each local authority within ONS classification Groups is shown in Figure 9.5. With the exception of just one local authority, all areas in the *Ports and Industry* Group exceeded the average for Great Britain. In contrast, the incidence of the majority of areas within the *Rural Amenity* and *Growth Area* Groups were below the average.

There is a well-known gradient of rising lung cancer by level of material deprivation.[6] The sharp rise in incidence across the deprivation groups is clearly illustrated for Great Britain as a whole and for each country and region of England in Figure 9.6. In all areas and for both sexes, the ratio of incidence in the most deprived group compared with the least deprived group was around 2:1. The incidence for the least deprived in Scotland was substantially higher than for the other areas of Great Britain, and 6 per cent higher than in the North East of England.

Map 9.1

Age-standardised lung cancer incidence rates by local authority grouped in quintiles, males all ages
Great Britain 1991-1993

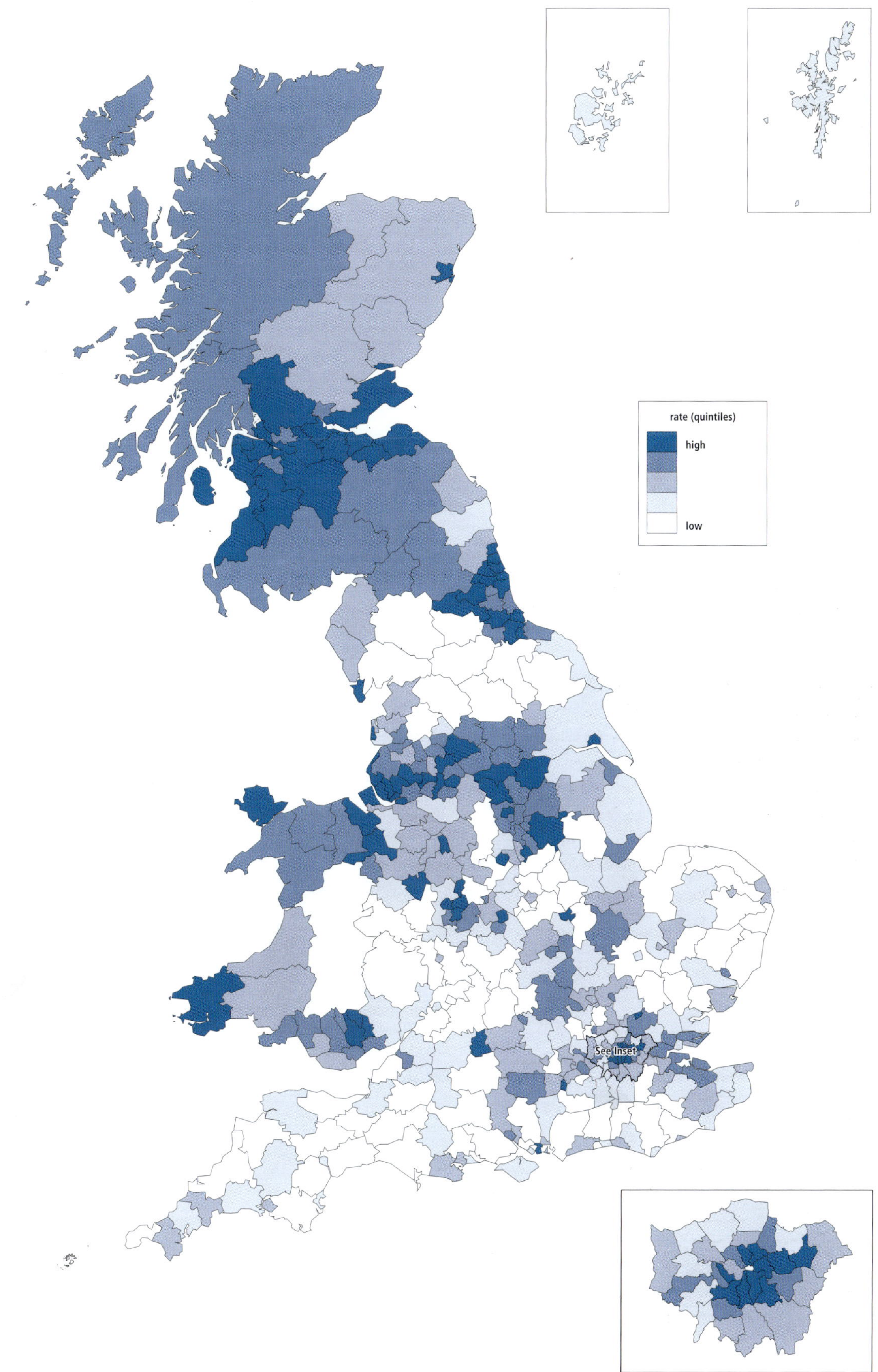

Map 9.2

Age-standardised lung cancer incidence rates by local authority, males all ages
Great Britain 1991-1993

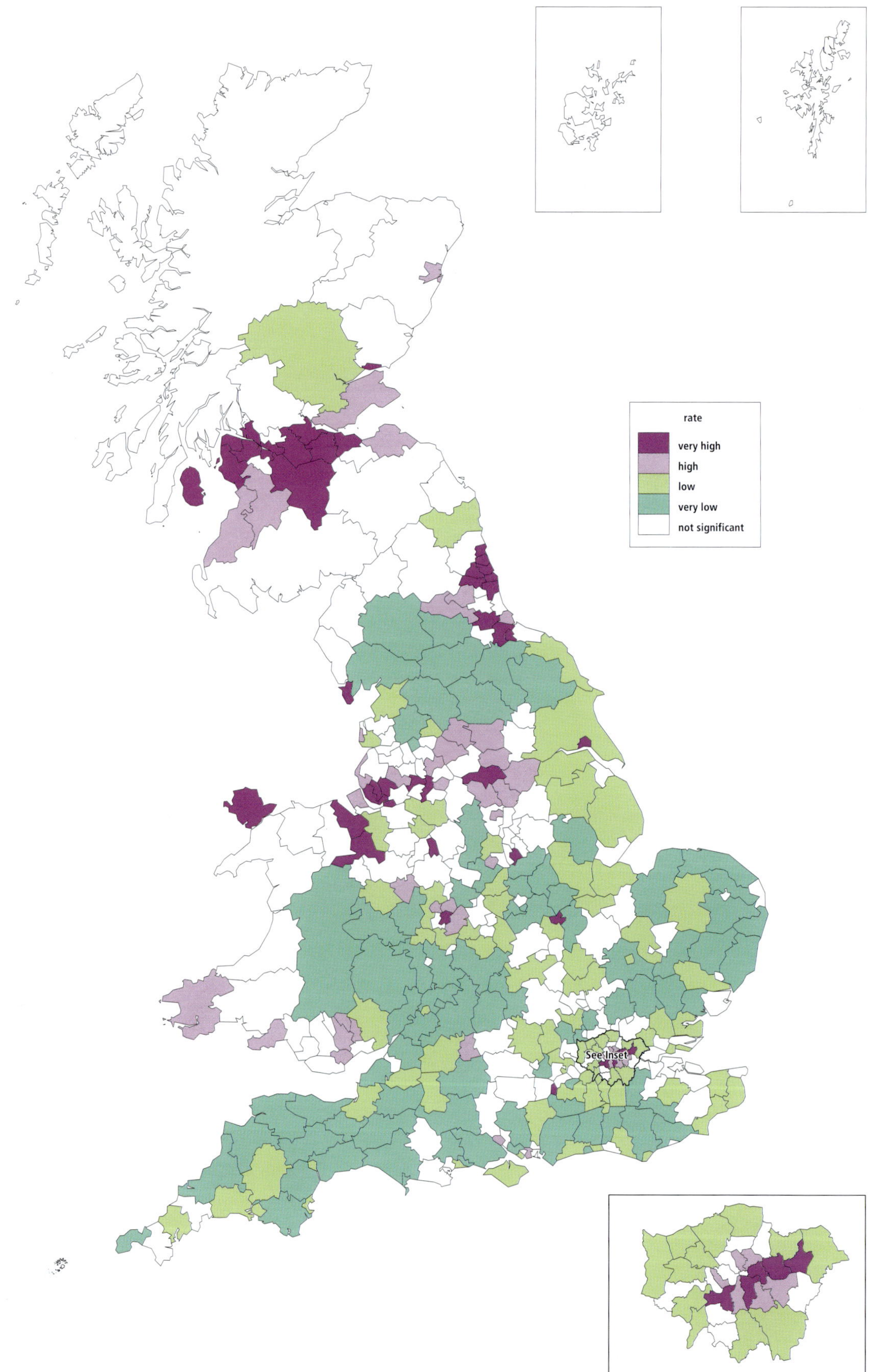

Map 9.3

Age-standardised lung cancer incidence rates by local authority grouped in quintiles, females all ages
Great Britain 1991-1993

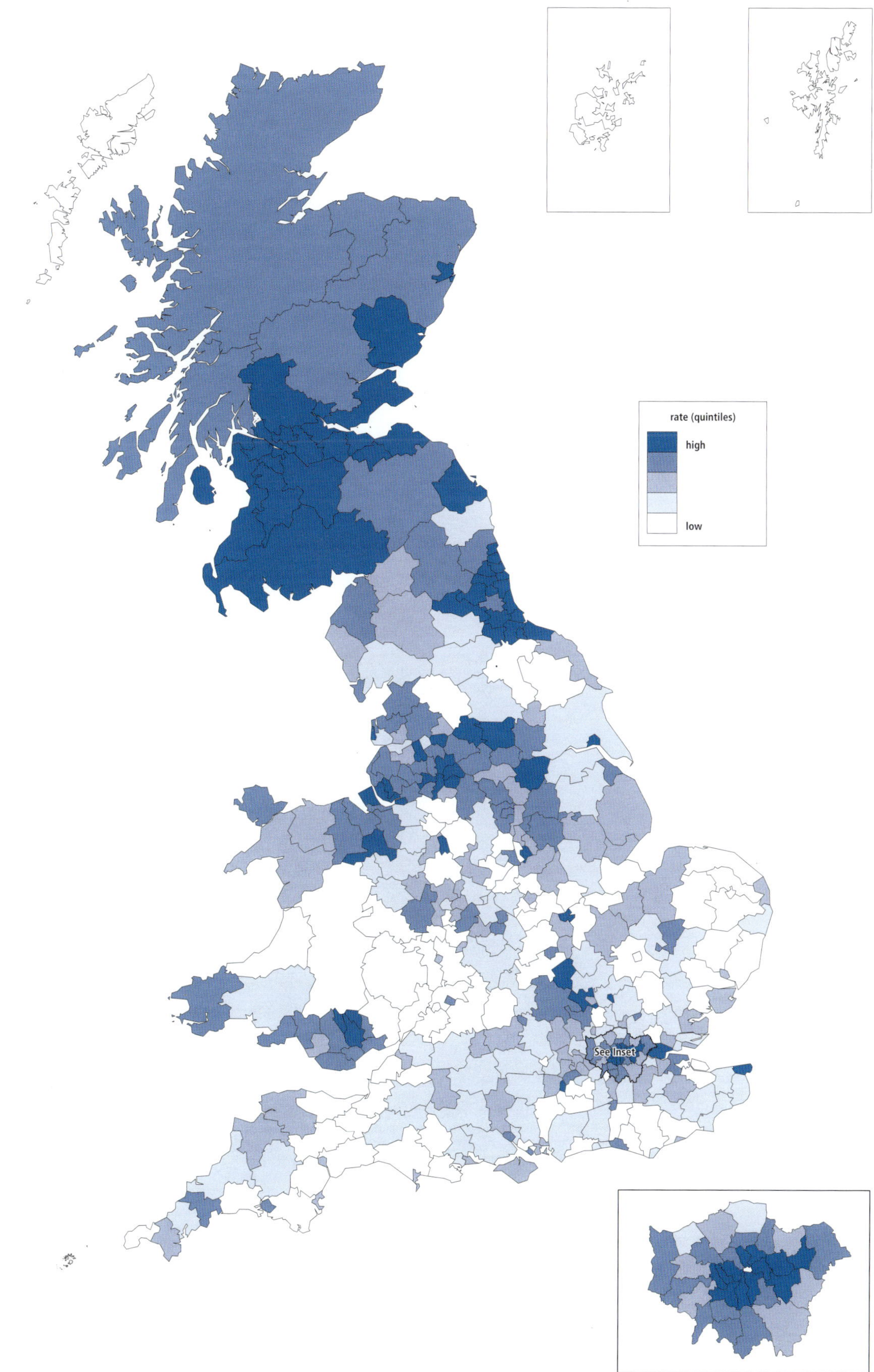

Map 9.4

Age-standardised lung cancer incidence rates by local authority, females all ages
Great Britain 1991-1993

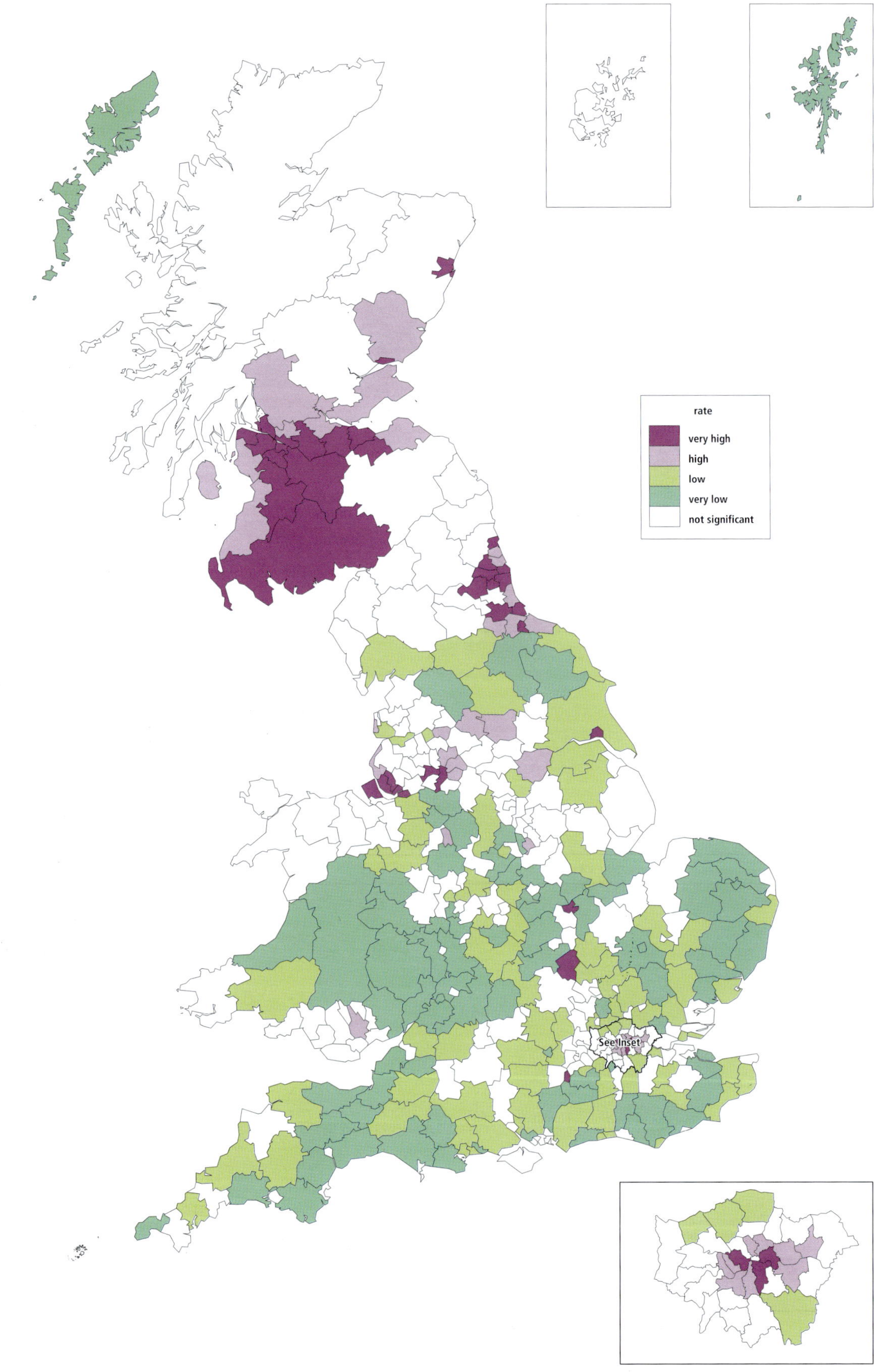

Figure 9.6

Lung cancer ASR by deprivation, all ages
Great Britain 1991-1993

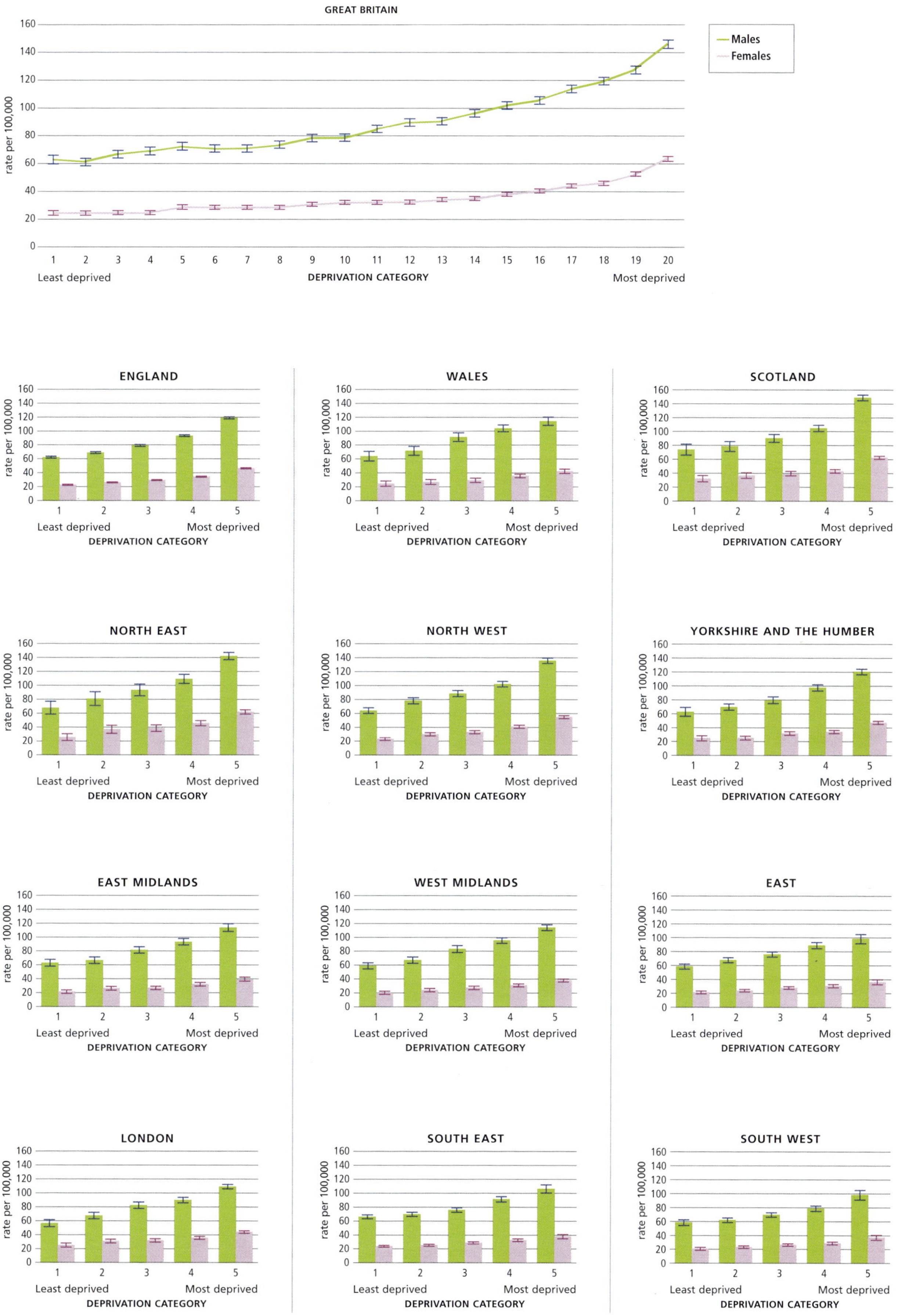

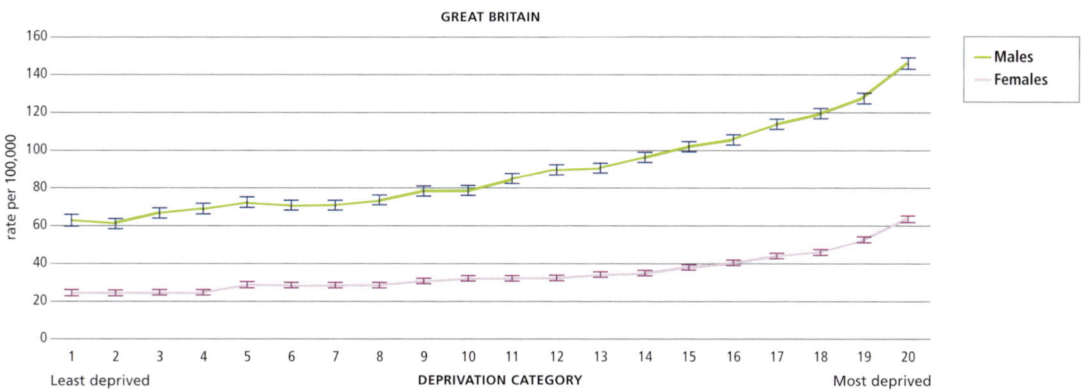

9.4 Breast cancer

There were on average 35,100 new cases of breast cancer diagnosed in the United Kingdom in 1991-1993, with 29,200 in England, 3,200 in Scotland, just under 2,000 in Wales and around 800 cases in Northern Ireland (Table 9.2). Of the countries in the United Kingdom, the highest incidence rate was in Wales, at 110 per 100,000, followed by Scotland (107), compared with the average of 105 for the United Kingdom as a whole. The lowest rate occurred in Northern Ireland at 99 per 100,000.

Within England, breast cancer incidence was higher in the southern regions and lower in the northern parts (Figure 9.7). The highest incidence occurred in the South West at almost 112 per 100,000 (Table 9.2) (around 7 per cent above the average for the United Kingdom), compared with the low of 90 per 100,000 in the North East of England (14 per cent below the average). The incidence of breast cancer increases with age in all regions except the North East region, where incidence was lower for women aged 65-74 than for those aged 45-64 and 75 and over; the incidence of breast cancer in elderly women in the North East was actually lower than for the 45-64 age group in all other regions and countries.

The range of local authority rates is shown in Figure 9.8. Few areas in the East Midlands, West Midlands and South West had an incidence of breast cancer below the average, while most did in the North East. The geographic pattern of incidence is also illustrated in Maps 9.5 and 9.6. Map 9.5 gives the directly age-standardised incidence rates of breast cancer by local authority (grouped into quintiles) and shows a band of authorities with high incidence running through the southern and central parts of England, as well as high levels in northern Wales and in Scotland. Lower incidence occurred in authorities in northern England. Only about a third of local authority areas had incidence which is significantly different from the average for Great Britain, but the areas of higher incidence remain clear in Map 9.6.

The ONS classification Groups with higher incidence included *New and Developing Areas* and *Growth Areas*, as well as *Coast and Country Resorts* and *Most Prosperous*, with rates around 5 per cent greater than average (Figure 9.9). Lower incidence occurred in *Coalfields, Manufacturing Centres, Ports and Industry* and *East Inner London*, around 5 per cent below the average for Great Britain.

The incidence of breast cancer *decreases* with increasing material deprivation, as shown in Figure 9.10. The incidence rates fall from around 115 per 100,000 in the least deprived to below 100 per 100,000 in the most deprived. The inverse gradient was apparent in most regions and countries of Great Britain but was not significant in all areas. There was virtually no gradient in Yorkshire and the Humber, and for a number of regions there appears to be a small rise between the first and second quintiles before incidence falls in the more deprived groups (Scotland, East Midlands, East of England and London).

Table 9.2

Incidence of breast cancer: average annual number of new cases and rates per 100,000 population United Kingdom 1991-1993

Females

Country/Region	Average annual number of cases	Crude Rate	ASR[1]	CIR[2]	15-44[1]	45-64[1]	65-74[1]	75+[1]
United Kingdom[3]	35,120	118.4	104.8	100.0	33	242	255	309
England	29,150	118.1	104.4	99.6	33	241	255	306
North East	1,330	99.4	90.2	86.0	31	218	197	221
North West	4,030	113.9	101.1	96.4	34	232	248	282
Yorkshire and the Humber	2,860	112.3	99.7	95.1	32	232	242	283
East Midlands	2,450	119.0	104.9	100.1	34	241	249	326
West Midlands	3,120	116.7	105.6	100.8	34	249	251	286
East	3,170	120.7	105.9	101.1	31	248	259	320
London	3,760	106.0	102.0	97.3	33	230	259	312
South East	5,030	127.9	109.8	104.8	36	250	271	326
South West	3,390	139.3	111.8	106.7	34	257	279	345
Wales	1,960	132.0	110.2	105.2	31	255	279	347
Scotland	3,200	121.2	107.3	102.4	35	249	250	329
Northern Ireland[4]	820	97.3	99.2	94.7	31	237	224	283

1   Directly age-standardised rate per 100,000 using the European standard population.
2   Comparative incidence ratio: the ratio of the region ASR and the ASR for the United Kingdom multiplied by 100.
3   The United Kingdom figure is an estimate as data prior to 1993 are not available for Northern Ireland (see note 4).
4   The data for Northern Ireland are for years 1993-1995.
The age-standardised rate in children aged under 15 is 0.1 per 100,000 or less in all countries and regions.

Figure 9.7

**Breast cancer CIR by country and region (United Kingdom = 100), females all ages
United Kingdom 1991-1993**

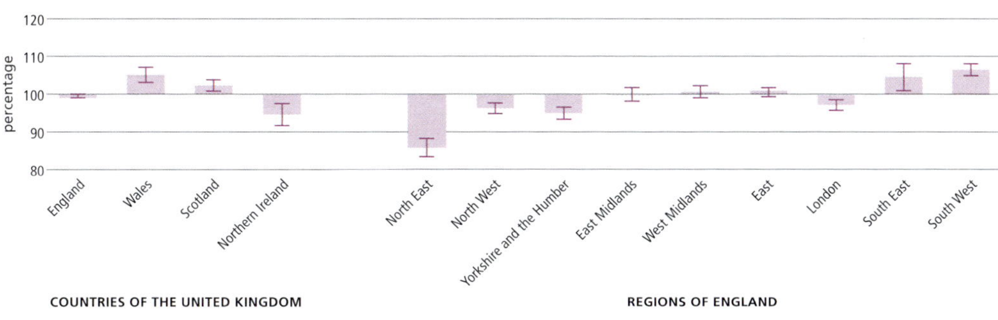

Figure 9.8

**Breast cancer ASR by local authority within countries and regions, females all ages
Great Britain 1991-1993**

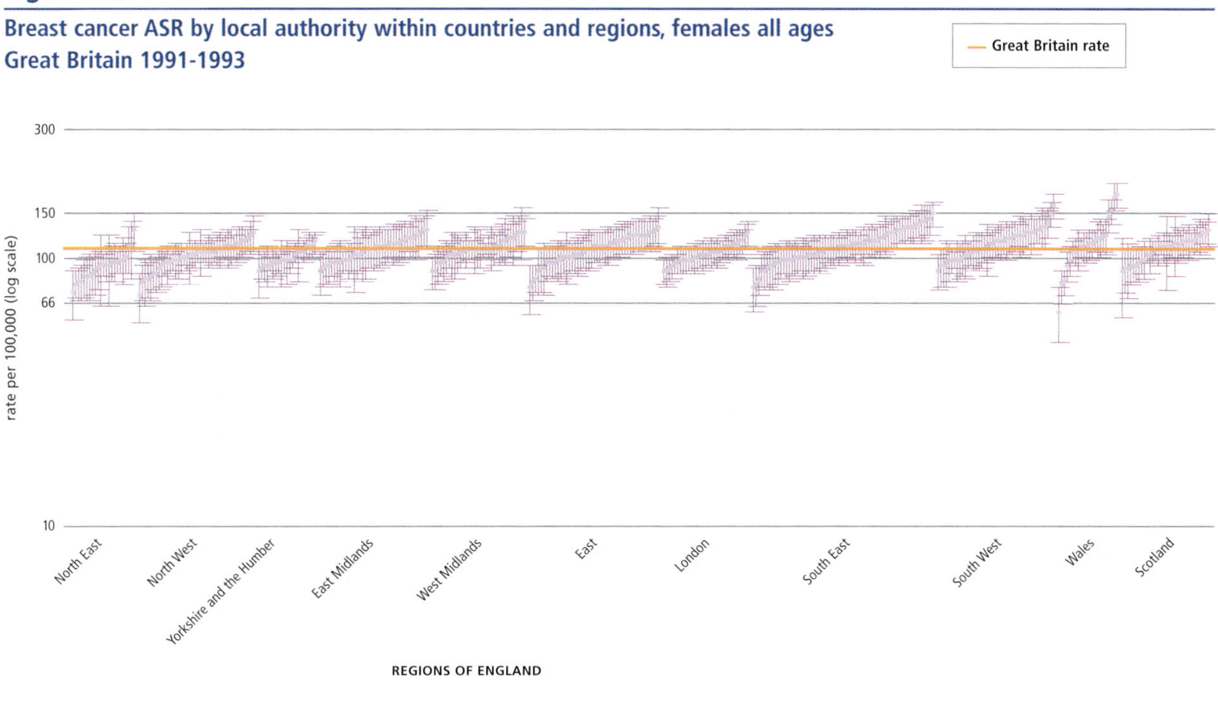

Figure 9.9

**Breast cancer CIR by ONS classification Group (Great Britain = 100), females all ages
Great Britain 1991-1993**

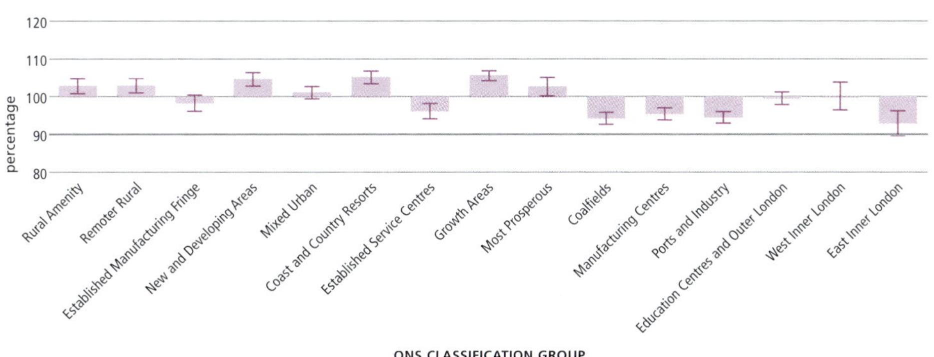

Map 9.5

Age-standardised breast cancer incidence rates by local authority grouped in quintiles, females all ages
Great Britain 1991-1993

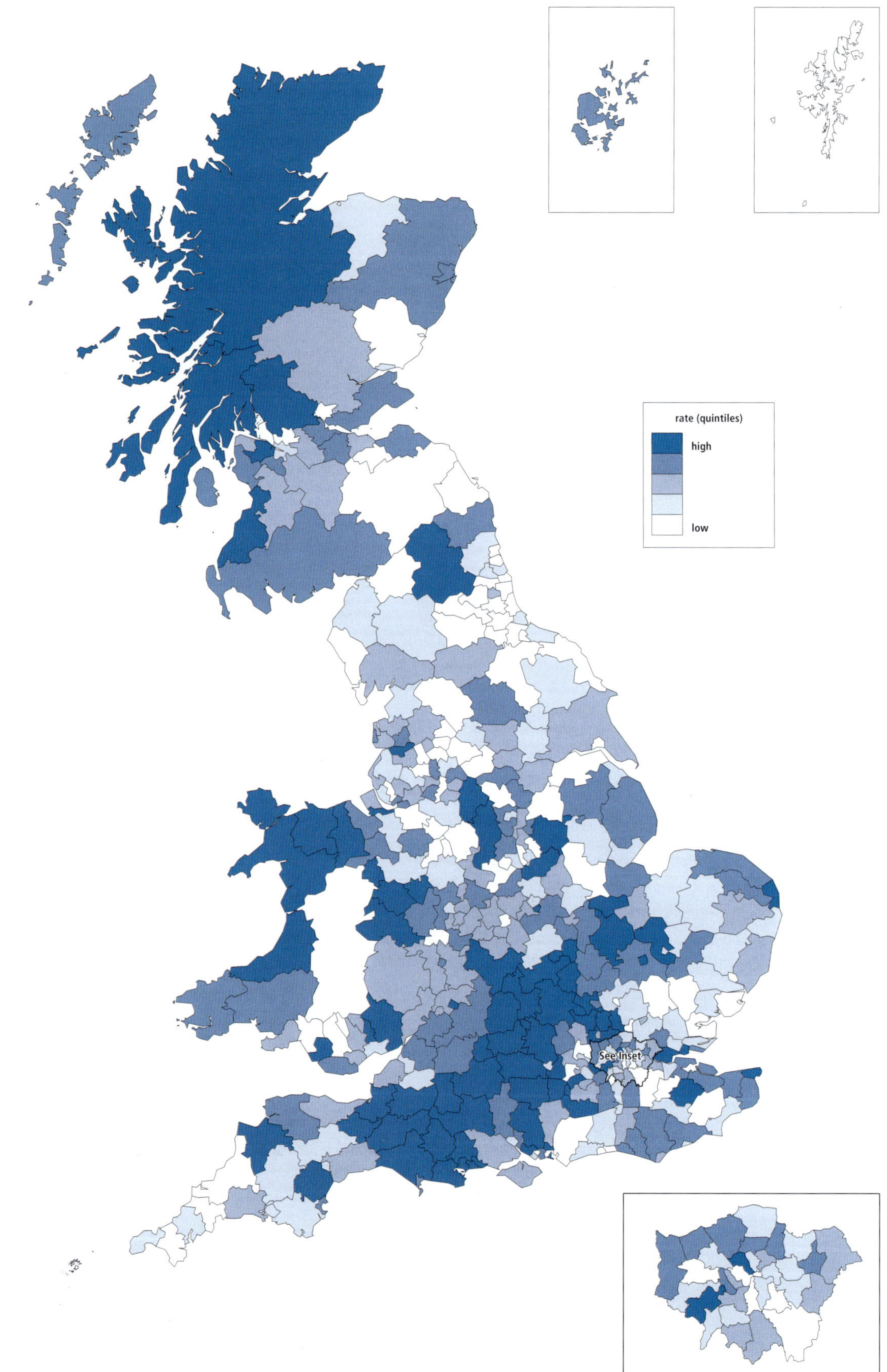

Map 9.6

Age-standardised breast cancer incidence rates by local authority, females all ages
Great Britain 1991-1993

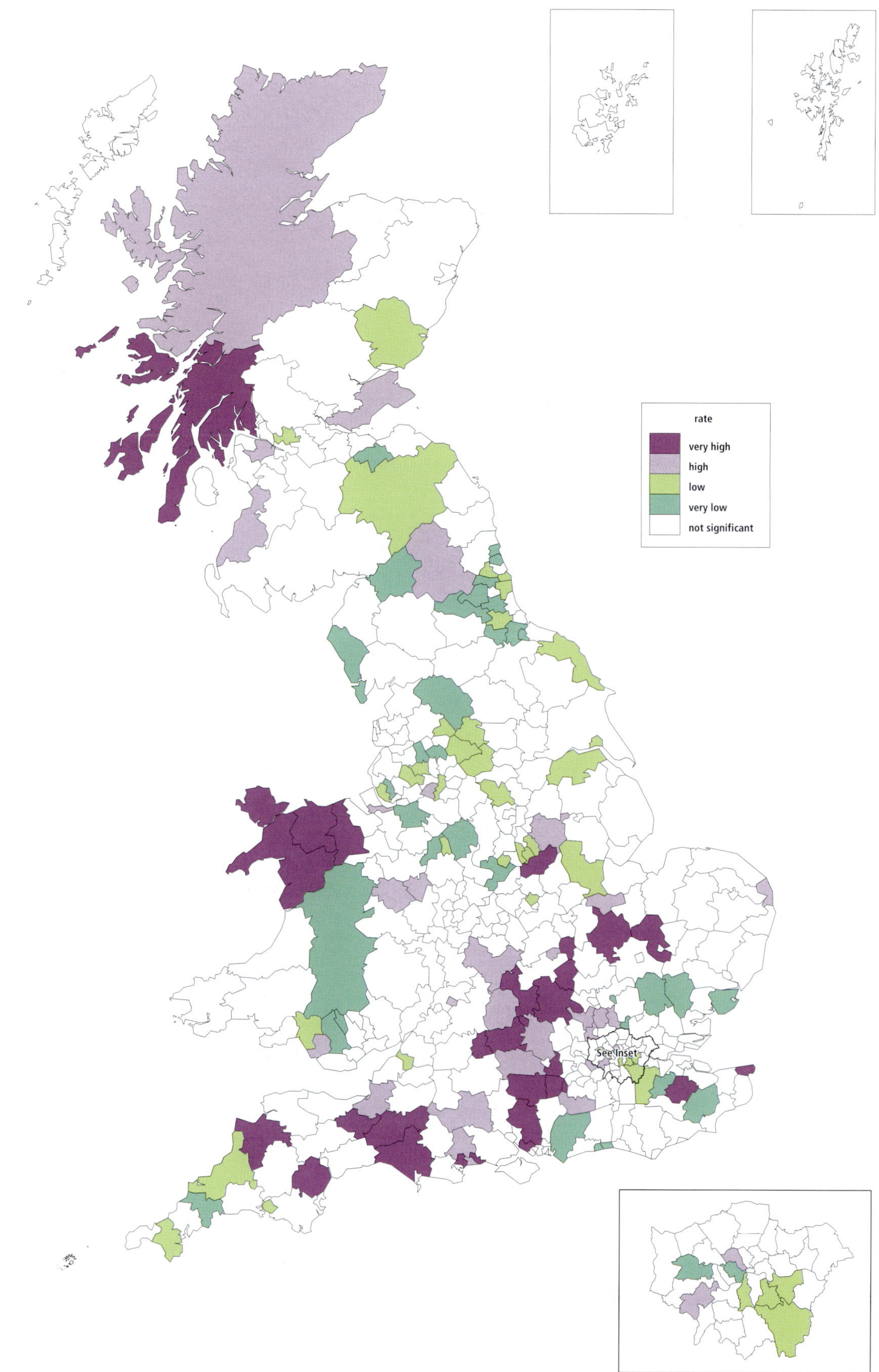

Figure 9.10

Breast cancer ASR by deprivation, females all ages
Great Britain 1991-1993

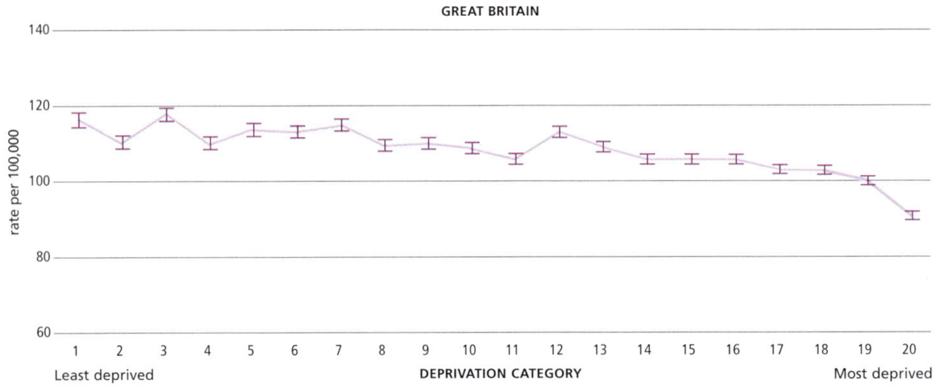

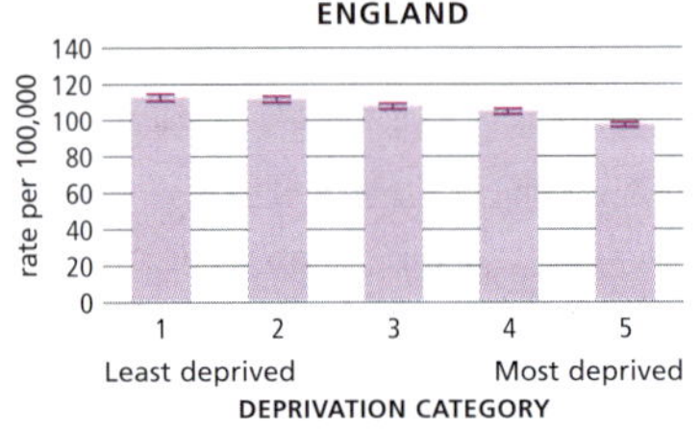

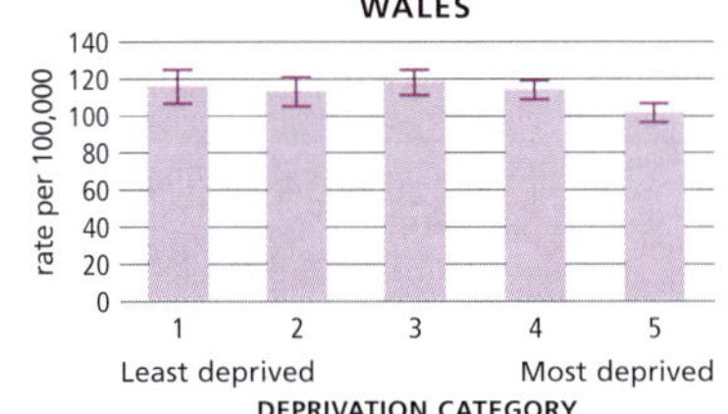

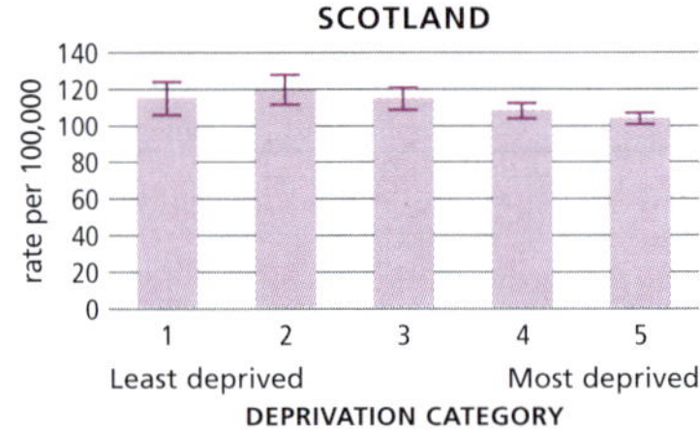

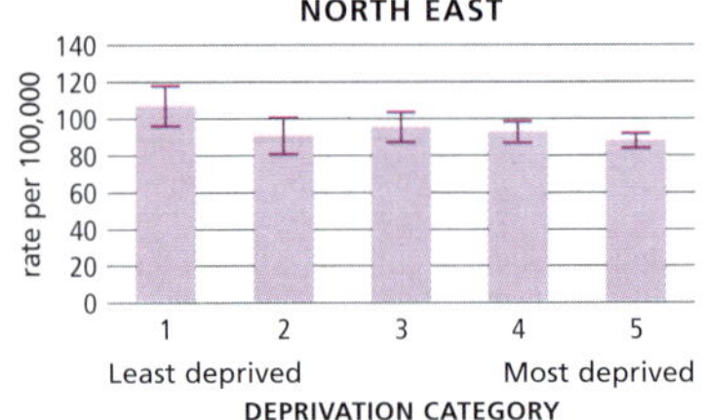

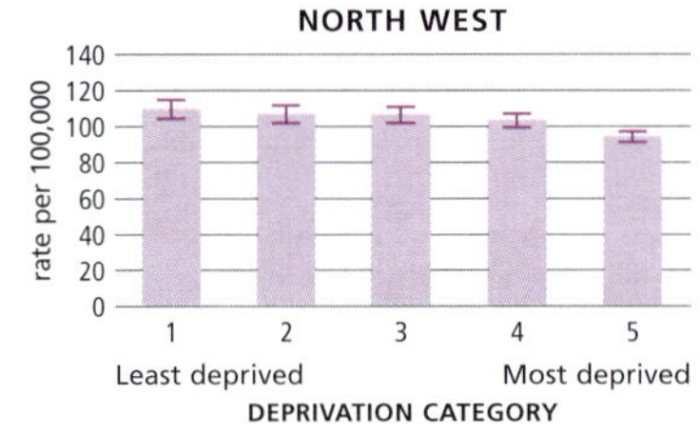

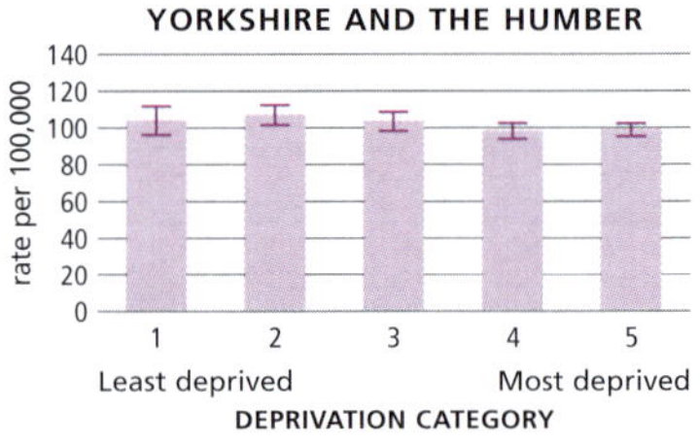

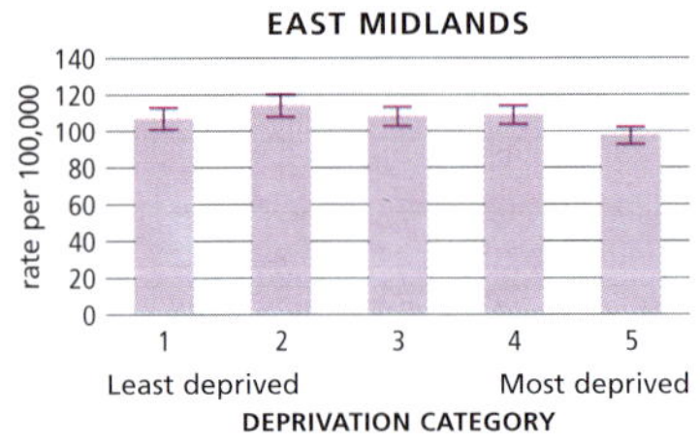

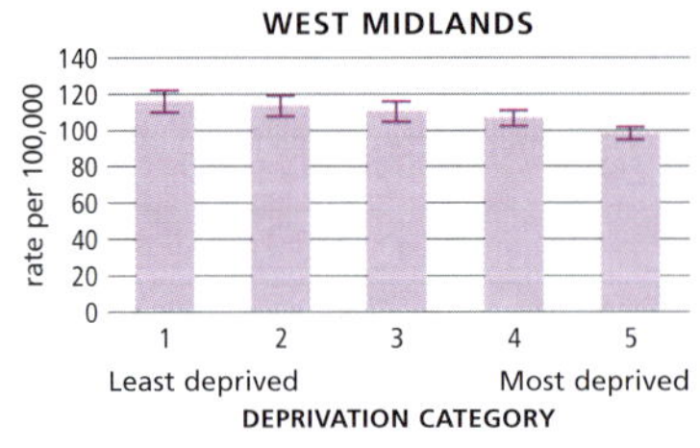

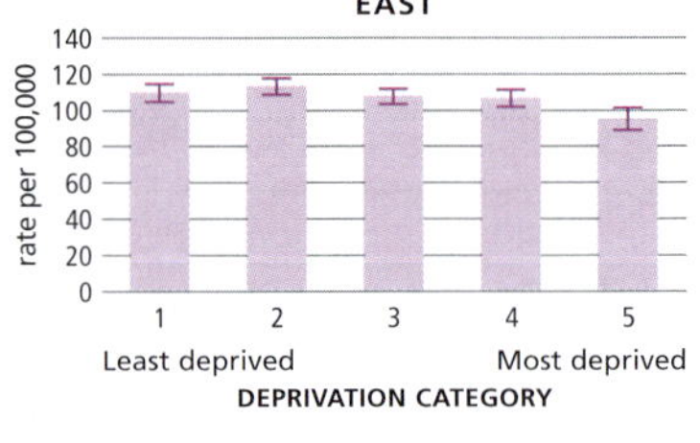

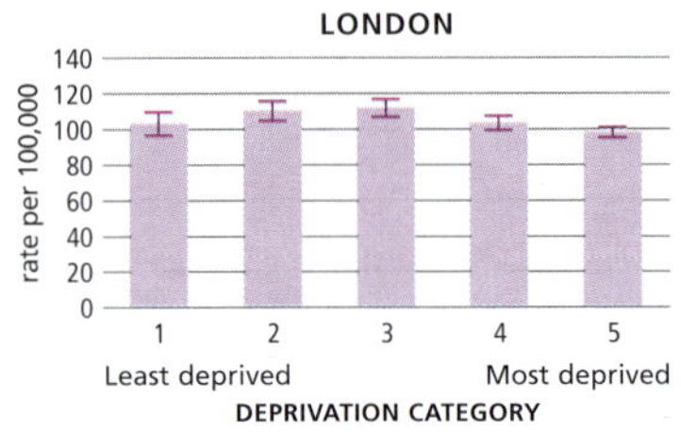

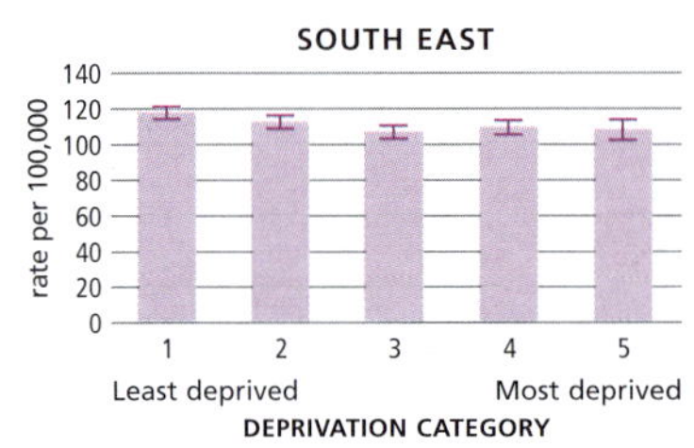

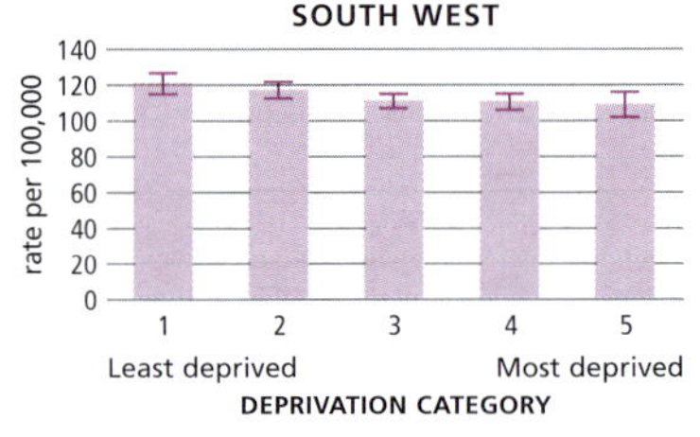

9.5 Prostate cancer

On average, there were 17,700 new cases of prostate cancer diagnosed in the United Kingdom in 1991-1993 (Table 9.3). Of these, 14,700 occurred in England, nearly 1,500 in Scotland, 1,000 in Wales and 450 in Northern Ireland. The age-standardised incidence rate of prostate cancer was almost 60 per 100,000 in Northern Ireland, 59 per 100,000 in Wales and 57 per 100,000 in Scotland. The rate for England was the lowest of the countries at 54 per 100,000.

Prostate cancer was more common in the southern parts of England than in the northern parts (Figure 9.11). The highest regional incidence in England occurred in the South West at almost 61 per 100,000 (Table 9.3), close to the levels in Northern Ireland, and more than 10 per cent higher than the average for the United Kingdom. The second highest incidence in England was in the South East at 59 per 100,000, around 8 per cent higher than the average. The lowest incidence occurred in the North East at 41 per 100,000, substantially lower than in the second lowest, the North West with a rate of almost 50 per 100,000. The incidence in the North East was almost 25 per cent lower than the average for the United Kingdom as a whole.

Prostate cancer is a disease of the elderly and is extremely rare in men aged under 45 in all regions and countries. The highest rate (in men aged 75 or over) in the North East was 529 per 100,000 compared with 805 per 100,000 in men of the same age in the South West.

The distribution of local authority prostate cancer rates by region are shown in Figure 9.12. The geographic pattern of prostate cancer incidence by local authority across Great Britain is also shown in Maps 9.7 and 9.8. Map 9.7 gives the directly age-standardised incidence rates (grouped into quintiles), and shows a band of high incidence from the South West across the south of England to the eastern coastline, as well as high levels in the northern and south western parts of Wales and areas in the north and west of Scotland. Many of these areas show a statistically significant variation from the average incidence for Great Britain as a whole (Map 9.8).

Figure 9.13 presents the ratio of the directly age-standardised prostate cancer incidence rates (CIR) by ONS classification Group compared with the rate for Great Britain. The types of area that showed higher incidence rates include *Coast and Country Resorts, New and Developing Areas* and the *Most Prosperous* (5-10 per cent above the average). Lower incidence occurred in groups including *Coalfields, East Inner London* and *Ports and Industry*, around 10 per cent below the average.

Prostate cancer tends to occur more frequently in men living within affluent areas than in deprived areas. The deprivation gradient for Great Britain shows a gradual reduction in incidence from around 60 per 100,000 to around 50 per 100,000 in the most deprived (Figure 9.14). The decline was steeper in the lower part of the distribution of deprivation (groups 11 to 20). The inverse gradient occurred in Wales and Scotland, as well as England as a whole, and in most regions of England (although the gradient was not always significant) but not in the South West. The inverse gradient was most pronounced in the North East and North West of England.

Table 9.3

Incidence of prostate cancer: average annual number of new cases and rates per 100,000 population United Kingdom 1991-1993

Males

| | Average annual number | Rate per 100,000 | | | | | | |
| | | Crude | | | | Age group | | |
Country/Region	of cases	Rate	ASR[1]	CIR[2]	15-44[1]	45-64[1]	65-74[1]	75+[1]
United Kingdom[3]	17,670	62.3	54.8	100.0	0.2	31	270	700
England	14,740	62.2	54.3	99.0	0.1	31	269	691
North East	570	45.1	41.3	75.3	0.2	24	201	529
North West	1,830	54.6	49.5	90.2	0.1	30	252	603
Yorkshire and the Humber	1,450	59.0	51.9	94.7	0.1	30	261	653
East Midlands	1,250	62.4	54.1	98.8	0.2	29	263	710
West Midlands	1,570	60.1	54.6	99.6	0.2	30	283	684
East	1,680	66.0	55.8	101.7	0.0	30	274	725
London	1,780	52.9	52.4	95.6	0.1	32	263	652
South East	2,660	70.6	59.0	107.6	0.2	35	295	738
South West	1,940	83.9	60.7	110.8	0.3	33	286	805
Wales	1,000	70.9	58.6	106.9	0.3	29	266	812
Scotland	1,480	59.9	57.0	103.9	0.1	34	283	715
Northern Ireland[4]	450	55.9	59.8	109.1	0.5	35	293	756

1   Directly age-standardised rate per 100,000 using the European standard population.
2   Comparative incidence ratio: the ratio of the region ASR and the ASR for the United Kingdom multiplied by 100.
3   The United Kingdom figure is an estimate as data for years prior to 1993 are not available for Northern Ireland (see note 4).
4   The data for Northern Ireland are for years 1993-1995.
The age-standardised rate in children aged under 15 is 0.1 per 100,000 or less in all countries and regions.

Figure 9.11

Prostate cancer CIR by country and region (United Kingdom = 100), all ages
United Kingdom 1991-1993

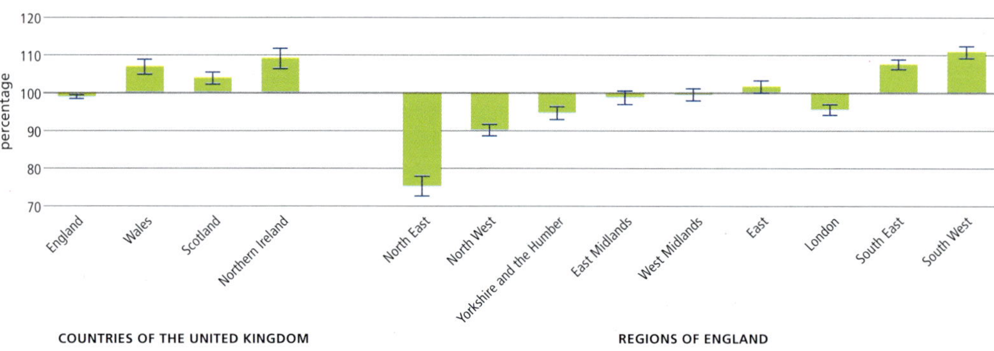

Figure 9.12

Prostate cancer ASR by local authority within countries and regions, all ages
Great Britain 1991-1993

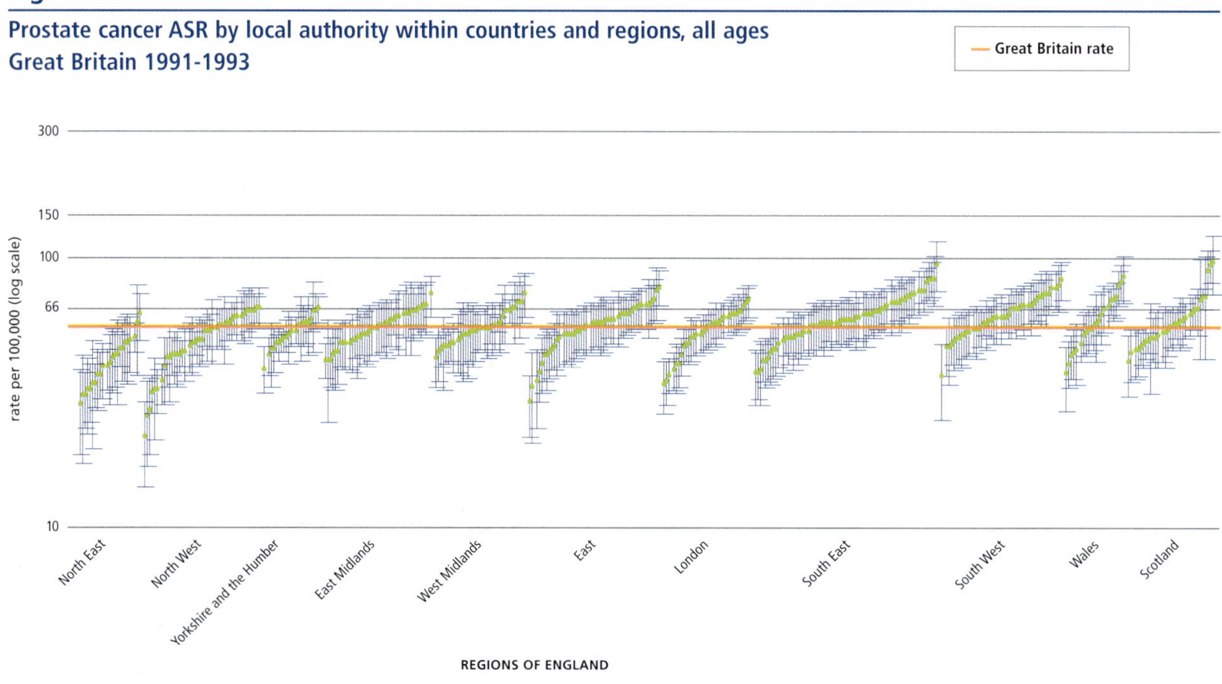

Figure 9.13

Prostate cancer CIR by ONS classification Group (Great Britain = 100), all ages
Great Britain 1991-1993

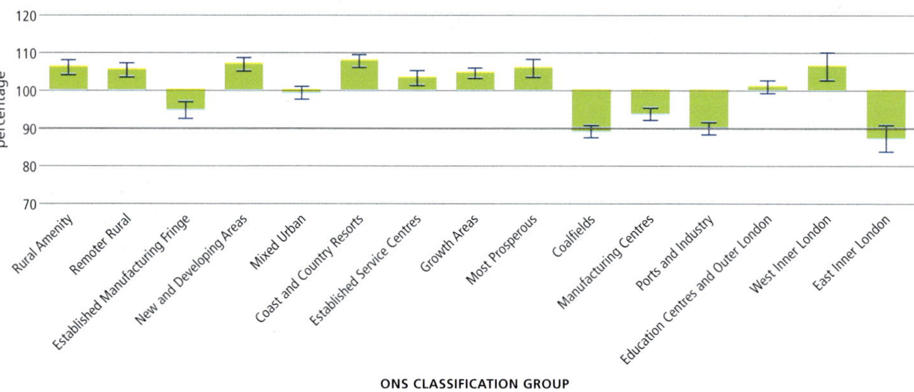

Map 9.7

Age-standardised prostate cancer incidence rates by local authority grouped in quintiles, all ages
Great Britain 1991-1993

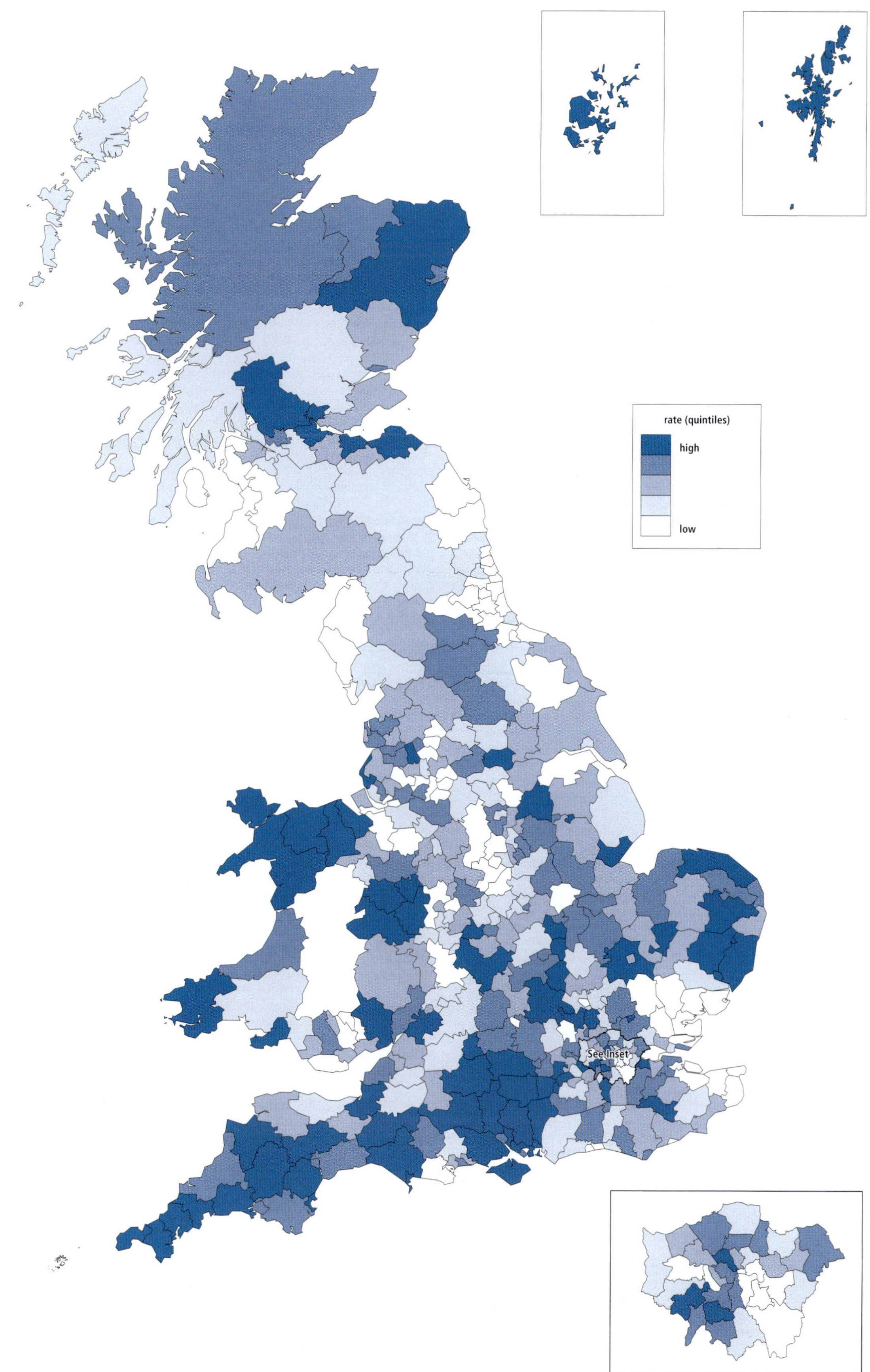

Map 9.8

**Age-standardised prostate cancer incidence rates by local authority, all ages
Great Britain 1991-1993**

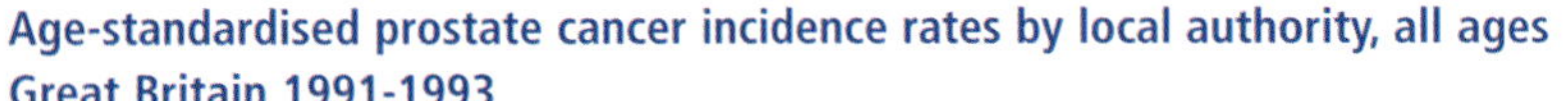

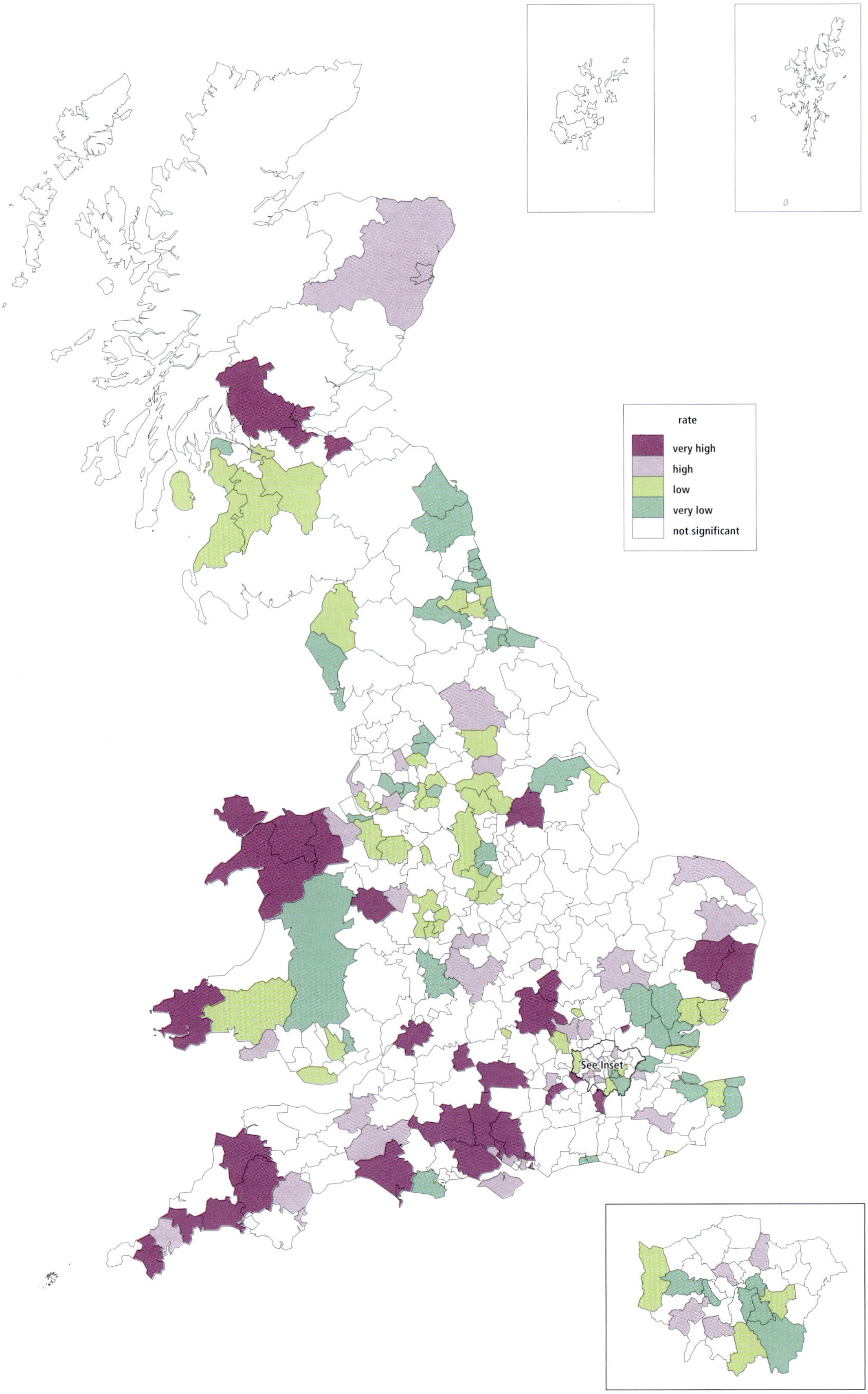

Figure 9.14

Prostate cancer ASR by deprivation, all ages
Great Britain 1991-1993

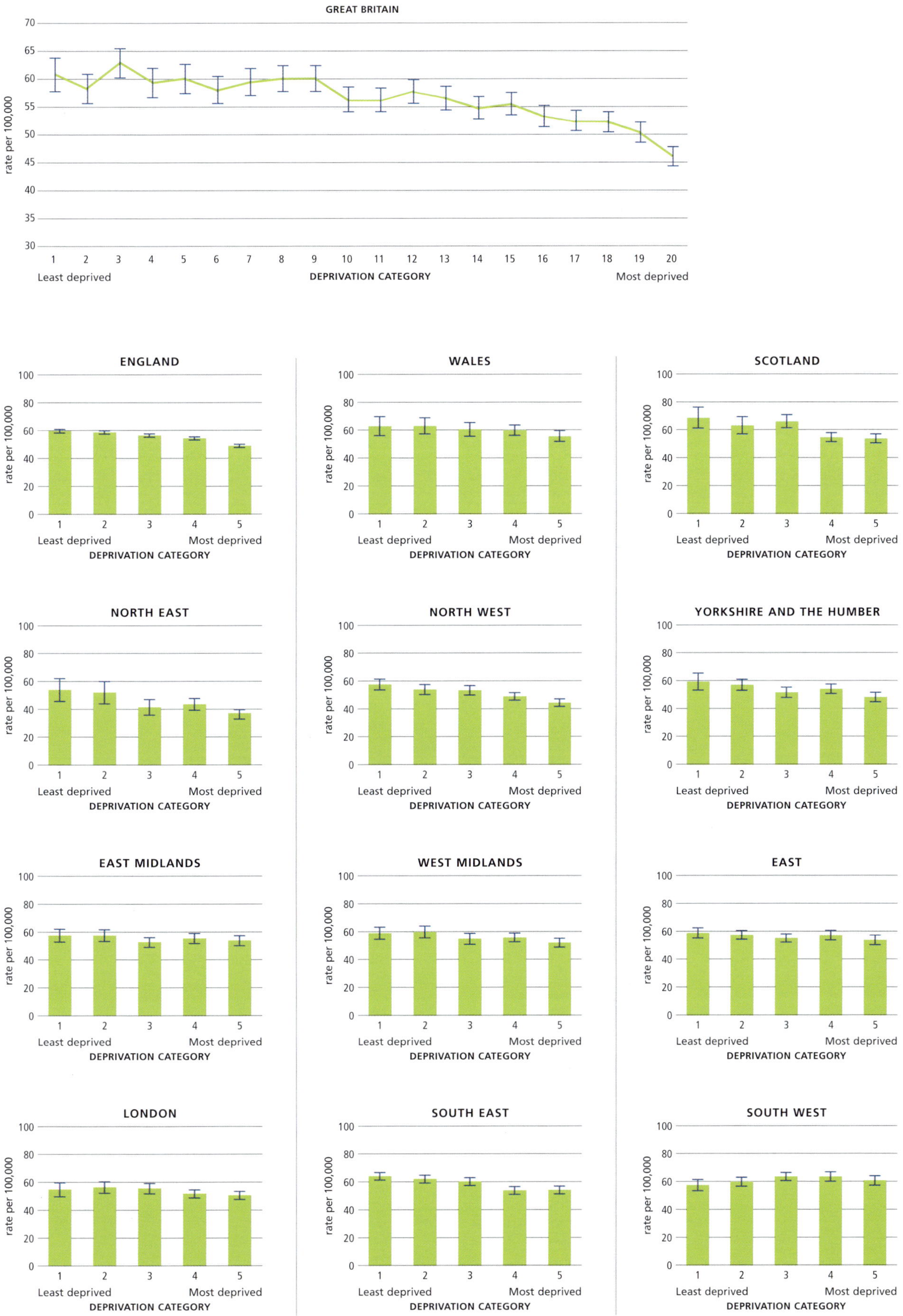

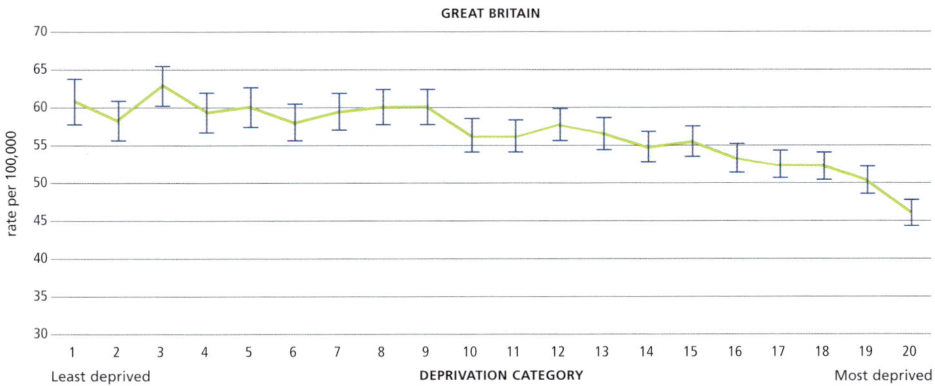

9.6 Colorectal cancer

There were on average 33,000 cases per annum in the United Kingdom in 1991-1993 (almost 16,700 in males and 16,300 in females). Table 9.4 shows that 82 per cent of cases occurred in England, 10 per cent in Scotland, 6 per cent in Wales, and 3 per cent in Northern Ireland. The age-standardised rates of colorectal cancer in 1991-1993 in the United Kingdom were just over 54 and 37 per 100,000 in males and females, respectively. Rates were significantly lower in England than for the United Kingdom as a whole for both males and females while rates were significantly and substantially higher in Northern Ireland, Scotland and Wales. Across the regions and constituent countries, the highest rates occurred in Wales, Scotland and Northern Ireland at over 60 cases per 100,000 in males and around 40 per 100,000 in females.

The incidence rates in the countries of the United Kingdom and the regions of England, compared with the United Kingdom average, are illustrated in Figure 9.15. In England, the highest rates for males were in West Midlands (59 per 100,000) and for females in the South West (40 per 100,000) (Table 9.4).

Table 9.4

Incidence of colorectal cancer: average annual number of new cases and rates per 100,000 population United Kingdom 1991-1993

Males

| Country/Region | Average annual number of cases | Rate per 100,000 | | | | | | |
		Crude Rate	ASR[1]	CIR[2]	15-44[1]	45-64[1]	65-74[1]	75+[1]
United Kingdom[3]	16,670	58.7	54.4	100.0	3.6	72	252	433
England	13,620	57.5	52.9	97.3	3.5	70	245	421
North East	730	57.6	53.8	99.0	3.4	73	246	421
North West	1,990	59.3	55.5	102.1	3.5	73	267	429
Yorkshire and the Humber	1,440	58.6	54.4	100.0	3.5	73	255	420
East Midlands	1,130	56.1	50.8	93.4	2.5	63	241	427
West Midlands	1,640	63.1	59.2	108.9	4.1	80	274	456
East	1,400	54.9	49.6	91.3	3.3	68	220	395
London	1,480	43.9	45.2	83.1	3.3	56	207	382
South East	2,230	58.9	52.8	97.1	3.6	68	249	422
South West	1,590	68.8	55.0	101.1	3.8	75	242	442
Wales	990	70.3	60.9	112.0	3.2	82	277	492
Scotland	1,580	63.9	62.3	114.5	4.8	79	291	505
Northern Ireland[4]	480	59.3	65.7	120.8	3.5	88	312	512

Females

| Country/Region | Average annual number of cases | Rate per 100,000 | | | | | | |
		Crude Rate	ASR[1]	CIR[2]	15-44[1]	45-64[1]	65-74[1]	75+[1]
United Kingdom[3]	16,250	54.8	36.9	100.0	3.2	51	159	293
England	13,310	53.9	36.0	97.7	3.1	49	157	288
North East	650	48.8	32.8	88.8	3.1	42	147	269
North West	1,910	53.9	35.8	97.0	3.3	48	158	287
Yorkshire and the Humber	1,350	52.9	35.1	95.1	3.0	47	156	282
East Midlands	1,040	50.7	34.4	93.3	2.8	47	147	281
West Midlands	1,460	54.4	38.1	103.4	3.1	54	164	295
East	1,380	52.8	35.8	97.0	2.9	48	159	283
London	1,540	43.6	32.0	86.8	2.4	44	136	265
South East	2,290	58.2	37.7	102.4	3.4	53	163	292
South West	1,680	69.0	40.2	108.9	3.8	55	170	321
Wales	920	62.1	39.1	106.2	3.3	55	163	315
Scotland	1,570	59.7	41.6	112.9	3.3	58	182	324
Northern Ireland[4]	460	54.1	44.4	120.5	4.7	68	169	343

1   Directly age-standardised rate per 100,000 using the European standard population.
2   Comparative incidence ratio: the ratio of the region ASR and the ASR for the United Kingdom multiplied by 100.
3   The United Kingdom figure is an estimate as data for years prior to 1993 are not available for Northern Ireland (see note 4).
4   The data for Northern Ireland are for years 1993-1995.
The age-standardised rate in children aged under 15 is 0.2 per 100,000 or less in all countries and regions.

Figure 9.15

Colorectal cancer CIR by country and region (United Kingdom = 100), all ages United Kingdom 1991-1993

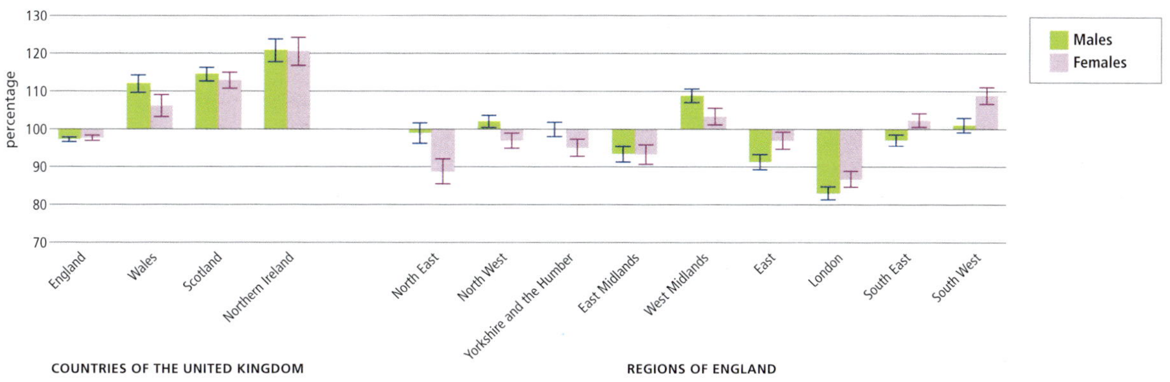

Figure 9.16

Colorectal cancer ASR by local authority within countries and regions, males all ages Great Britain 1991-1993

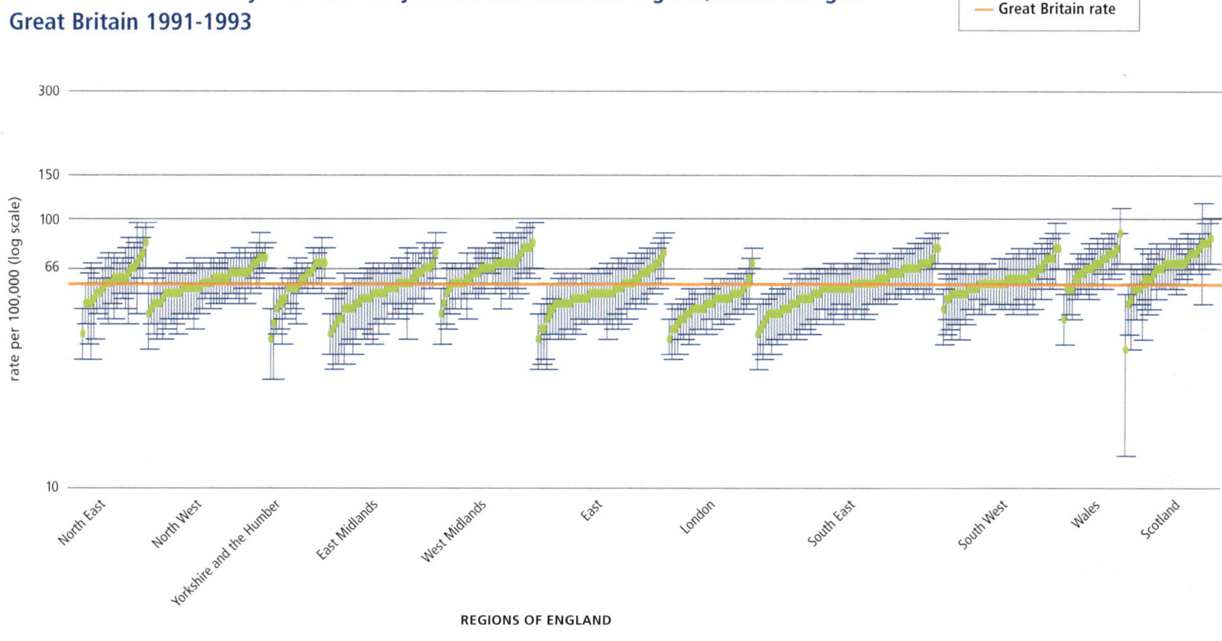

The rates in the other regions of England were generally between 50 and 55 per 100,000 for males and between 32 and 38 per 100,000 for females. Rates were low in London for both sexes (45 and 32 per 100,000 for males and females respectively) and in the North East in females (33 per 100,000) and in the East of England for males (50 per 100,000).

Incidence rates were highest in the 75 and over age group in every region and country for both males and females (Table 9.4). Northern Ireland, Scotland and Wales each had high rates across all the age groups for both males and females. The South West region of England had amongst the highest rates for females. The lowest rates in each age group were in London, around a third lower than for the highest region and country and more than 10 per cent below the average. The all-ages incidence rates by local authority within each region and country are shown in Figures 9.16 and 9.17 for males and for females, respectively. The majority of local authorities within

both Wales and Scotland can be seen to exceed the average for the United Kingdom – many of them significantly, while none of the London boroughs were significantly above the average.

Maps of the age-standardised incidence rates of colorectal cancer are not shown as there was very little statistically significant variation by local authority from the average for Great Britain (as can be seen from Figures 9.16 and 9.17).

Figure 9.18 presents the ratio of the directly age-standardised colorectal cancer incidence rates (CIR) by ONS classification Group compared with the rate for Great Britain. The highest incidence for males occurred in the *Ports and Industry, Coalfields* and *Established Service Centres* Groups, at about 6-7 per cent above the average. For females, the highest incidence was in the *Remoter Rural* Group at over 10 per cent above the average. The incidence in the two Inner London areas were substantially lower than the average (10-20 per cent) for both

Figure 9.17

**Colorectal cancer ASR by local authority within countries and regions, females all ages
Great Britain 1991-1993**

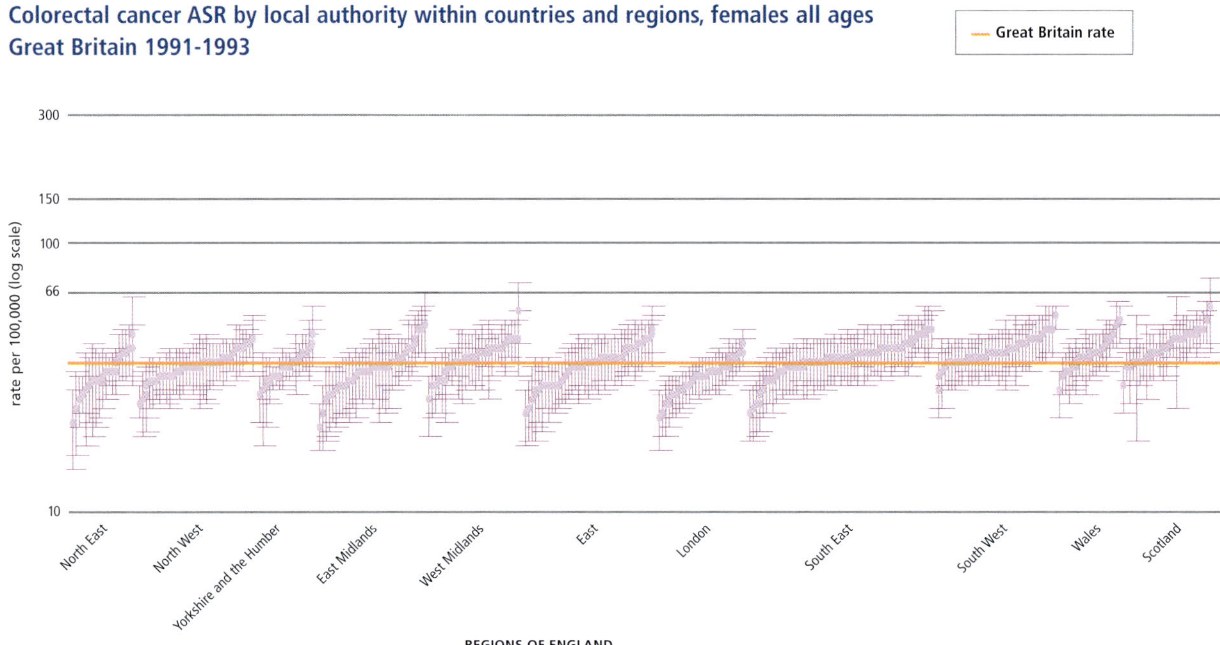

Figure 9.18

**Colorectal cancer CIR by ONS classification Group (Great Britain = 100), all ages
Great Britain 1991-1993**

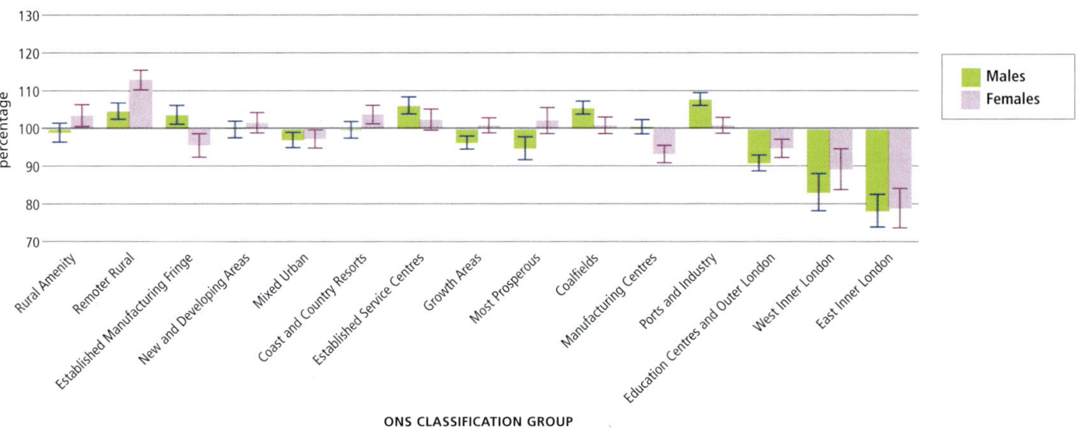

sexes, particularly in *East Inner London*. Other Groups with
relatively low incidence were for males in *Education Centres and
outer London* and for females in *Manufacturing Centres*, almost
10 per cent below the average for Great Britain.

There was a slight rise in incidence of colorectal cancer across
the deprivation groups in males in Great Britain, from around
50 per 100,000 in the least deprived to around 55 per 100,000
in the most deprived – but not in females (Figure 9.19).
Gradients with deprivation were noticeable only in the East
Midlands and North West regions of England and in Wales.

9.7 Discussion

The geographic variation in the incidence of each of lung,
breast and prostate cancers is greatly influenced by the patterns
of incidence with socio-economic deprivation. The North East
of England and Scotland have generally higher levels of socio-
economic deprivation than elsewhere in the United Kingdom,
and the incidence of lung cancer is around 30 per cent higher
than average in males and 45 per cent higher in females.
Smoking is the most significant risk factor in the development
of lung cancer and is more prevalent in manual and unskilled
socio-economic groups.[7] The regional incidence patterns reflect
the regional variation in smoking, shown in chapter 3 of this
volume (Figure 3.23). Not only was there a greater incidence of
lung cancer in the north, but survival from lung cancer also has
been shown to be lower in a number of these regions.[1,8]

Figure 9.19

Colorectal cancer ASR by deprivation, all ages
Great Britain 1991-1993

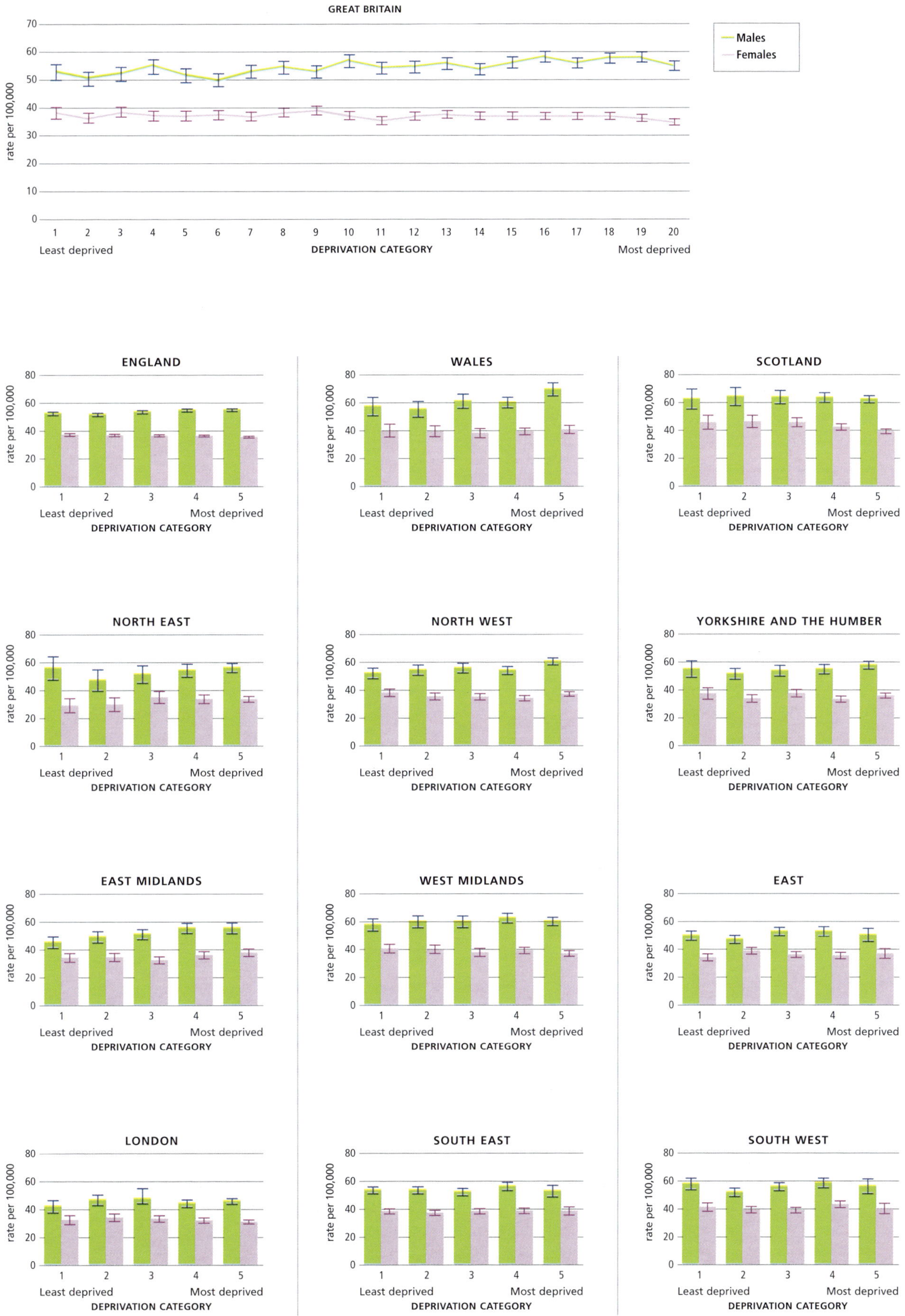

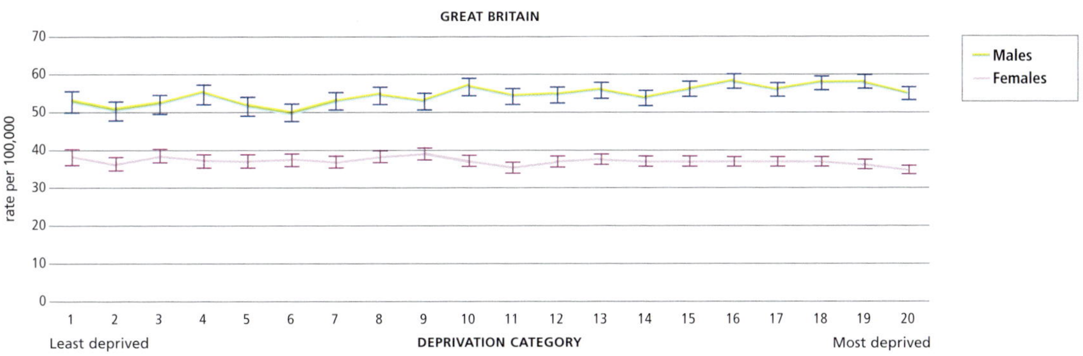

Breast and prostate cancer were similar in their geographic and deprivation patterns. Incidence was higher in the southern regions of England and there was an *inverse* deprivation gradient: incidence is higher in the less deprived groups than in the more deprived groups. The strength of the gradient for each of these cancers, however, was much less than for lung cancer. Also, the relationship of incidence with deprivation does not appear to be linear, with only small differences between the least deprived (categories 1-10) but then rates decreasing more rapidly in the more deprived groups.

In contrast to the negative relationship of incidence with deprivation, mortality from breast cancer was not related to deprivation (cases diagnosed in 1993).[2] As for most other cancers, survival from breast cancer is higher in the most affluent: for patients diagnosed in 1986-90 in England and Wales, the gap in survival between the most affluent and most deprived groups was almost 8 per cent.[1] Mortality from prostate cancer, however, shows an inverse gradient (higher risk for the least deprived) but this relationship is not as steep as for incidence and is a result of the smaller gap in survival by deprivation (a 3 per cent advantage for patients living in the least deprived areas).[1,2]

While the causes of prostate cancer are not well understood, the main risk factors for breast cancer relate to a woman's reproductive history: early menarche, late first pregnancy, low parity, and late menopause; endogenous hormones, both oestrogens and androgens, probably have an important role. Low childbearing has been associated with the development of breast cancer.[9] The fertility comparisons in chapter 5 of this volume (Figure 5.36) also indicate that the mean age of mothers at the birth of their child is higher in the southern regions of England – areas also associated with higher incidence of breast cancer. People in professional occupations, including lawyers, doctors and teachers (defined by mother's occupation), also have been shown to have higher mean ages at childbirth, compared with occupations such as packers and sorters and leather and shoe workers.[10]

The national breast screening programme was introduced in 1988 in England and Wales and Scotland for women aged 50-64 years. There was a phased introduction in many areas and the incidence rates presented here were influenced by the impact of the screening programme in those areas in which the first round (during which cases in the age groups screened, which are present but as yet undiagnosed, are identified through screening) was nearing completion. The incidence in England and Wales peaked in 1992, although the first round of screening was not complete in all areas until 1994/95.[2,5] In Scotland, while the first screening centres opened in 1988, national coverage was not attained until 1991.[11]

Local variations in the incidence of prostate cancer will be partly attributable to regional differences in diagnostic techniques. The rise in prostate cancer incidence during the 1980s has been attributed to the identification of latent carcinomas in investigations of benign conditions using transurethral resections of the prostate, and in autopsy, while the rapid increase in incidence during the early 1990s was associated with the rise in prevalence of PSA testing.[11,12]

The regional and deprivation patterns in the incidence of colorectal cancer were quite different from those for lung, breast and prostate cancers. There was far less variation across the regions of England. The absence of a strong relationship with deprivation is striking for a disease in which diet may play an important aetiological role.

The above analyses demonstrate the variability in the incidence for four of the major cancers across the country and for lung cancer the importance of socio-economic deprivation and its associated pattern of smoking. The results help to identify groups and areas in which smoking cessation activity could be most usefully directed.

References

1 Coleman MP, Babb P, Damiecki P, Grosclaude P, Honjo S, Jones J, Knerer G, Pitard A, Quinn MJ, Sloggett A and De Stavola BL. *Cancer survival trends in England and Wales, 1971-1995: deprivation and NHS region.* Studies in Medical and Population Subjects No.61. The Stationery Office (London: 1999).

2 Quinn MJ, Babb P, Brock A, Kirby L and Jones J. *Cancer trends in England and Wales 1950-1999.* Studies in Medical and Population Subjects No.66. The Stationery Office (London: 2001).

3 Harris V, Sandridge AL, Black RJ, Brewster DH and Gould A. *Cancer registration statistics Scotland 1986-1995.* Information & Statistics Division (Edinburgh: 1998).

4 Gavin AT and Reid J. (eds). *Cancer incidence in Northern Ireland 1993-95.* The Stationery Office (London: 1999).

5 Office for National Statistics. Press Release. 26 January 2001. *Cancer registrations in England, 1995-1997.*

6 Drever F and Bunting J. Patterns and trends in male mortality. In: Drever F and Whitehead M. (eds). *Health inequalities.* Series DS No.15. The Stationery Office (London: 1997), 95-107.

7 Drever F, Fisher K, Brown J and Clark J. *Social inequalities 2000.* The Stationery Office (London: 2000).

8 Scottish Cancer Intelligence Unit. *Trends in cancer survival in Scotland 1971-1995.* Information & Statistics Division (Edinburgh: 2000).

9 Beral V. Long term effects of childbearing on health. *Journal of Epidemiology and Community Health* 39 (1985), 343-346.

10 Babb P. Occupation and fertility. In Drever F. (ed.) *Occupational Health.* Series DS No.10. The Stationery Office (London: 1995), 232-234.

11 Swerdlow AJ, dos Santos Silva I, Reid A, Qiao Z, Brewster DH and Arrundale J. Trends in cancer incidence and mortality in Scotland: description and possible explanations. *British Journal of Cancer* 77 (suppl 3) (1998), 1-16.

12 Quinn MJ, Babb P, Kirby L and Brock A. Report: Registrations of cancer diagnosed in 1994-1997, England and Wales. *Health Statistics Quarterly* 7 (2000), 71-82.

Descriptive analysis of geographic variations in adult mortality by cause of death

Justine Fitzpatrick, Clare Griffiths, Mike Kelleher and Stan McEvoy

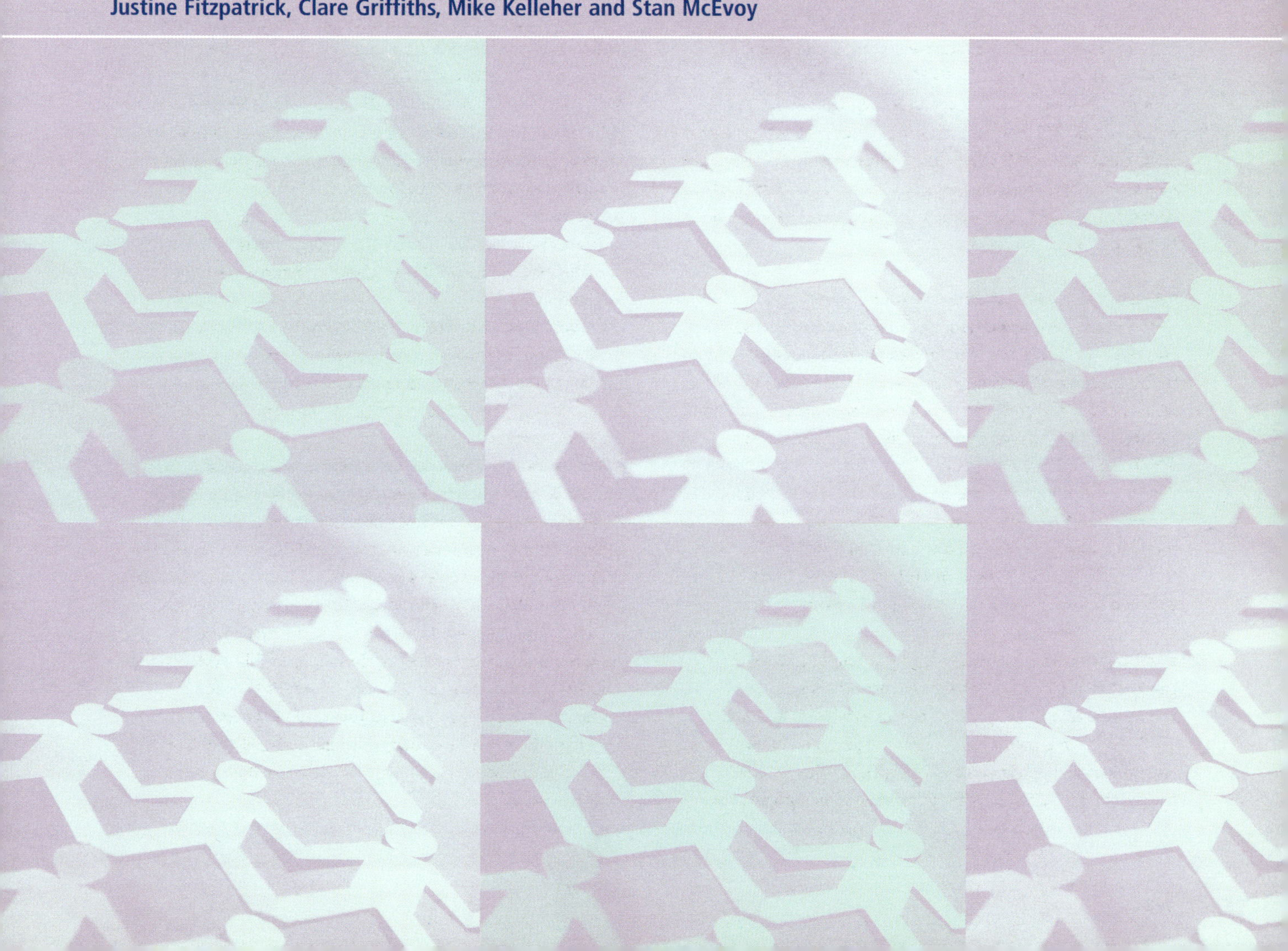

Chapter 10

Descriptive analysis of geographic variations in adult mortality by cause of death

Summary

• Scotland, Wales and Northern Ireland had higher all-cause mortality rates than England for most age groups studied and analysis of regional all-cause mortality within England shows that regions in the north had higher mortality than the southern regions.

• There were substantial differences in all-cause mortality rates by local authority within countries and regions. Authorities with the highest rates tended to be located in urban and industrial areas.

• Males aged 45-64 in London had much lower rates for ischaemic heart disease mortality given the pattern for all causes of death.

• The pattern for cancer and lung cancer mortality was very similar to that for all causes of death.

• There was no clear north-south pattern in colorectal cancer mortality and local authorities with high rates were less concentrated in urban areas than for other causes of death.

• There was little geographic variation in mortality from breast cancer and little variation in prostate cancer mortality by country. However, within England it was the southern regions and local authorities with characteristics associated with affluence that experienced the highest rates.

• There was no north-south pattern in all-age mortality from infectious diseases. London had particularly high mortality from both respiratory and infectious diseases.

• The geographic pattern of mortality from infectious disease varied considerably by age group. The pattern for those aged 65 and over was very similar to the pattern for all causes of death.

• Areas with high mortality rates from accidents were less concentrated in urban areas than for all causes of death. Those areas classified as *Remoter Rural* had the highest mortality.

• Areas with high mortality rates from suicide were largely confined to Scotland, Wales, the North West, London and the south coast of England.

• Areas with high mortality from drug-related poisonings were largely confined to inner London, Glasgow and Manchester.

• Areas with high mortality rates from alcohol-related deaths were largely confined to Scotland, London and Manchester.

| 10.1 Introduction

There has been a long-standing interest in geographic inequalities in mortality and reducing such inequalities is high on the current Government's agenda.[1,2,3,4,5] The report to the Prime Minister by the Cabinet Office, entitled *Sharing the Nation's Prosperity*,[6] produced in December 1999, also focused on inequalities and drew attention to a north-south divide in mortality - with higher mortality in the north of England, Wales, Scotland and Northern Ireland, and lower mortality in the south of England - but also pointed out that within each region and country there are local authorities which have mortality levels that are higher than the United Kingdom average and local authorities with lower than average mortality.

Drever and Whitehead[7] and Charlton[8] showed that within England and Wales, local authorities that had the highest mortality tended to be urban areas, particularly those with purpose-built inner city estates and deprived industrial areas. Both rural and prosperous areas tended to be the most healthy and also made the biggest health gains during the 1980s.

Recent work from the New Policy Institute and the Joseph Rowntree Foundation[9] found that of all the local authorities within Great Britain with mortality rates more than 10 per cent greater than Great Britain as a whole, more than a quarter were in Scotland, just under half in the north of England and just under a quarter in London. None were located in the south of England (outside London). Shaw and colleagues[10] have used parliamentary constituencies to illustrate inequalities in mortality by area. They found that the six constituencies within Great Britain with the highest mortality under age 65 were located in Glasgow, and only one from the highest 15 was outside Scotland or the north of England. Of the 15 areas with the lowest under-65 mortality rates, only one, Sheffield Hallam, was located outside the south of England.

This chapter provides further evidence of geographic inequalities in mortality at country, region and local authority level during the 1990s, expanding on previous work by including data for the whole of the United Kingdom. It looks at the patterns for both males and females separately, and focuses specifically on particular age groups if the geography of mortality in that age group is different from the geography of all-age mortality.

As well as all-cause mortality, this chapter examines geographic variation in mortality from particular causes of death. The following additional underlying causes of death are examined:
• Circulatory diseases (ischaemic heart disease and stroke)
• Cancers (all cancers, lung, breast, prostate, colorectal)
• Respiratory diseases

- Infectious diseases
- Accidents
- Suicide
- Drug-related poisonings and alcohol-related deaths

These causes were identified using the International Classificiation of Diseases, Ninth Revision (ICD9). They were chosen for two reasons. Either they are included as areas for health improvement in the Government's strategy for health in England, *Saving Lives: Our Healthier Nation*,[1] and are subsequently identified in the recently published NHS Plan,[2] and the strategy for Scotland *Towards a Healthier Scotland*,[3] or they account for a large proportion of total deaths every year. We have ensured consistency in definitions between countries as far as possible throughout this chapter, but differences in coding of cause of death may contribute to some of the variations seen between countries.

The recently revised ONS classification of local authorities[11] (presented in chapter 4 of this volume) is used as an indicator of the characteristics of areas and mortality rates for groups of authorities with similar characteristics are presented. The relative contribution of country and region of location and the ONS classification to differences in mortality rates by local authority is assessed for each cause of death using analysis of variance.

We have used age-standardised mortality rates throughout this chapter, unless otherwise stated. When presenting trends, we have used 3-year moving averages to smooth out yearly fluctuations in the data. Consequently trends are shown for 1992 to 1996 throughout the chapter. Maps have been used to describe the data at local authority level and a guide to how they have been constructed can be found in Appendix A.

10.2 All-cause mortality

This section looks at variations in all-cause mortality by country, region of England and local authority in the United Kingdom.

Variations between countries and regions

Tables 10.1 and 10.2 show age-standardised mortality rates for males and females respectively, over the period 1991 to 1997, for countries of the United Kingdom and regions of England. For both males and females, there was substantial geographic variation in mortality, between both the countries of the United Kingdom and the regions of England.

Males in Scotland, Wales and Northern Ireland had higher mortality than males in England and in the United Kingdom as a whole, for all age groups (Table 10.1). For male children, the pattern of country-level variation was the same as in the other age groups, but only Northern Ireland's rate was significantly higher than the United Kingdom's. For females, Scotland had substantially higher mortality than the United Kingdom at all ages, including childhood (Table 10.2). Wales and Northern Ireland had significantly higher mortality than the United Kingdom for all ages, and for those aged 45-64 and 65 and over. England had lower mortality than the United Kingdom as a whole for all ages and all the adult age groups.

For both males and females, within England, there was evidence of a clear north-south divide in mortality. Regions in the north had high mortality and regions in the south had low mortality for all ages, 45-64 and those aged 65 and over. The North East and the North West were the regions with the highest mortality and the South East, South West and East of England the regions with the lowest mortality in these age groups. The only major exception to this was that males in London, who had lower mortality than the United Kingdom as a whole at all ages and at ages 65 and over, had higher than average mortality at ages 45-64. For boys and girls aged 1-14, Yorkshire and the Humber had the highest mortality rate.

Although there was a steady decline in all-age mortality and in the mortality of those aged 45 and over in every country and region between 1992 and 1996, the geographic differences described above were maintained throughout the period. The North East had the largest percentage decline in all-age mortality of the regions of England and the South East the smallest for both males and females, so a small narrowing of the differences between the regions was seen. The differences between the countries remained relatively stable over this period.

For all countries there was also a decline in mortality for boys and girls aged 1-14 over the 1992 to 1996 period (Figure 10.1 and 10.2). For both males and females there was an overall narrowing of the difference between countries of the United Kingdom. For the regions of England, the mortality rates for children aged 1-14 were very variable over time and no real trend was apparent.

For males aged 15-44 the country-level pattern of mortality was the same as for all ages (Table 10.1). All countries except England had higher mortality than the United Kingdom rate. For females, although the overall pattern was the same as for all ages with Scotland, Wales and Northern Ireland having higher mortality than England, Scotland was the only country to have a rate significantly higher than the United Kingdom rate (Table 10.2).

Figures 10.3 and 10.4 show age-specific mortality rates for males and females aged 15-44 by country and 5-year age band. For males in the youngest two age groups shown here (aged 15-19 and 20-24) Northern Ireland and Scotland had similar mortality rates, with Northern Ireland's rate being slightly higher, continuing the pattern seen in children for males. Wales had higher mortality than England in the 15-29 age groups, but its rates were similar at ages 30-44. Northern Ireland's rate fell towards the rates in England and Wales in the 25-34 age groups and by the 35-39 age group its rate was almost the same. In contrast, Scotland had high mortality in all the age groups, beginning to differ dramatically from the other countries from the 25-29 age group onwards. For females, Scotland had a higher mortality rate in all the age groups, except 15-19, and its rate diverged from the others with increasing age.

For adults aged 15-44 there was a different geographic pattern of mortality within England than for all-age mortality, with the north-south divide not as clearly visible (Tables 10.1 and 10.2). For males, the North West and London had higher mortality rates than the United Kingdom for the 15-44 age group and all the other regions had lower rates. For females, the North West was the only region with a significantly higher mortality rate than the United Kingdom rate. The North East, which had the highest mortality at older ages, had lower mortality than the United Kingdom as a whole for the 15-44 age group for both males and females, although for females the rate did not differ significantly from the United Kingdom rate.

Although London had the highest rate overall in those aged 15-44, it had the lowest rates in those aged 15-19 and 20-24, but

the highest rates in those aged between 30 and 44 (Figure 10.5). Its rate continued to diverge from the other regions with increasing age. The North West had the highest mortality up to age 25-29. Figure 10.6 shows that for females, there was little variation by region in the rates at younger ages within the 15-44 age group, with marked differences only really becoming clear at older ages.

Figures 10.7 and 10.8 show trends in male and female mortality for those aged 15-44 by country. For males, the rate in Scotland increased between 1992 and 1996, leading to a widening of the difference between countries over time. The mortality rate for males and females aged 15-44 in Wales also increased over this time period while mortality in England remained relatively

Table 10.1

Age-standardised mortality rates for all causes of death by country and region, males
United Kingdom 1991-1997

			rates per 100,000		
	overall	1-14	15-44	45-64	65+
United Kingdom	976	23	113	806	6,468
England	~957	22	~109	~777	~6,374
North East	*1,101	24	~108	*948	*7,285
North West	*1,064	*25	*124	*921	*6,955
Yorkshire and the Humber	*999	*25	~105	*821	*6,650
East Midlands	~955	22	~103	~751	6,430
West Midlands	*1,000	23	~105	810	*6,686
East	~874	~20	~93	~649	~5,997
London	~967	22	*129	*833	~6,262
South East	~874	~19	~97	~666	~5,938
South West	~866	20	~103	~670	~5,822
Wales	*999	24	*117	*834	*6,599
Scotland	*1,141	25	*144	*1,046	*7,301
Northern Ireland	*1,019	*26	*124	*877	*6,649

* significantly higher than the United Kingdom rate
~ significantly lower than the United Kingdom rate

Table 10.2

Age-standardised mortality rates for all causes of death by country and region, females
United Kingdom 1991-1997

			rates per 100,000		
	overall	1-14	15-44	45-64	65+
United Kingdom	624	17	60	491	4,215
England	~611	17	~59	~474	~4,143
North East	*702	18	58	*578	*4,729
North West	*679	18	*66	*552	*4,551
Yorkshire and the Humber	*637	*20	60	500	*4,297
East Midlands	~616	17	59	~480	~4,176
West Midlands	*630	17	60	485	*4,265
East	~570	16	~53	~417	~3,937
London	~600	17	61	~479	~4,015
South East	~567	~14	~54	~415	~3,906
South West	~552	16	~56	~416	~3,761
Wales	*635	17	63	*507	*4,272
Scotland	*733	*19	*74	*618	*4,865
Northern Ireland	*642	20	59	*525	*4,292

* significantly higher than the United Kingdom rate
~ significantly lower than the United Kingdom rate

Figure 10.1

**Trends in age-standardised mortality rates for all causes of death by country, males aged 1-14
United Kingdom 1992-1996***

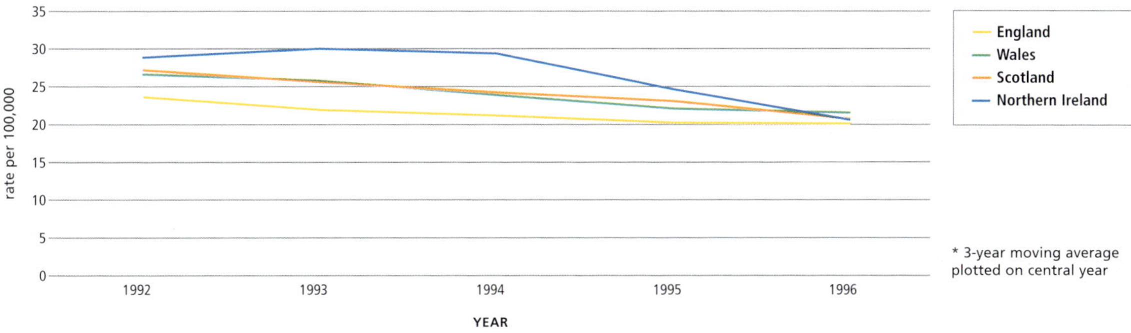

Figure 10.2

**Trends in age-standardised mortality rates for all causes of death by country, females aged 1-14
United Kingdom 1992-1996***

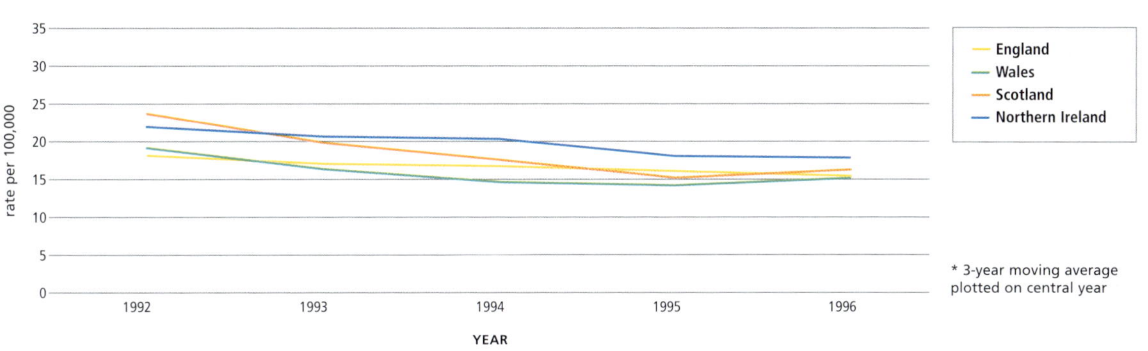

Figure 10.3

**Age-specific mortality rates for all causes of death by country, males aged 15-44
United Kingdom 1991-1997**

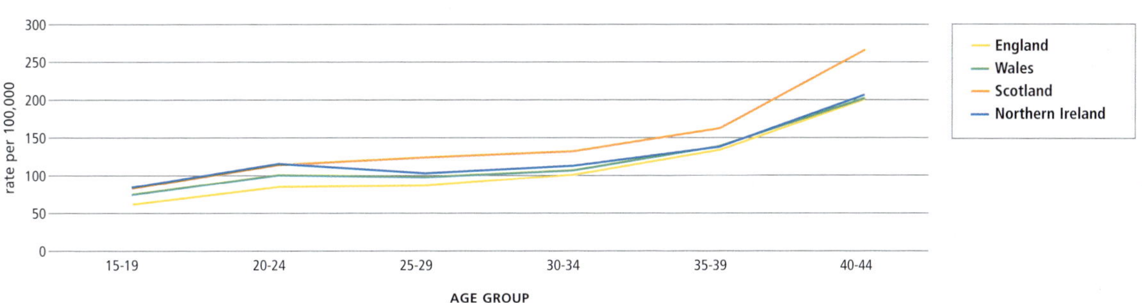

Figure 10.4

**Age-specific mortality rates for all causes of death by country, females aged 15-44
United Kingdom 1991-1997**

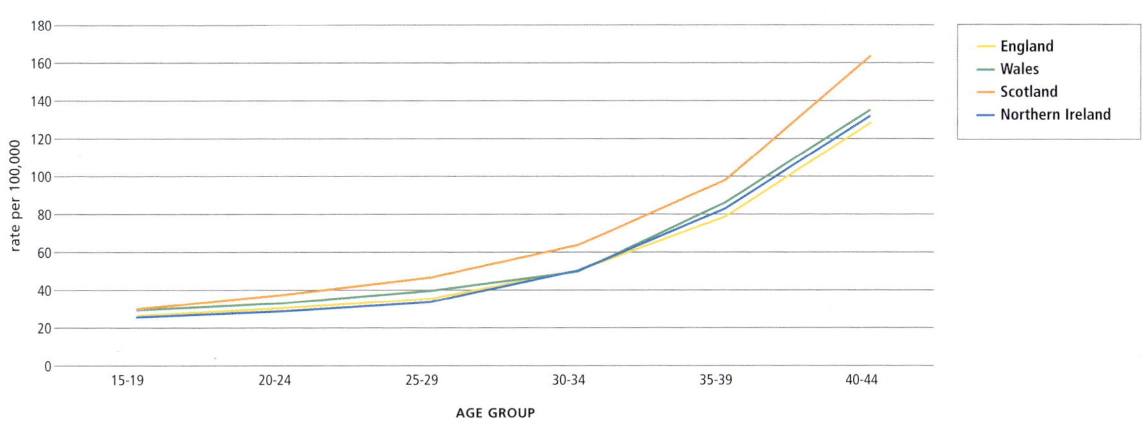

Figure 10.5

Age-specific mortality rates for all causes of death by region, males aged 15-44
England 1991-1997

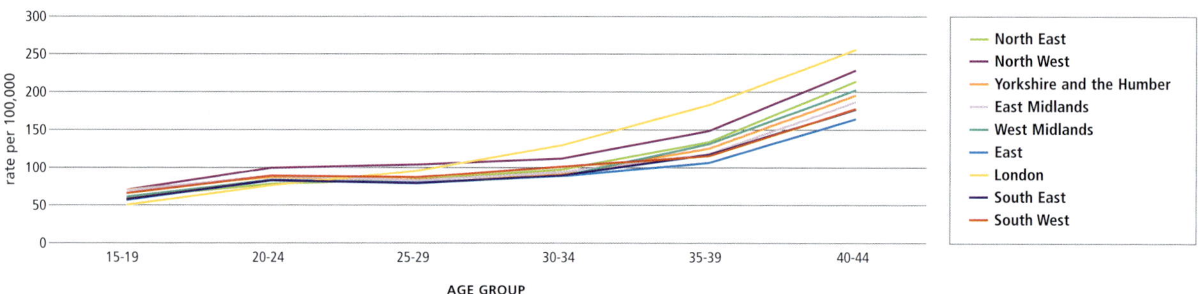

Figure 10.6

Age-specific mortality rates for all causes of death by region, females aged 15-44
England 1991-1997

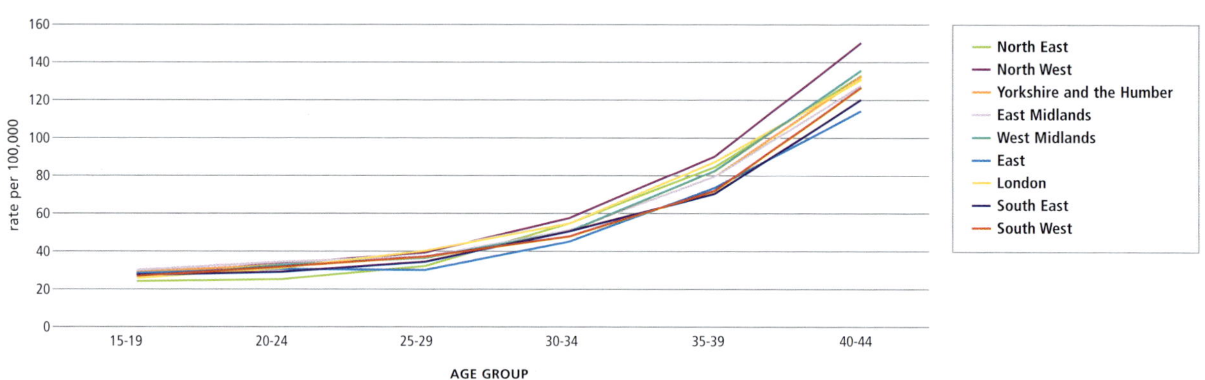

Figure 10.7

Trends in age-standardised mortality rates for all causes of death by country, males aged 15-44
United Kingdom 1992-1996*

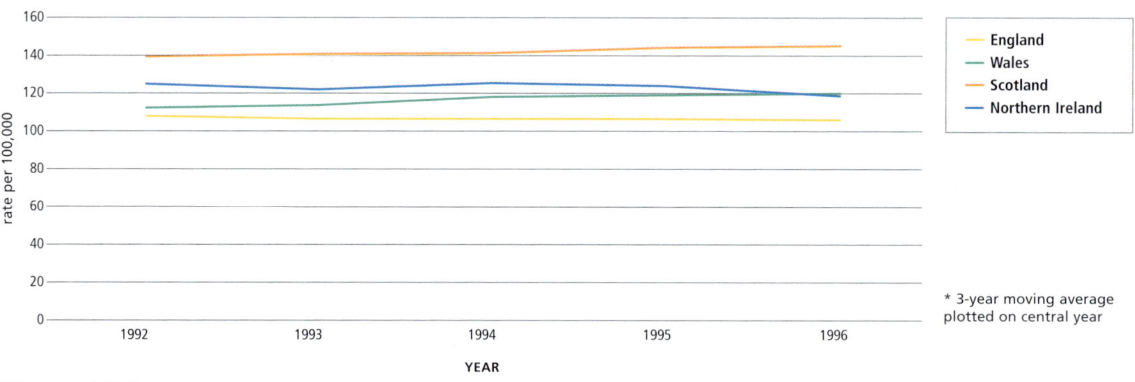

Figure 10.8

Trends in age-standardised mortality rates for all causes of death by country, females aged 15-44
United Kingdom 1992-1996*

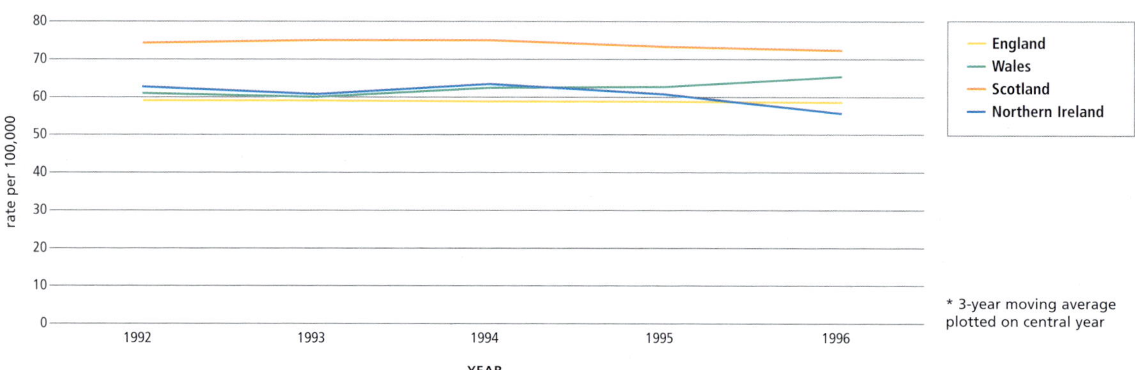

Figure 10.9

Trends in age-standardised mortality rates for all causes of death by region, males aged 15-44 England 1992-1996*

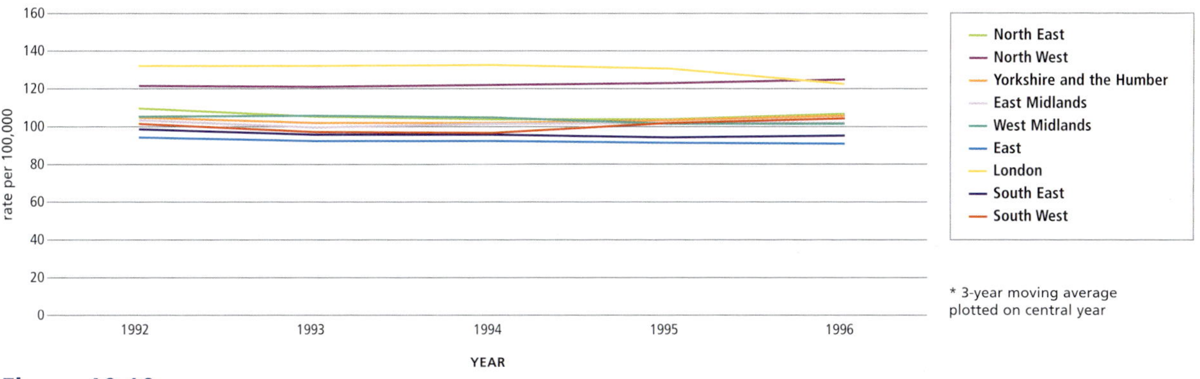

Figure 10.10

Trends in age-standardised mortality rates for all causes of death by region, females aged 15-44 England 1992-1996*

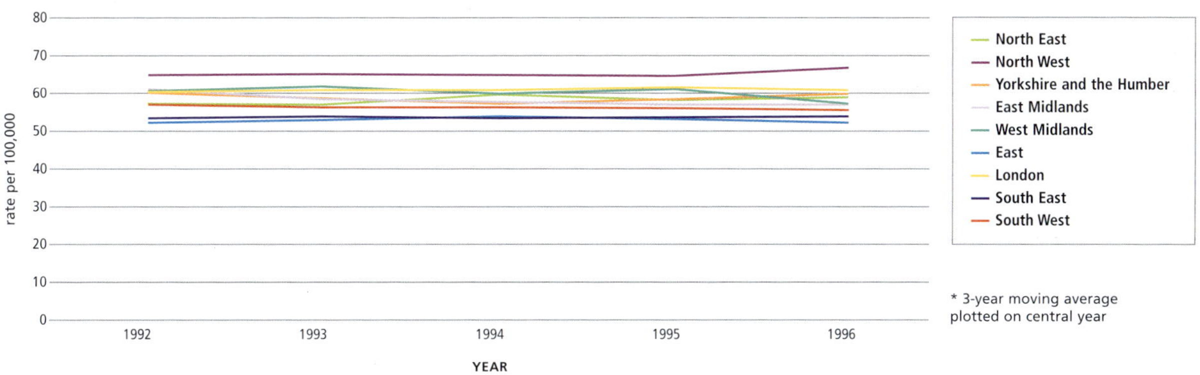

stable and mortality in Northern Ireland declined. At regional level, the North West had consistently higher mortality than the other regions for females and the rate in London was consistently higher for males until 1996 when it fell below the North West (Figures 10.9 and 10.10). There was little sign of a decline in the other regions of England.

Variations between local authorities

Map 10.1 presents the variation in age-standardised mortality rates for males by local authority across the United Kingdom. For all ages, there was a general pattern of high mortality in the majority of authorities in Scotland, the south and west of Northern Ireland, a group of authorities in the North East, a band of authorities from Merseyside to the Humber and south Wales. In addition, some authorities in London had high mortality rates, in contrast to the mortality rates for the London region as a whole shown in Table 10.1.

Areas with mortality rates classed as very high tended to be found in urban and early industrial areas. Outside London and Northern Ireland there were 60 authorities with very high mortality rates. Using the ONS classification of local authorities,[11] 49 of these authorities were classified as *Coalfields, Manufacturing Centres* or *Ports and Industry*. Other areas with very high mortality included two island councils in Scotland,

the Shetland Islands and Eilean Siar. These were classified as *Remoter Rural*. No *Remoter Rural* areas outside Scotland had very high mortality rates.

There was a general pattern of low mortality in authorities throughout the south and east of England. With the exception of authorities in outer London, authorities with mortality rates classed as very low were located away from major urban areas. Many different types of areas in terms of the ONS classification had very low mortality rates including: *Growth Areas, Most Prosperous, Rural Amenity* and *Remoter Rural*. Only three authorities in Scotland, East Renfrewshire, Aberdeenshire and the Scottish Borders, had low mortality rates. Areas with very high mortality rates surround these authorities.

The pattern of mortality across the United Kingdom for all-age mortality for females was similar to that seen for males (Map 10.2). However, there were some notable exceptions. In Scotland, slightly more authorities had very high mortality for females than for males (18 and 16 respectively) although fewer authorities had rates that differed significantly from the United Kingdom as a whole. Although the general pattern of all-age mortality in London was very similar for the two sexes, fewer authorities had very high mortality for females than for males.

Map 10.1

Age-standardised mortality rates for all causes of death by local authority, males all ages
United Kingdom 1991-1997

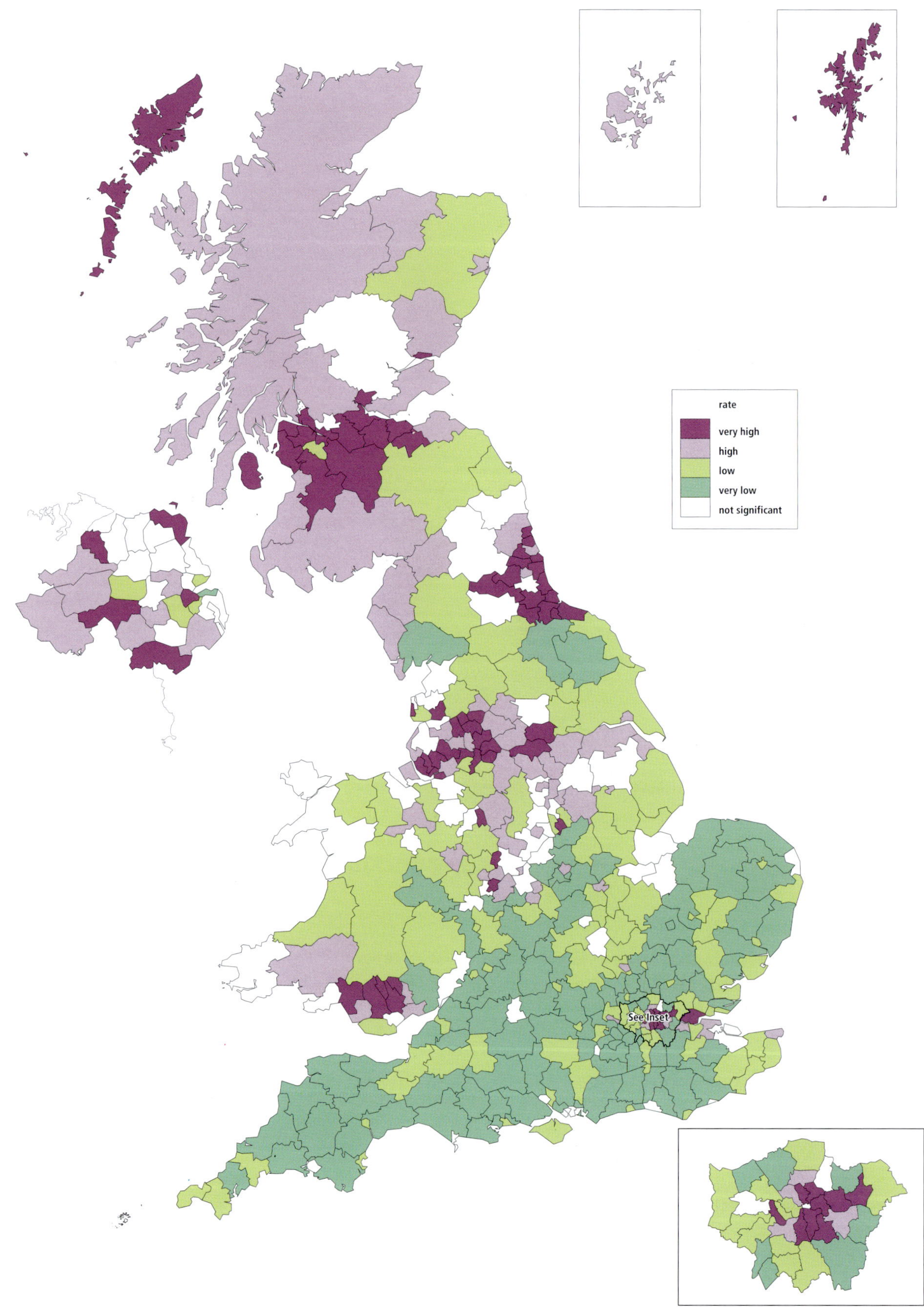

Map 10.2

Age-standardised mortality rates for all causes of death by local authority, females all ages
United Kingdom 1991-1997

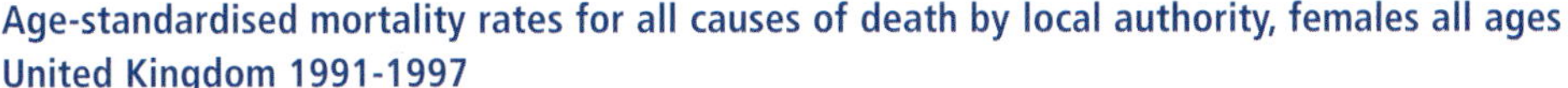

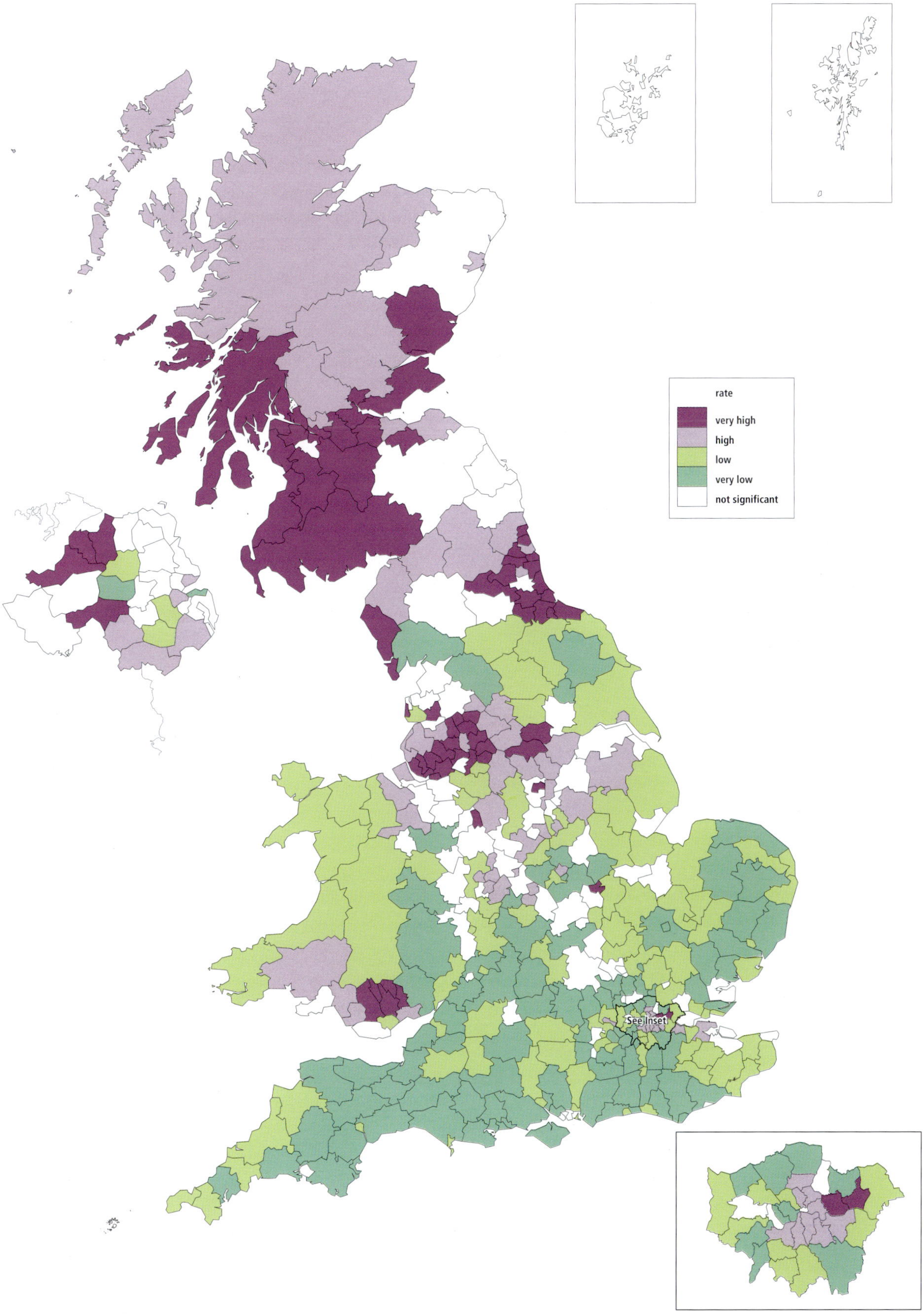

For both males and females there was considerable variation in mortality rates by local authority within all countries and regions. In addition, Figures 10.11 and 10.12 show that every country and region had some local authorities with similar mortality rates to authorities in all other countries and regions.

Figures 10.13 and 10.14 show the distribution of all-age all-cause mortality rates for males and females separately within the 15 ONS classification Groups. For both males and females there was variation in mortality rates by local authority within the Groups, with the most variation in the *Ports and Industry* Group. Generally there were some authorities within most ONS classification Groups which had similar mortality rates to authorities in all other Groups. The exception to this was authorities in the *Coalfields, Manufacturing Centres* and *Ports*

and Industry Groups which, for males, had higher mortality rates than all authorities in the *Most Prosperous* Group.

These differences were examined using analysis of variance to determine how much of the variation in all-age mortality rates by local authority in Great Britain was accounted for by the country or region of location (country/region) and how much was accounted for by the ONS classification Group to which the local authority belonged. The analysis showed that these two factors accounted for 83 per cent of the variation in rates by local authority for both males and females. It showed that both country/region of location and ONS classification Group contributed to the variation in mortality rates by local authority.

Figure 10.11

Age-standardised mortality rates for all causes of death by local authority within countries and regions, males all ages United Kingdom 1991-1997

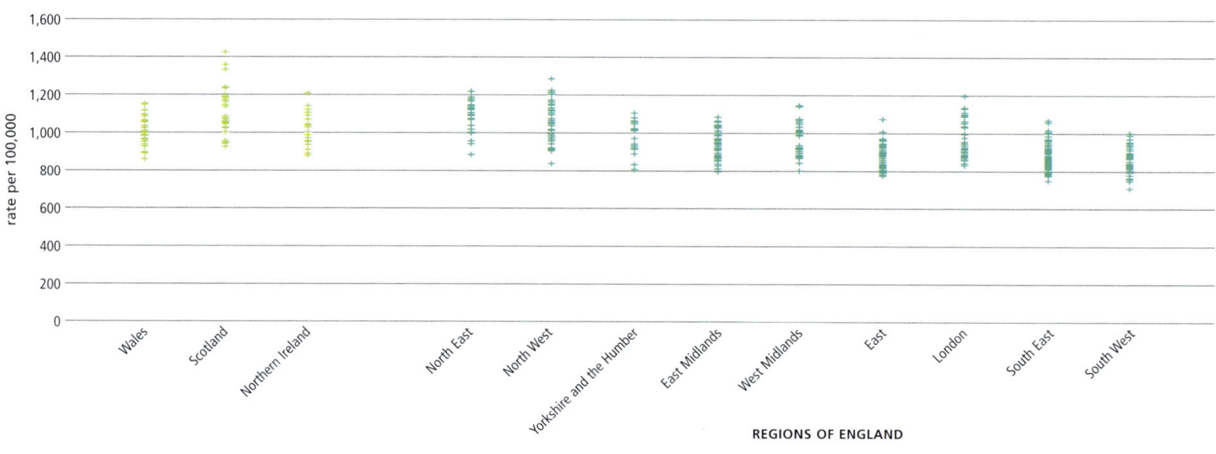

Figure 10.12

Age-standardised mortality rates for all causes of death by local authority within countries and regions, females all ages United Kingdom 1991-1997

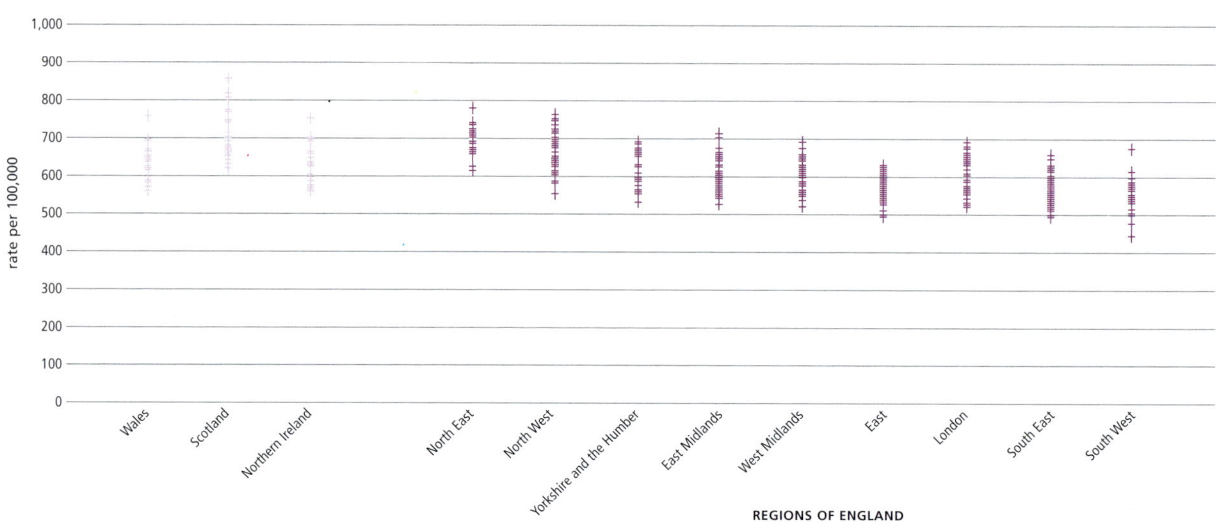

The average all-age mortality rates for males and females for the 15 classification Groups show that the *Ports and Industry* Group had the highest mortality rates for both males and females, followed by the *East Inner London, Manufacturing Centres* and *Coalfields* Groups which all had much higher mortality rates than Great Britain as a whole (Figure 10.15). The *Most Prosperous, Growth Areas* and *Rural Amenity* Groups had the lowest mortality rates for both males and females.

Due to the small number of deaths in childhood we have not mapped mortality rates for those aged 1-14 for individual local authorities. Mortality rates for those aged 1-14 by ONS classification Group show a very similar pattern to that presented for all-age mortality in Figure 10.15, but as the number of deaths in this age group was small, fewer Groups had a significantly different rate to Great Britain as a whole.

Maps 10.3 and 10.4 show mortality rates for males and females aged 15-44. Fewer authorities had mortality levels that differed significantly from the United Kingdom as a whole as there were only a small number of deaths in this age group in a single authority. There were some other notable differences between the pattern of mortality rates for males of all ages and the pattern for those aged 15-44. The authorities with the most favourable mortality rates were more geographically concentrated and were located in a band around the periphery of London. Some isolated authorities on the south coast of England had high mortality rates, for example Brighton and Hove, Bournemouth, Torbay and Hastings, whereas there were no authorities with high all-age mortality anywhere on this coast. Nevertheless, as for all ages, the majority of authorities with very high rates outside London and Northern Ireland (15 out of 20 authorities) were

Figure 10.13

Age-standardised mortality rates for all causes of death by local authority within ONS classification Groups, males all ages Great Britain 1991-1997

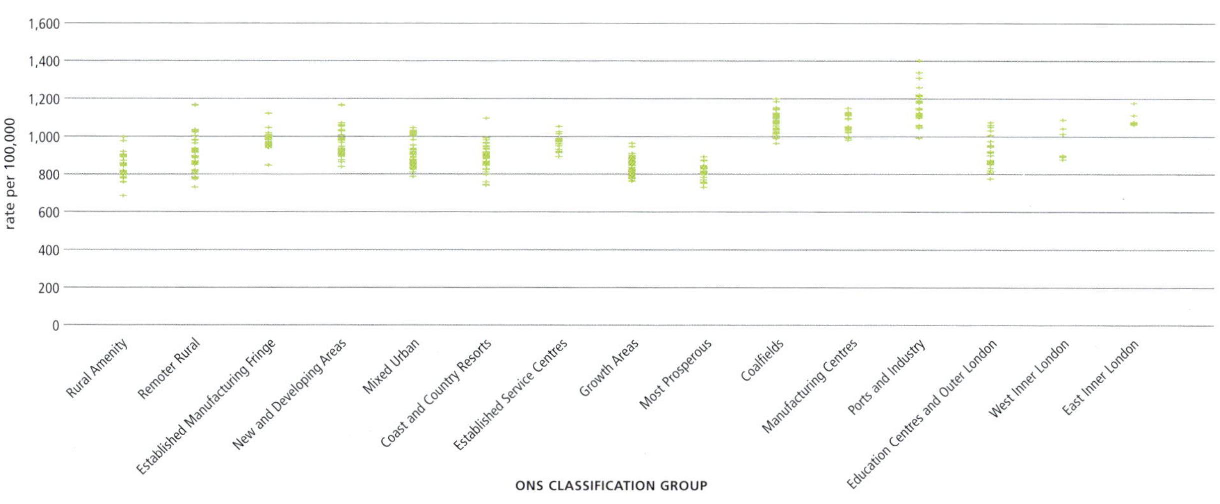

Figure 10.14

Age-standardised mortality rates for all causes of death by local authority within ONS classification Groups, females all ages Great Britain 1991-1997

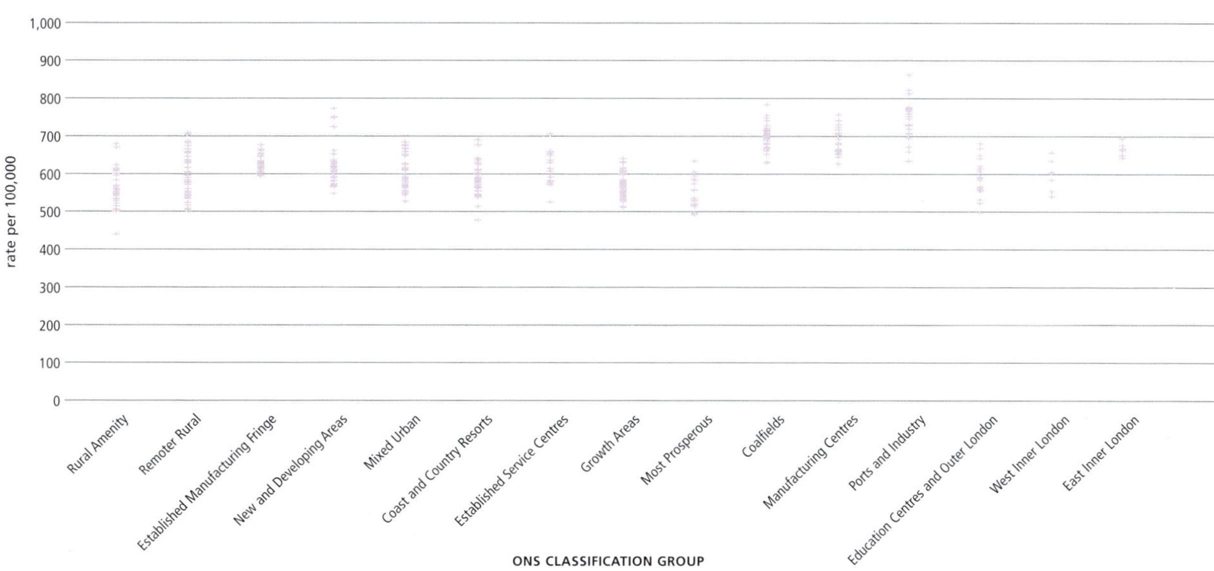

Map 10.3

Age-standardised mortality rates for all causes of death by local authority, males aged 15-44
United Kingdom 1991-1997

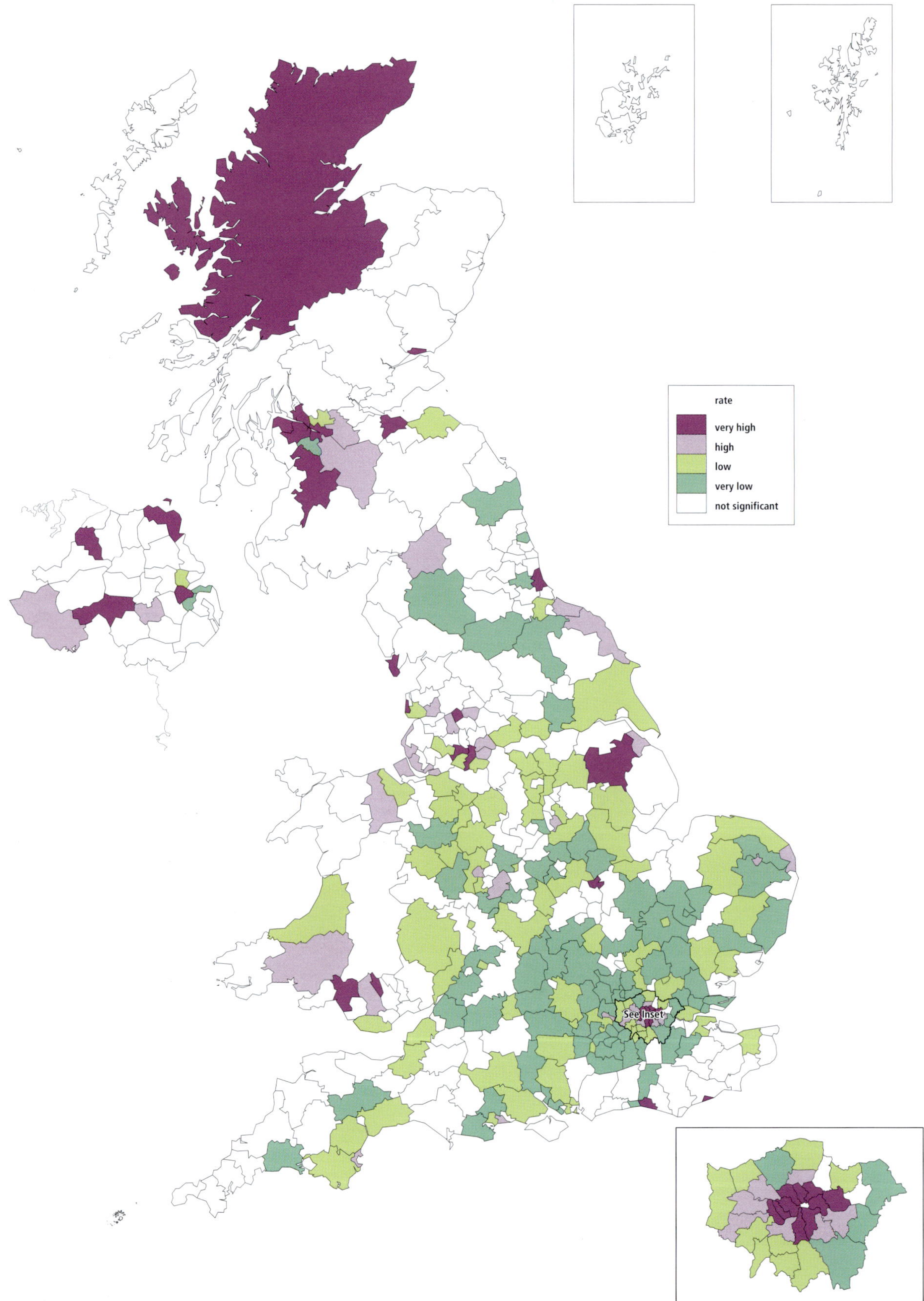

Map 10.4

Age-standardised mortality rates for all causes of death by local authority, females aged 15-44
United Kingdom 1991-1997

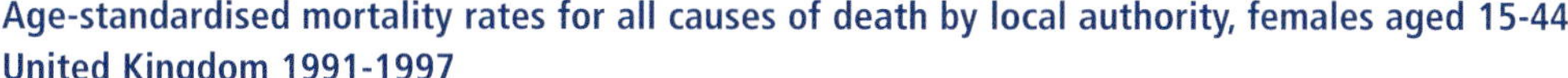

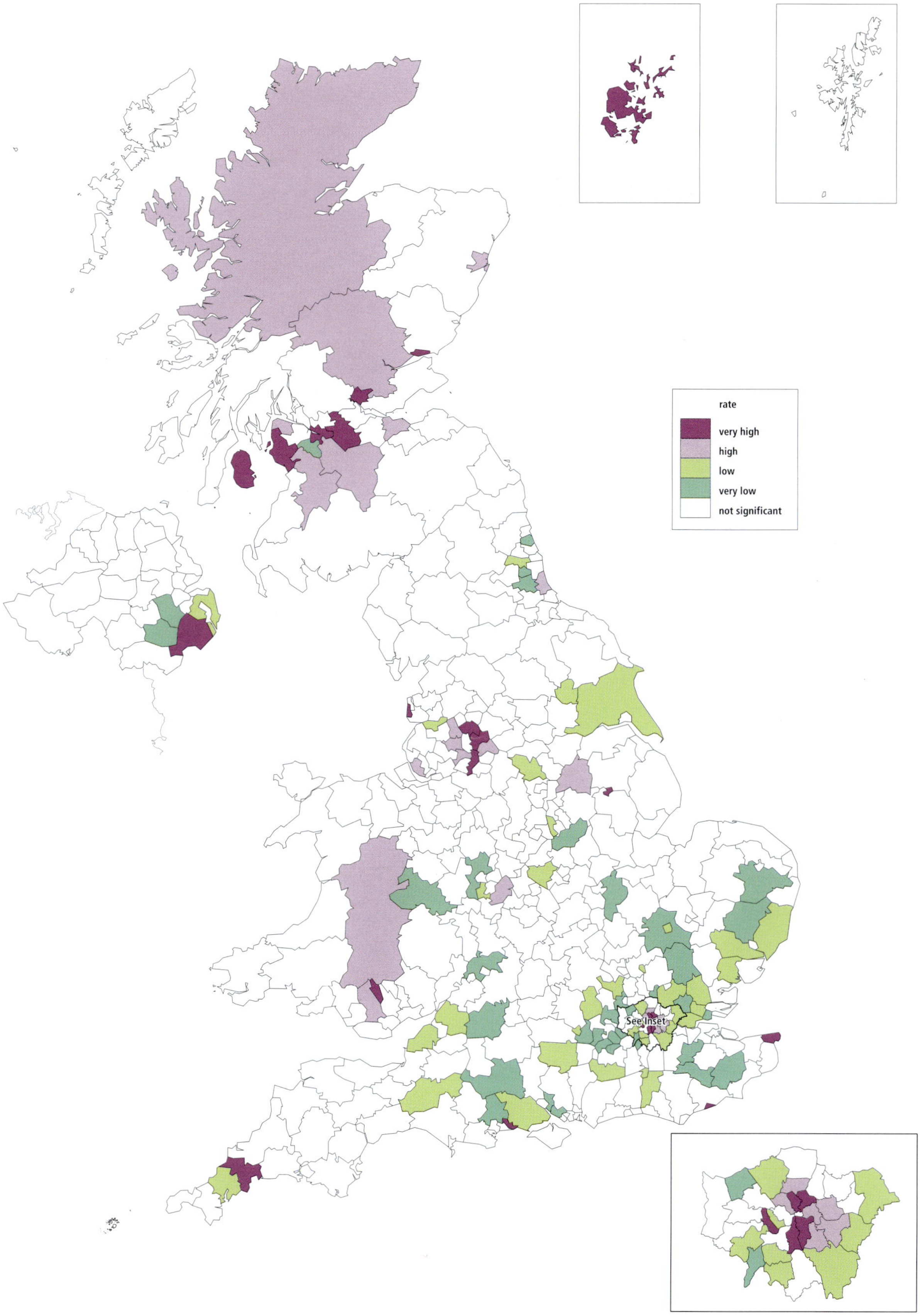

classified as *Coalfields, Manufacturing Centres* or *Ports and Industry*.

For females, as for males, there were a few authorities on the south coast of England with high mortality rates, for example Hastings and Christchurch. Sixteen authorities outside London and Northern Ireland had high mortality rates. Half of these were classified as *Coalfields, Manufacturing Centres* and *Ports and Industry*. However, a further six were classified as *Coast and Country Resorts* or *Established Service Centres*. This was a much larger proportion in these two groups than for males and females of all ages. For males aged 15-44, however, a large number of authorities in these groups had mortality rates classed as high instead of very high.

Figure 10.16 shows mortality rates for males and females aged 15-44 by ONS classification Group. For males aged 15-44, although the same Groups as for all ages had low mortality rates, the *West Inner London* Group had the highest mortality rates, followed closely by the *East Inner London* Group. For females aged 15-44, although the *West Inner London* Group did not have high mortality rates, in other respects the rest of the pattern was similar to that for males in this age group.

The pattern of mortality by local authority described for all ages was found to be similar for people aged 45-64 and aged 65 and over and therefore detailed analysis of the geographic patterns in these age groups is not presented.

Figure 10.15

Age-standardised mortality rates for all causes of death by ONS classification Group, all ages
Great Britain 1991-1997

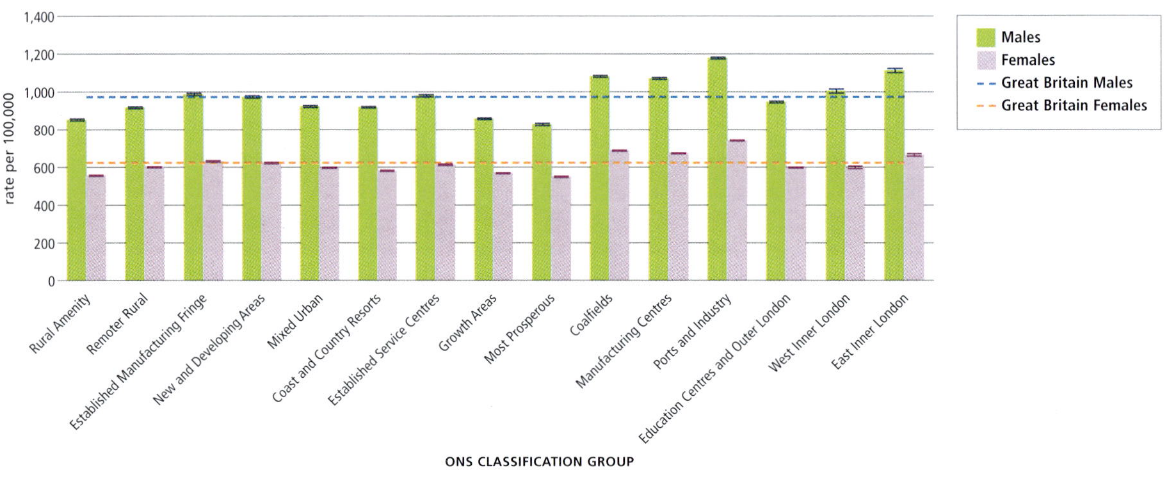

Figure 10.16

Age-standardised mortality rates for all causes of death by ONS classification Group, ages 15-44
Great Britain 1991-1997

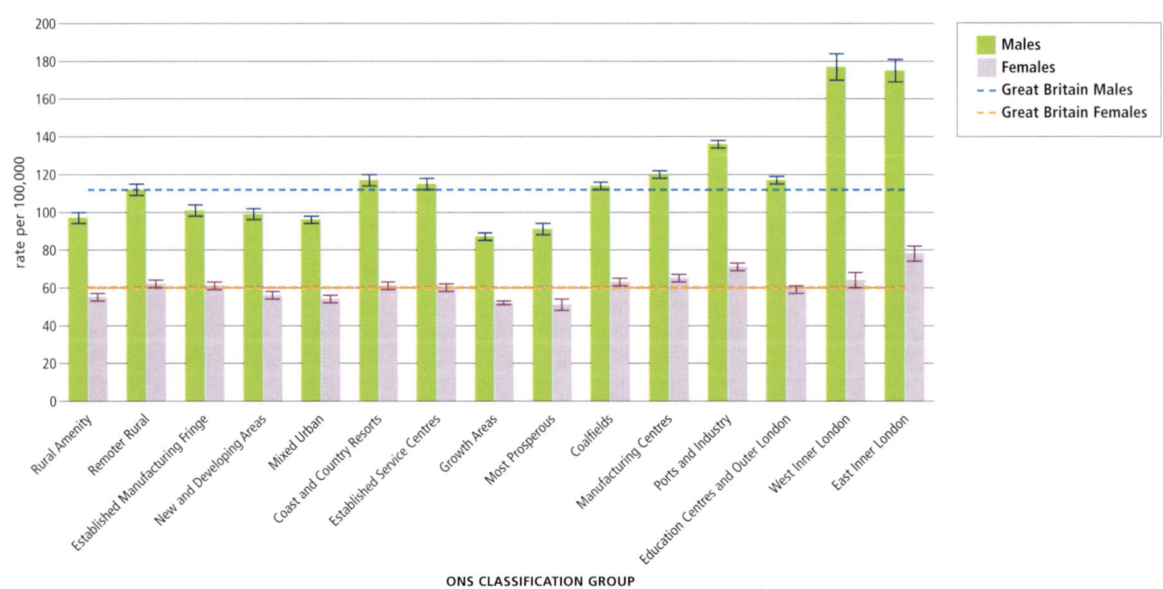

10.3 Circulatory diseases

This section looks at geographic variations in ischaemic heart disease (IHD) (ICD9 410-414) and stroke (ICD9 430-438) mortality. These two causes together account for nearly 40 per cent of all deaths in the United Kingdom every year. The Government's strategies for health[1, 3] identified heart disease and stroke as key target areas for health improvement.

Certain key risk factors for stroke and IHD have already been identified including smoking, poor diet, lack of physical activity, obesity and alcohol consumption.[12, 13, 14] However, the prevalence of these risk factors has varied over time and through different groups of the population. Chapter 3 of this volume presents geographic variation in nutritional intake, smoking and alcohol consumption by country of the United Kingdom and region of England. There was little geographic variation in nutritional intake, but some variation in alcohol consumption and smoking was seen (Figures 3.23 and 3.24). In 1996/7 people in Scotland, Northern Ireland and the northern regions of England were more likely to smoke than people in the southern regions of England. There was little difference in alcohol consumption by country, but men in the northern regions of England and women in the North West were shown to consume more than those in the southern regions of England.

The Government's strategy for health in England identifies smoking as the single biggest preventable cause of poor health.[1]

Table 10.3

Age-standardised mortality rates for ischaemic heart disease by country and region, males United Kingdom 1991-1997

| | rates per 100,000 | | | |
	overall	15-44	45-64	65+
United Kingdom	268	10	260	1,805
England	~261	10	~248	~1,765
North East	*315	*13	*323	*2,079
North West	*302	*13	*305	*2,000
Yorkshire and the Humber	*287	11	*280	*1,932
East Midlands	~262	10	~248	~1,776
West Midlands	*276	11	*269	*1,854
East	~232	~8	~202	~1,620
London	~246	10	~243	~1,647
South East	~226	~8	~198	~1,568
South West	~238	~8	~210	~1,655
Wales	*285	11	*281	*1,907
Scotland	*321	*13	*342	*2,093
Northern Ireland	*303	10	*308	*2,016

* significantly higher than the United Kingdom rate
~ significantly lower than the United Kingdom rate

Table 10.4

Age-standardised mortality rates for ischaemic heart disease by country and region, females United Kingdom 1991-1997

| | rates per 100,000 | | | |
	overall	15-44	45-64	65+
United Kingdom	127	2	72	984
England	~123	2	~67	~955
North East	*159	*3	*101	*1,203
North West	*147	*3	*90	*1,122
Yorkshire and the Humber	*138	2	*80	*1,068
East Midlands	~124	2	70	~963
West Midlands	*130	2	74	*1,002
East	~108	~1	~49	~866
London	~112	~2	~64	~868
South East	~103	~1	~47	~828
South West	~106	~2	~50	~844
Wales	*134	2	*80	*1,024
Scotland	*161	*3	*108	*1,205
Northern Ireland	*149	2	*93	*1,135

* significantly higher than the United Kingdom rate
~ significantly lower than the United Kingdom rate

The NHS Plan[2] for England proposes to *"set up smoking cessation services and to improve the diet of young people by making fruit freely available in schools for 4-6 year olds"* as part of achieving a reduction in health inequalities. A similar plan is evident in *Towards a Healthier Scotland.*[3]

As ischaemic heart disease and stroke account for such a high proportion of total deaths in the United Kingdom, it is likely that the geographic distribution of mortality from these causes closely resembles the geographic distribution of mortality from all causes of death.

Variations between countries and regions

Tables 10.3 and 10.4 show the variations by country and region in mortality from IHD for 1991 to 1997. Tables 10.5 and 10.6 show the figures for stroke. The geographic variation was similar to that described for all-cause mortality. Scotland, Northern Ireland and Wales all had higher mortality from IHD and stroke than England for both males and females. Across age groups the pattern was very similar to this, although the rates were small for those aged 15-44, particularly for females. Although there was a decline in mortality from both IHD and stroke in all the countries, this geographic pattern was maintained throughout 1992 to 1996, with no narrowing of the differences between countries over time.

Within England, there was a north-south divide in mortality from both IHD and stroke, similar to that seen for all cause mortality.

Table 10.5

Age-standardised mortality rates for stroke by country and region, males
United Kingdom 1991-1997

| | rates per 100,000 | | | |
	overall	15-44	45-64	65+
United Kingdom	82	3	41	639
England	~79	3	~39	~618
North East	*95	4	*49	*741
North West	*90	*4	*49	*691
Yorkshire and the Humber	*84	3	42	*657
East Midlands	81	3	39	632
West Midlands	*88	3	43	*687
East	~72	~2	~30	~574
London	~71	3	44	~533
South East	~72	3	~31	~570
South West	~72	3	~31	~577
Wales	82	4	43	636
Scotland	*110	*4	*58	*857
Northern Ireland	*87	4	*47	*667

* significantly higher than the United Kingdom rate
~ significantly lower than the United Kingdom rate

Table 10.6

Age-standardised mortality rates for stroke by country and region, females
United Kingdom 1991-1997

| | rates per 100,000 | | | |
	overall	15-44	45-64	65+
United Kingdom	73	3	31	582
England	~70	3	~29	~561
North East	*81	3	*39	*633
North West	*79	*4	*36	*621
Yorkshire and the Humber	73	3	31	585
East Midlands	~72	3	30	~570
West Midlands	*75	3	31	*599
East	~66	~2	~24	~534
London	~61	3	~29	~474
South East	~67	~3	~24	~541
South West	~66	~2	~23	~543
Wales	*75	3	31	*595
Scotland	*99	*4	*45	*780
Northern Ireland	*78	4	33	*622

* significantly higher than the United Kingdom rate
~ significantly lower than the United Kingdom rate

The geographic pattern by age group within England was similar to all ages for those aged 45-64, but less apparent for those aged 15-44. One point to note is that London had low mortality from IHD for those aged 15-44 and 45-64, whereas for all causes of death London had high mortality in these age groups. As seen for the countries, there was a decline in mortality from IHD and stroke in all the regions of England and the geographic pattern of variation was maintained throughout 1992 to 1996, similar to the trends already described for all causes of death.

Variations between local authorities

For all ages, for males there was a general pattern of high mortality from IHD in the majority of authorities in Scotland and Northern Ireland as shown in Map 10.5. This pattern is not surprising given the high rates for the countries as a whole (Tables 10.3 and 10.4). Within England, a large number of authorities in the north of England - particularly authorities in and surrounding Tyne and Wear and Greater Manchester - had high mortality. Within Wales, only a group of authorities in south Wales had high rates of death, despite the high mortality in Wales as a whole.

For stroke, fewer authorities in Northern Ireland had high mortality than for IHD. All but one authority in Scotland had high mortality from stroke (Map 10.6). In addition, a group of English authorities bordering Scotland had high stroke mortality. Fewer authorities in south Wales had high rates of death from stroke than for IHD as reflected in the fact that Wales as a whole did not have a significantly higher rate of death from stroke than the United Kingdom (Table 10.5).

As for the pattern of mortality from all causes of death, areas with mortality rates from IHD classed as very high in Map 10.5 tended to be found in urban and early industrial areas outside London. Outside London and Northern Ireland there were 59 authorities with very high IHD mortality rates. Fifty of these authorities were classified as *Coalfields, Manufacturing Centres* or *Ports and Industry*. Three *Remoter Rural* areas had very high IHD mortality: the Shetland Islands, Eilean Siar and Argyll and Bute. The first two of these also had high all-cause mortality. No *Remoter Rural* areas outside Scotland had very high mortality rates from IHD. However, for stroke, areas with very high mortality rates were not as concentrated in urban and industrial areas. Outside London and Northern Ireland there were 47 authorities with very high mortality rates. Only 23 of these authorities were classified as *Coalfields, Manufacturing Centres* or *Ports and Industry*, 10 were classified as *Remoter Rural* areas. Nine of these were in Scotland and the other was Eden in the North West region.

As with all causes, there was a general pattern of low mortality from IHD and stroke in authorities throughout the south and east of England. Authorities with very low mortality rates were located away from major urban areas, with the exception of authorities in London. No authorities in Scotland, Northern Ireland or Wales had very low mortality rates from IHD and only four had low mortality rates: the Scottish Borders, East Dunbartonshire, Monmouthshire and Ceredigion. No authorities in Scotland had lower mortality rates from stroke than the United Kingdom as a whole and only two authorities in each of Wales and Northern Ireland had low stroke mortality. Authorities with low mortality

from both causes are found in many different ONS classification Groups, however a large proportion were classified as *Growth Areas* or *Most Prosperous*.

The pattern of mortality across the United Kingdom for all-age mortality from IHD and stroke for females was broadly similar to that seen for males (Map 10.7 and 10.8), particularly for stroke. However there are some notable differences between the pattern for males and females. A number of authorities in Northern Ireland had lower IHD mortality rates than the United Kingdom as a whole for females, whereas no authorities in Northern Ireland had lower rates for males. For females, no authorities in Scotland had lower IHD mortality rates than the United Kingdom as a whole, whereas two had lower mortality rates for males. As for males, a large number of authorities which had very high rates from IHD or stroke were classified as *Coalfields, Manufacturing Centres* or *Ports and Industry*.

The distribution of all-age IHD mortality rates for males and females separately within the 15 ONS classification Groups and within countries and regions was similar to that seen for all causes of death presented in Figures 10.13 and 10.14. However, for male stroke mortality there were more local authorities within different classification Groups which had similar mortality rates (Figure 10.17). In addition, mortality rates from IHD and stroke for the 15 classification Groups showed a very similar pattern to that shown in Figure 10.15 for all causes. The main exception to this is that the *West Inner London* Group had much lower IHD mortality than the United Kingdom as a whole. For stroke mortality this Group and the *East Inner London* Group were the exceptions and had much lower mortality than the United Kingdom as a whole. These patterns were clearly visible by local authority in Maps 10.5-10.8.

An analysis of variance was conducted to examine how much of the local authority variation in all-age mortality rates for IHD and stroke in Great Britain was accounted for by the country or region (country/region) in which the authority was located and how much by the ONS classification Group to which the local authority belonged. The analysis showed that differences in these two factors accounted for more than 80 per cent of the variation in IHD mortality by local authority for both males and females and more than 70 per cent of the variation in stroke mortality by local authority for males and females. It showed that for IHD mortality both country/region and ONS classification Group significantly contributed to the variation. For stroke mortality, as indicated by the maps presented, the correlation with country/region was much greater than the correlation with ONS classification Group. In particular, for females, ONS classification Group was no longer significant after controlling for region or country.

For males and females aged 15-44, few authorities had mortality rates from IHD or stroke that differed significantly from the rate for the United Kingdom as a whole. The pattern of IHD and stroke mortality in males and females aged 65 and over, and IHD mortality in males and females and females aged 45-64 was broadly similar to the pattern for all ages.

Map 10.5

Age-standardised mortality rates for ischaemic heart disease by local authority, males all ages
United Kingdom 1991-1997

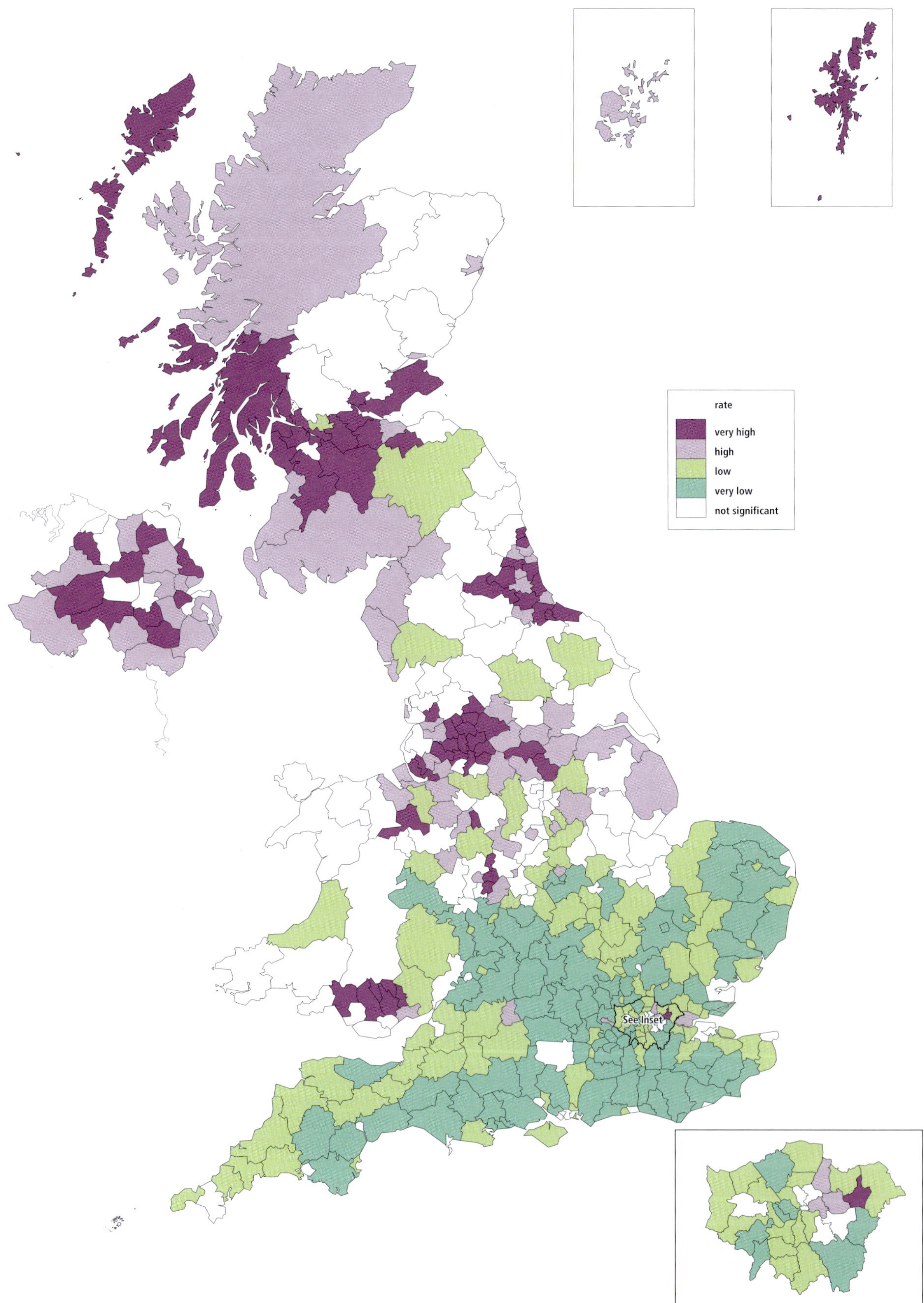

Map 10.6

Age-standardised mortality rates for stroke by local authority, males all ages
United Kingdom 1991-1997

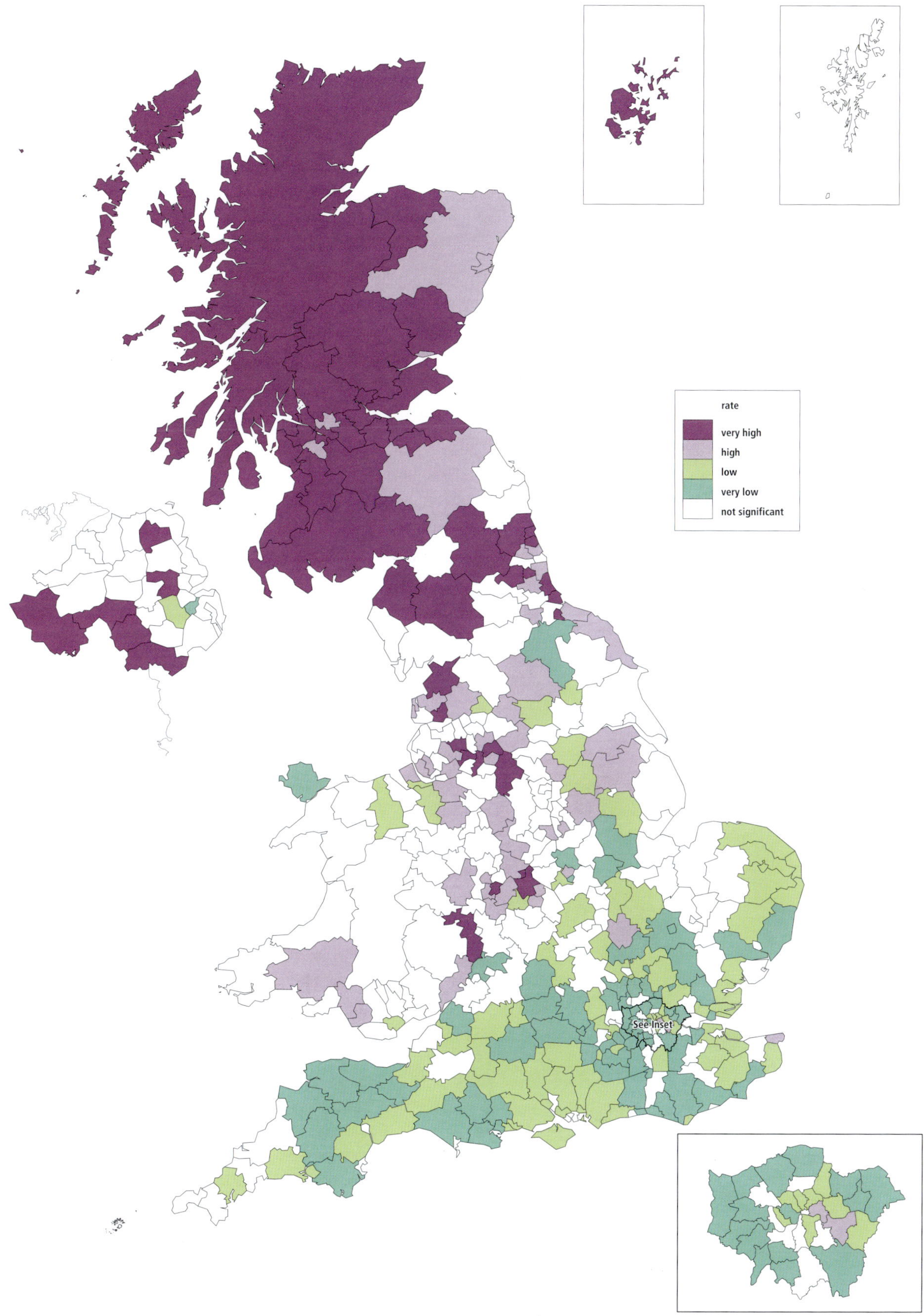

Map 10.7

Age-standardised mortality rates for ischaemic heart disease by local authority, females all ages United Kingdom 1991-1997

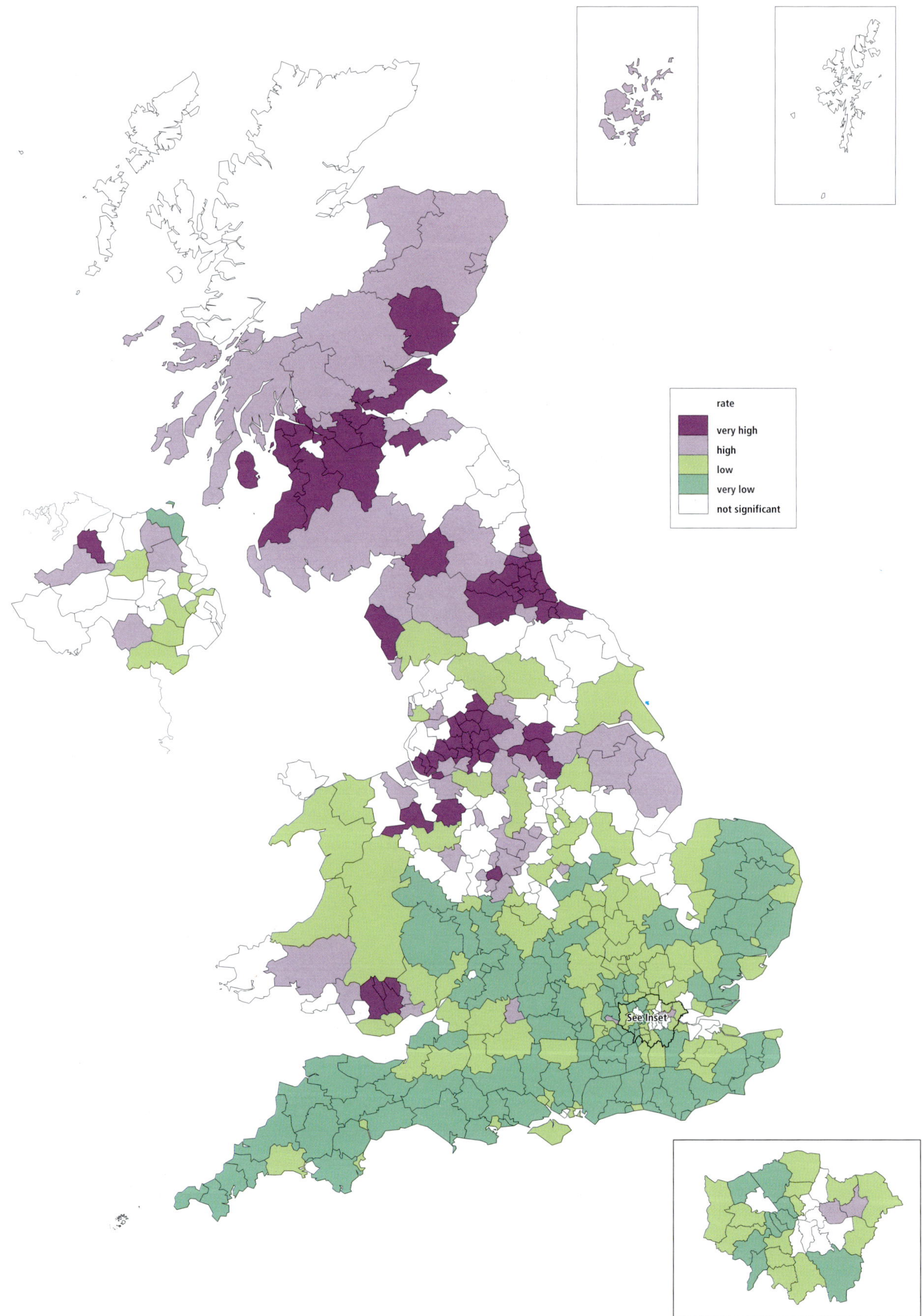

Map 10.8

Age-standardised mortality rates for stroke by local authority, females all ages
United Kingdom 1991-1997

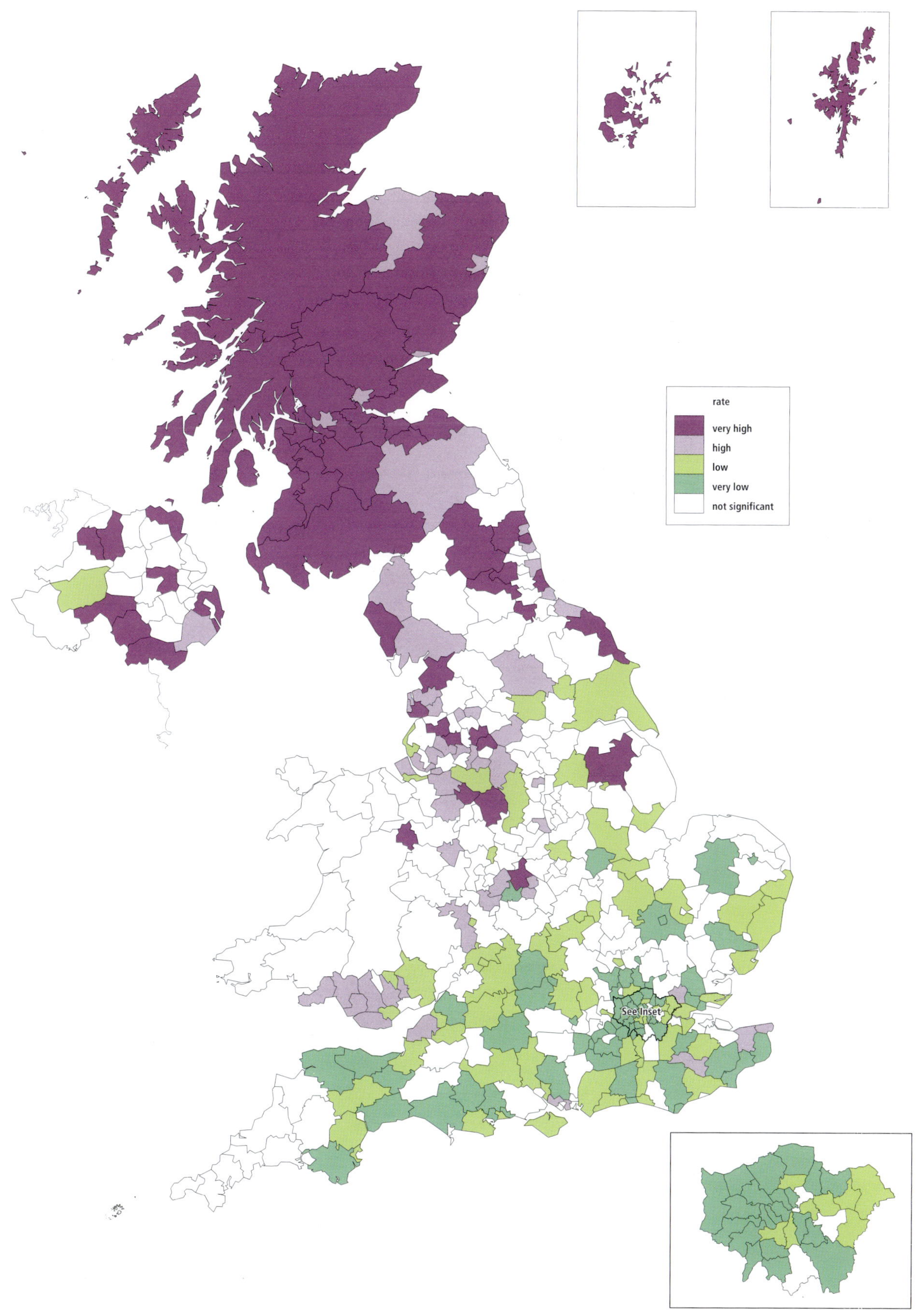

Map 10.9

**Age-standardised mortality rates for stroke by local authority, males aged 45-64
United Kingdom 1991-1997**

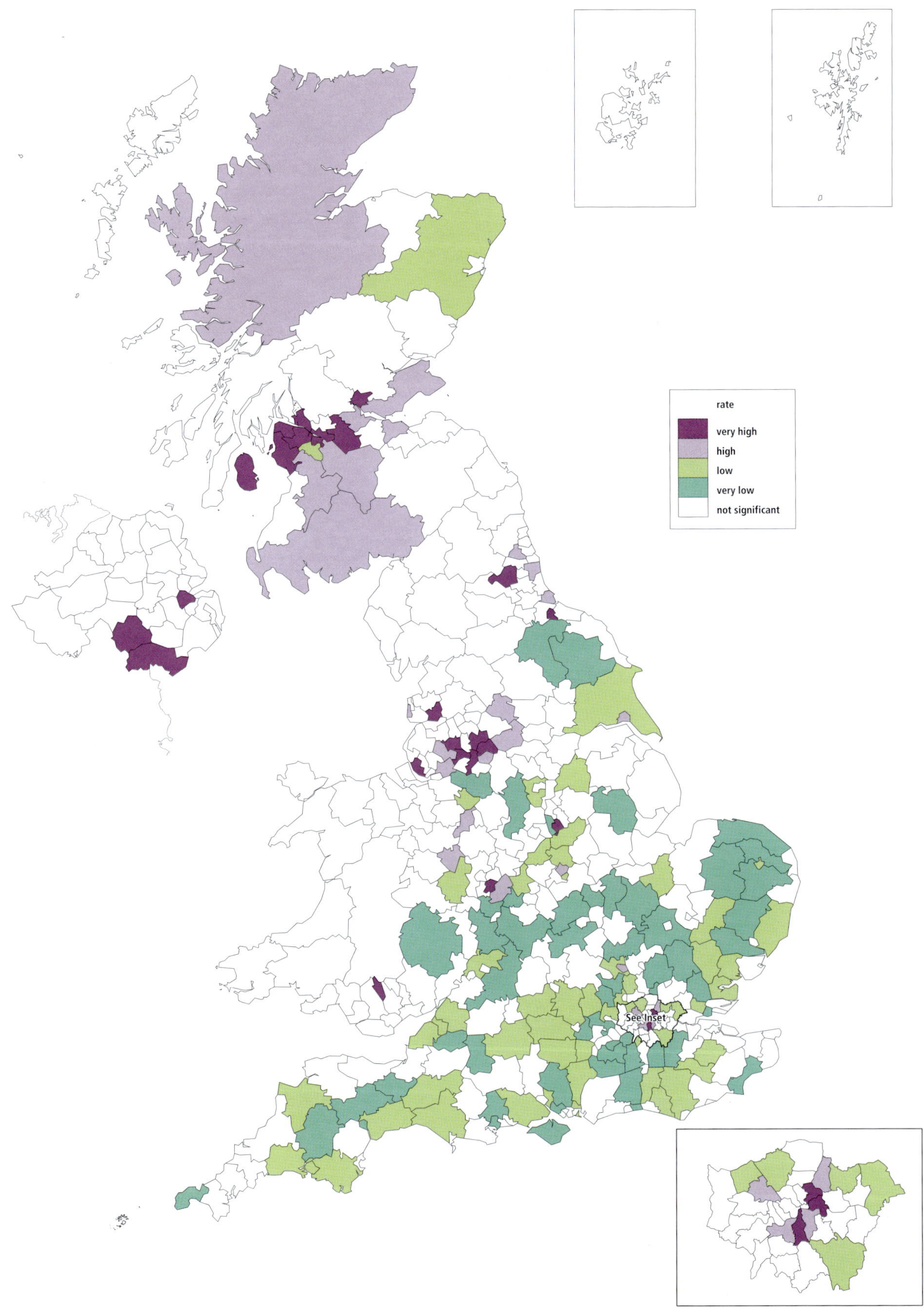

However for stroke mortality in males aged 45-64, areas with very high rates were more geographically concentrated than for all-age stroke mortality and were largely confined to urban and industrial areas (Map 10.9). This was similar to the pattern seen for all causes of death in this age group. Nineteen authorities outside London and Northern Ireland had very high rates, all of which were classified as *Coalfields, Manufacturing Centres* and *Ports and Industry*. More than half of the authorities with low rates were classified as *Growth Areas* or *Most Prosperous*.

Figure 10.18 shows mortality rates from stroke for males and females aged 45-64 by ONS classification Group. Although the pattern of mortality between Groups was very similar to that seen for all-age mortality from all causes of death and all-age stroke mortality, the magnitude of the differences between rates within different Groups was much greater for mortality from stroke in males and females aged 45-64. For example, for all-cause mortality for males aged 45-64, the *Ports and Industry* Group had the highest mortality. Mortality in this Group was 1.9 times higher than in the *Most Prosperous* Group. For stroke mortality in males aged 45-64, the difference between these two Groups was 2.7. In addition, unlike for all-age stroke mortality, the London Groups did not have low stroke mortality at ages 45-64.

For stroke mortality among males and females aged 45-64, an analysis of variance showed that both country and region and ONS classification contributed to the variation in mortality rates by local authority. The effect of ONS classification Group was much stronger than for all-age stroke mortality.

Figure 10.17

Age-standardised mortality rates for stroke by local authority within ONS classification Groups, males all ages Great Britain 1991-1997

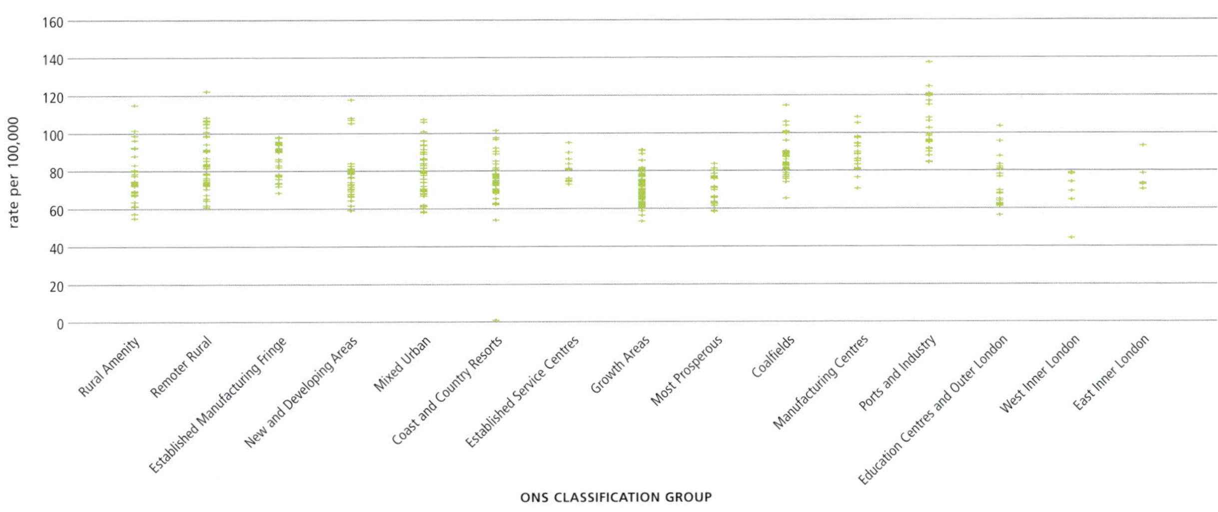

Figure 10.18

Age-standardised mortality rates for stroke by ONS classification Group, ages 45-64 Great Britain 1991-1997

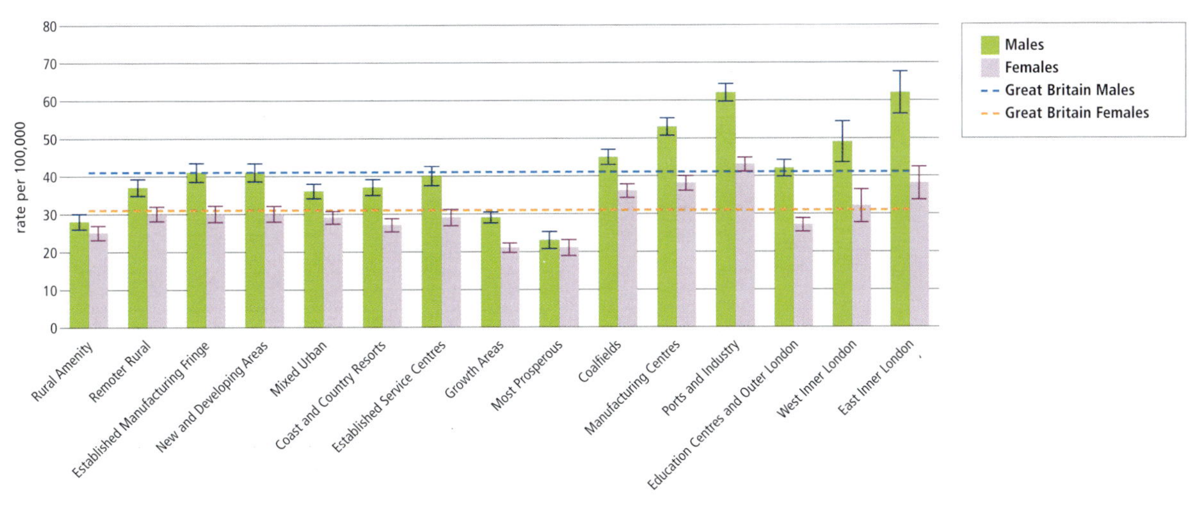

10.4 Cancer

Since 1950, deaths from major causes such as ischaemic heart disease and stroke have declined dramatically, but cancer mortality has declined at a much slower rate in both men and women. In England and Wales, cancer became the most important cause of death in females in 1969 and in males in 1995. Overall, cancer accounts for 25 per cent of all deaths in the United Kingdom. Cancer is identified as a high priority for health improvement in both England and Scotland.[1,2,3]

This section examines geographic variation in mortality for all cancers combined (all malignant neoplasms ICD9 140-208) as well as for the top three cancers in men (lung, prostate and colorectal) and in women (breast, colorectal and lung), accounting for just over 50 per cent of all cancers. The variation in the incidence of these cancers is presented in chapter 9. Trends in both the incidence, mortality and survival from the major cancers are discussed in more detail in the volume *Cancer trends in England and Wales, 1950-1999.*[15]

Variations between countries and regions
All cancers
All-age mortality from cancer showed a similar, but not identical, geographic pattern to all-cause mortality (Tables 10.7 and 10.8). For both males and females Scotland had the highest and Northern Ireland the lowest mortality from cancer of the countries of the United Kingdom. There was a decline in all-age

Table 10.7

Age-standardised mortality rates for all cancers by country and region, males
United Kingdom 1991-1997

| | rates per 100,000 | | | |
	overall	15-44	45-64	65+
United Kingdom	261	17	281	1,658
England	~257	17	~275	~1,639
North East	*307	18	*341	*1,938
North West	*281	18	*317	*1,762
Yorkshire and the Humber	*266	17	*292	*1,682
East Midlands	~252	16	~263	~1,625
West Midlands	263	17	280	*1,685
East	~237	~15	~243	~1,536
London	~256	*18	~273	~1,634
South East	~241	16	~248	~1,560
South West	~235	16	~248	~1,501
Wales	263	17	287	1,670
Scotland	*297	17	*336	*1,864
Northern Ireland	~253	17	284	~1,576

* significantly higher than the United Kingdom rate
~ significantly lower than the United Kingdom rate

Table 10.8

Age-standardised mortality rates for all cancers by country and region, females
United Kingdom 1991-1997

| | rates per 100,000 | | | |
	overall	15-44	45-64	65+
United Kingdom	176	23	250	940
England	~174	23	~246	~928
North East	*197	24	*283	*1,050
North West	*186	24	*268	*991
Yorkshire and the Humber	178	24	252	948
East Midlands	~173	23	247	~913
West Midlands	175	24	246	932
East	~165	~21	~232	~885
London	~174	~21	~243	942
South East	~165	22	~231	~886
South West	~163	22	~230	~865
Wales	177	24	253	936
Scotland	*199	24	*282	*1,074
Northern Ireland	~169	22	250	~876

* significantly higher than the United Kingdom rate
~ significantly lower than the United Kingdom rate

mortality from cancer through the period 1992 to 1996 for both males and females in every country, however, Scotland had the highest mortality in every year for both sexes. Within England for all ages, regions which had high mortality were those located in the north. The regions with low cancer mortality were the southern regions (Tables 10.7 and 10.8). This geographic pattern was maintained throughout 1992 to 1996, with a decline in mortality from cancer being seen in all regions. The geographic pattern of cancer mortality for those aged 15-44, 45-64 and 65 and over was similar to that for all ages.

Lung Cancer

Lung cancer (ICD9 162) accounts for 29 per cent of all cancer deaths in the United Kingdom every year in males and 16 per cent in females. Therefore, geographic patterns in lung cancer are more likely to follow the pattern for all cancer mortality in men than women.

As for all cancers, Scotland had the highest mortality from lung cancer of all the countries and Northern Ireland had the lowest rates for both sexes (Tables 10.9 and 10.10). Wales and England also had significantly lower mortality than the United Kingdom from lung cancer. The trends in male mortality from lung cancer by country are very similar to those seen for all cancers, with a decline in every country. For females the trend was different; mortality rates from lung cancer increased in Scotland and in Northern Ireland between 1992 and 1996, but remained the same in Wales and declined in England (Figure 10.19).

Table 10.9

Age-standardised mortality rates for lung cancer by country and region, males
United Kingdom 1991-1997

| | rates per 100,000 | | |
	overall	45-64	65+
United Kingdom	76	85	491
England	~74	~82	~480
North East	*103	*114	*667
North West	*88	*106	*552
Yorkshire and the Humber	*81	*90	*519
East Midlands	~71	~77	~468
West Midlands	77	86	495
East	~63	~64	~424
London	76	82	501
South East	~63	~65	~417
South West	~60	~66	~390
Wales	~74	85	~473
Scotland	*100	*117	*630
Northern Ireland	~71	88	~436

* significantly higher than the United Kingdom rate
~ significantly lower than the United Kingdom rate

Table 10.10

Age-standardised mortality rates for lung cancer by country and region, females
United Kingdom 1991-1997

| | rates per 100,000 | | |
	overall	45-64	65+
United Kingdom	31	42	178
England	~29	~39	~172
North East	*46	*65	*260
North West	*37	*53	*209
Yorkshire and the Humber	*33	*47	*191
East Midlands	~26	~36	~151
West Midlands	~27	~36	~156
East	~24	~30	148
London	*32	41	*194
South East	~24	~30	~147
South West	~22	~28	~131
Wales	~29	40	~165
Scotland	*44	*62	*252
Northern Ireland	~27	40	~147

* significantly higher than the United Kingdom rate
~ significantly lower than the United Kingdom rate

Within England, the regions with the highest rates of mortality from lung cancer than the United Kingdom were those in the north, and the regions which had lower mortality than the United Kingdom were located in the south, as seen for all cancers (Tables 10.9 and 10.10). The North East had markedly higher mortality than the other regions. There was a decline in lung cancer mortality during 1992 to 1996 for males in all regions, although the smallest decline was found in the North East. For females, rates remained relatively stable in most regions, with some experiencing a decline, for example the East Midlands, and some experiencing an increase, for example Yorkshire and the Humber (Figure 10.20).

Mortality among those aged 45-64 and 65 and over had a

similar geographic pattern to that presented for all ages. In addition, the country and regional level pattern presented for mortality from lung cancer was similar to the pattern presented for the incidence of lung cancer in chapter 9. This is likely to be due to the fact that survival from lung cancer is poor.[16]

Colorectal Cancer

Colorectal cancer (ICD9 152-153) accounts for 12 per cent of all cancer deaths in the United Kingdom every year. The geographic pattern in mortality from colorectal cancer was slightly different from that seen for all cancers and more like the pattern for all causes of death. Wales, Scotland and Northern Ireland had higher mortality than England for both sexes (Tables 10.11 and 10.12). All the countries showed an

Figure 10.19

Trends in age-standardised mortality rates for lung cancer by country, females all ages United Kingdom 1992-1996*

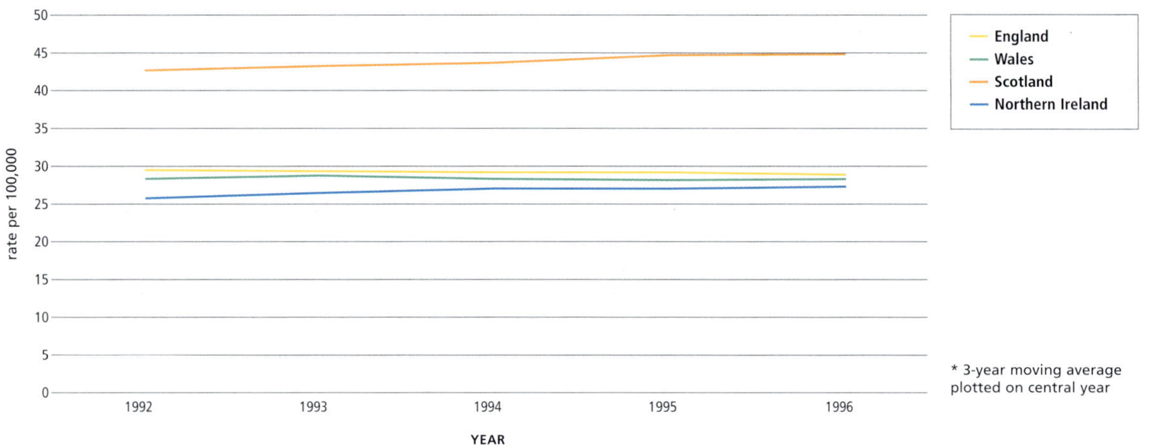

Figure 10.20

Trends in age-standardised mortality rates for lung cancer by region, females all ages England 1992-1996*

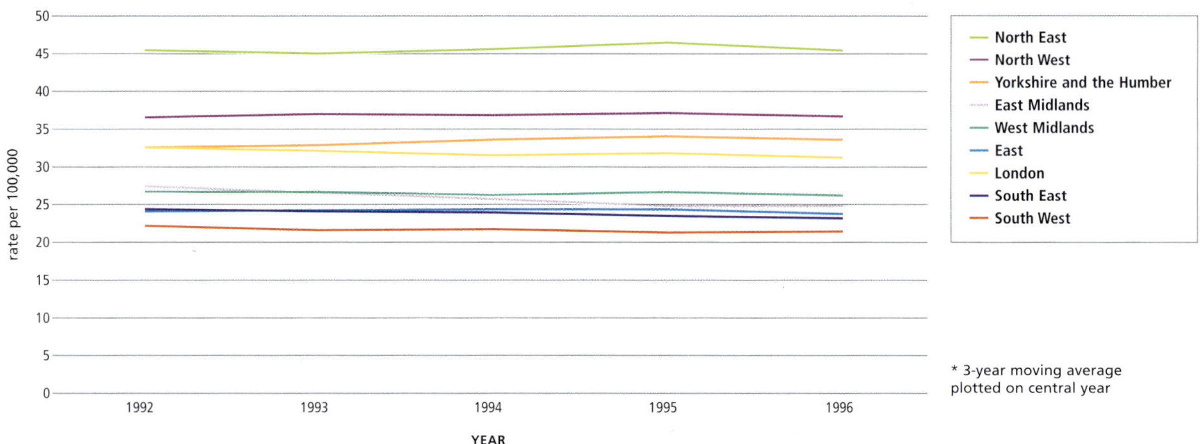

Table 10.11

**Age-standardised mortality rates for colorectal cancer by country and region, males
United Kingdom 1991-1997**

		rates per 100,000	
	overall	45-64	65+
United Kingdom	29	33	185
England	~29	32	~182
North East	*34	*40	*213
North West	*32	*36	*205
Yorkshire and the Humber	29	34	181
East Midlands	29	32	186
West Midlands	*31	34	*200
East	~26	31	~162
London	~25	~28	~160
South East	~27	~30	~174
South West	~27	31	~173
Wales	*32	36	*201
Scotland	*34	*38	*214
Northern Ireland	30	34	189

* significantly higher than the United Kingdom rate
~ significantly lower than the United Kingdom rate

Table 10.12

**Age-standardised mortality rates for colorectal cancer by country and region, females
United Kingdom 1991-1997**

		rates per 100,000	
	overall	45-64	65+
United Kingdom	19	22	119
England	~19	22	117
North East	20	23	123
North West	*20	23	*125
Yorkshire and the Humber	~18	21	115
East Midlands	~18	21	~114
West Midlands	20	23	122
East	~18	21	~113
London	~17	~19	~108
South East	18	22	~114
South West	18	21	118
Wales	*20	25	123
Scotland	*22	*25	*136
Northern Ireland	*21	25	124

* significantly higher than the United Kingdom rate
~ significantly lower than the United Kingdom rate

Figure 10.21

**Trends in age-standardised mortality rates for colorectal cancer by country, males all ages
United Kingdom 1992-1996***

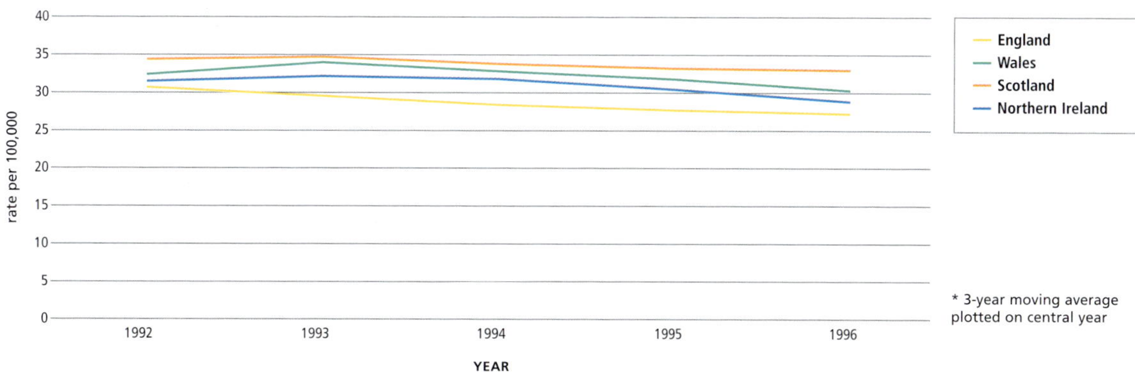

overall decline in mortality from colorectal cancer for both males and females over this time period. The difference in rates between Scotland and England widened through the 1990s for males (Figure 10.21), but remained similar for females. At regional level the pattern of colorectal cancer mortality was also similar to all causes of death, however, fewer areas had rates that differed significantly from the United Kingdom rate. All the regions had a decline in mortality from colorectal cancer, for both males and females. Mortality among those aged 45-64 and 65 and over showed a very similar geographic pattern to that described above.

Prostate Cancer

The geographic pattern of mortality from prostate cancer (ICD9 185) was completely different from that seen for all-cause and all-cancer mortality. There were no countries with a rate significantly higher than the United Kingdom as a whole and Scotland, Wales and Northern Ireland had a significantly lower mortality rate than the United Kingdom as a whole (Table 10.13). This is interesting as Wales and Scotland had a

higher than average incidence of prostate cancer between 1991 and 1993 as presented in chapter 9. Previous studies have shown that those living in Scotland have better survival from prostate cancer than the rest of the United Kingdom.[17] There was an increase in the rates in Wales and Northern Ireland between 1992 and 1996 and an increase followed by a slight decline in Scotland. England had a decrease in mortality through the period and was the only country to experience an overall decline (Figure 10.22).

At regional level within England it was the Midlands and southern regions that had the highest rates of death from prostate cancer (Table 10.13). The lowest rates were found in the North East and North West. This pattern was similar to that presented for the incidence of prostate cancer in chapter 9. All the regions of England had a decline in rates between 1992 and 1996.

The geographic pattern of prostate cancer mortality by age group for those aged 45 and over was similar to that described for all ages.

Table 10.13

**Age-standardised mortality rates for prostate cancer by country and region, males
United Kingdom 1991-1997**

	rates per 100,000		
	overall	45-64	65+
United Kingdom	29	11	236
England	29	11	239
North East	~26	10	~215
North West	~27	11	~219
Yorkshire and the Humber	28	11	230
East Midlands	*30	11	*249
West Midlands	*30	10	*247
East	*30	11	*247
London	*30	12	*248
South East	*30	11	*248
South West	29	10	236
Wales	~25	~8	~213
Scotland	~28	11	~226
Northern Ireland	~27	10	~222

* significantly higher than the United Kingdom rate
~ significantly lower than the United Kingdom rate

Figure 10.22

**Trends in age-standardised mortality rates for prostate cancer by country, males all ages
United Kingdom 1992-1996***

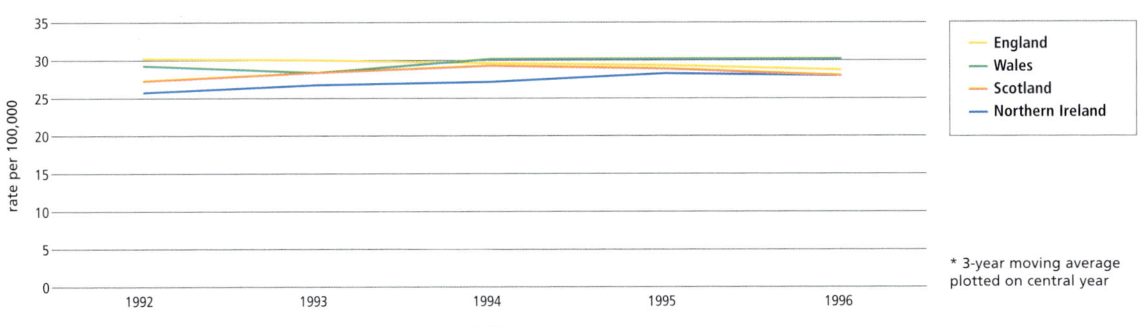

Breast Cancer

Breast cancer (ICD9 174) accounts for 19 per cent of all cancer deaths in women in the United Kingdom. Geographic variation in breast cancer mortality was less marked than that for all cancers (Table 10.14). Northern Ireland had significantly lower breast cancer mortality than the United Kingdom. There were declines in breast cancer mortality in each country between 1992 and 1996 (Figure 10.23).

Within England at a regional level, the East and West Midlands and the East of England had significantly higher rates than the United Kingdom and the North West and Yorkshire and the Humber lower, a different pattern to all-cause and all-cancer mortality (Table 10.14). It is interesting to see that the South East, South West and North East regions all had average levels of breast cancer mortality over this time period despite differences in incidence rates between 1991 and 1993 (see chapter 9). The South East and South West had a high incidence of breast cancer, whereas the North East a very low

incidence. Previous geographic analysis has shown that those in the South East have higher survival from breast cancer.[16] Each region had a decline in mortality from breast cancer from 1992 to 1996, the largest being found in the South East, London and the North East. The region with the smallest decline was the North West (Figure 10.24), the region previously shown to have the lowest survival within England.[16]

Variations between local authorities

For all ages, for males there was a general pattern of high mortality from cancer and lung cancer in groups of authorities in Scotland and the north of England - particularly among authorities in and surrounding Tyne and Wear, Glasgow, Manchester and Liverpool (Map 10.10 and 10.11). As for all causes of death, areas with very high mortality rates from cancer and lung cancer tended to be found in urban and early industrial areas. Outside London and Northern Ireland there were 44 authorities with very high cancer mortality rates. Thirty-eight of these authorities were

Table 10.14

Age-standardised mortality rates for breast cancer by country and region, females
United Kingdom 1991-1997

		rates per 100,000		
	overall	15-44	45-64	65+
United Kingdom	37	8	68	150
England	37	8	68	151
North East	36	8	69	~143
North West	~36	8	67	~142
Yorkshire and the Humber	~35	8	~64	~143
East Midlands	*39	8	71	*160
West Midlands	*38	8	69	*159
East	*38	8	69	*157
London	37	~7	68	154
South East	37	8	67	151
South West	37	7	68	152
Wales	37	7	69	150
Scotland	37	8	69	146
Northern Ireland	~35	9	69	~126

* significantly higher than the United Kingdom rate
~ significantly lower than the United Kingdom rate

Figure 10.23

Trends in age-standardised mortality rates for breast cancer by country, females all ages
United Kingdom 1992-1996*

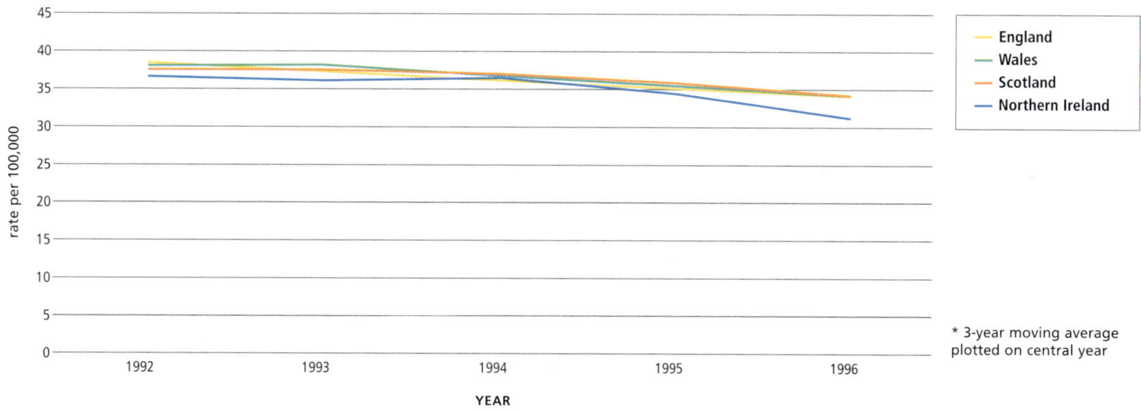

classified as *Coalfields, Manufacturing Centres* or *Ports and Industry*. This was a similar pattern to the incidence of lung cancer presented in chapter 9.

For colorectal cancer, for males of all ages a very different geographic pattern emerged. A number of authorities in Scotland (including rural areas) and the north of England and south Wales had high rates (Map 10.12). Authorities with high rates from this cause of death were not as highly centred around urban areas as those with high rates from other causes. However, although those with very high rates from colorectal cancer appeared to be less concentrated in urban areas, 18 of the 28 authorities with very high rates outside London and Northern Ireland were classified as *Coalfields, Manufacturing Centres* or *Ports and Industry*.

For prostate cancer the picture was very different to that for all cancers; authorities with high rates were scattered in the south of England and Northern Ireland (Map 10.13). Unlike all causes of death and all cancers, areas with very high mortality rates from prostate cancer tended to be located away from urban and industrial areas. Outside London and Northern Ireland there were 22 authorities with very high mortality rates. None of these authorities were classified as *Coalfields, Manufacturing Centres* or *Ports and Industry* and nine were classified as *Growth Areas* or *Most Prosperous*.

As with all causes, there was a general pattern of low mortality from cancer and lung cancer in authorities throughout the south and east of England. Authorities with very low mortality rates were located away from major urban areas. Unlike all causes of death a number of authorities in Northern Ireland and Wales had very low mortality rates from cancer. Of the 92 authorities with very low cancer mortality rates, 44 were classified as *Most Prosperous* or *Growth Areas* and 35 were classified as *Rural Amenity* or *Remoter Rural*.

Authorities with low mortality rates from colorectal cancer were scattered throughout England, particularly in the south and east and were classified in many different ONS classification Groups. Authorities with low rates from prostate cancer were mainly located in central and northern England. Of the 20 authorities with very low mortality rates, nine were classified as *Coalfields, Manufacturing Centres* or *Ports and Industry*. This is the opposite to that seen for all cancers and lung cancer where the majority of authorities with very high rates were in these ONS classification Groups.

The pattern of mortality across the United Kingdom for all-age mortality from cancer and lung cancer for females was broadly similar to that seen for males (Maps 10.14 and 10.15), although particularly for all cancers fewer authorities had very high rates.

The pattern of mortality across the United Kingdom for all-age mortality from colorectal cancer for females was slightly different to that seen for males (Map 10.16). The main difference between males and females was in the pattern by ONS classification Group. There are 19 authorities outside London and Northern Ireland with very high rates from colorectal cancer. Seven of these authorities were classified as *Coalfields, Manufacturing Centres* or *Ports and Industry* and seven were classified as *Remoter Rural*. This is a much larger proportion in this Group than for males.

For all ages, for females there was little geographic variation in breast cancer mortality (Map 10.17). Unlike all cancers, areas with very high mortality rates were generally not located in urban or industrial areas and were found in many different ONS classification Groups. In addition, areas with low rates were found in many different classification Groups. The map presented here is also very different to that showing the incidence of breast cancer in chapter 9. Groups of areas in central and south west England had a very high incidence of breast cancer, yet the mortality levels in Map 10.17 are average, indicating that these areas are likely to have higher than average survival.

Figure 10.24

Trends in age-standardised mortality rates for breast cancer by region, females all ages England 1992-1996*

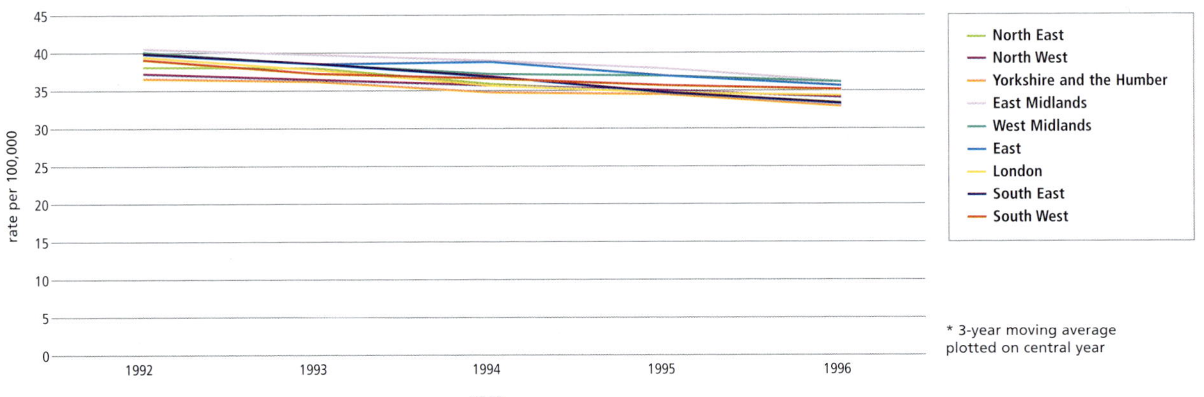

Map 10.10

Age-standardised mortality rates for all cancers by local authority, males all ages
United Kingdom 1991-1997

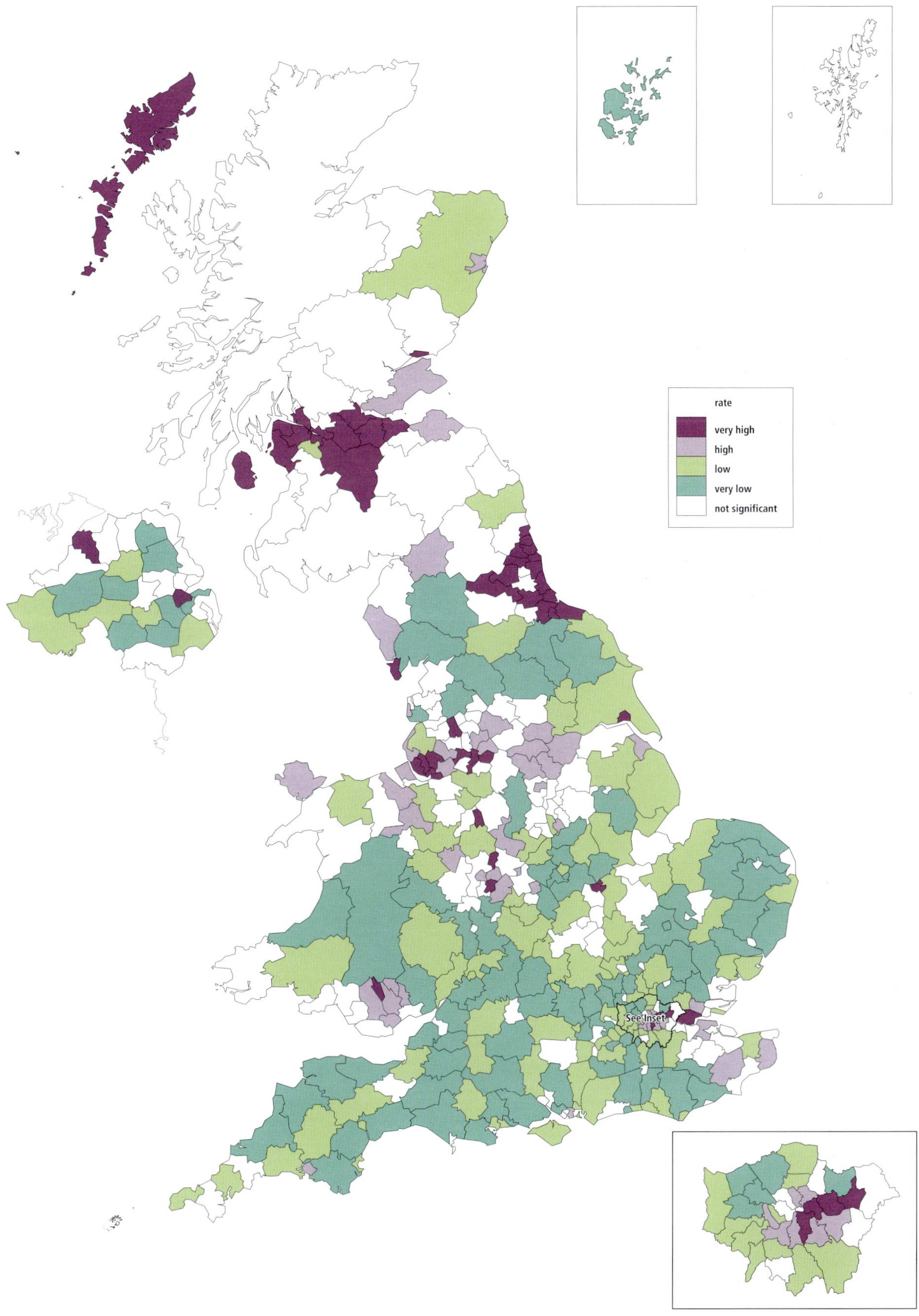

Map 10.11

Age-standardised mortality rates for lung cancer by local authority, males all ages
United Kingdom 1991-1997

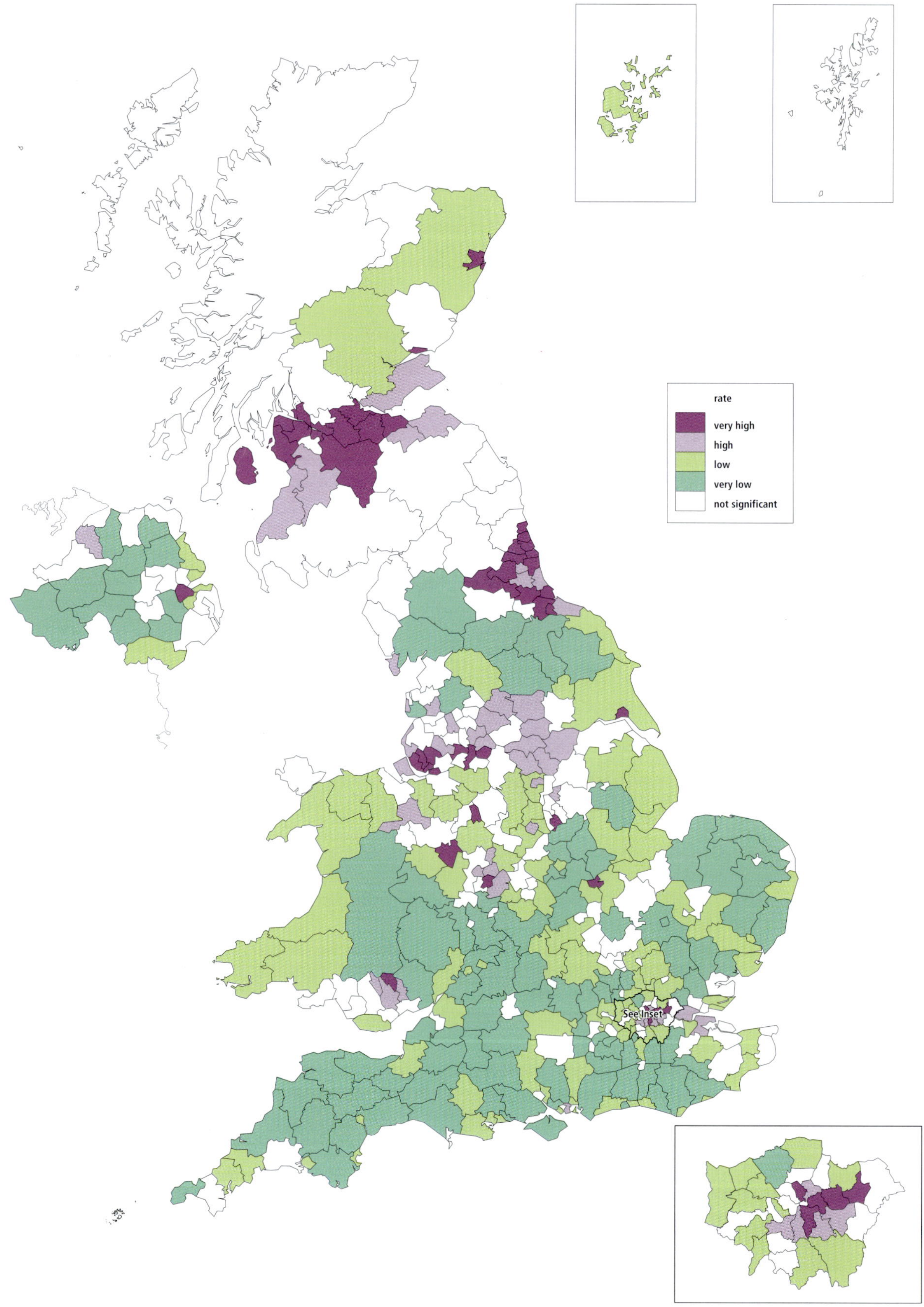

Map 10.12

Age-standardised mortality rates for colorectal cancer by local authority, males all ages
United Kingdom 1991-1997

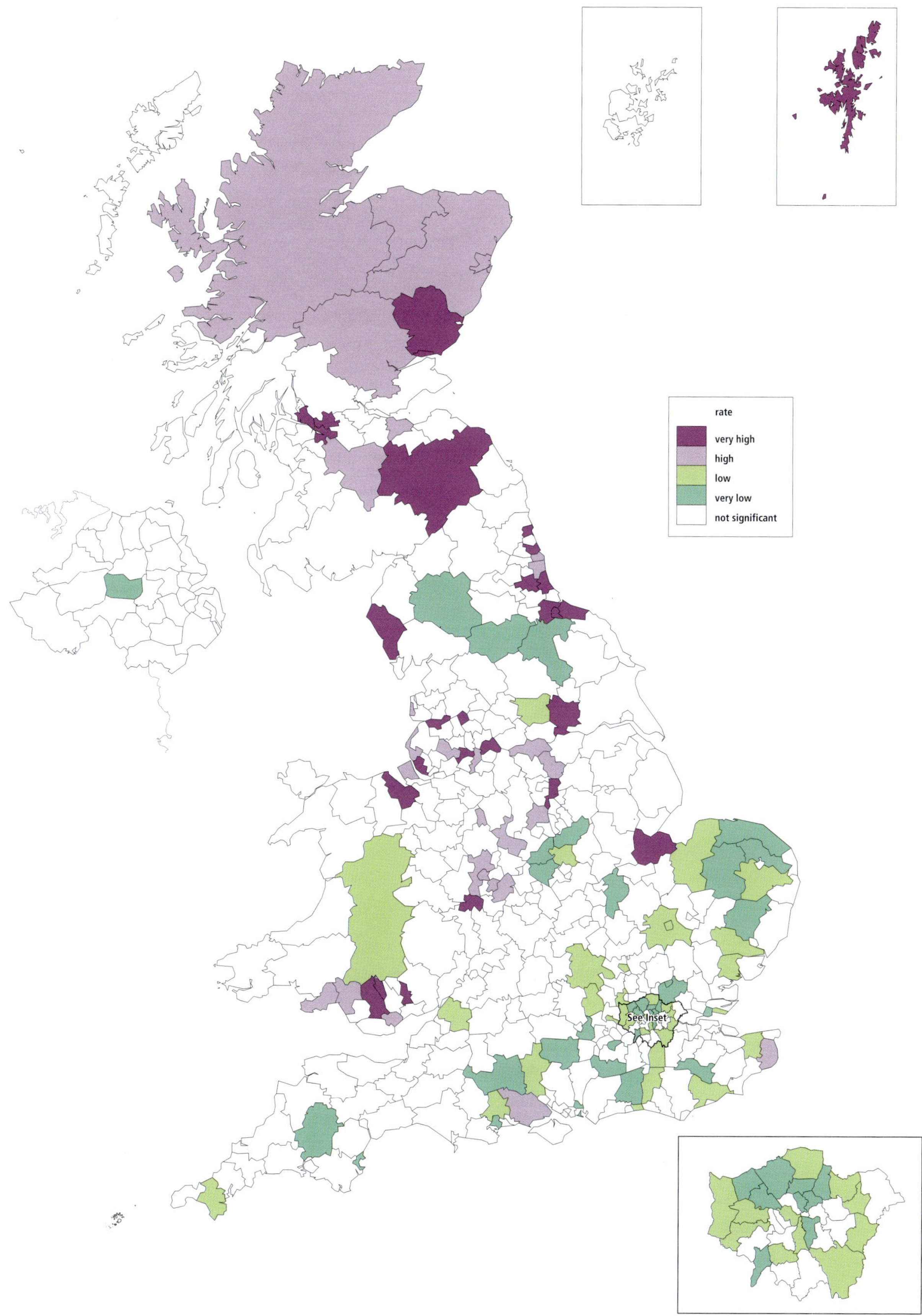

Map 10.13

Age-standardised mortality rates for prostate cancer by local authority, males all ages
United Kingdom 1991-1997

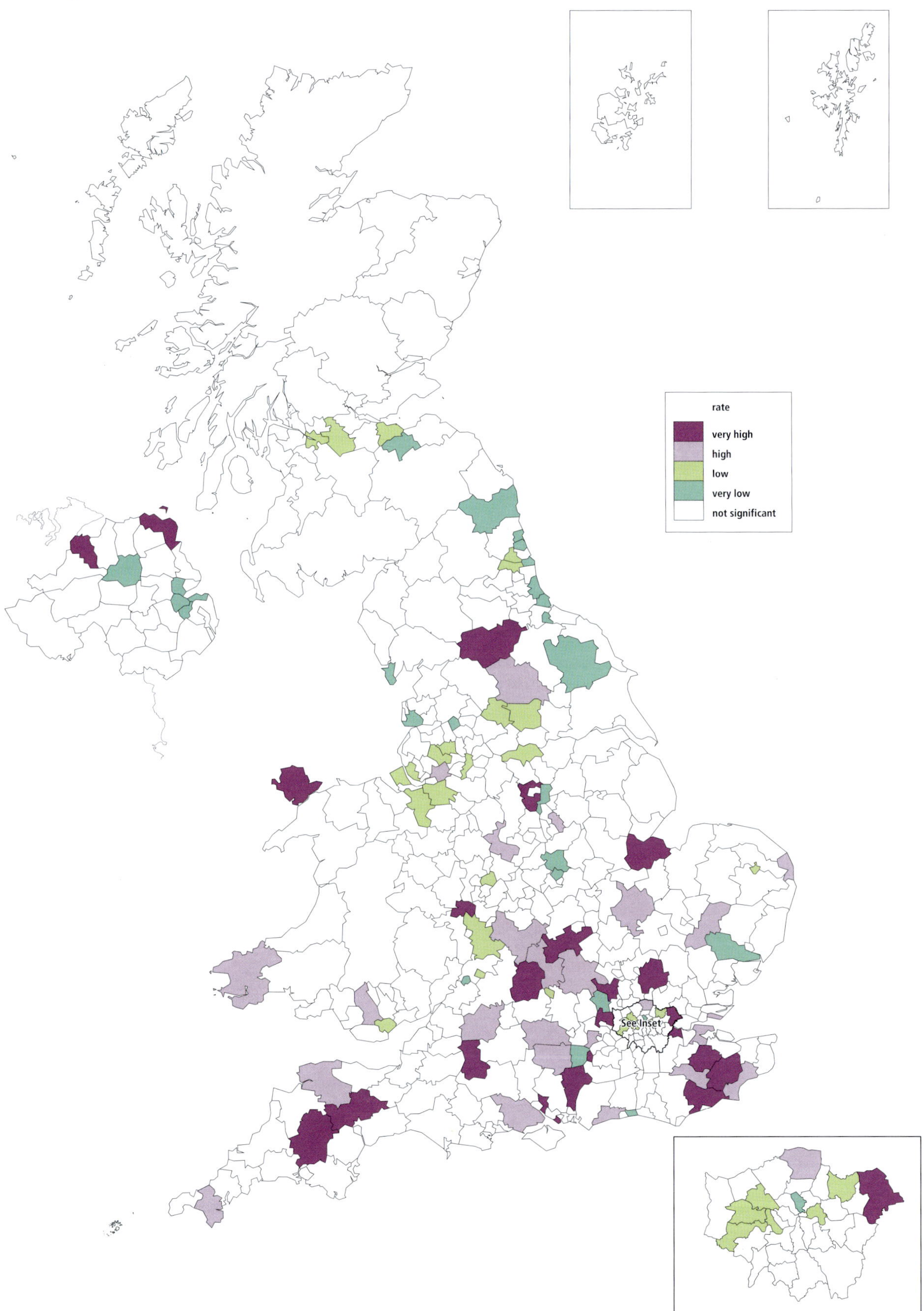

Map 10.14

Age-standardised mortality rates for all cancers by local authority, females all ages
United Kingdom 1991-1997

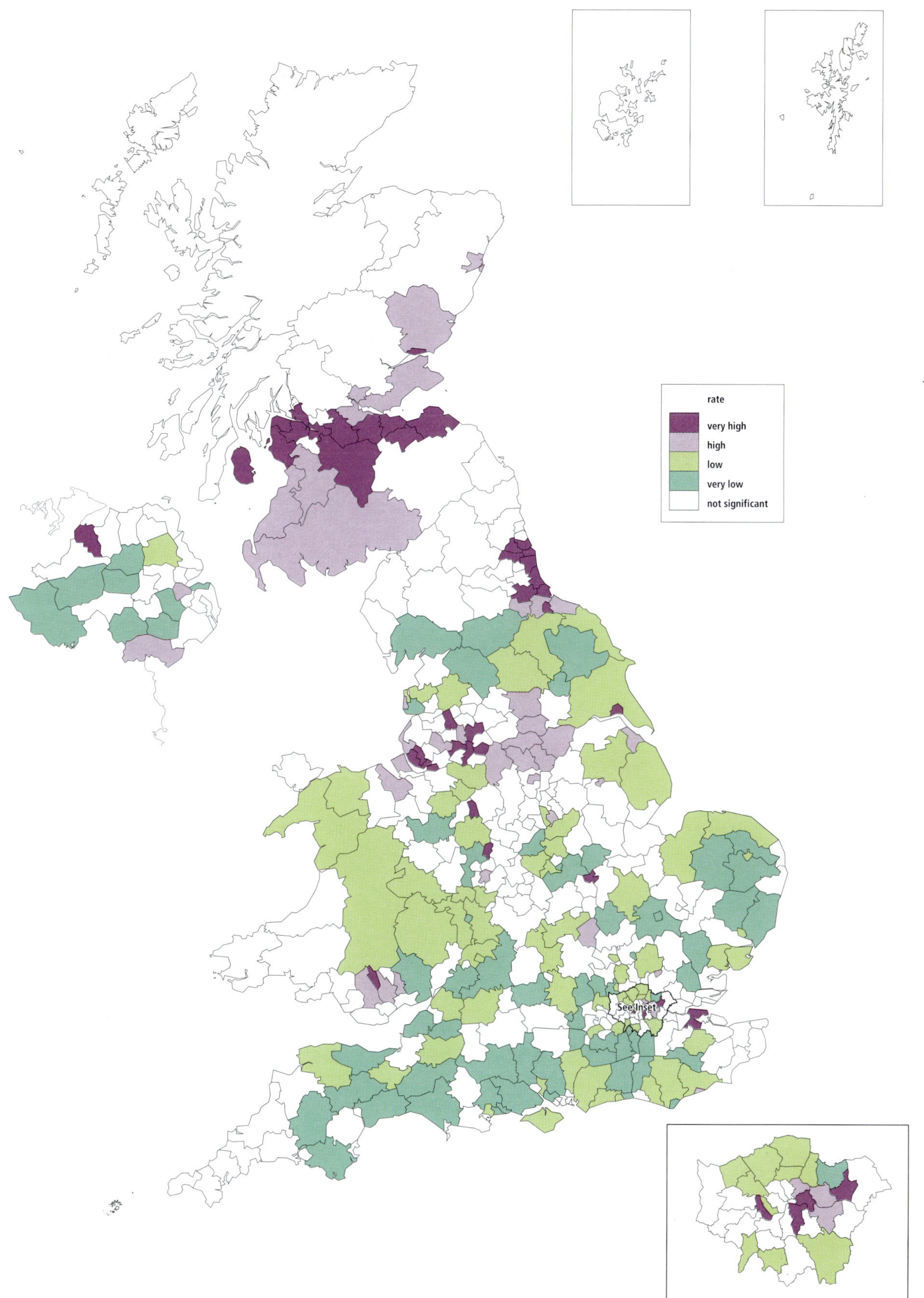

Map 10.15

**Age-standardised mortality rates for lung cancer by local authority, females all ages
United Kingdom 1991-1997**

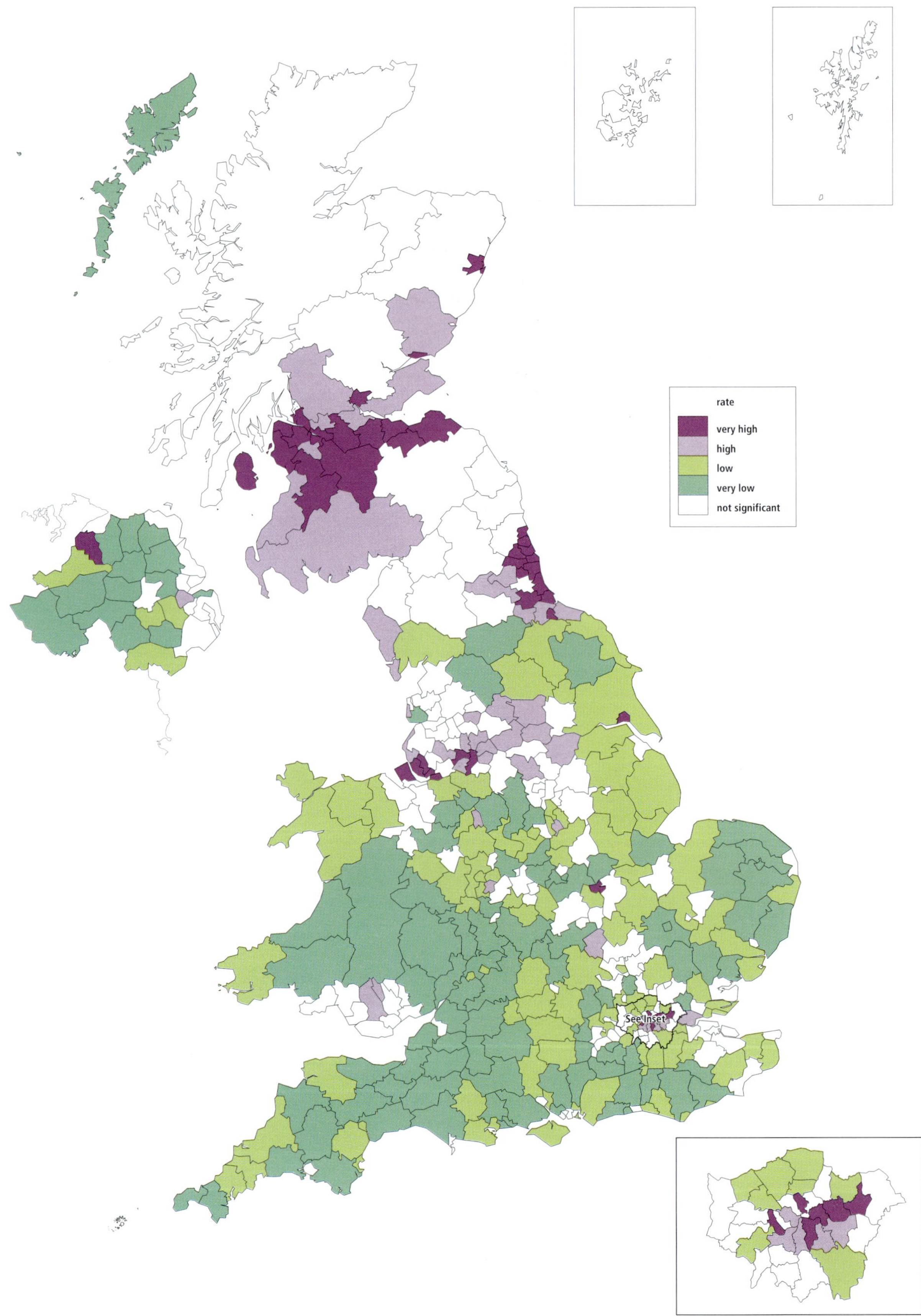

Map 10.16

Age-standardised mortality rates for colorectal cancer by local authority, females all ages
United Kingdom 1991-1997

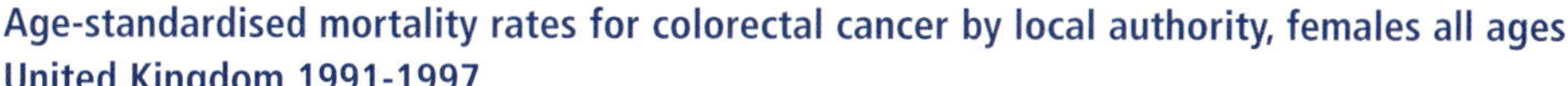

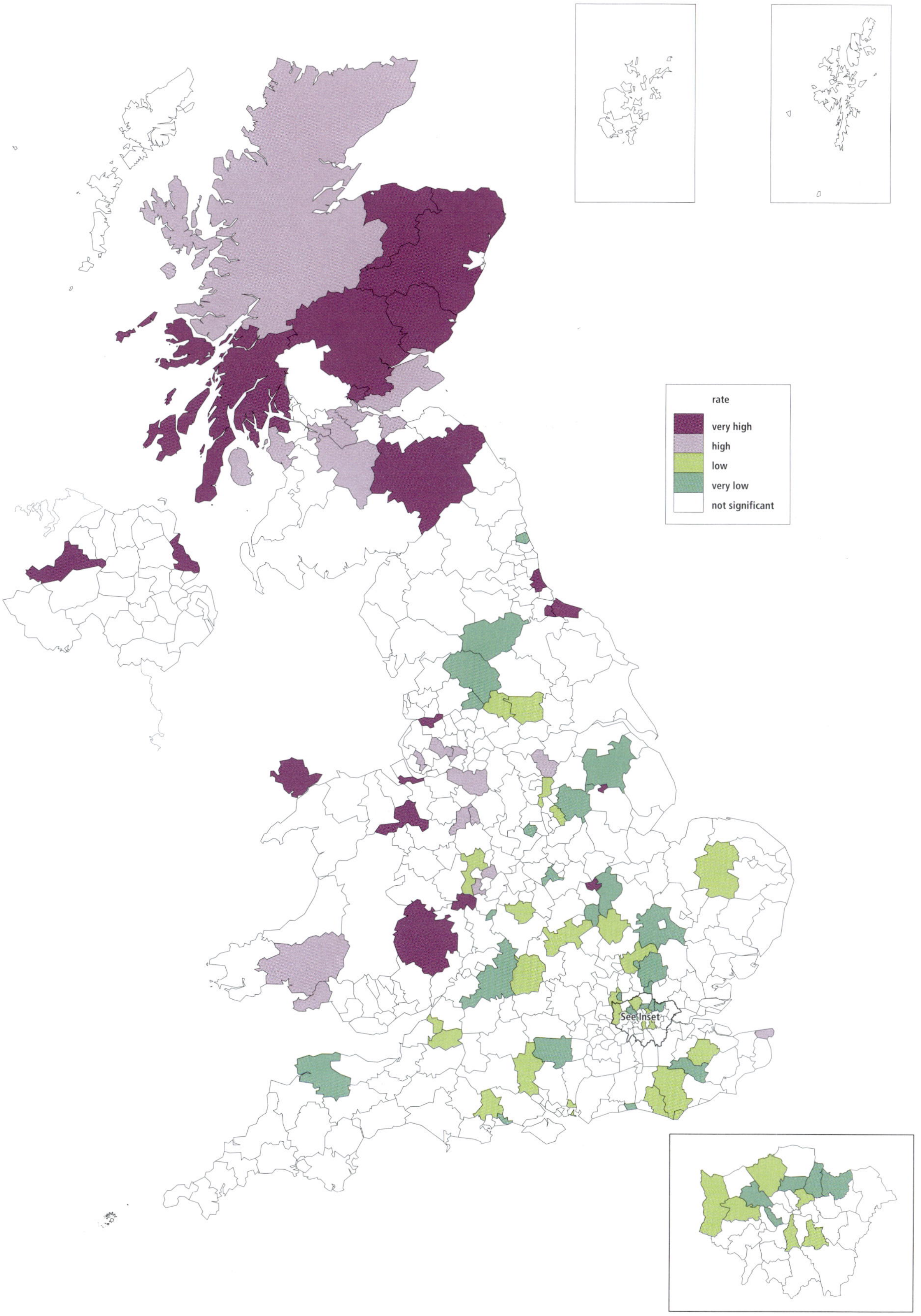

Map 10.17

Age-standardised mortality rates for breast cancer by local authority, females all ages
United Kingdom 1991-1997

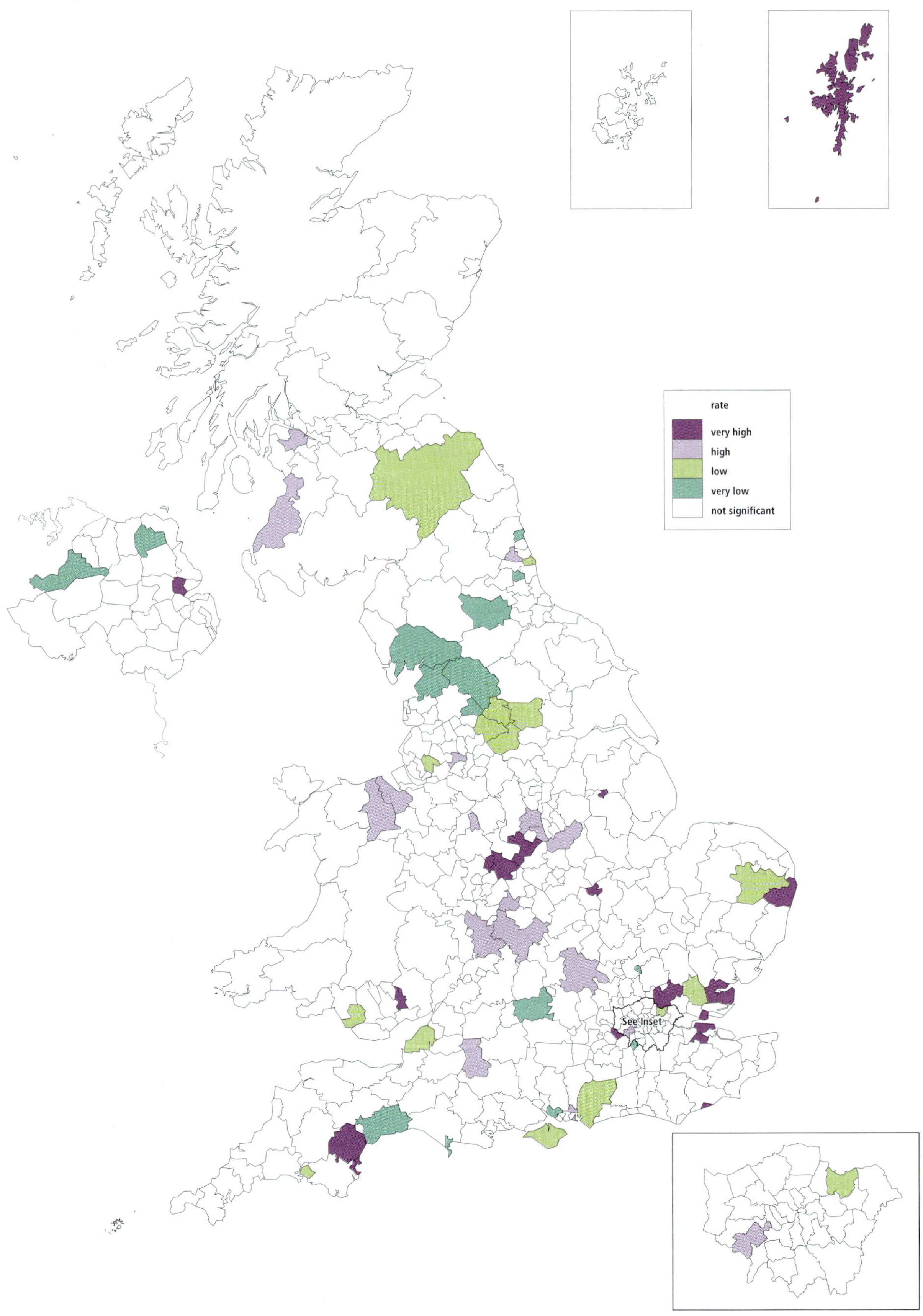

Figure 10.25

Age-standardised mortality rates for lung cancer by ONS classification Group, all ages Great Britain 1991-1997

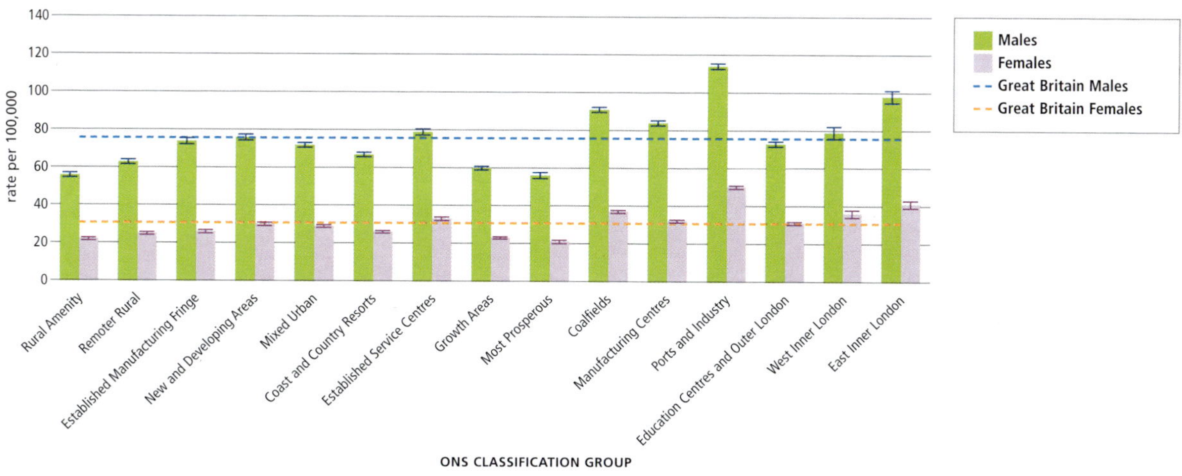

Figure 10.26

Age-standardised mortality rates for colorectal cancer by ONS classification Group, all ages Great Britain 1991-1997

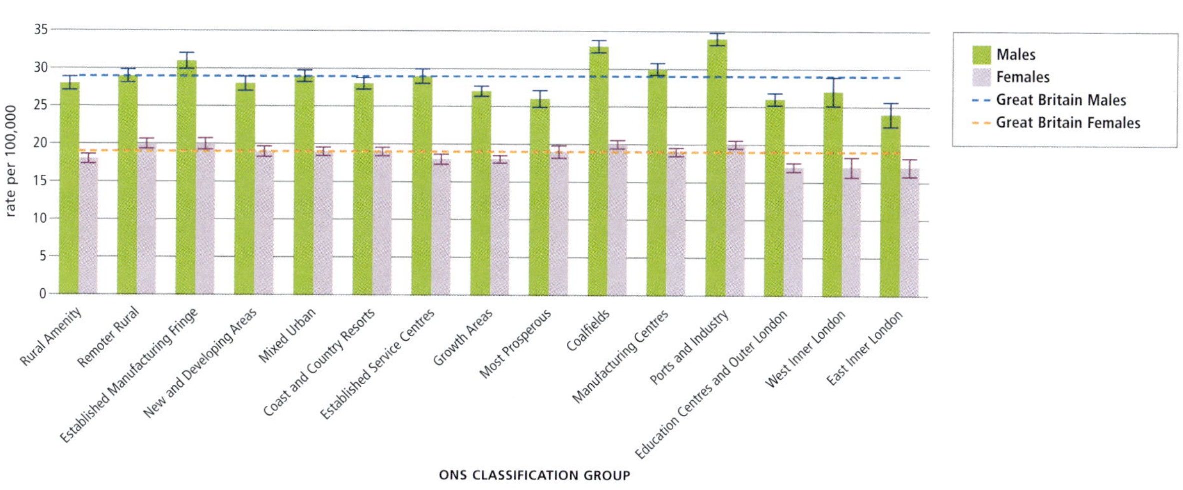

Figure 10.27

Age-standardised mortality rates for prostate cancer by ONS classification Group, males all ages Great Britain 1991-1997

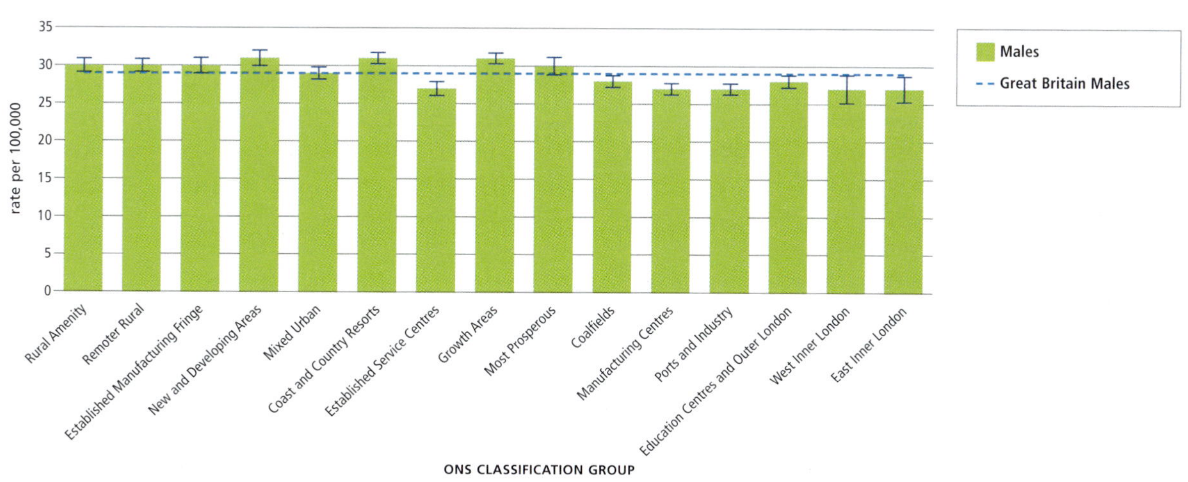

The pattern of cancer and lung cancer mortality by ONS classification Group was very similar to that seen for all causes of death with *Coalfields, Manufacturing Centres, Ports and Industry* and *East Inner London* having the highest rates and *Growth Areas* and *Most Prosperous* the lowest. However, for lung cancer the absolute difference between the classification Groups was much larger for both males and females (Figure 10.25).

For colorectal cancer in males and females, a slightly different pattern by ONS classification Group to that presented for lung cancer emerged (Figure 10.26). Generally there was little variation in mortality from colorectal cancer by ONS classification Group. Although high rates were still found in the *Coalfields* and *Ports and Industry* Groups, the *East Inner London* Group had lower mortality than Great Britain as a whole. In addition the *Remoter Rural* Group had high rates for females and the *Established Manufacturing Fringe* Group had high rates for both males and females.

As expected the pattern of prostate cancer mortality by ONS classification Group was very different to that seen for all cancers (Figure 10.27). Generally there was little variation in mortality rates between the different classification Groups. It is one of the few causes of death where the *Coalfields, Manufacturing Centres* and *Ports and Industry* Groups had lower mortality than average. In addition, it is one of the few causes of death where the *Most Prosperous* and the *Growth Areas* Groups had higher mortality than average. The picture for breast cancer was also very different to the picture for all causes. All Groups had similar rates to Great Britain as a whole.

An analysis of variance was conducted to examine how much of the variation in all-age cancer mortality rates by local authority in Great Britain was accounted for by the country or region of location (country/region) and how much was accounted for by the ONS classification Group to which the local authority belonged. The analysis showed that differences in these two factors accounted for between 70 and 80 per cent of the variation in rates by local authority for males and females. It showed that both country and region, and ONS classification Group contributed to the variation in cancer mortality rates by local authority. Similar results were found for lung cancer mortality.

A similar analysis was conducted for colorectal cancer. Although the results obtained were very similar to that for all cancer, less of the variation in mortality rates by local authority was found to be explained by country/region and ONS classification Group - around 60 per cent for males and 40 per cent for females.

For female breast cancer, country and region of residence was found to be the only factor contributing to the variation in mortality rates by local authority. There was no effect of ONS classification Group after controlling for country and region. However, country and region only explained around 30 per cent of the variation in breast cancer mortality by local authority. Similar results were found for prostate cancer for males.

10.5 Respiratory diseases

This section examines geographic variation in mortality from respiratory diseases (ICD9 460-519). Respiratory diseases account for 14 per cent of all deaths in the United Kingdom every year. In 1993 in England and Wales, the ONS introduced a new system for processing mortality data. This introduced changes in the way that mortality data are coded. For most causes of death, this had only a small impact on the number of deaths recorded, however, the changes resulted in a large increase in the number of deaths allocated to respiratory diseases.[18, 19] Therefore, we have only looked at mortality between 1993 and 1997 and have not looked at trends.

Variations between countries and regions

Tables 10.15 and 10.16 show mortality rates from respiratory diseases by country of the United Kingdom and region of England between 1993 and 1997.

Scotland and Northern Ireland had higher all-age mortality from respiratory diseases than England and Wales for both males and females between 1993 and 1997. At regional level within England there was evidence of a north-south divide in respiratory disease mortality with the North East and North West having higher rates than regions in the south for both males and females. The exception to this is that London had high rates of death from respiratory diseases.

For those aged 15-44 Scotland had the highest rates for both males and females. At regional level within England, only London had higher mortality from respiratory diseases than the United Kingdom as a whole for males aged 15-44 and all the other regions except the North West had lower rates. In London, respiratory disease accounted for just under 10 per cent of all male deaths in this age group and the rate in London was 3.5 times greater than the rate in the East of England, the region with the lowest rate. For females, there was little variation in mortality in this age group.

For respiratory disease mortality in those aged 45-64 and aged 65 and over, the picture was more similar to the all-age one, especially for males. The main exception was that London did not have high respiratory disease mortality for females aged 45-64. For those aged 65 and over, the rates in Scotland and Northern Ireland were much higher than the rate in other countries, with a dramatically higher rate in Scotland for males.

Variations between local authorities

For all ages, for males the pattern of mortality from respiratory diseases was very similar to that seen for all causes of death (Map 10.18), with concentrations of authorities with high rates around south Wales, Liverpool, Manchester and the east of London. Authorities in central Scotland had very high rates. In Northern Ireland a large number of authorities on the border with the Republic of Ireland and the east coast had high mortality. This pattern was similar for females (Map 10.19).

As for all causes, areas with mortality rates classed as very high in Map 10.18 tended to be found in urban and early industrial areas. Outside London and Northern Ireland there were 61 authorities with very high mortality rates. About half of these authorities were classified as *Coalfields, Manufacturing Centres* or *Ports and Industry*.

The distribution of mortality rates from respiratory diseases by local authority within ONS classification Groups was very similar to that seen for all causes of death. Figure 10.28 shows the pattern of all-age mortality rates by ONS classification Group. The pattern was similar to the all-cause pattern in that high rates were found in the *Coalfields, Manufacturing Centres* and *Ports and Industry* Groups. However, the rates for *West*

Inner London and *East Inner London* were relatively higher than the all-cause rates in these Groups and the rates in the *Remoter Rural* Group were relatively lower than the all-cause rates.

An analysis of variance was conducted to examine how much of the variation in all-age respiratory mortality rates by local authority in Great Britain was accounted for by the country or region of location (country/region) and how much was accounted for by the ONS classification Group to which the local authority belonged. The analysis showed that differences in these two factors accounted for between 60 and 70 per cent of the variation in rates by local authority for males and females. It showed that ONS classification Group was more highly correlated with respiratory disease mortality than country/region.

Table 10.15

**Age-standardised mortality rates for respiratory diseases by country and region, males
United Kingdom 1993-1997**

| | rates per 100,000 | | | |
	overall	15-44	45-64	65+
United Kingdom	144	5	55	1,155
England	~139	5	~52	~1,118
North East	*155	~4	*63	*1,243
North West	*160	6	*67	*1,275
Yorkshire and the Humber	144	~4	53	1,170
East Midlands	~139	~4	~50	~1,128
West Midlands	143	~4	52	1,156
East	~125	~3	~36	~1,033
London	*158	*11	*65	*1,238
South East	~126	~4	~43	~1,025
South West	~110	~4	~38	~893
Wales	145	~4	51	1,180
Scotland	*190	*6	*90	*1,496
Northern Ireland	*160	4	*62	*1,291

* significantly higher than the United Kingdom rate
~ significantly lower than the United Kingdom rate

Table 10.16

**Age-standardised mortality rates for respiratory diseases by country and region, females
United Kingdom 1993-1997**

| | rates per 100,000 | | | |
	overall	15-44	45-64	65+
United Kingdom	90	3	37	717
England	~87	3	~34	~694
North East	*99	3	*48	*781
North West	*102	4	*45	*804
Yorkshire and the Humber	91	3	40	720
East Midlands	~86	3	~34	~686
West Midlands	~84	~2	~33	~676
East	~80	3	~25	~650
London	*94	3	~35	*759
South East	~80	3	~28	~652
South West	~68	~2	~25	~547
Wales	90	3	*41	710
Scotland	*119	*5	*64	*910
Northern Ireland	*107	4	*45	*850

* significantly higher than the United Kingdom rate
~ significantly lower than the United Kingdom rate

　　　

Map 10.18

Age-standardised mortality rates for respiratory diseases by local authority, males all ages
United Kingdom 1993-1997

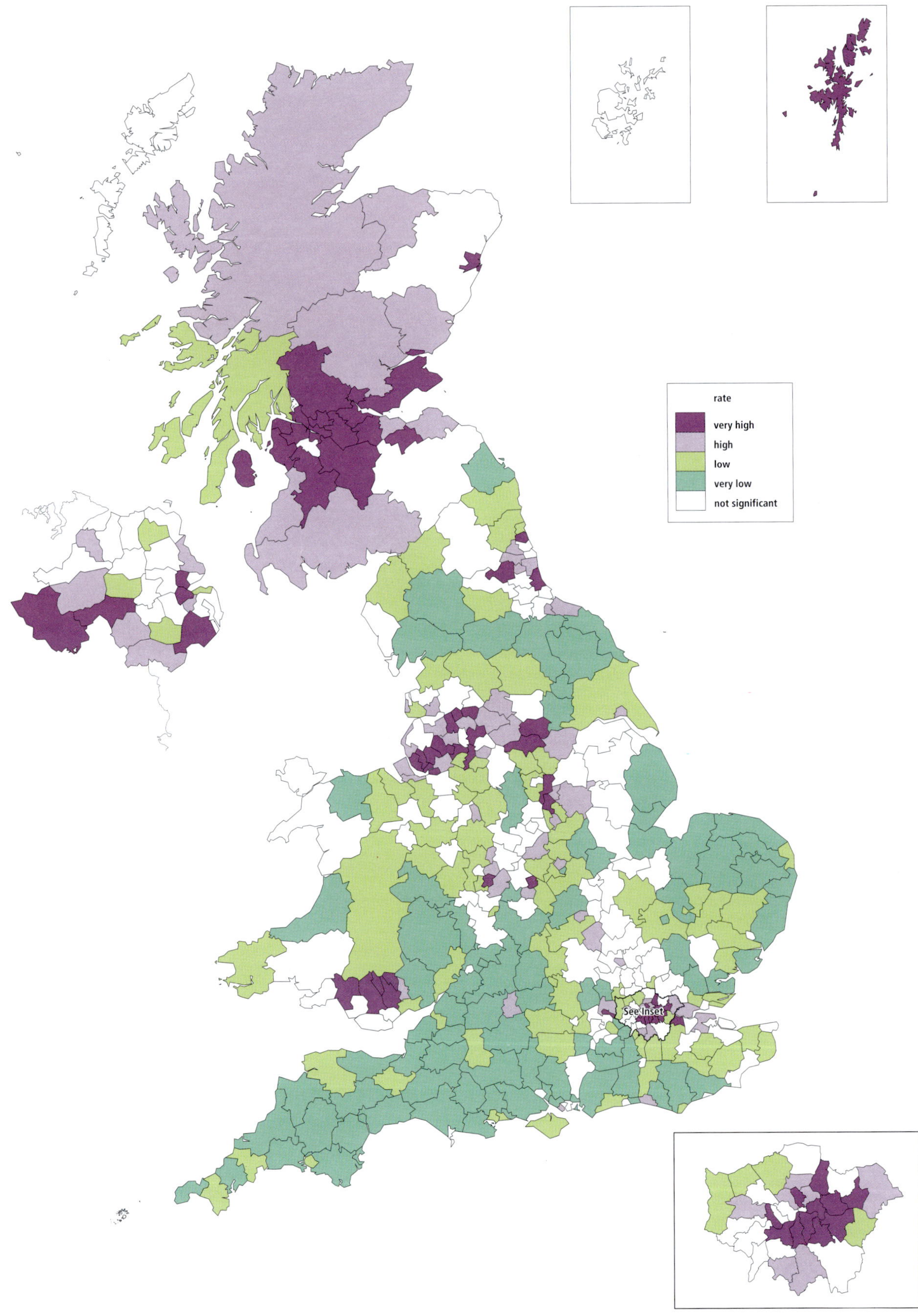

Map 10.19

Age-standardised mortality rates for respiratory diseases by local authority, females all ages
United Kingdom 1993-1997

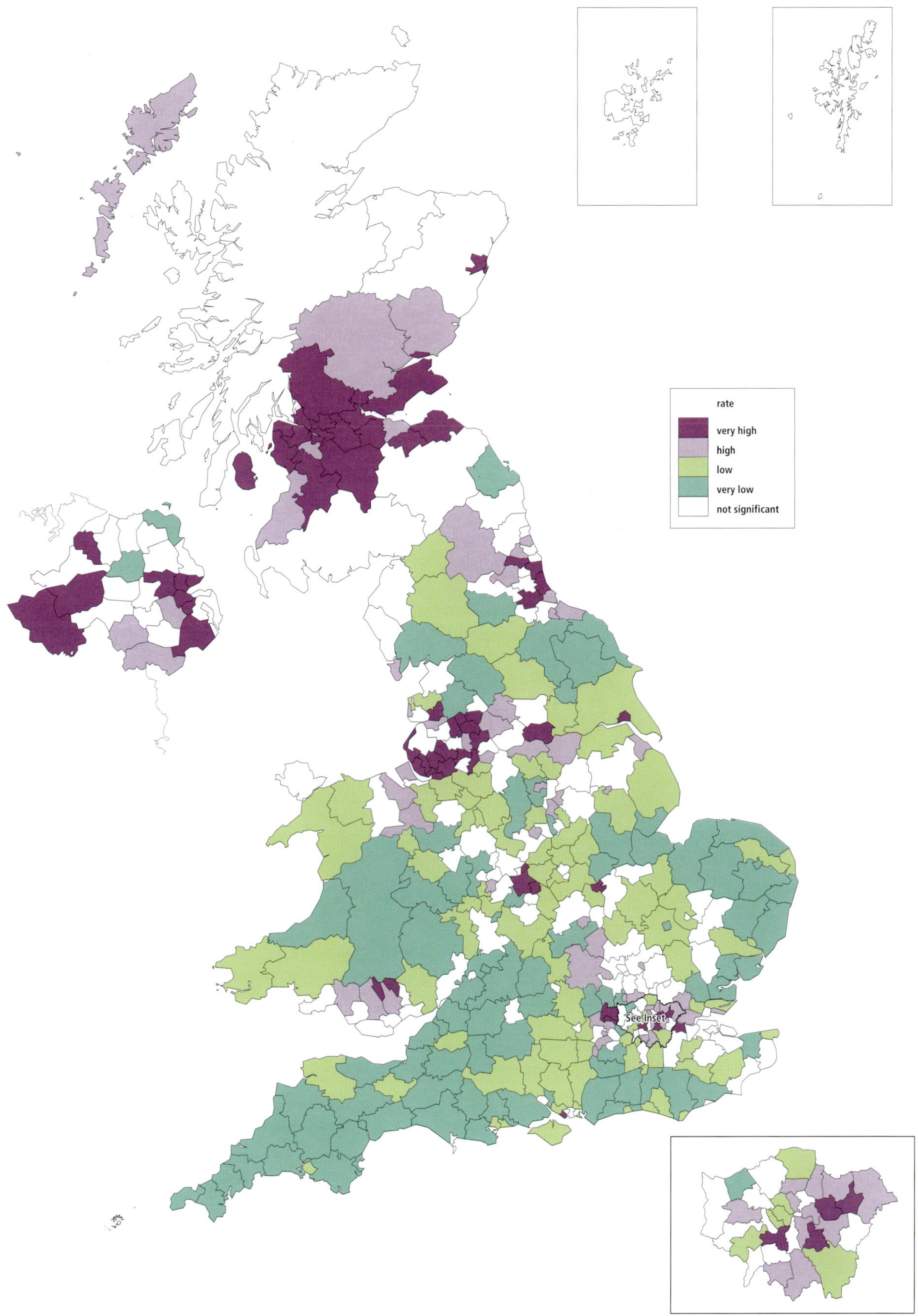

The pattern of mortality from respiratory diseases in males and females aged 45-64 and 65 and over were broadly similar to all ages. However, the average mortality rates for the 15 ONS classification Groups for those aged 15-44 were very different from the all-age pattern presented above, particularly for males (Figure 10.29). For males, the *East Inner London* and the *West Inner London* Groups had much higher than average rates, with *West Inner London* the highest. Mortality in the *West Inner London* Group was 13 times that of the *Remoter Rural* Group, the Group with the lowest rate.

10.6 Infectious diseases

This section examines geographic variation in mortality from infectious diseases (ICD9 001-139). Infectious diseases account for less than one per cent per cent of all deaths in the United Kingdom every year. The types of diseases included under this broad heading include: tropical diseases, meningitis, hepatitis and tuberculosis. However, this definition will exclude diseases such as pneumonia which are coded to the organ system chapters of ICD9. Therefore deaths from pneumonia are included with other diseases of the respiratory system.

From 1993 onwards in England and Wales and 1996 onwards in Scotland, AIDS-related deaths are included in the codes ICD9 001-139. In Northern Ireland these deaths are included within ICD9 001-139 throughout 1991 to 1997. In England and Wales, AIDS-related deaths were recorded under the ICD9 code 279.1 in 1991 and 1992. These deaths have therefore been included in the analysis in this chapter. In Scotland ICD9 279.1 was used up to and including 1995. These deaths have also been included in this analysis.

Figure 10.28

Age-standardised mortality rates for respiratory diseases by ONS classification Group, all ages Great Britain 1993-1997

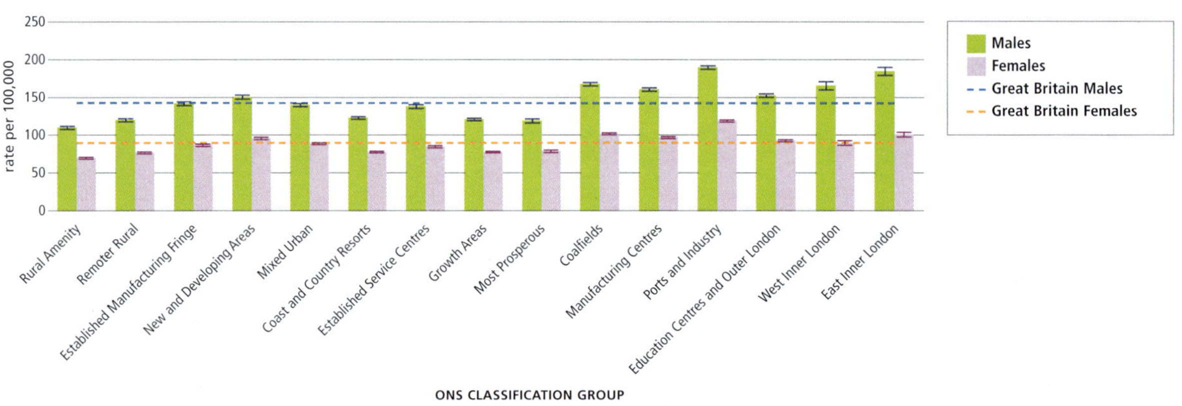

Figure 10.29

Age-standardised mortality rates for respiratory diseases by ONS classification Group, ages 15-44 Great Britain 1993-1997

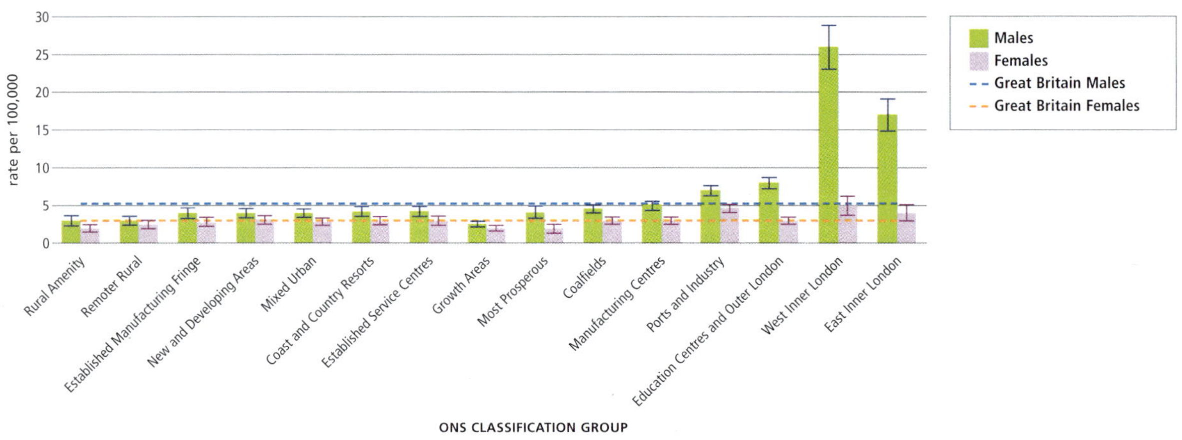

Variation between countries and regions

Tables 10.17 and 10.18 show age-standardised mortality rates from infectious diseases, including AIDS, by country of the United Kingdom and region of England between 1991 and 1997. Mortality from infectious diseases had a quite different geographic pattern to all-cause mortality.

Tables 10.17 and 10.18 show that Scotland had a significantly higher all-age mortality rate from infectious diseases than the United Kingdom as a whole and Northern Ireland had a significantly lower rate for both males and females. Both England and Wales had a similar mortality level to the United Kingdom as a whole for both males and females. This geographic pattern was maintained across the period 1992 to 1996, however, there is evidence of an increase in infectious disease mortality in Scotland, England and to a lesser extent Wales (Figures 10.30 and 10.31).

Within England, for males and females, London was the only region that had a significantly higher all-age mortality rate from infectious diseases than the United Kingdom as a whole. For males, the lowest rate was in the East Midlands and East of England; London's mortality rate was 2.8 times greater. For females, the lowest rates were in the East Midlands, South East and South West. However, London's rate was only 1.7 times greater. The difference between London and the rest of England was maintained throughout 1992 to 1996. There was some evidence of an increase in rates in all regions for females, however, the rate in London increased more rapidly than elsewhere (Figures 10.32 and 10.33).

Table 10.17

Age-standardised mortality rates for infectious diseases by country and region, males
United Kingdom 1991-1997

	rates per 100,000			
	overall	15-44	45-64	65+
United Kingdom	7	5	7	25
England	7	5	7	24
North East	~6	~2	6	*30
North West	~6	~3	~6	26
Yorkshire and the Humber	~6	~3	~5	25
East Midlands	~5	~3	~5	~22
West Midlands	~6	~3	6	24
East	~5	~3	~5	23
London	*14	*14	*16	*29
South East	~6	~4	7	~21
South West	~6	~4	~5	~21
Wales	7	~3	~5	*31
Scotland	*9	*6	8	*34
Northern Ireland	~3	~1	~4	~15

* significantly higher than the United Kingdom rate
~ significantly lower than the United Kingdom rate

Table 10.18

Age-standardised mortality rates for infectious diseases by country and region, females
United Kingdom 1991-1997

	rates per 100,000			
	overall	15-44	45-64	65+
United Kingdom	4	2	3	17
England	4	2	3	~16
North East	4	~1	3	19
North West	4	~1	3	17
Yorkshire and the Humber	4	1	3	15
East Midlands	~3	~1	3	~15
West Midlands	4	1	4	17
East	4	~1	3	18
London	*5	*3	*5	*19
South East	~3	~1	~3	~14
South West	~3	2	~3	~14
Wales	4	~1	4	*21
Scotland	*5	2	*4	*26
Northern Ireland	~2	~0	3	~9

* significantly higher than the United Kingdom rate
~ significantly lower than the United Kingdom rate

Figure 10.30

**Trends in age-standardised mortality rates for infectious diseases by country, males all ages
United Kingdom 1992-1996***

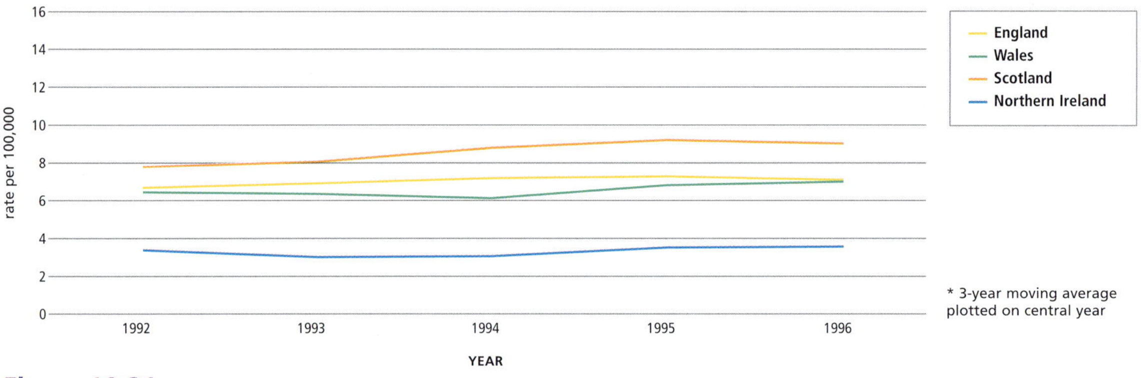

Figure 10.31

**Trends in age-standardised mortality rates for infectious diseases by country, females all ages
United Kingdom 1992-1996***

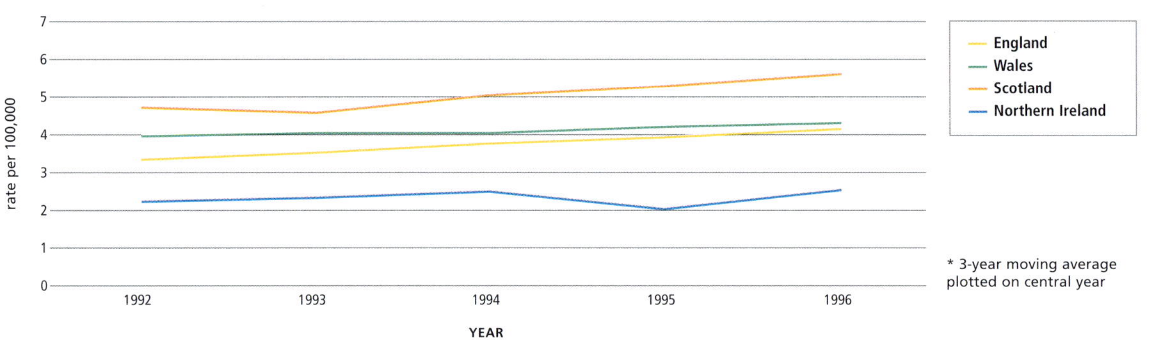

Figure 10.32

**Trends in age-standardised mortality rates for infectious diseases by region, males all ages
England 1992-1996***

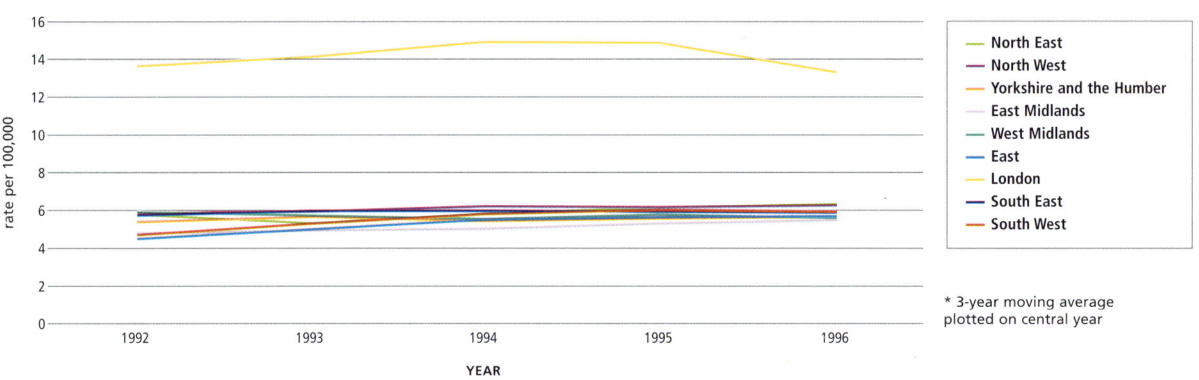

Figure 10.33

**Trends in age-standardised mortality rates for infectious diseases by region, females all ages
England 1992-1996***

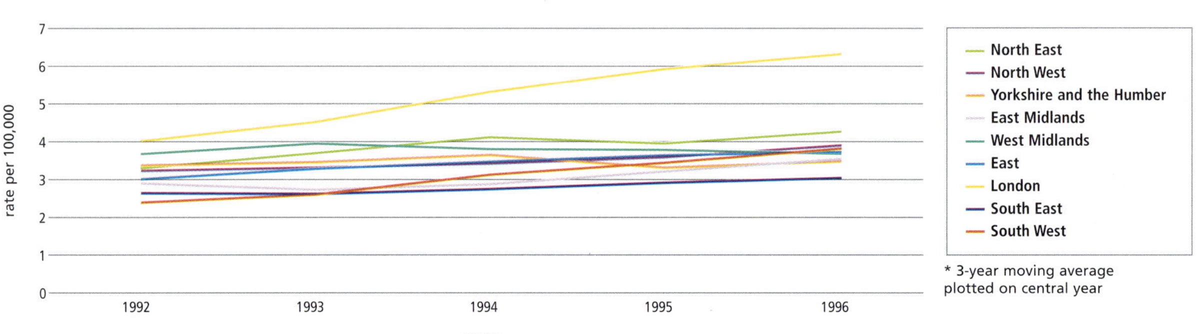

The geographic pattern for infectious disease mortality in younger adults aged 15-44 and adults aged 45-64 by country and region was broadly similar to all ages. For males and females aged 65 and over, Wales also had higher mortality from infectious diseases than the United Kingdom as a whole. Within England, for those aged 65 and over the high rates in London were maintained, however, the rate in the North East was equally as high. Trends in mortality for males and females by age group, country and region were similar to those already presented for all ages.

Variations between local authorities

The pattern of mortality from infectious diseases for males was very different to that seen for all causes of death (Map 10.20). Few authorities had rates that were higher than the rate for the United Kingdom as a whole. This is because the distribution of infectious disease mortality rates is very skewed, with high rates in a few authorities bringing up the average rate for the United Kingdom as a whole. Only 28 authorities had high rates, of which 18 were found within the London region. There were 14

authorities with mortality rates from infectious diseases classed as very high. Twelve of these authorities were within the London region and the other two, City of Edinburgh and Brighton and Hove, were within the *Education Centres and Outer London* Group. No other types of area had very high rates of mortality from infectious diseases. Authorities with low rates were scattered through the rest of England, Wales and Scotland, with only one in Northern Ireland.

The pattern of mortality across the United Kingdom for all-age mortality from infectious diseases for females was slightly different to that seen for males (Map 10.21). Fewer authorities had rates that were significantly lower than the rate in the United Kingdom as a whole, whereas slightly more authorities had rates that were higher than the United Kingdom as a whole. This demonstrates that the distribution of rates by local authority for females is less skewed than that for males. Concentrations of authorities around London, south Wales, Manchester, Glasgow and Edinburgh had high rates. Eighteen authorities had very high rates of death from infectious

Figure 10.34

Age-standardised mortality rates for infectious diseases by local authority within ONS classification Groups, males all ages Great Britain 1991-1997

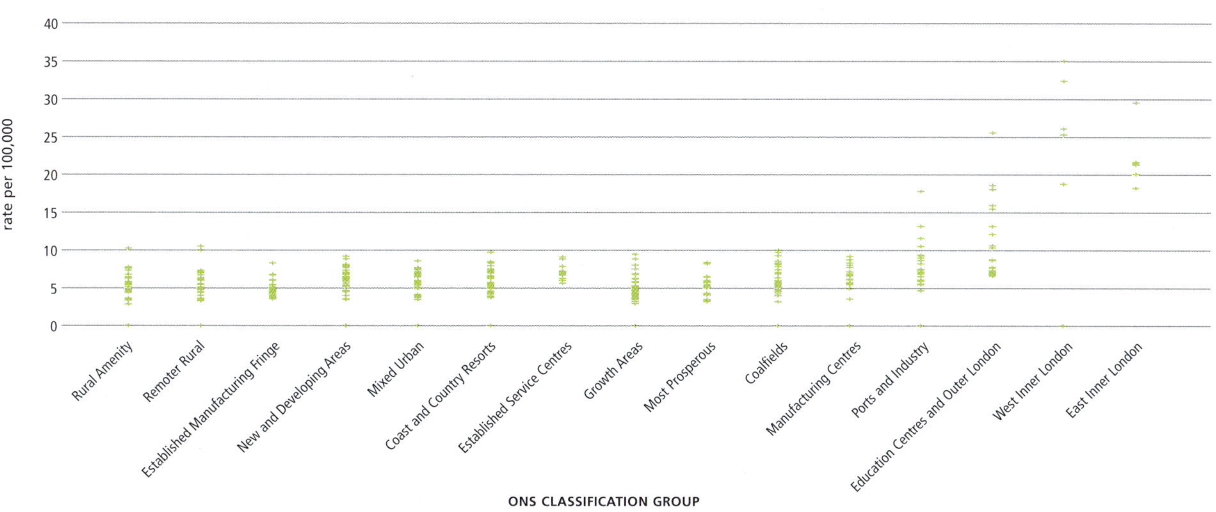

Figure 10.35

Age-standardised mortality rates for infectious diseases by ONS classification Group, all ages Great Britain 1991-1997

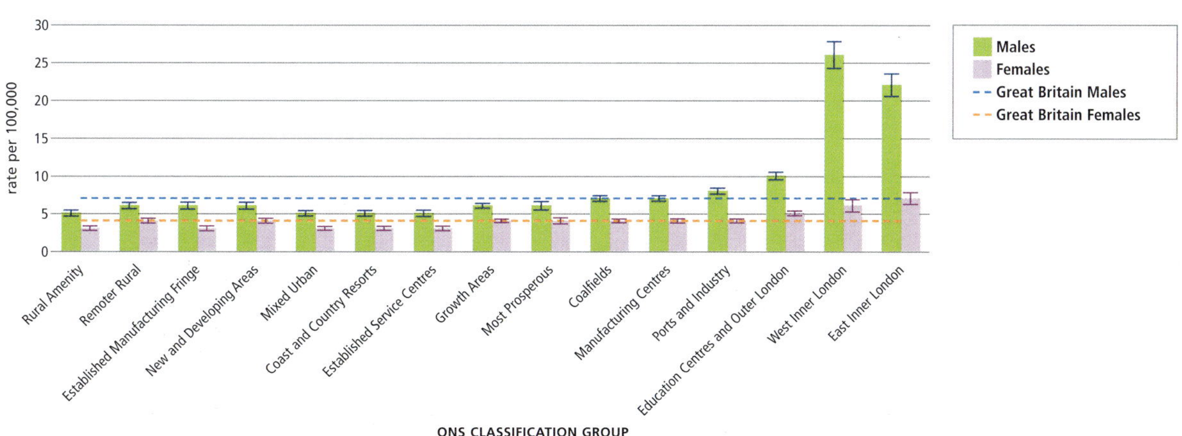

Map 10.20

Age-standardised mortality rates for infectious diseases by local authority, males all ages
United Kingdom 1991-1997

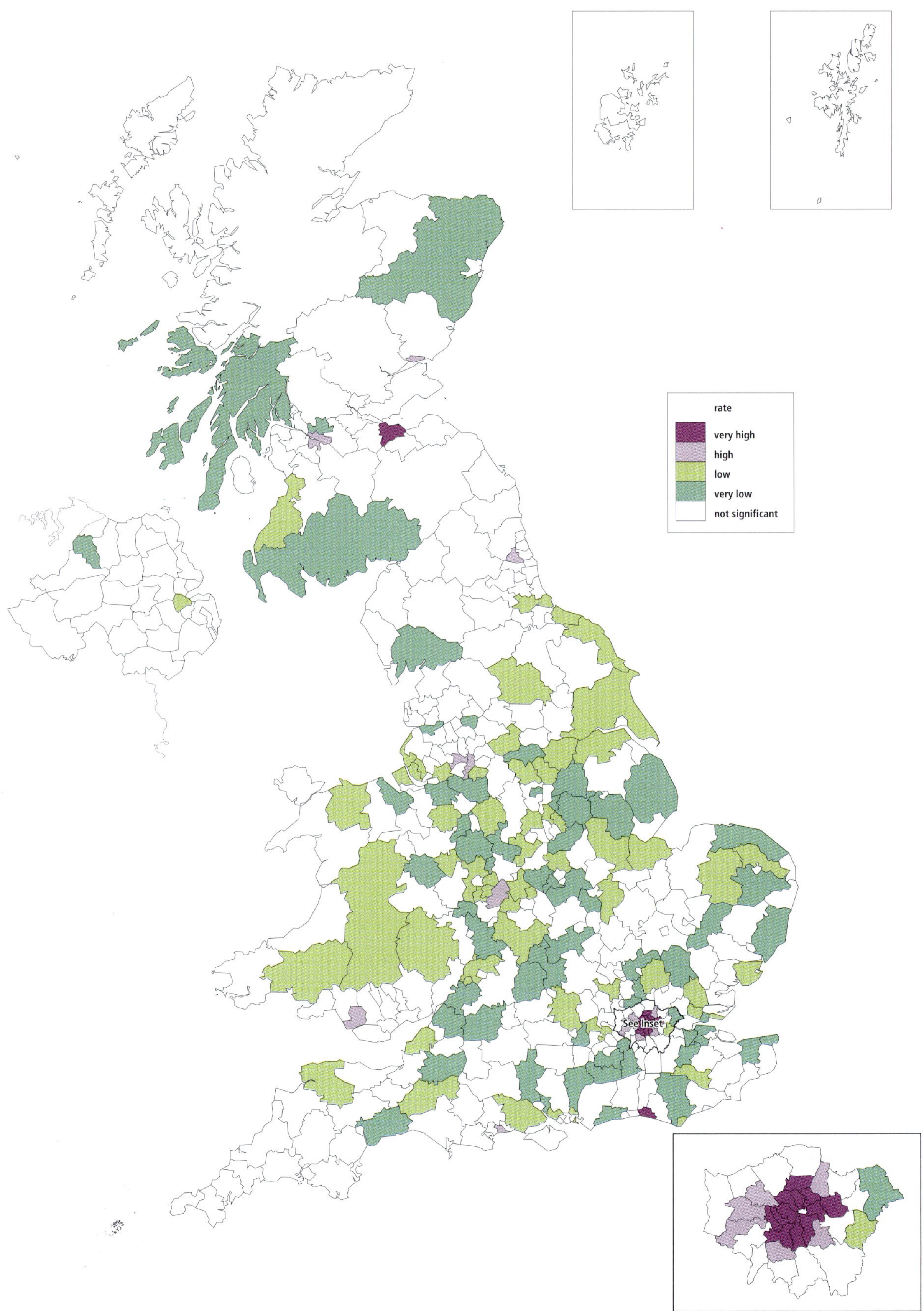

Map 10.21

Age-standardised mortality rates for infectious diseases by local authority, females all ages
United Kingdom 1991-1997

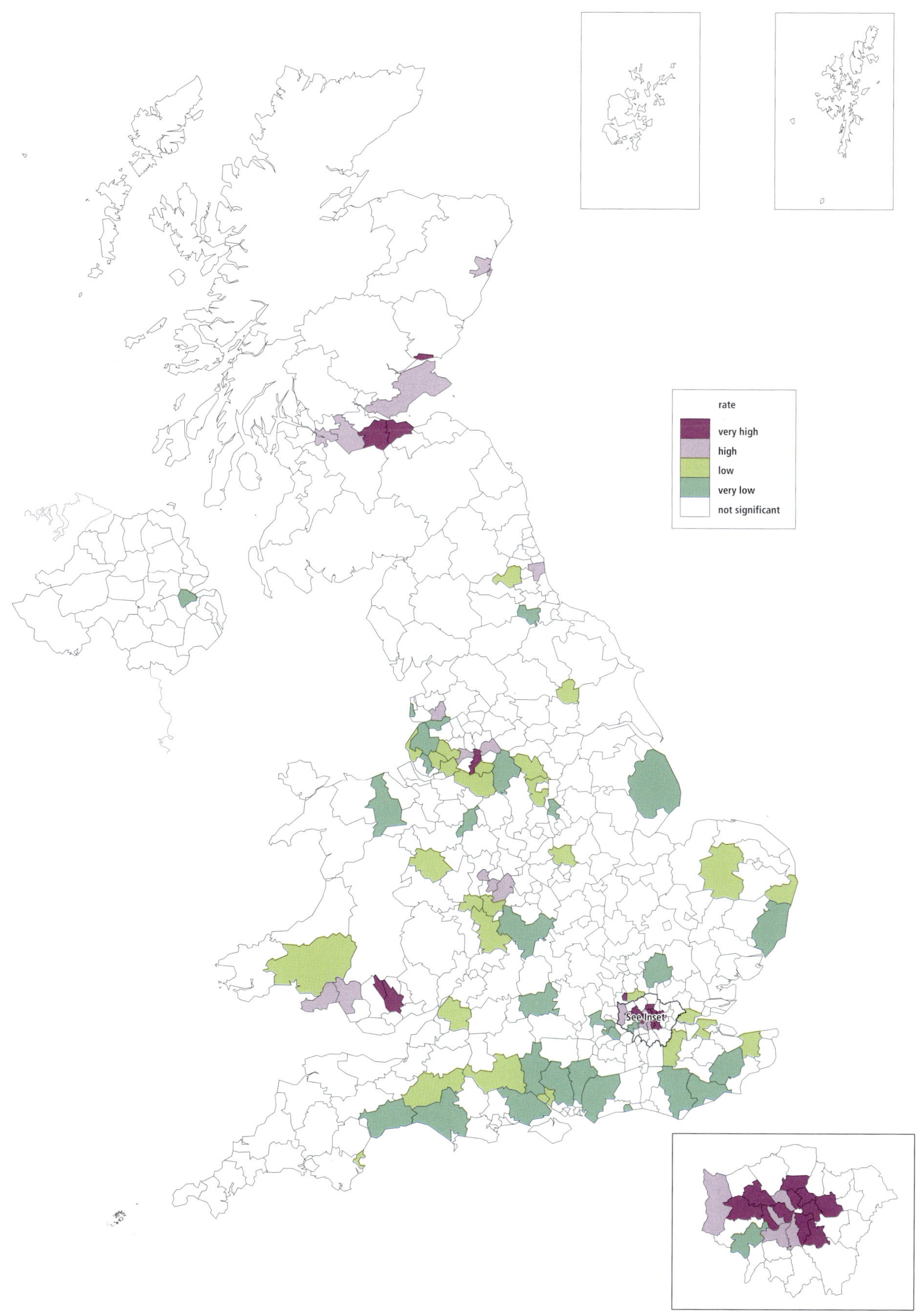

diseases. Only seven of these were outside London, however, they belonged to many different ONS classification Groups.

Figure 10.34 shows the distribution of all-age mortality rates from infectious diseases for males within the 15 ONS classification Groups. For males, all Groups had similar ranges and values except for *West Inner London* and *East Inner London*. In these Groups the range in rates was smaller and authorities with the lowest mortality had much higher rates than authorities with the highest mortality in most other Groups. Figure 10.35 shows the average all-age mortality rates from infectious diseases for males and females by the 15 classification Groups. The pattern identified in Figure 10.34 and in the regional analysis is apparent in these charts. The *West Inner London* and *East Inner London* Groups had much higher mortality rates than all other Groups. However, the *Education Centres and Outer London* Group and the *Ports and Industry* Group also had high rates.

An analysis of variance was conducted to examine how much of the variation in all-age infectious disease mortality rates by local authority in Great Britain was accounted for by the country or region of location (country/region) and how much was accounted for by the ONS classification Group to which the local authority belonged. Together these two factors explained only 45 per cent of the variation in females and 62 per cent of the variation in males. Both country/region and ONS classification Group contributed to the variation.

For males and females in particular age groups, few authorities had mortality rates from infectious diseases that differed significantly from the rates for the United Kingdom as a whole. Therefore, we have not presented maps for particular age groups. The pattern of mortality by ONS classification Group in those aged 15-44 and 45-64 was similar to that for all ages. Figure 10.36 shows the pattern of mortality from infectious diseases among those aged 65 and over by ONS classification

Group. A very different pattern to that presented for all ages emerged. Although the *West Inner London* and *East Inner London* Groups had high rates of death, the rates in the *Ports and Industry* and *New and Developing Areas* Groups were almost as high for both males and females.

10.7 Accidents

This section examines geographic variation in deaths from accidents (ICD9 E800-E949) in the United Kingdom between 1991 and 1997. The Government's strategies for health in England and Scotland identified accidents as a key area for health improvement.[1,3] Accidents are responsible for two per cent of all deaths every year in the United Kingdom and were until recently the leading cause of death in children, however, death rates from accidents in children have been decreasing steadily throughout the last 30 years. In addition, accidental falls are a substantial cause of death in older people.

A previous study looking at deaths from road traffic accidents in England and Wales showed that rates in metropolitan areas were lower than the average for England and Wales and that rates in rural areas, particularly in East Anglia and parts of the Midlands were higher than the average for England and Wales.[20] However, road traffic accidents are just a sub-section of the deaths included in the analysis in this section. Other types include accidental falls, accidental poisonings and those caused by fire and environmental factors. Deaths from accidental poisoning by drugs and alcohol are also analysed in section 10.9 of this chapter which examines all drug-related poisonings and alcohol-related causes. Different types of accidents may have very different geographic patterns, however in most cases the number of deaths were too small to analyse separately.

The countries of the United Kingdom have different registration and coding systems for deaths from accidents which may

Figure 10.36

Age-standardised mortality rates for infectious diseases by ONS classification Group, ages 65 and over Great Britain 1991-1997

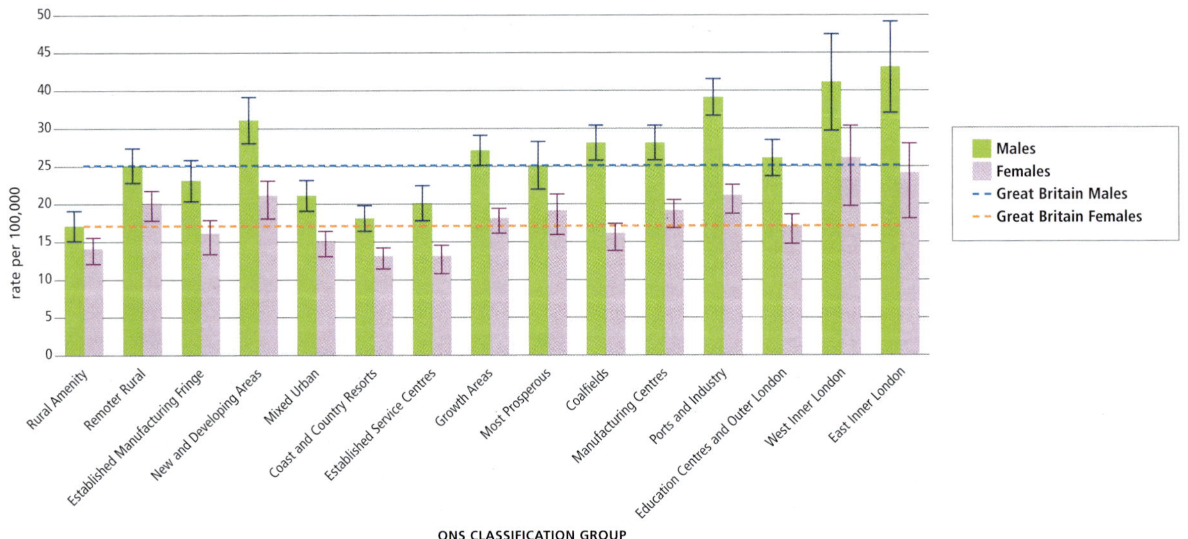

introduce artificial variations in mortality. Unfortunately, the effect of these differences is difficult to quantify. Box 10.1 explains the registration and coding system for deaths from accidents and suicide in the constituent countries of the United Kingdom.

Variations between countries and regions

Tables 10.19 and 10.20 show age-standardised mortality rates from accidents for males and females by country and region of the United Kingdom. For all-age mortality, Wales, Scotland and Northern Ireland had higher mortality rates from accidents than the United Kingdom rate for both males and females, and England had a lower rate. Between 1992 and 1996, significant declines in accident mortality were seen in Scotland for both males and females, and in Northern Ireland for females. Within England, at regional level the North West and East Midlands had the highest mortality from accidents in males and the regions in the south had the lowest (Table 10.19). The pattern was similar for females except only the East Midlands had a significantly higher rate than the United Kingdom (Table 10.20). In general, rates for the regions of England remained fairly static between 1992 and 1996.

Accidents form about a quarter of all deaths in children aged 1-14 and show a geographic pattern similar to all-age mortality from accidents (Tables 10.19 and 10.20). All countries experienced a decline in male mortality from accidents in this age group between 1992 and 1996 (Figure 10.37). The trend at regional level is not as clear, however, there were substantial declines in some regions including the West Midlands, North East and London (Figure 10.38).

For those aged 15-44, 45-64 and 65 and over the geographic pattern and trend by country was similar to the all-age pattern of mortality from accidents for both males and females. Within England the pattern for those aged 15-44 was similar to the all-age pattern, however, the difference between the regions with the highest and lowest male mortality from accidents widened between 1992 and 1996 (Figure 10.39). For those aged 45-64 no region had a significantly higher accident mortality rate than the United Kingdom as a whole. For those aged 65 and over, the regional geographic pattern was different from the pattern for all ages. The West Midlands was the only region with a significantly higher rate than the United Kingdom as a whole for males, for females the North East also had a significantly high rate (Tables 10.19 and 10.20). However, the rate in the West Midlands declined for males in the later part of the period (Figure 10.40).

Variations between local authorities

The previous section highlighted the higher mortality from accidents in Wales, Scotland and Northern Ireland than in England. For all ages, for males, Map 10.22 shows that there was a general pattern of high mortality from accidents in the majority of authorities in Scotland and Northern Ireland and a large number of authorities in Wales. A cluster of authorities in eastern England including King's Lynn and West Norfolk, Fenland, East Cambridgeshire and South Holland also had high rates of mortality from accidents. This is a similar cluster within England to that seen in a previous analysis of road traffic accidents.[20]

Forty-six authorities in the United Kingdom had very high rates. Sixteen of these were in Northern Ireland. Of the 27 with very high rates outside Northern Ireland and London, 13 were areas classified as *Remoter Rural*. All of these were in Scotland or in the two main clusters in England - bordering Scotland and on the east coast. Another 12 of those with high rates were

Box 10.1

Registration and coding of suicide and accidents in England, Wales, Scotland and Northern Ireland

In England and Wales deaths suspected to be from accidents or suicide are referred to the coroner. The coroner will investigate the death and certify the cause of death after a post mortem, an inquest or both. Unless a post mortem shows that the death was due to natural causes the coroner must open an inquest. If an inquest is necessary, a death can usually be registered only after the inquest.

Scotland does not have a system of coroners and inquests and there is no delay in the initial registration of a death which in England and Wales would be referred to a coroner. The death is registered using the doctor's certificate of cause of death. The cause of death is coded by the General Register Office for Scotland (GROS) using information provided at the time of registration. This information may indicate the death was accidental or that the death was due to suicide or self-inflicted injury and could immediately attract an appropriate code. In the absence of such information the death would be given a code indicating injury undetermined whether accidentally or purposely inflicted.

The certifying doctor or registrar reports such deaths to the Procurator Fiscal at the same time as the death is registered. When the Procurator Fiscal has examined the case he informs the GROS of any changes to the information originally recorded on the death certificate, including clarification of the cause of death. If necessary, GROS will then change the underlying cause of death.

GROS also consult with the forensic departments that carried out any post mortem, the Crown Office and the Scottish Executive Home and Health Departments on a regular basis to ensure that any information that these organisations hold is used to allocate the correct codes to suicides and other deaths (e.g. homicides). However, no changes are made to the records after about the end of March in the year following that in which the death was originally registered.

In Northern Ireland coroners do not record verdicts on accidents and suicide as they do in England and Wales, instead they forward a summary of 'findings' to the Registrar. From these findings staff at the General Register Office for Northern Ireland (GRONI) decide if the death is a suicide, accident etc. GRONI consult with coroners on findings where it is unclear whether the death was a suicide or not and then code the death accordingly.

Figure 10.37

**Trends in age-standardised mortality rates for accidents by country, males aged 1-14
United Kingdom 1992-1996***

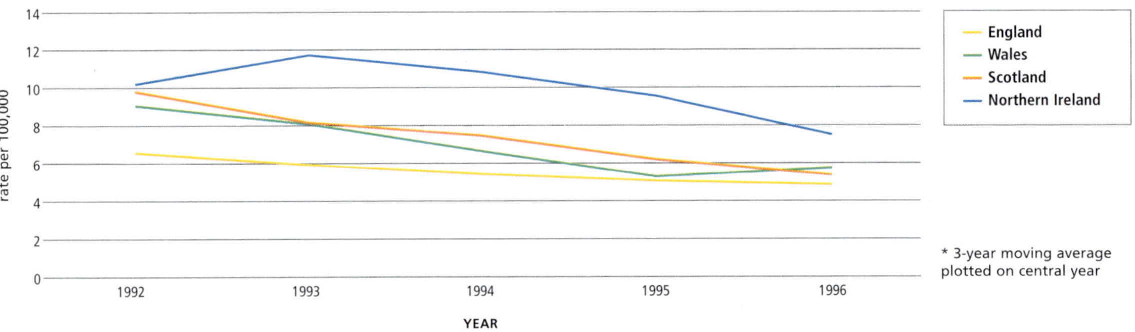

Figure 10.38

**Trends in age-standardised mortality rates for accidents by region, males aged 1-14
England 1992-1996***

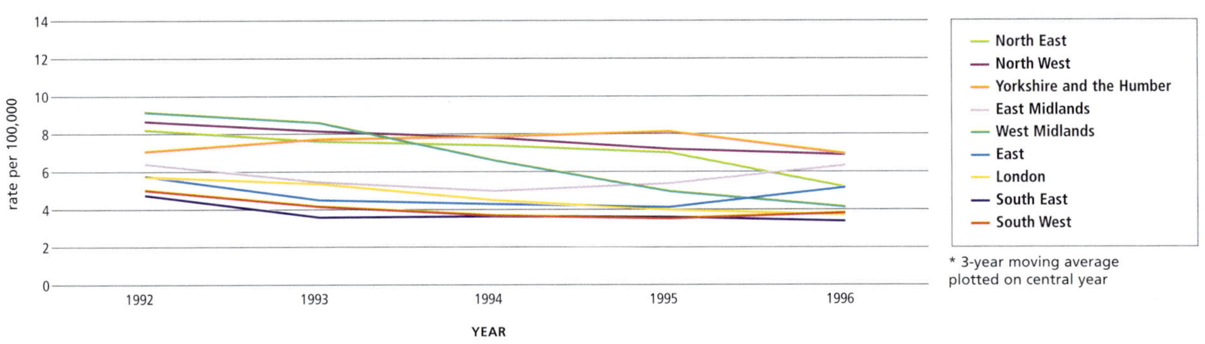

Figure 10.39

**Trends in age-standardised mortality rates for accidents by region, males aged 15-44
England 1992-1996***

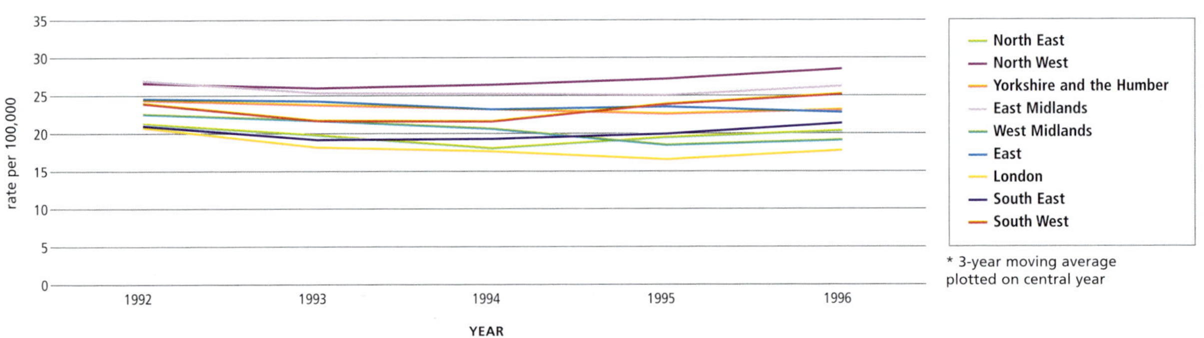

Figure 10.40

**Trends in age-standardised mortality rates for accidents by region, males aged 65 and over
England 1992-1996***

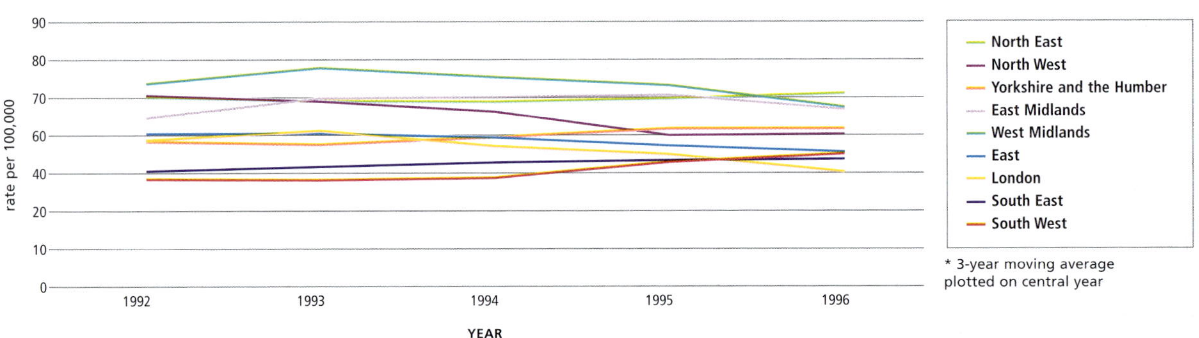

classified as *Coalfields*, *Manufacturing Centres* or *Ports and Industry*. Areas with low mortality from accidents were located on the periphery of London and other parts of south and central England. No authorities in Scotland or Wales and only one authority in Northern Ireland had lower rates of death from accidents than the United Kingdom as a whole.

The pattern of mortality across the United Kingdom for all-age mortality from accidents for females was broadly similar to that seen for males (Map 10.23), with Scotland and Northern Ireland dominating the authorities with high rates.

Figure 10.41 shows the distribution of all-age accident mortality rates for males within the 15 ONS classification Groups. There was wide variation in rates by local authority within the Groups;

the most variation was in the *Remoter Rural* Group. This distribution was very different to that seen for all causes in Figure 10.13. Unlike the pattern for all causes of death, some authorities in every classification Group had mortality rates that were similar to authorities in all other classification Groups.

Figure 10.42 shows all-age accident mortality rates for males and females for the 15 classification Groups. Unlike all causes of death the *Remoter Rural* Group had the highest mortality rates for both males and females, followed by the *Ports and Industry* Group. The pattern was different from other causes of death in that the rate in the *Ports and Industry* Group was very different from other similar areas: *Manufacturing Centres* and *Coalfields*.

Table 10.19

Age-standardised mortality rates for accidents by country and region, males
United Kingdom 1991-1997

			rates per 100,000		
	overall	1-14	15-44	45-64	65+
United Kingdom	24	6	24	21	65
England	~23	6	~23	~19	~61
North East	23	7	~21	19	71
North West	*26	*8	*28	21	66
Yorkshire and the Humber	24	8	24	20	~60
East Midlands	*25	6	*27	19	68
West Midlands	23	7	~21	20	*73
East	~23	~5	24	~18	~59
London	~21	~5	~19	22	~56
South East	~20	~4	~21	~17	~53
South West	~22	~4	25	~ 18	~53
Wales	*27	8	*29	22	71
Scotland	*33	*8	*27	*32	*104
Northern Ireland	*34	*10	*33	*32	*87

* significantly higher than the United Kingdom rate
~ significantly lower than the United Kingdom rate

Table 10.20

Age-standardised mortality rates for accidents by country and region, females
United Kingdom 1991-1997

			rates per 100,000		
	overall	1-14	15-44	45-64	65+
United Kingdom	11	3	6	9	53
England	~11	3	6	8	~48
North East	11	4	~5	~7	*58
North West	12	3	7	9	51
Yorkshire and the Humber	~10	4	6	8	~44
East Midlands	*12	3	*8	9	56
West Midlands	11	4	~5	9	*57
East	11	3	7	8	~47
London	~10	3	6	9	~41
South East	~10	~2	~5	~7	~46
South West	~10	3	7	~8	~44
Wales	*13	3	*8	9	*61
Scotland	*17	*5	*7	*12	*92
Northern Ireland	*15	*5	*8	*14	*61

* significantly higher than the United Kingdom rate
~ significantly lower than the United Kingdom rate

Map 10.22

Age-standardised mortality rates for accidents by local authority, males all ages
United Kingdom 1991-1997

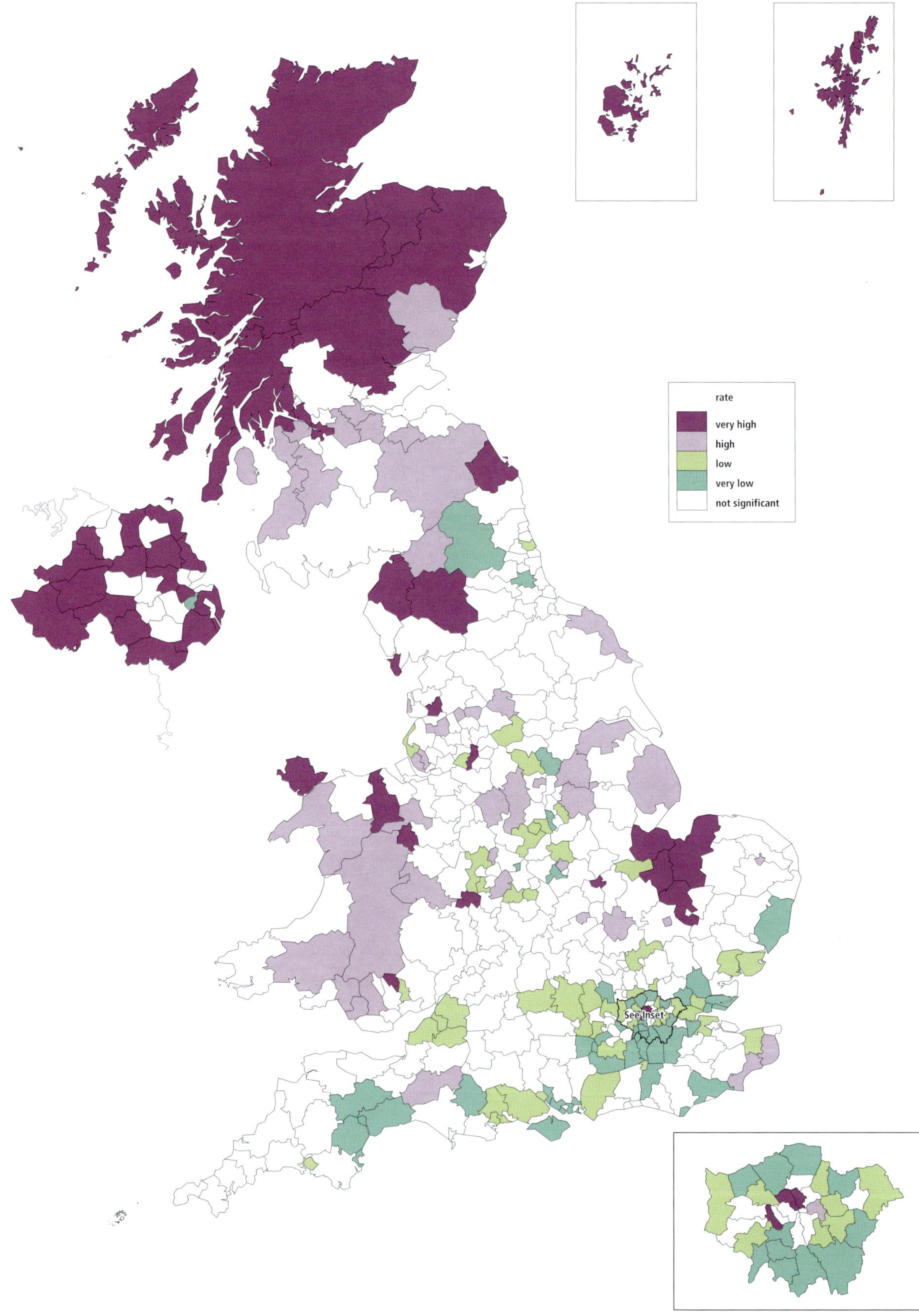

Map 10.23

Age-standardised mortality rates for accidents by local authority, females all ages
United Kingdom 1991-1997

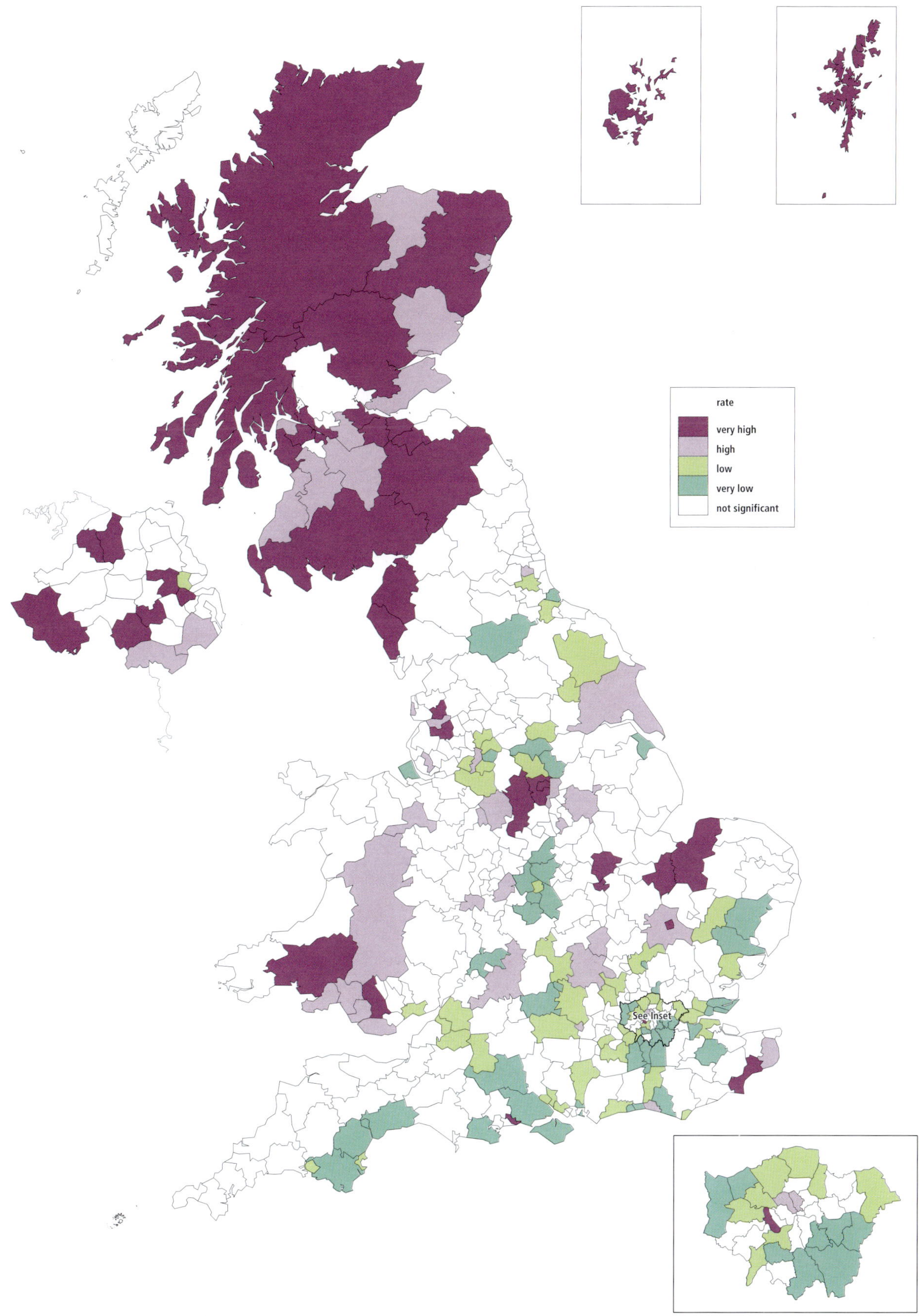

Figure 10.41

Age-standardised mortality rates for accidents by local authority within ONS classification Groups, males all ages
Great Britain 1991-1997

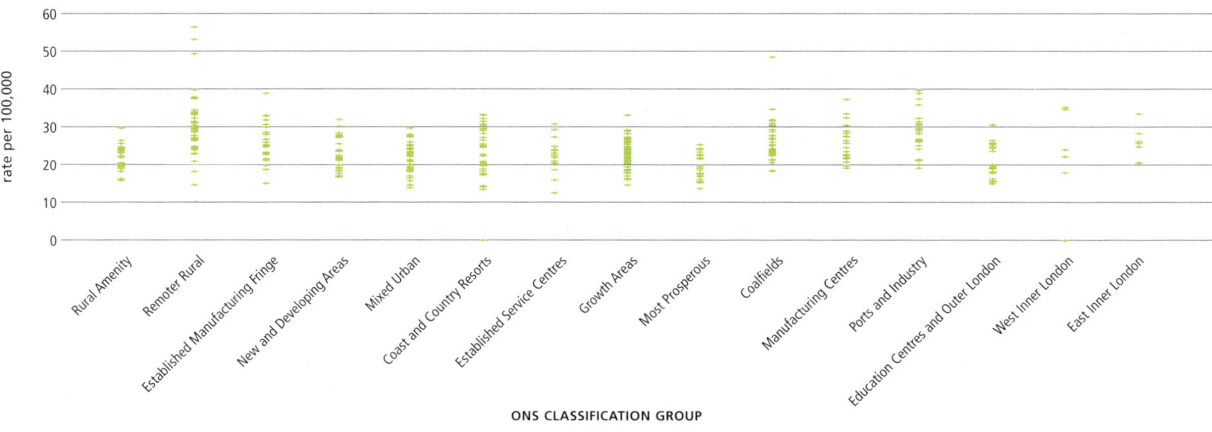

Figure 10.42

Age-standardised mortality rates for accidents by ONS classification Group, all ages
Great Britain 1991-1997

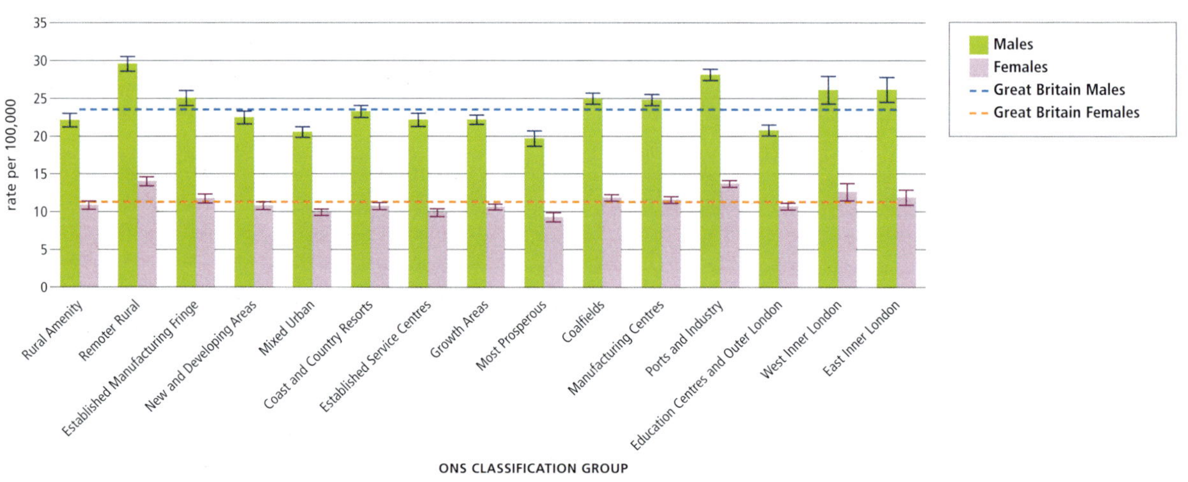

Figure 10.43

Age-standardised mortality rates for accidents by ONS classification Group, males aged 1-14
Great Britain 1991-1997

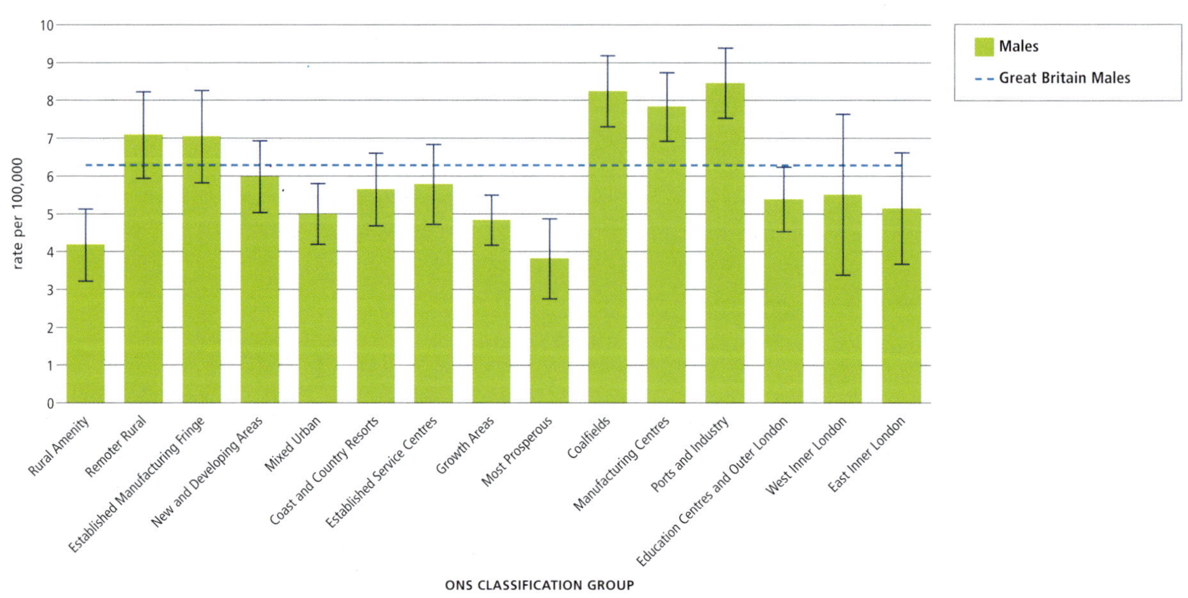

As demonstrated by Figure 10.41, not all authorities within the *Remoter Rural* Group had high rates. However, three authorities in particular had exceptionally high rates, the Shetland Islands, the Orkney Islands and Eilean Siar. The population of the *Remoter Rural* Group is very geographically concentrated with nearly 40 per cent in Scotland and over 20 per cent in the South West of England. In addition, authorities in Scotland make up over 40 per cent of the population of the *Ports and Industry* Group.

An analysis of variance was conducted to examine how much of the variation in all-age accident mortality rates by local authority in Great Britain was accounted for by the country or region of location (country/region) and how much was accounted for by the ONS classification Group to which the local authority belonged. The analysis showed that differences in these two factors accounted for around 40 per cent of the variation in rates by local authority for males and females. It showed that both country/region, and ONS classification Group contributed to the variation in accident mortality rates by local authority. However, unlike the analysis of all-cause mortality, country/region and ONS classification Group explain equal amounts of the variation in accident mortality. Thus, country/region was more strongly correlated with accident mortality than with all-cause mortality.

Figure 10.43 shows accident mortality rates for males aged 1-14 by ONS classification Group. Although the number of deaths in this age group was small, the pattern of mortality was very different to that seen for all-age accident mortality and more closely resembles the pattern for all-age all-cause mortality. The *Coalfields, Manufacturing Centres* and *Ports and Industry* Groups had higher mortality than Great Britain for males in this age group.

10.8 Suicide and undetermined injury

This section examines geographic variation in mortality from suicides (ICD9 E950-959, E980-989) in the United Kingdom. Throughout this chapter 'suicides' are defined as deaths from suicide and 'deaths from injury and poisoning undetermined whether accidentally or purposely inflicted'. It is likely that most undetermined deaths (or open verdicts) are cases where the harm was self-inflicted but there was insufficient evidence to prove that the deceased deliberately intended to kill themselves.[21] Therefore, these deaths are usually included in any analysis of suicide mortality.

For England and Wales, we have excluded all deaths assigned to the code E988.8. This code is used in cases where a coroner adjourns an inquest awaiting prosecution in a higher court. The coroner is able to register these deaths before other legal proceedings have been completed. As a large proportion of these cases are subsequently found to be homicides these deaths are excluded from our analysis. Their inclusion would present an inaccurate picture of suicide mortality.

The countries of the United Kingdom have different registration and coding systems for deaths from suicide which may introduce artificial variations in mortality. Unfortunately, the effect of these differences is difficult to quantify. Box 10.1 describes the registration and coding system for deaths from suicide in the constituent countries of the United Kingdom.

Deaths from suicide and undetermined injury account for one per cent of deaths every year in the United Kingdom. The Government's strategies for health in England and Scotland identified mental health as a key area for health improvement.[1,3] Risk factors for mental illness and suicide include: poverty, unemployment, bereavement, relationship problems and social isolation. This leads to considerable socio-economic and geographic variation in suicide mortality. Previous studies have identified that death rates from suicide in Scotland are much higher than in the other constituent countries of the United Kingdom although the differences have not been consistent over time.[22] In addition large regional and local differences in suicide rates have been reported. Areas with high suicide rates tended to be those characterised as having higher than average levels of deprivation.[22]

Variations between countries and regions

Tables 10.21 and 10.22 show suicide mortality rates by country of the United Kingdom and region of England between 1991 and 1997. For all ages, males in Scotland and Wales had higher rates than the United Kingdom as a whole and England and Northern Ireland had lower rates, whereas for females, Scotland was the only one of the countries which had a higher suicide rate than the United Kingdom as a whole. Over the period studied, there was a general decline in suicides in England, Wales and Northern Ireland, whereas in Scotland there was a slight increase for both males and females (Figures 10.44 and 10.45). This resulted in a widening of the difference between Scotland and the rest of the United Kingdom.

None of the regions of England had significantly higher mortality from suicide for males or females than the United Kingdom as a whole, although for males generally the regions in the north had higher rates than the regions in the south (Tables 10.21 and 10.22). In general rates for the regions of England remained fairly static or declined between 1992 and 1996.

For those aged 15-44, the geographic pattern by country was similar to all-age mortality from suicide in both males and females. However, due to small numbers of deaths in this age group, particularly for females, the rates were often not significantly different from the United Kingdom as a whole. Both Scotland and Wales had an increase in male suicide rates between 1992 and 1996. England had a decline and the rate in Northern Ireland remained virtually the same. There were no consistent trends by country for females aged 15-44.

The North West had higher mortality than any other region for both males and females aged 15-44. Figure 10.46 shows that for males the rate in the North West was consistently higher than the other regions over the period 1992-1996 and that, although its rate declined, the difference between the North West and the region with the lowest male mortality, the East of England, widened over this period. By contrast, the

North East and Yorkshire and the Humber had an increase in suicide rates over this time period, so that the gap between the North West and these regions declined.

For those aged 45-64 and those aged 65 and over, the geographic variation between countries was very similar to all ages for suicide. However, for males in both of these age groups, Scotland's rate diverged from the other countries between 1992 and 1996, especially for those aged 65 and over (Figure 10.47). Tables 10.21 and 10.22 show that there was little regional variation in suicide mortality for those aged 45-64 and 65 and over.

Variations between local authorities

Map 10.24 shows male suicide mortality rates by local authority. A number of authorities in Scotland and Wales had high mortality from suicide, reflecting the pattern at country level. Within England, few authorities had high mortality, except a concentration of authorities in the North West of England, in London and on the south coast including Brighton and Hove, Hastings and the Isle of Wight.

Unlike mortality from all causes of death, areas with mortality rates from suicide classed as very high were located mainly in Scotland and Wales, although many were found in the *Remoter Rural, Coalfields, Manufacturing Centres* and *Ports and Industry*. From these maps it would appear that differences in suicide rates between local authorities were more closely related to the regional location of the authority than to the characteristics of areas.

Table 10.21

**Age-standardised mortality rates for suicide and undetermined injury by country and region, males
United Kingdom 1991-1997**

| | rates per 100,000 | | | |
	overall	15-44	45-64	65+
United Kingdom	15	21	19	18
England	~14	~19	~18	17
North East	15	20	18	18
North West	16	*23	19	~15
Yorkshire and the Humber	15	20	18	16
East Midlands	~14	~19	~17	19
West Midlands	~13	~18	~16	17
East	~14	~17	18	18
London	~14	~18	19	17
South East	~14	~18	18	18
South West	15	20	19	18
Wales	*17	*24	19	17
Scotland	*24	*33	*28	*24
Northern Ireland	~14	20	~15	~14

* significantly higher than the United Kingdom rate
~ significantly lower than the United Kingdom rate

Table 10.22

**Age-standardised mortality rates for suicide and undetermined injury by country and region, females
United Kingdom 1991-1997**

| | rates per 100,000 | | | |
	overall	15-44	45-64	65+
United Kingdom	5	5	7	7
England	~5	~5	7	7
North East	5	6	7	~5
North West	5	*6	7	~6
Yorkshire and the Humber	5	5	7	7
East Midlands	~4	~5	6	6
West Midlands	~4	~4	~5	8
East	~4	~4	~5	8
London	5	5	7	8
South East	5	5	8	8
South West	5	5	7	8
Wales	~4	5	6	6
Scotland	*8	*9	*11	*9
Northern Ireland	~4	5	7	~4

* significantly higher than the United Kingdom rate
~ significantly lower than the United Kingdom rate

Figure 10.44

Trends in age-standardised mortality rates for suicide and undetermined injury by country, males all ages
United Kingdom 1992-1996*

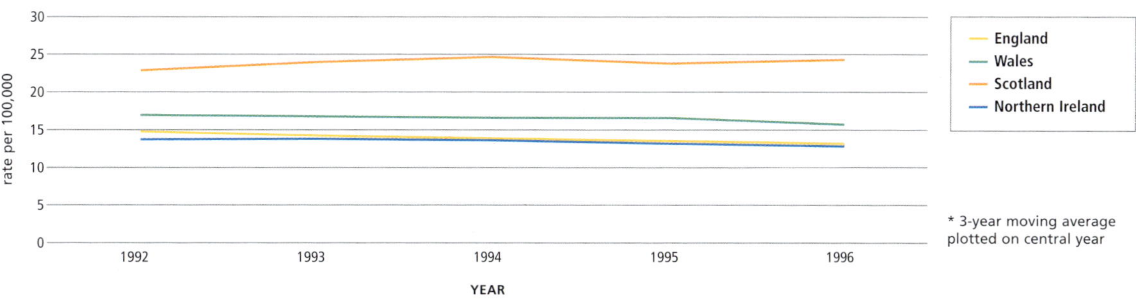

Figure 10.45

Trends in age-standardised mortality rates for suicide and undetermined injury by country, females all ages
United Kingdom 1992-1996*

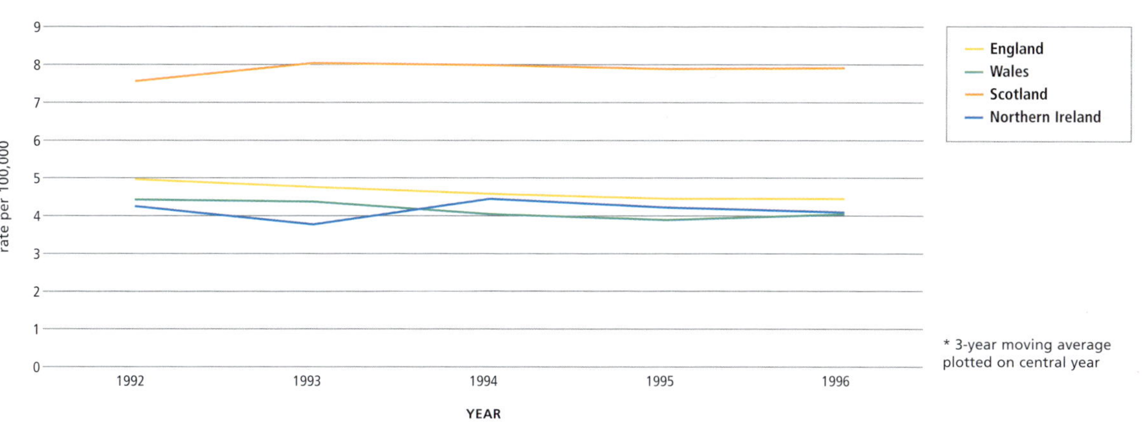

Figure 10.46

Trends in age-standardised mortality rates for suicide and undetermined injury by region, males aged 15-44
England 1992-1996*

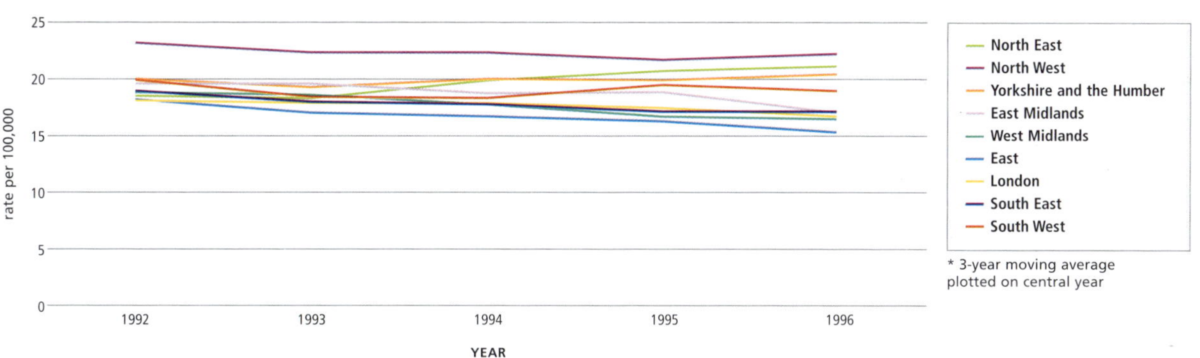

Figure 10.47

Trends in age-standardised mortality rates for suicide and undetermined injury by country, males aged 65 and over
United Kingdom 1992-1996*

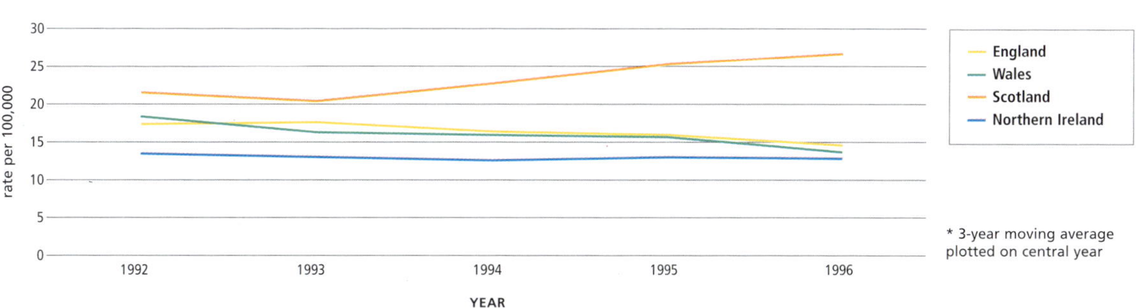

Map 10.24

Age-standardised mortality rates for suicide and undetermined injury by local authority, males all ages
United Kingdom 1991-1997

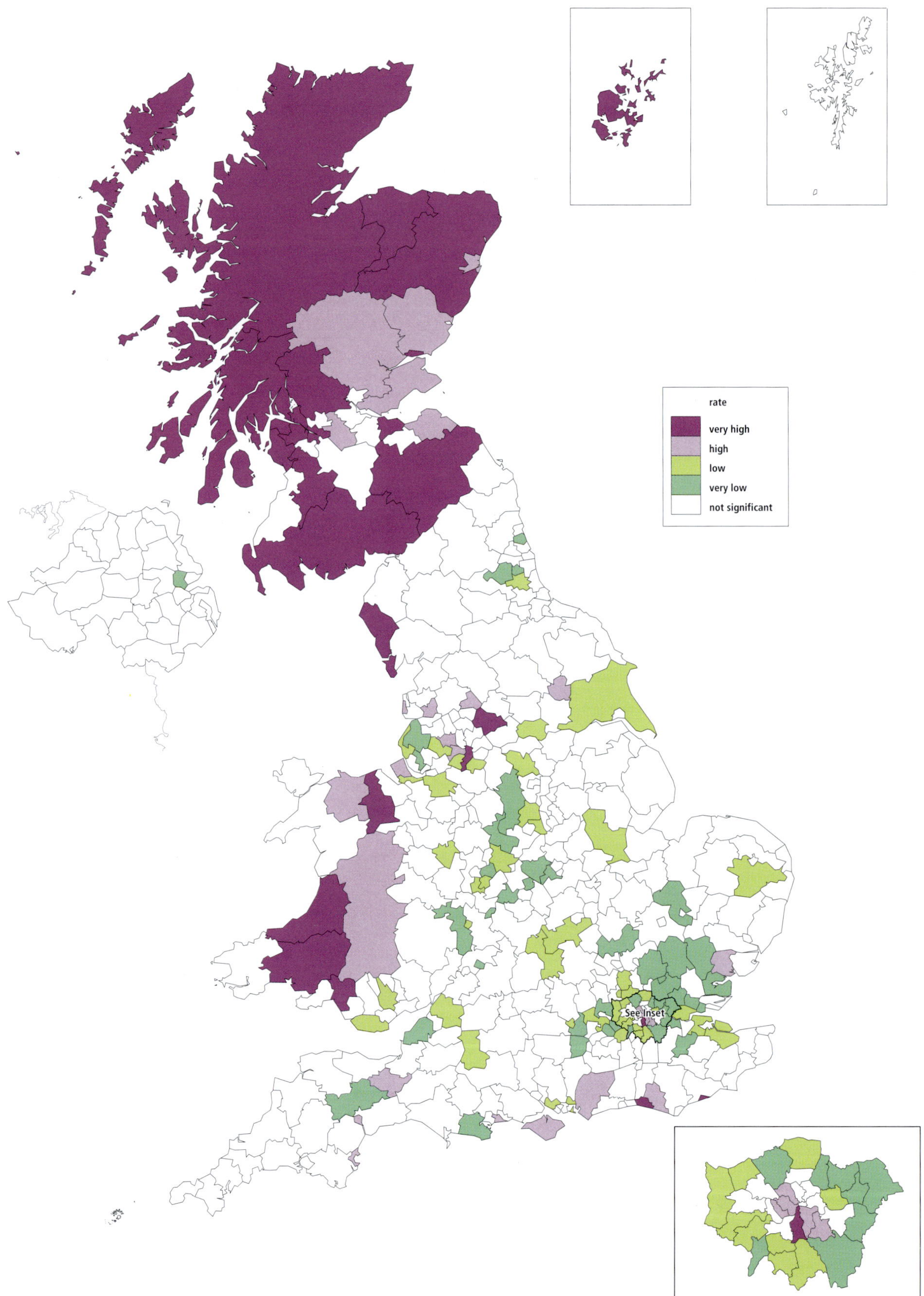

Map 10.25

Age-standardised mortality rates for suicide and undetermined injury by local authority, females all ages
United Kingdom 1991-1997

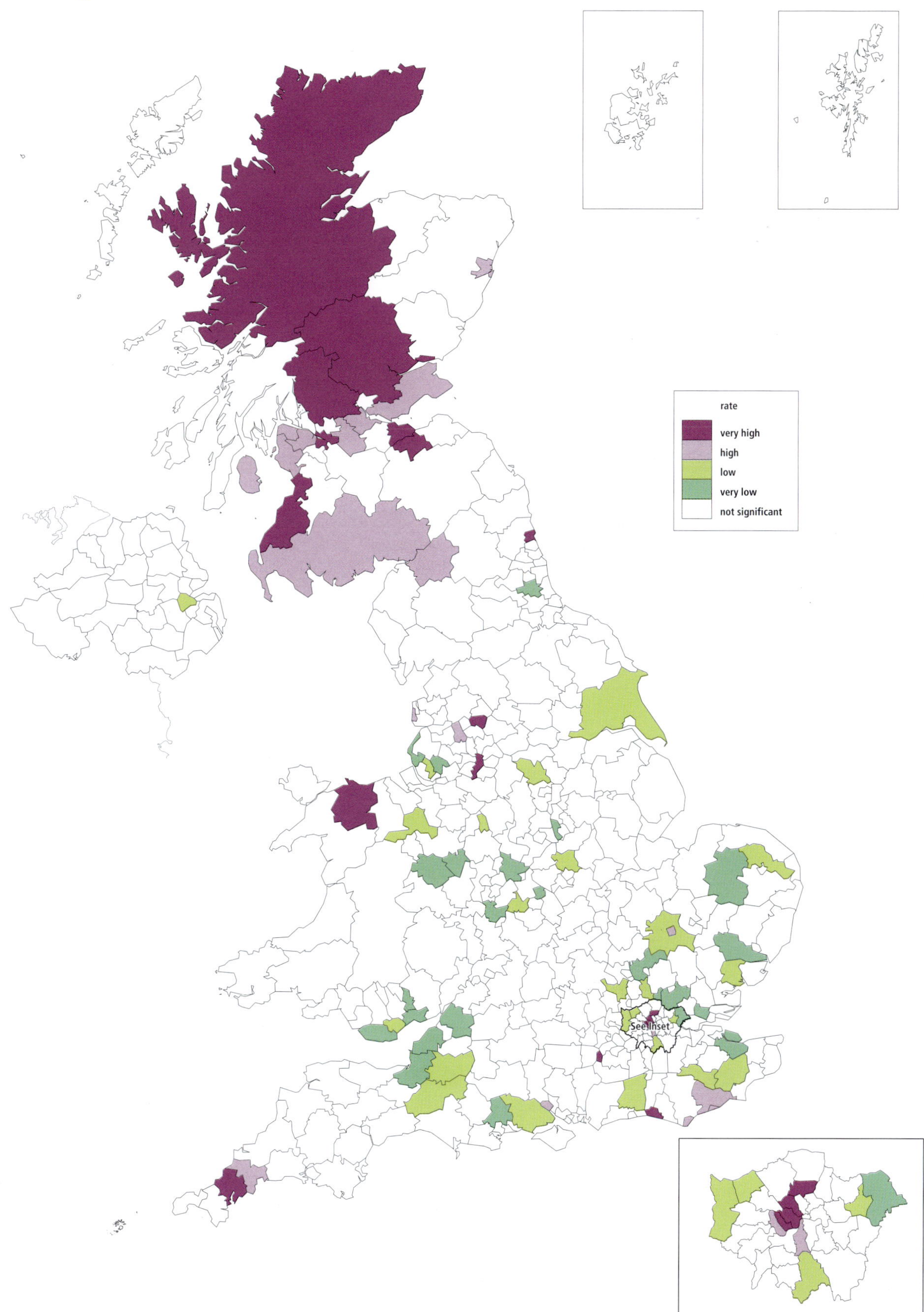

Map 10.26

Age-standardised mortality rates for suicide and undetermined injury by local authority, males aged 15-44
United Kingdom 1991-1997

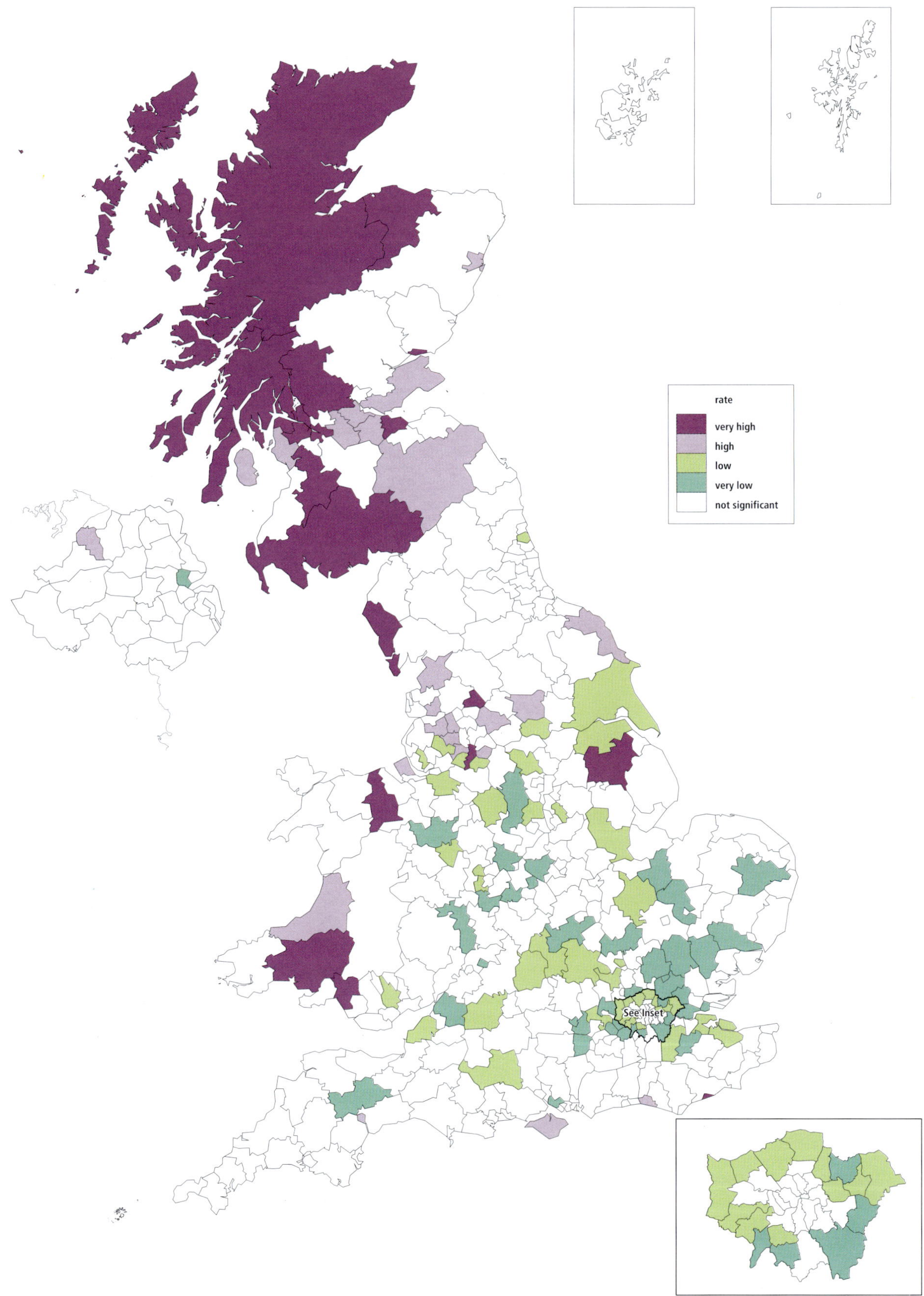

Figure 10.48

Age-standardised mortality rates for suicide and undetermined injury by local authority within ONS classification Groups, males all ages
Great Britain 1991-1997

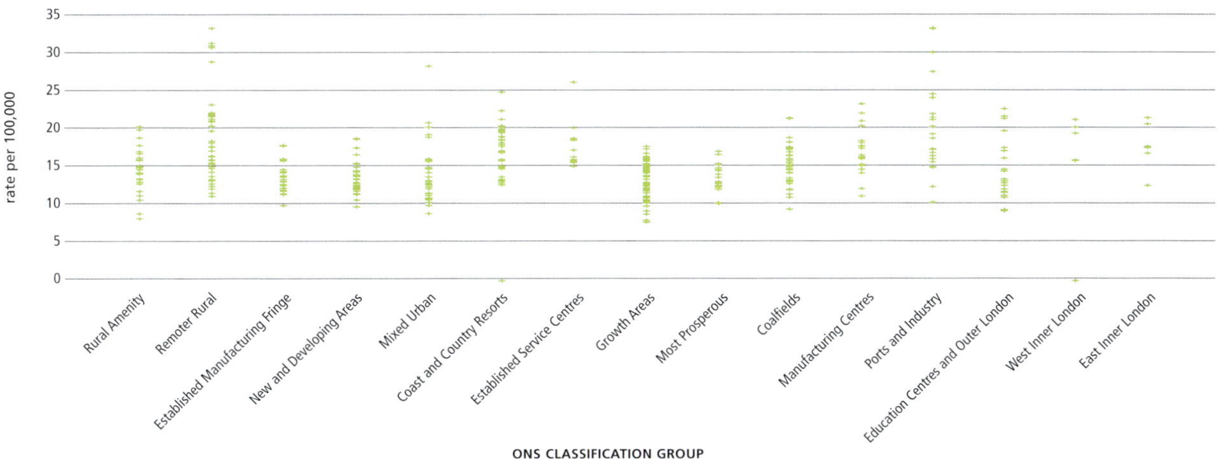

Figure 10.49

Age-standardised mortality rates for suicide and undetermined injury by ONS classification Group, all ages
Great Britain 1991-1997

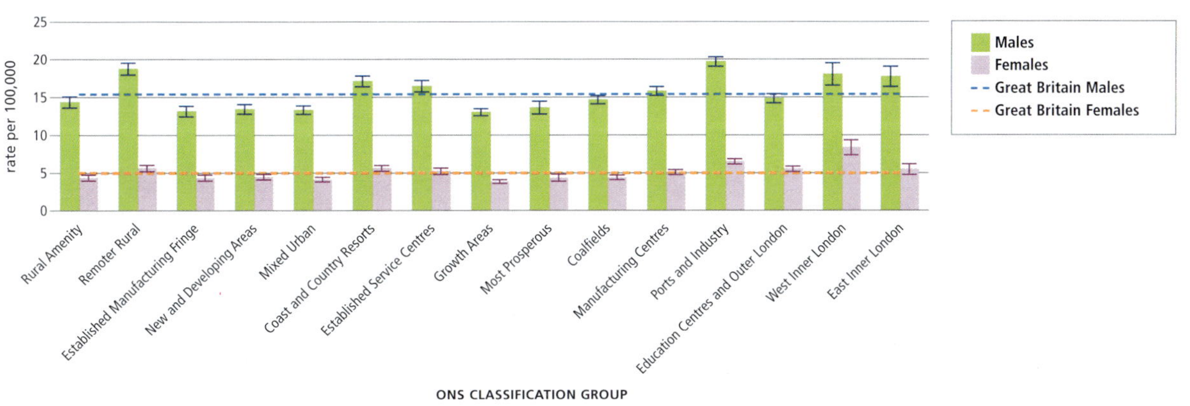

Figure 10.50

Age-standardised mortality rates for suicide and undetermined injury by ONS classification Group, ages 65 and over
Great Britain 1991-1997

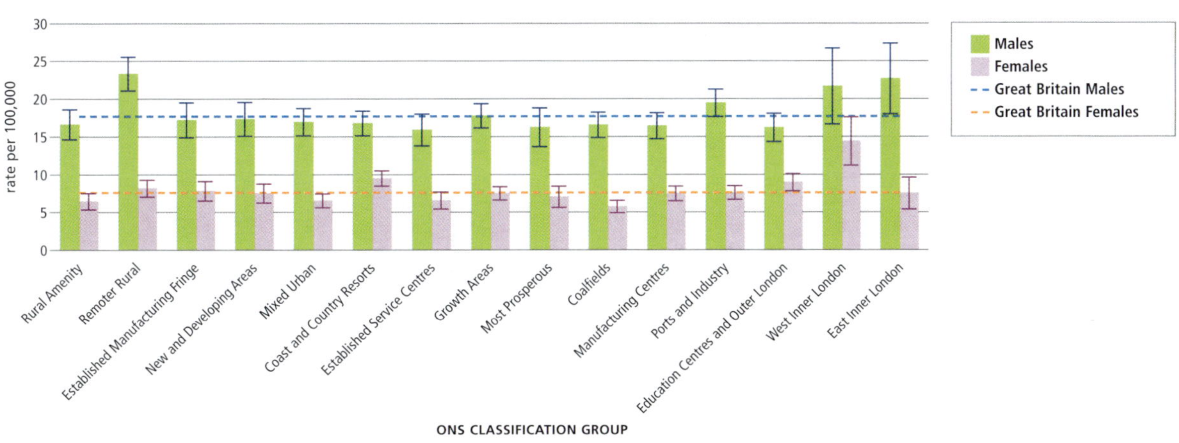

Areas with low mortality from suicide were located on the periphery of London and other parts of south and central England. No authorities in Scotland or Wales had very low rates of death from suicide. Although Northern Ireland as a whole had a lower mortality rate than the United Kingdom as a whole, due to the small number of deaths in any one local authority, only one authority in Northern Ireland had a mortality rate classed as very low in Map 10.24. Of the 40 authorities outside London and Northern Ireland with very low rates from suicide, 13 were classified as *Growth Areas*.

The pattern of mortality across the United Kingdom for all-age mortality from suicide for females was slightly different to that seen for males (Map 10.25). Fewer authorities in Wales and Scotland had high death rates from suicide. Only a small number of authorities in England had high rates of death, but these are in similar locations to authorities with high mortality for males.

There was large variation in mortality from suicide between local authorities within ONS classification Groups indicating that ONS classification Group is less closely associated with suicide than all-cause mortality. Figure 10.48 shows the picture for males. The widest range in mortality rates for males was seen in the *Remoter Rural* and *Ports and Industry* Groups. Figure 10.49 shows all-age suicide mortality rates for males and females by the 15 classification Groups. The pattern was slightly different to that seen for all causes of death. Although the *Ports and Industry, East Inner London* and *West Inner London* Groups still had higher than average mortality levels, high mortality was also evident in the *Remoter Rural, Coast and Country Resorts* and *Established Service Centres* Groups.

An analysis of variance was conducted to examine how much of the variation in all-age suicide mortality rates by local authority in Great Britain was accounted for by the country or region of location (country/region) and how much was accounted for by the ONS classification Group to which the local authority belonged. The analysis showed that differences in these two factors together accounted for around 50 per cent of the variation in rates by local authority for males and females. It showed that both country/region, and ONS classification Group contributed to the variation in suicide mortality rates by local authority, however, much of the variation was left unexplained.

For males aged 15-44, the pattern of suicide mortality rates by local authority across the United Kingdom was similar to that for all ages (Map 10.26). However, no authorities in London had high rates of death in this age group. Those authorities classified as *Remoter Rural, Coalfields, Manufacturing Centres* or *Ports and Industry* still dominate those with high rates. The average mortality rates by ONS classification Group reflected this pattern.

Figure 10.50 shows suicide mortality for those aged 65 and over by ONS classification Group. For females only the *West Inner London* Group and the *Coast and Country Resorts* Group had significantly higher than average mortality. For males, the *Remoter Rural* Group had the highest rates.

10.9 Alcohol-related mortality and deaths from drug-related poisonings

This section examines geographic variation in deaths from drug-related poisonings and alcohol-related causes. Deaths involving drugs and alcohol can occur under a range of circumstances with varying social and policy implications. The deceased may be a long term drug user or a recreational drug user; the drugs involved may be controlled drugs, prescribed substances, over-the-counter medication, or a mixture and alcohol may also be involved; the death may be due to an accident, suicide and in some cases possible homicide. Therefore, the collection of mortality data on drug-related poisonings and alcohol-related deaths is problematic, and these problems are well documented.[23, 24] Deaths from these causes that have been found to be accidents or suicide are also included in sections 10.7 and 10.8 of this chapter.

There has been an increase in public concern about drug usage, alcohol consumption and the associated risks in recent years. It is widely reported that drug and alcohol misuse are associated with poor health and in extreme cases an increased risk of death.[25, 26, 27, 28] Within England and Scotland, the Government has highlighted alcohol and drug misuse as part of its public health strategy.[1, 2, 3] Drug misuse in the United Kingdom is being tackled by the appointment of the first United Kingdom Anti-drug Co-ordinator, and being matched at a local level by Drug Action Teams. In May 1999 the United Kingdom Anti-drug Co-

---

Box 10.2   Deaths from drug-related poisonings, ONS definition

ICD9 Underlying cause code	Description
292	Drug psychoses
304	Drug dependence
305.2-305.9	Non dependent abuse of drugs
E850-E858	Accidental poisoning by drugs, medicaments and biologicals
E950.0-E950.5	Suicide and self-inflicted poisoning by solid or liquid substances
E980.0-E980.5	Poisoning by solid or liquid substances, undetermined whether accidentally or purposely inflicted
E962.0	Assault by poisoning - drugs and medicaments

ordinator also launched a 10-year strategy for tackling drug misuse.[29] Within England the public health strategy aims to encourage sensible drinking, protect individuals and communities from associated anti-social and criminal behaviour and provide services to enable people to overcome alcohol misuse problems.[1]

Previous studies have reported geographic variation in drug usage. Within England, recent results indicate that the proportion of the population aged 16-29 who have used any drug in the last year was greater in the northern and southern regions, and in London, than the Midlands and eastern England. Wales was reported to have similar levels of drug use to that of eastern England.[30] Previous analysis of drug-related poisonings by Government Office Region in England has

shown that high rates of death are found in the North West for women and men aged 15-44 and for women aged 45 and over. London was also found to have high rates of death for men and women aged 15-44 and for men aged 45 and over. At younger ages low rates of death were found in the Midlands regions and in the south and east of England for men.[23]

For this chapter deaths have been extracted using the current ONS definition of deaths from drug-related poisonings. The causes were selected using the ICD9 codes listed in Box 10.2. The drug-related poisoning deaths for Scotland and Northern Ireland for the basis of this report have been extracted using the same codes as we have used for England and Wales. This is not the standard method of compiling drug-related poisonings currently in use in Scotland and Northern Ireland. For this

Table 10.23

Age-standardised mortality rates for drug-related poisonings by country and region, males
United Kingdom 1991-1997

	rates per 100,000			
	overall	15-44	45-64	65+
United Kingdom	6	10	5	4
England	~6	~10	5	4
North East	~5	~8	5	5
North West	*8	*15	6	4
Yorkshire and the Humber	6	10	5	4
East Midlands	~4	~6	~4	4
West Midlands	~4	~6	4	4
East	~5	~8	4	4
London	*7	*12	*6	4
South East	~5	~8	~4	4
South West	~5	~9	5	3
Wales	~5	9	~3	~3
Scotland	*9	*17	*7	5
Northern Ireland	~4	~5	*7	6

* significantly higher than the United Kingdom rate
~ significantly lower than the United Kingdom rate

Table 10.24

Age-standardised mortality rates for drug-related poisonings by country and region, females
United Kingdom 1991-1997

	rates per 100,000			
	overall	15-44	45-64	65+
United Kingdom	3	4	4	4
England	~3	~4	4	4
North East	3	4	5	3
North West	*4	*5	5	4
Yorkshire and the Humber	3	4	5	4
East Midlands	~3	~3	4	~3
West Midlands	~3	~3	~3	5
East	~2	~3	~3	5
London	*4	5	5	*5
South East	~3	~3	4	5
South West	~3	~3	4	4
Wales	~3	4	4	4
Scotland	*5	*7	*6	4
Northern Ireland	3	~3	*7	~3

* significantly higher than the United Kingdom rate
~ significantly lower than the United Kingdom rate

reason differences between figures published in this report and those published by the General Register Office for Scotland (GROS) and the General Register Office for Northern Ireland (GRONI) may be observed. Although the method of extraction of deaths was the same for all four countries in this chapter, differences in the method of certifying and coding deaths from drug-related poisoning by country may bring about artificial differences in the level of mortality reported. In particular, in Scotland an active search for drug involvement in deaths is carried out which may inflate death rates in Scotland relative to the rest of the United Kingdom.

Noble examined the relationship between mortality and alcohol consumption from 1979 to 1992.[24] The results show that overall alcohol-related mortality rates for both men and women had barely increased over the period. The General Household Survey[31] and the Health Survey for England[32] both include questions related to alcohol consumption. The results from the 1984 to 1996 General Household Surveys show that alcohol consumption has remained relatively constant for men, but has gradually increased for women in the same period. Similar results were seen from the Health Survey for England for 1993 to 1996. Chapter 3 of this volume (Figure 3.24) shows alcohol consumption by country of the United Kingdom and region of England. There was little variation in alcohol consumption by country, but those in the North West of England and males in the North East were shown to consume more than those in the southern regions of England.

Table 10.25

Age-standardised mortality rates for alcohol-related deaths by country and region, males
United Kingdom 1991-1997

| | rates per 100,000 | | | |
	overall	15-44	45-64	65+
United Kingdom	11	5	23	24
England	~9	~4	~20	~22
North East	11	5	26	23
North West	*13	*6	*29	25
Yorkshire and the Humber	~8	~4	~16	~18
East Midlands	~7	~4	~14	~18
West Midlands	~10	5	~20	~22
East	~7	~3	~13	~19
London	*14	*6	*31	*30
South East	~8	~3	~17	24
South West	~8	~4	~16	~21
Wales	10	5	23	24
Scotland	*21	*9	*50	*44
Northern Ireland	11	5	25	20

* significantly higher than the United Kingdom rate
~ significantly lower than the United Kingdom rate

Table 10.26

Age-standardised mortality rates for alcohol-related deaths by country and region, females
United Kingdom 1991-1997

| | rates per 100,000 | | | |
	overall	15-44	45-64	65+
United Kingdom	6	2	13	15
England	~5	~2	~11	~14
North East	5	2	11	16
North West	*7	*3	*16	17
Yorkshire and the Humber	~4	~2	~9	~12
East Midlands	~5	~2	~10	14
West Midlands	6	2	11	15
East	~4	~1	~8	~12
London	*7	3	*15	17
South East	~5	~2	~10	14
South West	~4	~2	~9	~13
Wales	6	3	12	17
Scotland	*11	*4	*25	*22
Northern Ireland	6	3	14	15

* significantly higher than the United Kingdom rate
~ significantly lower than the United Kingdom rate

A description of the causes of death and the ICD9 codes that are used in this chapter to represent alcohol-related mortality are listed in Box 10.3.

Variations between countries and regions

Tables 10.23 to 10.26 show age-standardised mortality rates from drug-related poisoning and alcohol-related deaths in the United Kingdom by country and region 1991-1997. The geographic pattern of mortality was similar, though not identical for both drug-related poisoning and alcohol-related mortality.

Scotland had the highest rates of alcohol-related mortality in all the age groups for both males and females. Generally mortality rates in Scotland were around twice the rates in other countries. For drug-related poisoning, Scotland had the highest all-age rate and the highest rate in young adults aged 15-44 for both males and females. Male mortality in Scotland in the 15-44 age group was over three times the rate in Northern Ireland. Mortality from drug-related poisonings among 45-64 year old adults shows a different pattern, Northern Ireland had similar rates to Scotland. Mortality from both of these causes in England and Wales was either lower than or very similar to mortality in the United Kingdom as a whole for both sexes and for all age groups examined.

There was a large increase in both alcohol-related deaths and drug-related poisonings for males in every country over the period studied, but the geographic pattern has not changed substantially. In most cases, Scotland's rate appeared to diverge from the other countries. Smaller increases were seen for females (Figures 10.51-10.54). Due to the small number of deaths involved, the trends are not shown for individual age groups.

Tables 10.23 to 10.26 show that within England, generally the North West and London were the regions that had the highest levels of alcohol-related deaths and deaths from drug-related poisonings. Rates for alcohol-related deaths in the regions with the highest rates were about double the rates in the regions with the lowest rates across all age groups, although the difference was smaller in those aged 65 and over. For drug-related poisonings in those aged 65 and over, although rates in London are still high, other regions also had equally high rates.

These different geographic patterns by age group are likely to be due to differences in the percentage of deaths due to

different substances. Deaths involving drugs of abuse, antidepressants and paracetamol show different age-specific patterns. Previous analysis within England and Wales has shown that in the age groups below 45, death rates for males are higher for heroin and/or morphine, and methadone than for other substances. It is at these age groups where the most variation between countries and regions was seen in this analysis. For males over the age of 45, death rates are generally higher for paracetamol and antidepressants. For females, death rates from paracetamol and antidepressants are higher than drugs of abuse at every age group.[33] For females and for those aged over 45, results from this analysis show there was less variation in mortality between countries and regions.

Figures 10.55 to 10.58 show that mortality rates increased in the majority of regions over the period studied for both alcohol-related mortality and deaths from drug-related poisonings for males and for alcohol-related mortality for females. For drug-related poisonings for males, mortality rates in the regions in the rest of England, except the Midlands regions were becoming closer to those in London and the North West. It is difficult to discern trends for females, as the numbers involved are quite small (Figure 10.56), however, there is some evidence of a decline in female drug-related poisonings in London. Previous analysis showed that most of the increase in deaths from drug-related poisonings in England and Wales in the 1990s was due to an increase in deaths from heroin and/or morphine, and methadone poisoning.[33]

Variations between local authorities

For all ages, for males the pattern of mortality from drug-related poisonings was very different to that seen for all causes of death (Map 10.27). Reflecting the strong regional differences presented above, authorities with high rates of death were concentrated in inner London, and around Glasgow and Manchester. In addition, some authorities throughout the rest of England had high rates, particularly on the south coast. No authorities in Northern Ireland had higher rates than the United Kingdom as a whole.

For alcohol-related deaths the pattern of authorities with high rates was not dissimilar to that for drug-related poisonings in England. Generally more authorities in west London had high rates than for drug-related poisonings and fewer authorities around Manchester. However a larger number of authorities in Scotland had high alcohol-related death rates including the island councils and the Highlands (Map 10.28).

Box 10.3   Deaths from alcohol-related causes, ONS definition

ICD9 Underlying cause code	Description
291	Alcoholic psychoses
303	Alcohol dependence syndrome
305.0	Non-dependent abuse of alcohol
425.5	Alcoholic cardiomyopathy
571	Chronic liver disease and cirrhosis
E860	Accidental poisoning by alcohol

Figure 10.51

Trends in age-standardised mortality rates for drug-related poisonings by country, males all ages United Kingdom 1992-1996*

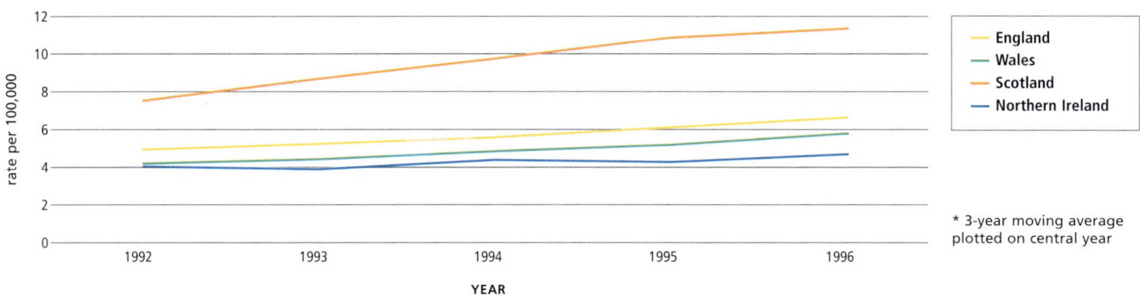

Figure 10.52

Trends in age-standardised mortality rates for drug-related poisonings by country, females all ages United Kingdom 1992-1996*

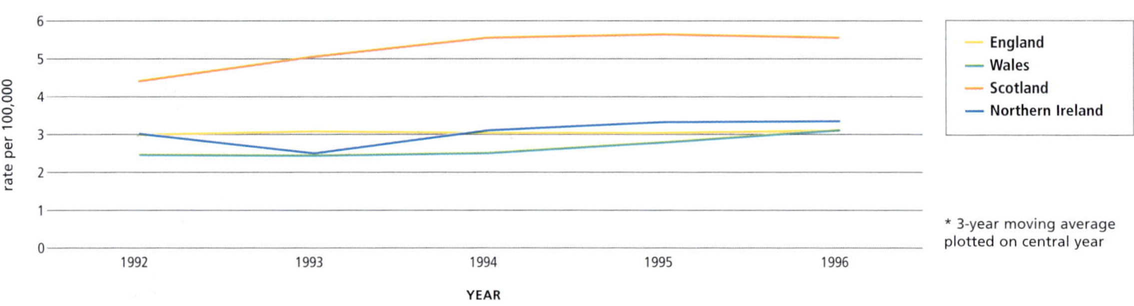

Figure 10.53

Trends in age-standardised mortality rates for alcohol-related deaths by country, males all ages United Kingdom 1992-1996*

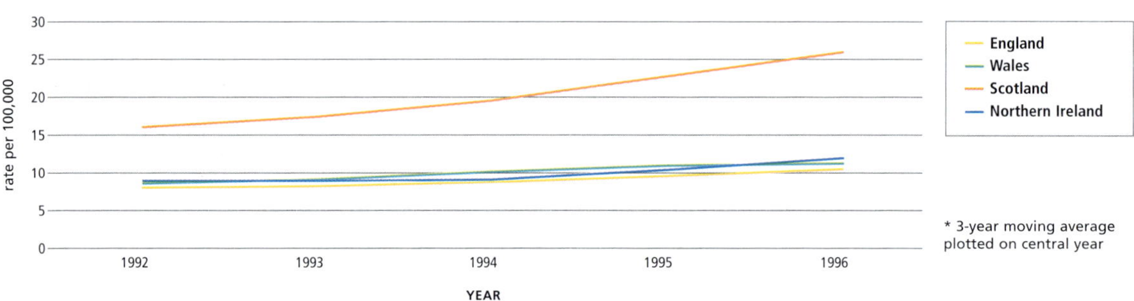

Figure 10.54

Trends in age-standardised mortality rates for alcohol-related deaths by country, females all ages United Kingdom 1992-1996*

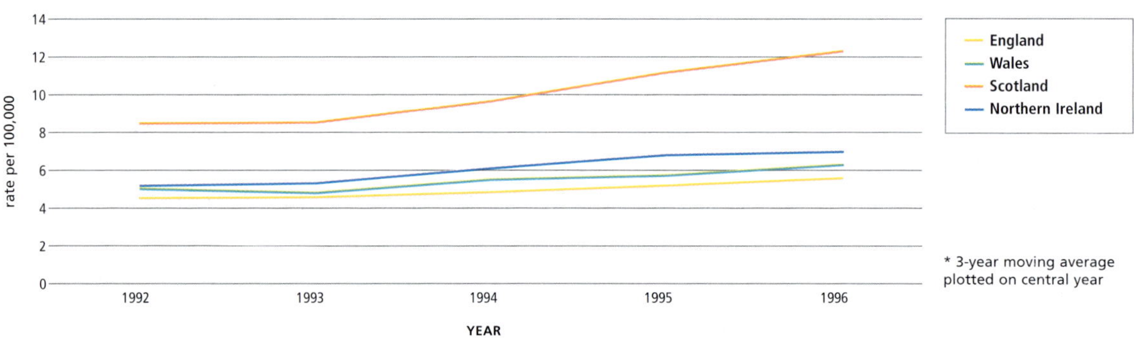

Figure 10.55

Trends in age-standardised mortality rates for drug-related poisonings by region, males all ages England 1992-1996*

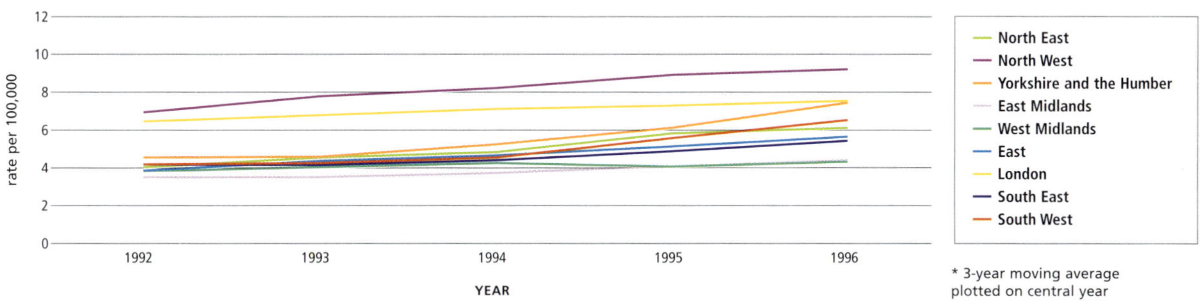

Figure 10.56

Trends in age-standardised mortality rates for drug-related poisonings by region, females all ages England 1992-1996*

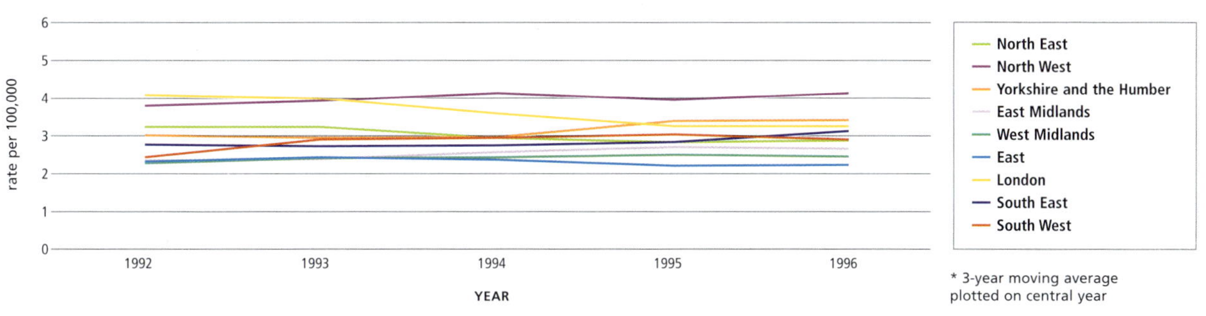

Figure 10.57

Trends in age-standardised mortality rates for alcohol-related deaths by region, males all ages England 1992-1996*

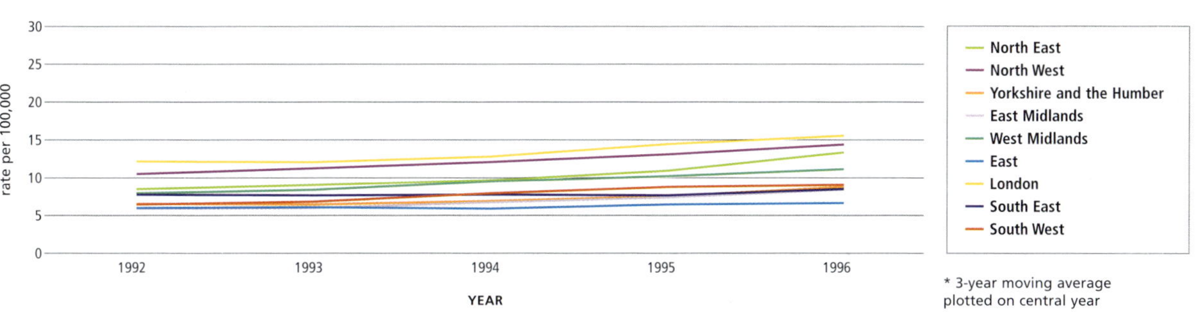

Figure 10.58

Trends in age-standardised mortality rates for alcohol-related deaths by region, females all ages England 1992-1996*

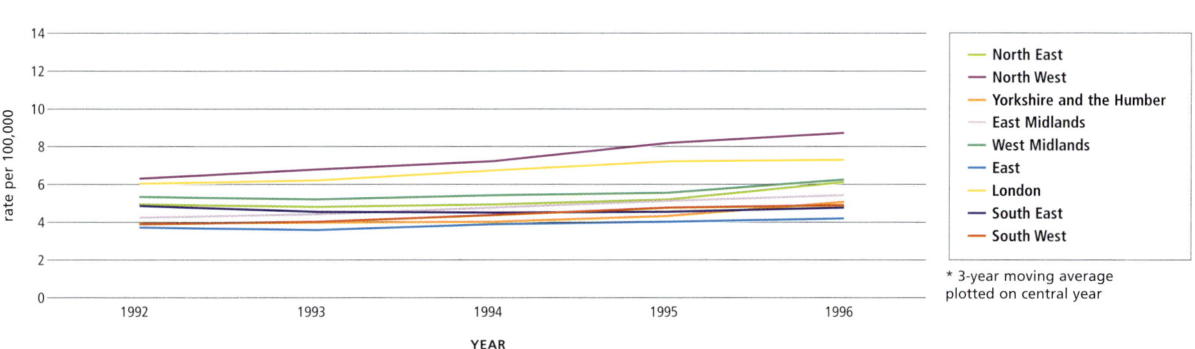

Map 10.27

Age-standardised mortality rates for drug-related poisonings by local authority, males all ages
United Kingdom 1991-1997

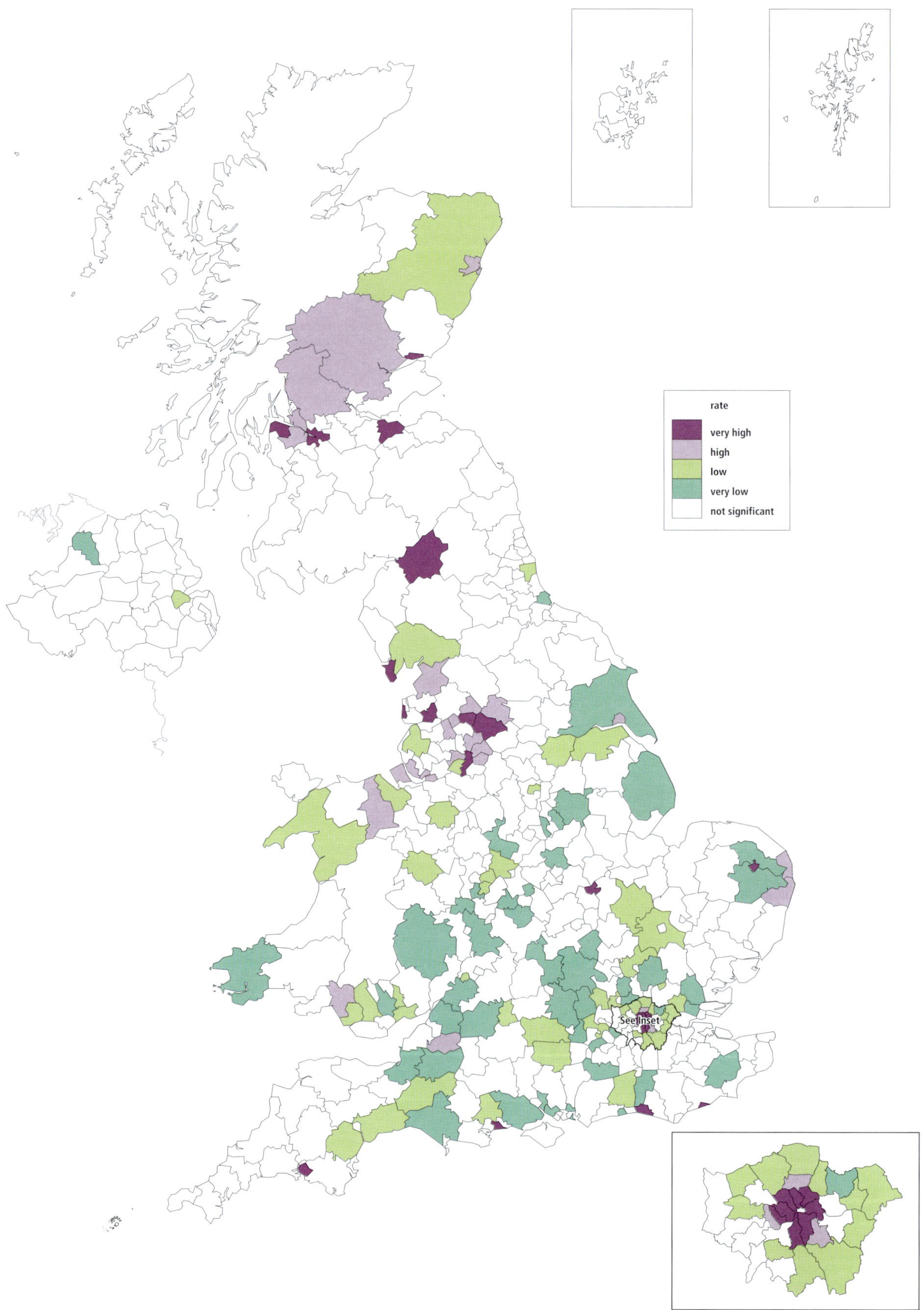

Map 10.28

Age-standardised mortality rates for alcohol-related deaths by local authority, males all ages
United Kingdom 1991-1997

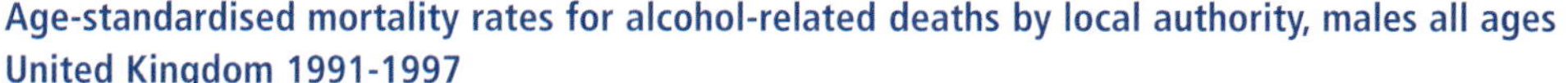

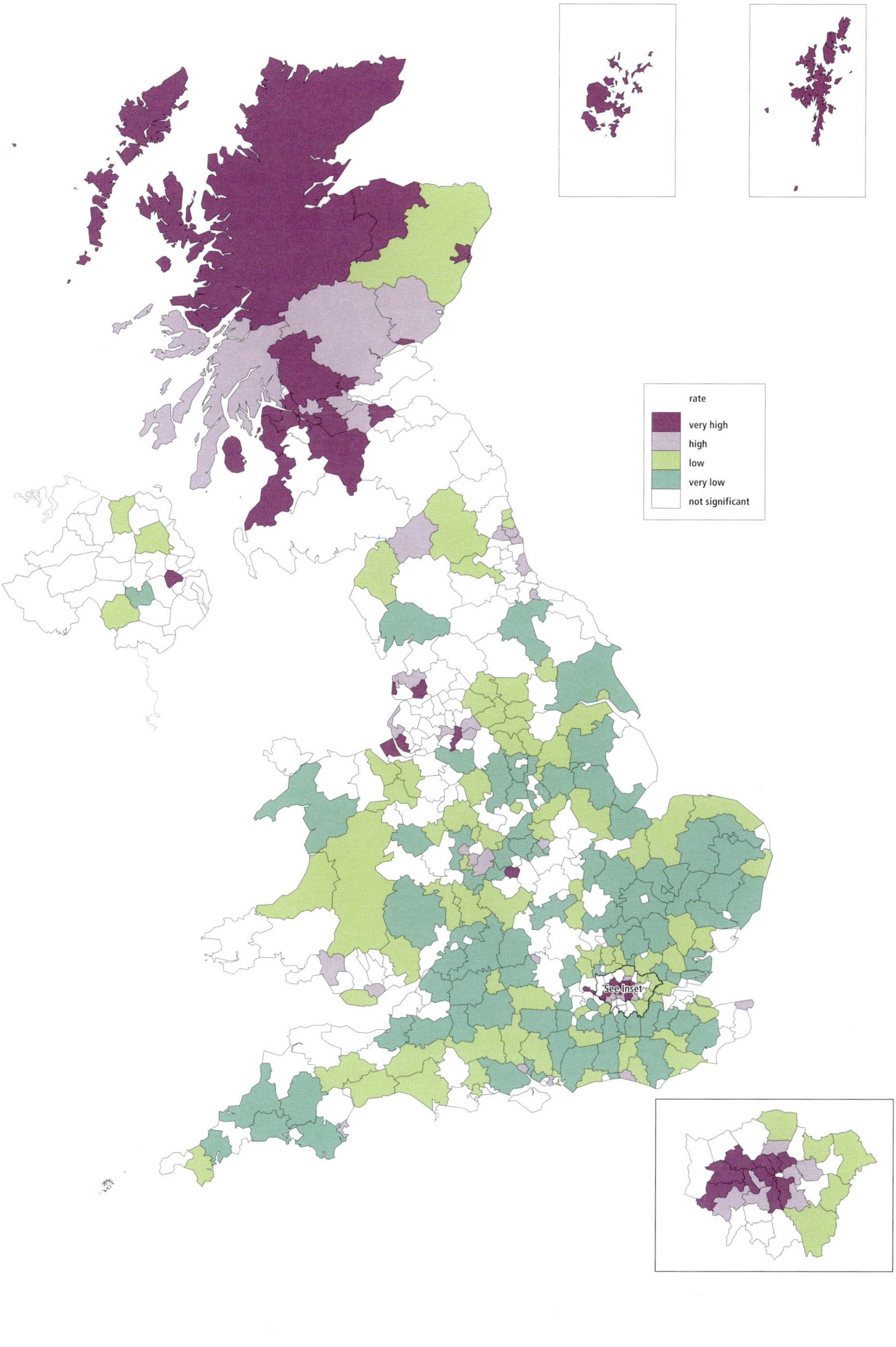

Map 10.29

Age-standardised mortality rates for drug-related poisonings by local authority, females all ages
United Kingdom 1991-1997

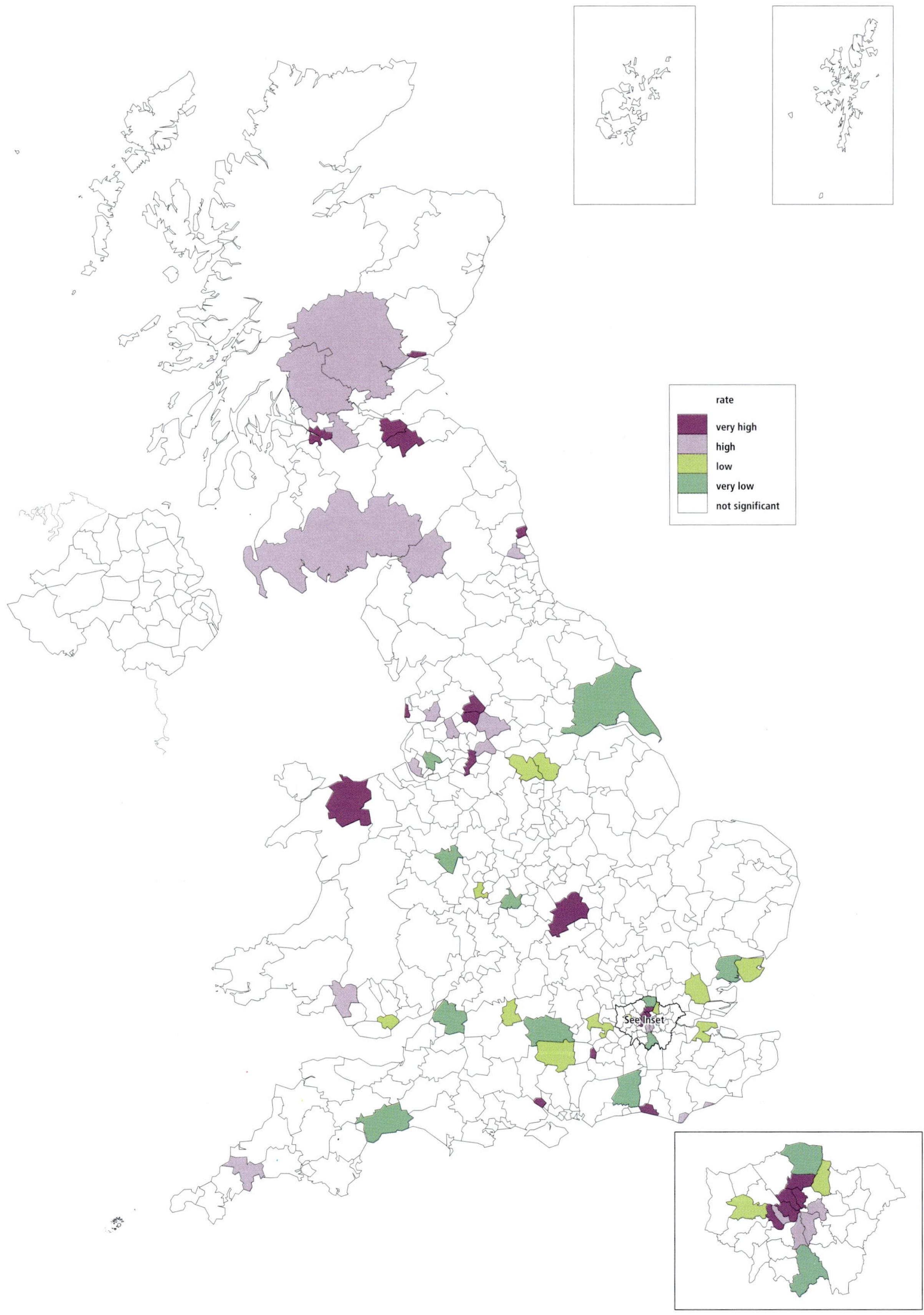

Map 10.30

Age-standardised mortality rates for alcohol-related deaths by local authority, females all ages
United Kingdom 1991-1997

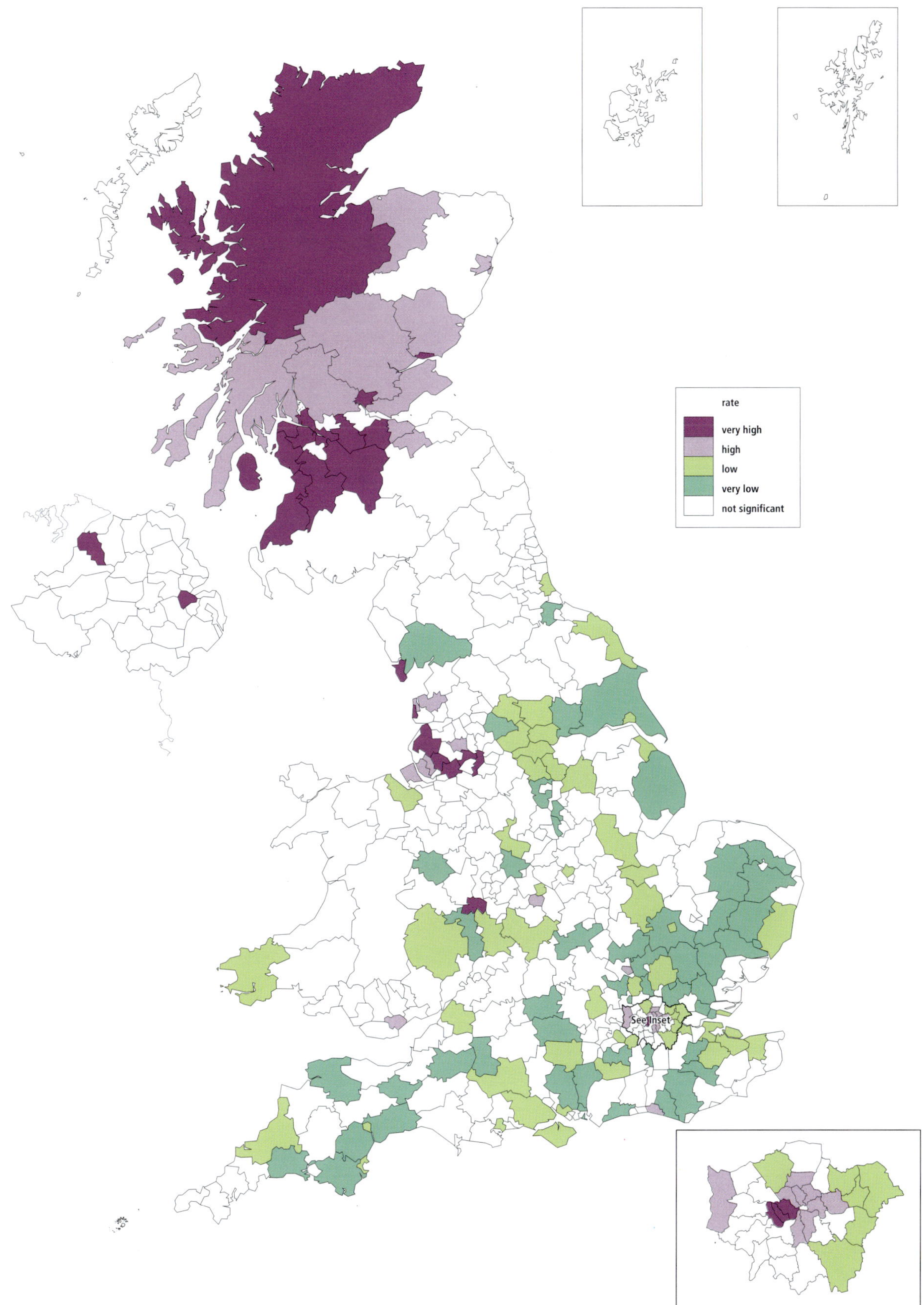

As for all causes, a large proportion of authorities with very high mortality rates were found in urban and early industrial areas. For both causes, half of the authorities with very high rates outside London and Northern Ireland were classified as *Coalfields*, *Manufacturing Centres* or *Ports and Industry*. However, unlike the pattern for all-cause mortality, no *Remoter Rural* areas had high mortality from drug-related deaths. For alcohol-related causes, three *Remoter Rural* areas in Scotland, the Shetland Islands, Orkney Islands and Eilean Siar, had very high mortality. No *Remoter Rural* areas outside Scotland had very high mortality rates from alcohol-related causes. In addition two authorities in the *Education Centres and Outer London* Group in Scotland had very high rates from alcohol-related causes, City of Edinburgh and Aberdeen City. No authorities in this Group outside Scotland had very high rates.

Authorities with low rates from both these causes were scattered mainly around England and Wales, away from major urban areas, although there was a ring of authorities with low rates in outer London from both of these causes. No authorities in Scotland had very low mortality rates from alcohol-related

causes and only one had low mortality rates, Aberdeenshire. Areas with low rates of drug and alcohol-related mortality were found in many different classification Groups, although around half of those with very low rates outside London and Northern Ireland were classified as *Growth Areas*.

The pattern of mortality across the United Kingdom for all-age mortality from alcohol and drug-related causes for females was broadly similar to that seen for males (Map 10.29 and 10.30) although fewer authorities had rates that differed significantly from the rate in the United Kingdom as a whole. No authorities in Scotland or Northern Ireland had low mortality rates for females from either of these causes. For drug-related causes, the clusters of authorities with high rates were in similar areas to those seen for males, however, there were fewer authorities on the south coast of England with high rates.

Despite the differences in the maps presented in this section, if we examine the level of mortality from drug-related and alcohol-related causes for the 15 ONS classification Groups for males and females separately a similar pattern emerges for the

Figure 10.59

Age-standardised mortality rates for drug-related poisonings by ONS classification Group, all ages Great Britain 1991-1997

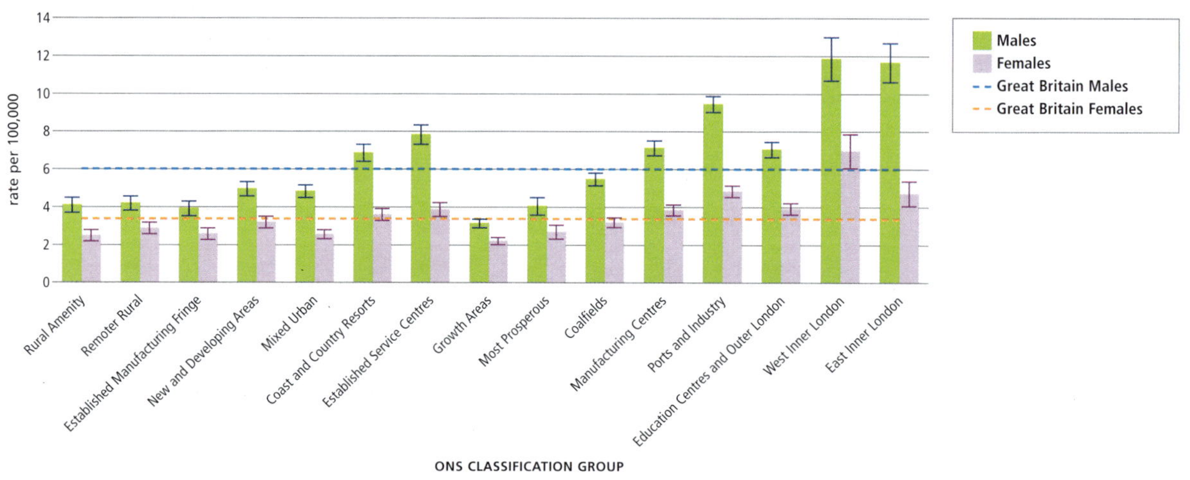

Figure 10.60

Age-standardised mortality rates for alcohol-related deaths by ONS classification Group, all ages Great Britain 1991-1997

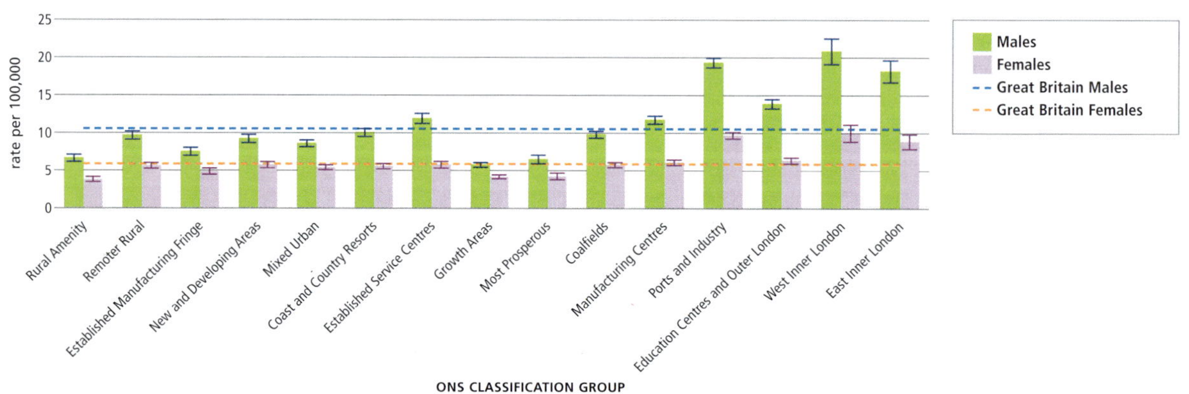

two causes (Figures 10.59 and 10.60). For both males and females the Groups with the highest rates are *Ports and Industry*, *West Inner London* and *East Inner London*. Generally the Groups with the lowest rates are *Growth Areas* and *Most Prosperous*. The pattern differs from the pattern for all causes of death where the *Coalfields* and the *Manufacturing Centres* Groups also had high mortality. The pattern by ONS classification Group is strongly related to the regional pattern. The *Ports and Industry* Group is one of the most geographically concentrated Groups with over 40 per cent of its population located in Scotland and a further 20 per cent in the North West. Authorities classified as *West Inner London* and *East Inner London* are entirely located within inner London. Scotland, the North West and London as a whole have been shown to have high mortality from drug-related poisonings and alcohol-related causes. It is the authorities in the Groups above that account for the excess mortality in these regions.

An analysis of variance was conducted to examine how much of the variation in all-age drug-related poisoning and alcohol-related mortality rates by local authority in Great Britain was accounted for by the country or region of location (country/region) and how much was accounted for by the ONS classification Group to which the local authority belonged. The analysis showed that differences in these two factors accounted for between 50 and 70 per cent of the variation in rates by local authority for males and females. It showed that both country/region, and ONS classification Group contributed to the variation in mortality rates from these causes by local authority, however, as expected the effect of ONS classification Group was much stronger than the effect of country/region.

10.10 Discussion

This chapter has demonstrated clear differences in all-cause mortality rates for various causes of death by country, region of England and local authority in the United Kingdom. In general, Scotland, Wales and Northern Ireland had higher mortality than England for most age groups studied and the analysis of regional mortality within England confirms findings from other studies of a north-south divide in mortality at this level.[34] However, we have also demonstrated that within the countries of the United Kingdom and within the regions of England there were substantial differences in the mortality rates for local authorities. The majority of authorities with the highest rates tended to be found in urban and industrial areas and classified as *Ports and Industry*, *Manufacturing Centres* and *Coalfields*. The characteristics of the authorities in these Groups include: a high percentage of the population that is unemployed, a high proportion of the population living in social housing and terraced housing and a high proportion of the population in Social Classes IV and V. Various studies looking at the mortality risk of individuals have found that those who are unemployed, those who live in rented accommodation and those in the lower Social Classes have higher than average mortality.[35, 36, 37]

Although both country and region of location, and ONS classification Group help to explain the variation in mortality

rates for local authorities in Great Britain, the effect of ONS classification Group explains much more of the variation than country/region. This indicates that the combination of factors measured by the ONS classification Groups such as type of housing, employment conditions and specific location factors (such as port, seaside or country) were more strongly correlated with mortality rates than the regional location of the local authority.

This is also evident if we compare the pattern of mortality to the socio-economic characteristics of the population presented in chapter 3. The pattern of mortality by local authority is very similar to the pattern of the percentage of the population in Social Class IV or V and high unemployment presented in Maps 3.6 and 3.7. Areas with a high proportion of the population in these classes or a high proportion unemployed tended to have higher than average mortality. In addition, there is some relationship to the geographic pattern of children living in lone parent households as presented in Map 3.12 in chapter 3. Areas with a high proportion of children living in lone parent households tended to have higher than average mortality, as did areas with a high proportion of the population without access to a car (Map 3.16). Chapter 12 examines the relationship between car access and mortality within countries and regions of the United Kingdom.

Therefore, some of the differences in mortality rates between countries of Great Britain and regions of England can be explained by the characteristics of the individual authorities within these countries and regions in terms of both the individuals living within the areas and characteristics of the areas themselves. Countries and regions with a high percentage of the population living in authorities which were classified as *Ports and Industry*, *Manufacturing Centres* and *Coalfields* had higher mortality than countries and regions with a low proportion of authorities in this Group. For example, the North East of England had the highest percentage of its population living in authorities classified to these Groups and the North East had the highest mortality rates of all the regions of England.

We have not been able to measure the effect of migration on the mortality rates presented in this chapter. Analysis in the previous Decennial Supplement on geography found that generally, on average, migrants have higher mortality than non-migrants. However, movers into more affluent areas tend to have similar or lower mortality than the area they moved into and therefore the pattern of mortality for migrants across the country and the effect of migration on mortality rates in the area of origin and destination is not straightforward.[38]

The geographic variation in IHD and stroke mortality was broadly similar to the patterns presented for all causes. However, there are some notable differences. Firstly, for IHD mortality, the main difference was that for males aged 45-64, London had lower mortality than the United Kingdom as a whole, whereas for all causes London had higher mortality than the United Kingdom as a whole. This was also demonstrated by the patterns for ONS classification Groups and local authorities.

Various studies have tried to explain the low mortality rates in London from heart disease in comparison with other causes of death. One such study concluded that this is likely to be due to differences in standards of living early in life and the fact that maternal health and nutrition in London was very good in the early part of the 20th century, principally due to the large numbers of women migrating to London and taking up jobs in domestic service.[39] However, another study has demonstrated that migrants to London also acquire low mortality rates from heart disease.[40] In addition, various studies have shown a negative association between water hardness and the risk of cardiovascular disease mortality and a positive association between temperature and rainfall and risk of cardiovascular disease.[41] Water in London and the South East is much harder than elsewhere in Great Britain,[42] but rainfall is around average for Great Britain.[42]

The reverse was true for stroke mortality in those aged 45-64; parts of London had very high rates of death. ONS classification Groups with high mortality rates from stroke in those aged 45-64 were *Ports and Industry, Manufacturing Centres, West Inner London* and *East Inner London*. Factors known to be associated with increased stroke mortality are socio-economic deprivation and ethnicity as well as other lifestyle factors such as smoking and drinking.[43, 44] All these ONS classification Groups mentioned here have a higher than average proportion of the population from minority ethnic groups and socio-economic characteristics associated with material deprivation.

The findings presented in this chapter are consistent with other studies of geographic variations in cancer mortality, with the incidence data presented in chapter 9 of this volume and with previous analysis of cancer survival.[16] Geographic variations in lung cancer presented here are similar to the pattern presented for all causes of death, however, there are some differences between the pattern for all causes and geographic variation in colorectal, prostate and breast cancer. At country and regional level, there was no clear north-south pattern in mortality from colorectal cancer and local authorities with high rates were less concentrated in urban areas.

For breast cancer there was little variation in mortality by country, region, local authority and ONS classification Group. The reasons for this are complex. Geographic variation in the incidence of breast cancer presented in chapter 9 shows that those in the more affluent parts of the United Kingdom had higher than average incidence of breast cancer. However, studies have shown that the more affluent areas also had higher than average survival from breast cancer, possibly resulting in less geographic variation in mortality from breast cancer.[16, 45, 46]

There was also little variation in prostate cancer mortality at country level, but within England it was the southern regions that experienced the highest rates. Local authorities with high mortality rates from prostate cancer are located away from

urban areas and analysis by ONS classification Group shows that those areas classified as *Most Prosperous* and *Growth Areas* had higher than average mortality. Further discussion of variations in cancer incidence and its relationship to mortality can be found in chapter 9.

For infectious and respiratory diseases the striking point to note is the high mortality in London. For infectious diseases the mortality rate in London also increased much faster than all other regions. For males aged 15-44, London stood out as having substantially higher mortality from infectious and respiratory diseases than the other regions of England. Analysis of the impact of HIV on mortality of men aged 15-54 in London has shown that in 1996 HIV was the leading cause of death in inner London. Excluding HIV-related deaths from analysis of trends reduced the increasing mortality in this age group in London to a flat trend showing no change over time.[47] The impact of HIV on mortality rates in London is therefore very important in this age group.

High accident mortality was experienced by the majority of authorities in Scotland and Northern Ireland and a large number in Wales indicating that higher than average mortality from accidents was less concentrated in urban areas than all cause mortality. Few local authorities in England had higher than average mortality, except for a cluster of authorities in the east of England, which was not seen for all causes of death. Unlike the analysis of all-cause mortality, country/region and ONS classification Group explained equal amounts of the variation in accident mortality. Thus, country/region was more highly correlated with accident mortality than with all-cause mortality.

The pattern of suicide mortality across the United Kingdom was different to that presented for all causes of death where authorities with high mortality were largely confined to urban and industrial areas. Local authorities with high suicide mortality were largely confined to Scotland and Wales, along with scattered authorities in the North West of England, London and the south coast of England. This is reflected in the pattern of mortality by ONS classification Group where many Groups, not just those containing urban authorities, had higher than average rates of suicide mortality. Previous analysis examining the association between suicide and area-based deprivation and social fragmentation (using an index comprised from private renting, single person households, unmarried persons and mobility) at the parliamentary constituency level showed that suicide mortality was more strongly associated with social fragmentation than deprivation, whereas deaths from other causes were more closely related to deprivation.[48] Therefore, suicide is unlikely to follow the same pattern by ONS classification Group as other causes of death.

Analysis by local authority indicates that high rates of drug-related poisonings were largely confined to inner London, Glasgow and Manchester. The pattern for alcohol-related mortality was similar, although authorities with higher than average mortality in Scotland were not confined to the area immediately surrounding Glasgow. Many other local authorities in Scotland also had high levels of alcohol-related mortality.

Chapters 11 and 12 of this volume extend the analysis presented in this chapter. Chapter 11 examines the relationship between deprivation and mortality within countries and regions of Great Britain. Chapter 12 looks at variation within countries and regions of the United Kingdom by individual Social Class and variation within England and Wales by alternative social classifications.

References

1 Department of Health. White Paper. *Saving Lives: Our Healthier Nation* The Stationery Office (London: 1999).

2 Department of Health. White Paper. *The NHS Plan*. The Stationery Office (London: 2000).

3 Scottish Executive. White Paper. *Towards a Healthier Scotland*. The Stationery Office (Edinburgh: 1999).

4 Department of Health, Social Security and Personal Services. *Investing for Health*. Department of Health, Social Security and Personal Services (Belfast: 2000).

5 Welsh Office. *Better Health Better Wales*. The Stationery Office (Cardiff: 1998).

6 Cabinet Office. Report. *Sharing the Nation's Prosperity. Variation in Economic and Social Conditions Across the United Kingdom*. Cabinet Office (London: 1999).

7 Drever F and Whitehead M. Mortality in regions and local authority districts in the 1990s: exploring the relationship with deprivation. *Population Trends* 82 (1995), 19-26.

8 Charlton J. Which areas are healthiest? *Population Trends* 83 (1996), 17-24.

9 Howarth C, Kenway P, Palmer G and Miorelli R. *Monitoring poverty and social exclusion 1999*. Joseph Rowntree Foundation (York: 1999).

10 Shaw M, Dorling D, Gordon D and Davey Smith G. *The widening gap. Health inequalities and policy in Britain*. The Policy Press (Bristol: 1999).

11 Office for National Statistics. *The ONS classification of local and health authorities: revised for authorities in 1999*. The Stationery Office (London: 1999).

12 Marmot MG. Life style and national and international trends in coronary heart disease mortality. *Postgraduate Medical Journal* 60 (1984), 3-8.

13 Barker DJ and Osmond C. Infant mortality, childhood nutrition and ischaemic heart disease in England and Wales. *Lancet* 8489 (1986), 1077-1081.

14 Marmot M and Wilkinson R (ed.) *Social determinants of health*. Oxford University Press (Oxford: 1999).

15 Quinn MJ, Babb P, Brock A, Kirby L and Jones J. *Cancer trends in England and Wales 1950-1999*. The Stationery Office (London: 2001).

16 Coleman MP, Babb P, Damiecki P, Grosclaude P, Honjo S, Jones J, Knerer G, Pitard A, Quinn M, Sloggett A and De Stavola B. *Cancer survival trends in England and Wales 1991-1995*. The Stationery Office (London: 1999).

17 Scottish Cancer Intelligence Unit. *Trends in cancer survival in Scotland 1971-1995*. ISD Publications (Edinburgh: 2000).

18 Office of Population Censuses and Surveys. Series DH2 1993/1994.

19 Rooney C and Devis T. Mortality Trends in England and Wales 1980-1994: the impact of introducing automated cause coding and related changes in 1993. *Population Trends* 86 (1996), 29-35.

20 Christophersen O, Dix D and Rooney C. Road traffic deaths: trends and comparisons with DETR figures. *Health Statistics Quarterly* 3 (1998), 14-23.

21 Charlton J, Kelly S, Dunnell K, Evans B, Jenkins R and Wallis R. Trends in suicide deaths in England and Wales. *Population Trends* 69 (1992), 10-16.

22 Bunting J and Kelly S. Geographic variations in suicide mortality, 1982-1996. *Population Trends* 93(1998), 7-18.

23 Christopherson O, Rooney C and Kelly S. (1998) Drug-related mortality: methods and trends. *Population Trends* 93 (1998), 1-9.

24 Noble B. Deaths associated with the use of alcohol, drugs, and volatile substances. *Population Trends* 76 (1994), 7-17.

25 Plant M. Trends in alcohol and illicit drug-related diseases, in Charlton J and Murphy M. (eds.) *The Health of Adult Britain 1841-1994, Volume 1*. The Stationery Office (London: 1997), 114-127.

26 Royal College of Physicians. *The great growing evil: the medical consequences of alcohol abuse*. Tavistock (London: 1999).

27 Vershuren P. (ed.) *Health issues related to alcohol consumption*. ILSI Press (Brussels: 1993).

28 Holder HD and Edwards G. *Alcohol and Public Policy: evidence and issues*. Oxford University Press (Oxford: 1995).

29 Cabinet Office. White Paper. *Tackling drugs to build a better Britain: The Government's 10-year strategy for tackling drugs misuse*. The Stationery Office (London: 1998).

30 Home Office. *Drug Misuse Declared in 1998: results from the British Crime Survey*. Home Office (London: 1999).

31 Office for National Statistics. *Living in Britain. Results from the 1996 General Household Survey*. The Stationery Office (London: 1998).

32 Department of Health. *Health Survey for England 1996*. The Stationery Office (London: 1998).

33 Office for National Statistics. Report: Deaths related to drug poisoning: results for England and Wales 1994-1998. *Health Statistics Quarterly* 7 (2000), 83-86.

34 Illsley R and Le Grand J. Regional inequalities in mortality. *Journal of Epidemiology and Community Health* 47 (1993), 444-449.

35 Drever F and Bunting J. Patterns and trends in male mortality. In Drever F and Whitehead M. (eds.) *Health Inequalities*. Series DS No. 15. The Stationery Office (London: 1997), 95-107.

36 Bethune A. Unemployment and mortality. In Drever F and Whitehead M. (eds.) *Health Inequalities*. Series DS No. 15. The Stationery Office (London: 1997), 156-167.

37 Goldblatt PO. Mortality and alternative social classifications. In Goldblatt PO. (ed.) *Longitudinal Study: mortality and social organisation 1971-1981*. Series LS No. 6. HMSO (London: 1990), 164-192.

38 Britton M, Goldblatt PO, Jones DR and Rosato M. The influence of migration on geographic variation in mortality. In Britton M. (ed.) *Mortality and Geography: a review in the mid 1980s. England and Wales*. Series DS No. 9. HMSO (London: 1990), 79-94.

39 Barker D, Osmond C and Pannett B. Why Londoners have low death rates from ischaemic heart disease and stroke. *British Medical Journal* 305 (1992), 1551-1553.

40 Strachan DP, Leon DA and Dodgeon B. Mortality from cardiovascular disease among interregional migrants in England and Wales. *British Medical Journal* 310 (1995), 423-427.

41 Shaper A. Geographic variations in cardiovascular mortality in Great Britain. *British Medical Bulletin* 40 (1984), 366-373.

42 Office for National Statistics. *Regional Trends* 34. The Stationery Office (London: 1999).

43 Maheswaran R, Elliott P and Strachan D. Socio-economic deprivation, ethnicity and stroke mortality in Greater London and south east England. J*ournal of Epidemiology and Community Health* 51 (1997), 127-131.

44 Balarajan R. Ethnic differences in mortality from ischaemic heart disease and cerebrovascular disease in England and Wales. *British Medical Journal* 302 (1991), 560-564.

45 Schrijvers J, Mackenbach J, Lutz J, Quinn M and Coleman M. Deprivation and survival from breast cancer. *British Journal of Cancer* 72 (1995), 738-743.

46 Goodwin J, Freeman J, Freeman D and Nattinger A. Geographic variations in breast cancer mortality: do higher rates imply elevated incidence or poorer survival? *American Journal of Public Health* 88 (1998), 458-460.

47 Hickman M, Bardsley M, De Angelis D and Ward H. Impact of HIV on adult (15-54) mortality in London: 1979-96. *Sexually Transmitted Infections* 75 (1999), 385-388

48 Whitley M, Gunnell D, Dorling D and Davey Smith G. Ecological study of social fragmentation, poverty and suicide. *British Medical Journa*l 319 (1999), 1034-1037.

Analysis of mortality by deprivation and cause of death

Zoe Uren and Justine Fitzpatrick

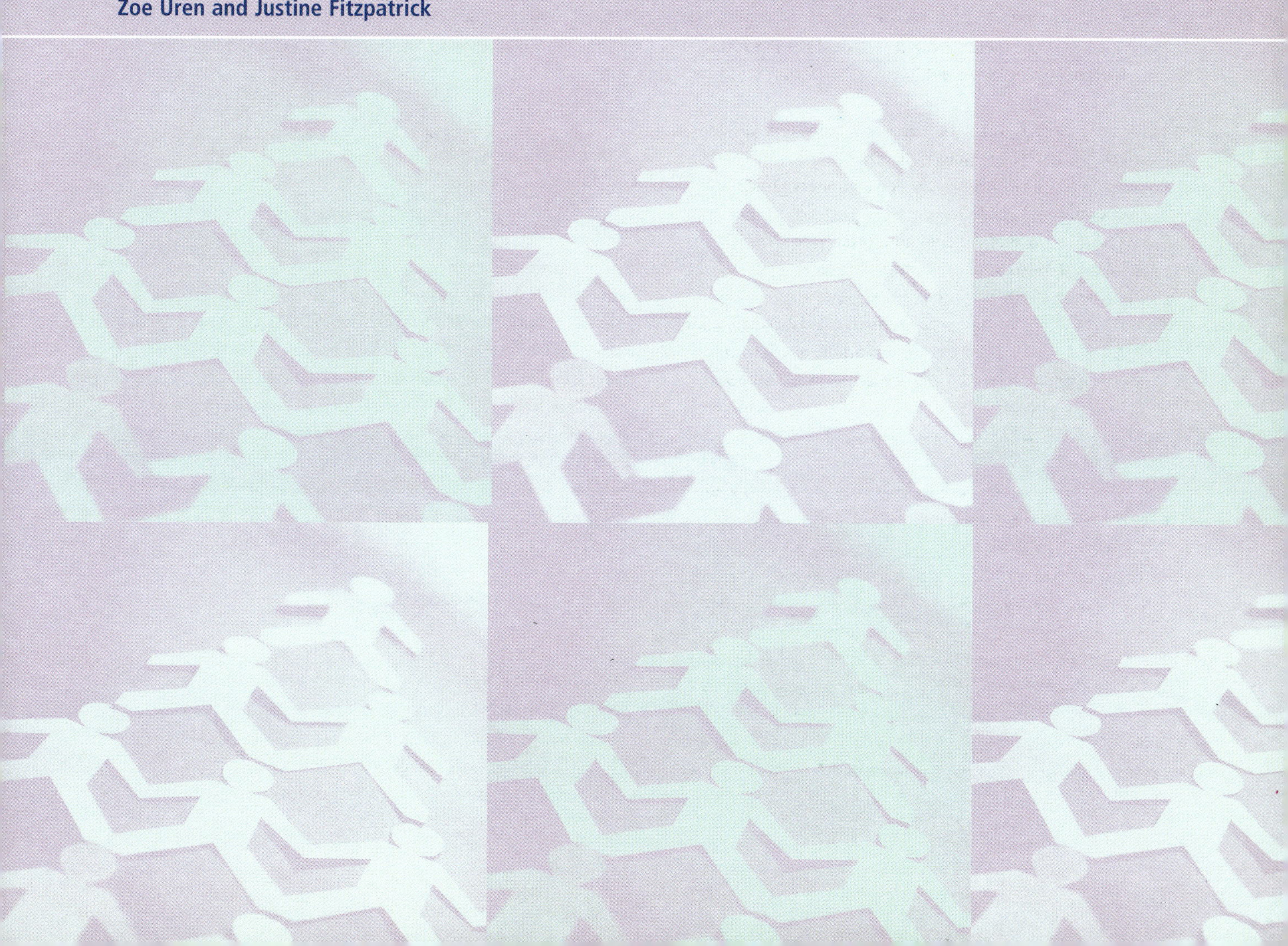

Chapter 11

Analysis of mortality by deprivation and cause of death

Summary

- There was a clear gradient of increasing all-cause mortality with increasing deprivation for all countries of the United Kingdom and regions of England.

- Deaths from ischaemic heart disease, stroke, cancer and lung cancer also followed this general pattern, however, the relationship was not so clear for deaths from suicide and accidents.

- The largest difference between mortality for the most and least deprived areas was seen for ischaemic heart disease and lung cancer.

- For all-cause mortality, for those living in areas of equal deprivation as measured by the Carstairs and Morris index of deprivation, regions in the north had higher mortality than regions in the south. This was also true for ischaemic heart disease, stroke and lung cancer.

- Deprivation was found to be more strongly correlated with mortality than country or region for all causes of death examined.

11.1 Introduction

The geographic relationship between mortality and deprivation has been analysed in a number of studies. Drever and Whitehead examined the relationship between deprivation (using the Department of the Environment's 1991 Index of Local Conditions) and mortality in 350 local authorities in England from 1989 to 1993.[1] The report outlined that there is a very strong relationship between mortality and deprivation at the local authority level. Areas with high deprivation scores tended to have higher mortality than those with lower deprivation scores. This relationship was most marked for males, but it was still strong for females.

The relationship between deprivation at the electoral ward level and mortality has also been very well researched. A positive linear relationship has been confirmed; with increasing deprivation there is an increase in mortality.[2] In addition, studies have shown that there is no threshold level beyond which increasing deprivation is no longer associated with increasing mortality.[3] However, the gradient in increasing mortality with deprivation has shown to be stronger for women than men in some studies, while in others the reverse is true.[2,3]

Some studies have looked at whether the relationship between mortality and deprivation varies throughout different parts of Great Britain. Eames and colleagues showed that there is a stronger correlation between mortality and deprivation in the northern regions - often because these areas experience a wider range of deprivation. However, in some areas - with a very narrow range of deprivation - a steeper gradient was observed.[3] In addition, some studies have examined the relationship between deprivation and mortality for specific causes of death separately and have found that the relationship is not constant for all causes.[3,4,5]

This chapter examines the relationship between deprivation measured at the area level and mortality within countries of Great Britain and the regions of England, for males and females aged 15-64, between 1991 and 1993. It looks at all causes of death and the following specific causes:

- Ischaemic heart disease

- Stroke

- Cancer

- Lung cancer

- Accidents

- Suicide and undetermined injury

Chapter 10 provides the International Classification of Diseases (Ninth Revision) codes for these causes and a discussion of the likely coding differentials between countries of the United Kingdom.

11.2 Methods and data

Death records of males and females aged 15-64 in Great Britain were extracted at electoral ward level (postcode sector level in Scotland) for the three years 1991-1993. Analysis was focused around 1991 as population data is only available for this year. All deaths were allocated a Carstairs and Morris deprivation score[6] for the electoral ward (postcode sector in Scotland) and areas were divided into quintiles and twentieths based on this score. The method of allocating wards and postcode sectors to quintiles and twentieths is explained in more detail in chapter 4. The data was analysed using directly age-standardised mortality rates, for all causes and specific causes of death. For more details see Appendix A.

11.3 All cause mortality

Figure 11.1 shows age-standardised mortality rates by deprivation twentieth within Great Britain for males and females separately. The chart shows clearly that mortality rates increase with increasing deprivation for both males and females. Not only was there a difference between the mortality experience of areas in the most and least deprived twentieths,

Figure 11.1

Age-standardised mortality rates for all causes of death by deprivation, country and region, ages 15-64 Great Britain 1991-1993

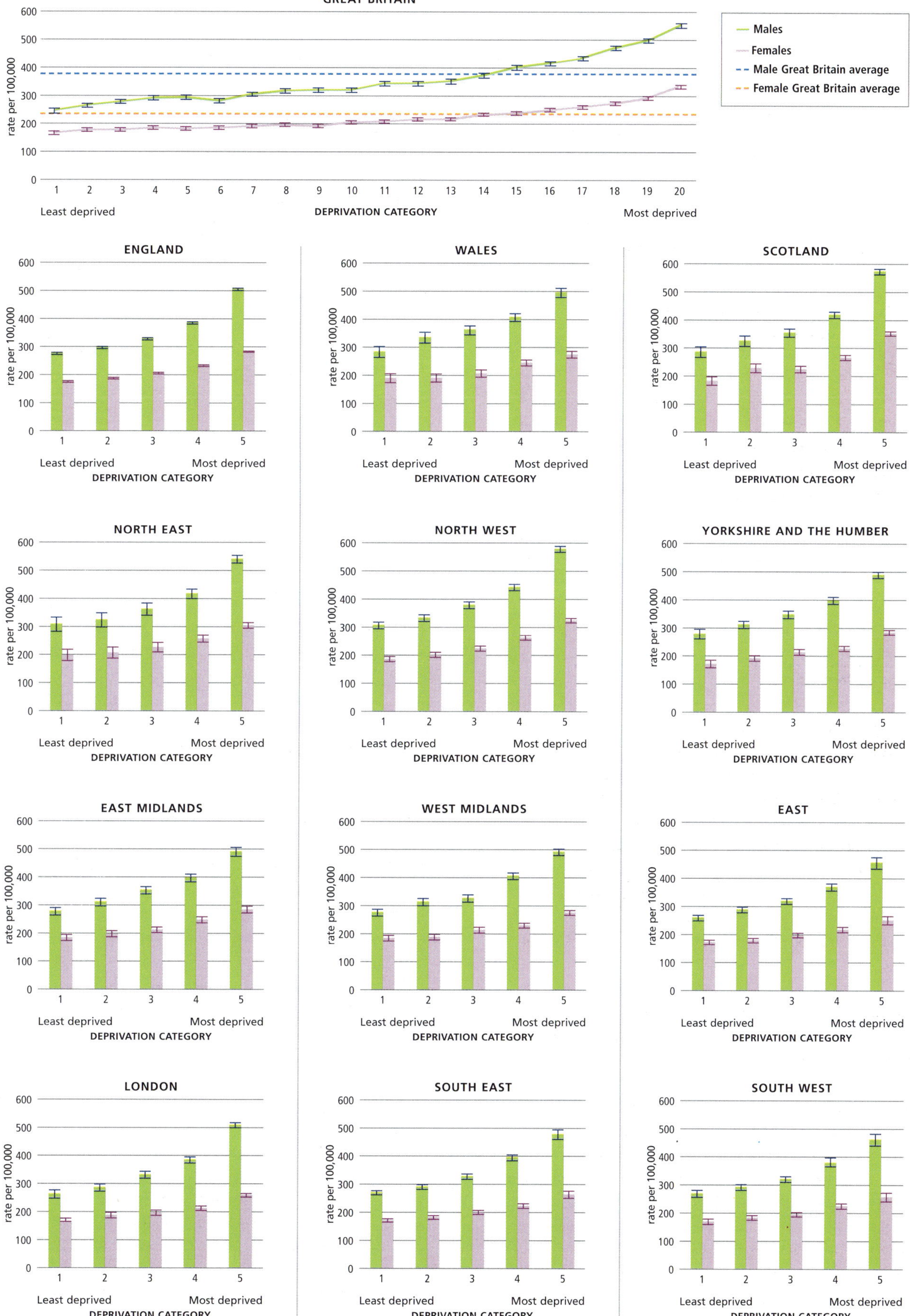

but also there was a gradual gradient of increasing mortality with increasing deprivation. This relationship was evident for both males and females where the ratio of mortality rates between the highest and lowest deprivation twentieths was 2.2 and 2.0 respectively, indicating that those living in the most deprived areas had double the mortality rates of those living in the least deprived areas.

Figure 11.1 also shows age-standardised mortality rates by deprivation quintiles for countries of Great Britain and regions of England. For every country and region there was an increase in mortality rates with increasing deprivation for both males and females. The relative difference in mortality between the most and the least deprived areas was higher for males than females in all countries and regions of Great Britain.

At country level, Scotland had the largest relative differences in the mortality experiences of the most and the least deprived (a ratio of 2.0 for males and 1.9 for females). The country with the smallest differences was Wales.

Within England, there was a difference in mortality both within and between deprivation quintiles for the different regions. The greatest relative difference in mortality between the most and least deprived was within London for males and the North West for females (a ratio of 1.9 and 1.7 respectively). Generally the southern regions, except London, had smaller differences between the most and least deprived areas than the northern regions. For the most deprived (deprivation quintile 5), the regions with the highest mortality rates for males and females were the North East and the North West. The lowest rates were found in the East of England, the South East and South West for both sexes. London also had low mortality rates for females in this deprivation quintile. For the least deprived (deprivation quintile 1) the areas with the lowest rates for both sexes were the South West, East of England, South East and London (and Yorkshire and the Humber for females) and those with the highest were the North East (and the North West for males). However within the North East and the North West mortality rates were consistently higher than England as a whole within all deprivation quintiles. In contrast mortality rates were consistently low in each deprivation quintile in the South West for both sexes. So generally there was a north-south divide in mortality rates within deprivation quintiles as regions in the north had higher mortality than regions in the south.

11.4 Ischaemic heart disease (IHD)

Figure 11.2 shows age-standardised mortality rates from IHD by deprivation twentieth within Great Britain. The gradient of increasing mortality with increasing deprivation was very clear for both males and females. The difference in mortality between the highest and lowest deprivation twentieths was 2.7 and 4.2 for males and females respectively, and was much greater than that seen for all-cause mortality presented in Figure 11.1. Although IHD mortality rates were higher for males, there was more variation in female mortality by deprivation twentieth.
The pattern of increasing mortality with increasing

deprivation by quintile within countries of Great Britain and regions of England closely resembles that for all causes of death. The countries with the greatest relative differences in IHD mortality between the deprivation quintile 1 and 5 were Wales and Scotland (difference of 2.2 and 3.1 for males and females respectively).

The geographic variation in female IHD mortality rates for areas of equal deprivation was greater than the variation for males. For example, the difference between the areas with highest and lowest mortality rates within deprivation quintile 5 was 1.4 for males and 1.7 for females, whereas for all causes of death these differences were similar for the two sexes. In addition, there appears to be a north-south divide within England when examining deprivation-specific IHD mortality rates. Areas in the north had higher IHD mortality than areas with equivalent deprivation in the south for both males and females.

11.5 Stroke

Figure 11.3 shows age-standardised mortality rates for stroke within Great Britain by deprivation twentieth. The gradient of increasing mortality with increasing deprivation is less clear than that presented for all causes of death. For example, for females, those that were least deprived had higher mortality rates than those with higher deprivation (twentieths 2 and 3).

The pattern by deprivation quintile presented in Figure 11.3 shows that as a rule the general pattern of increasing mortality with increasing deprivation existed for most countries of Great Britain and regions of England. However, there were some exceptions. For example, in the North East those considered the least deprived (quintile 1) had higher mortality than those that were more deprived (quintile 2 and 3) for both males and females. The gradient of increased mortality with increased deprivation was clearest in the North West and the East of England for males and the West Midlands for females. The greatest differences between the most and least deprived quintiles was in the West Midlands and the South West for females (a difference of 2.5) and Yorkshire and the Humber for males (2.5). As for IHD mortality, there was some evidence that, for areas of equal deprivation, areas in the north of England had higher mortality from stroke than areas in the south of England outside London.

11.6 All cancers

There was a clear gradient of increasing mortality with increasing deprivation, by deprivation twentieth in Great Britain for cancer (Figure 11.4). However, this gradient was less steep than for all cause mortality. For males, mortality rates in the most deprived were 1.9 times those in the least deprived and for females this was reduced to 1.4. This compares to 2.2 and 2.0 for males and females respectively for all causes. Thus, the differences between mortality rates for each deprivation twentieth were greater for males than for females. However, this is likely to be due to differences in the types of cancer dominating these all cancer

Figure 11.2

Age-standardised mortality rates for ischaemic heart disease by deprivation, country and region, ages 15-64
Great Britain 1991-1993

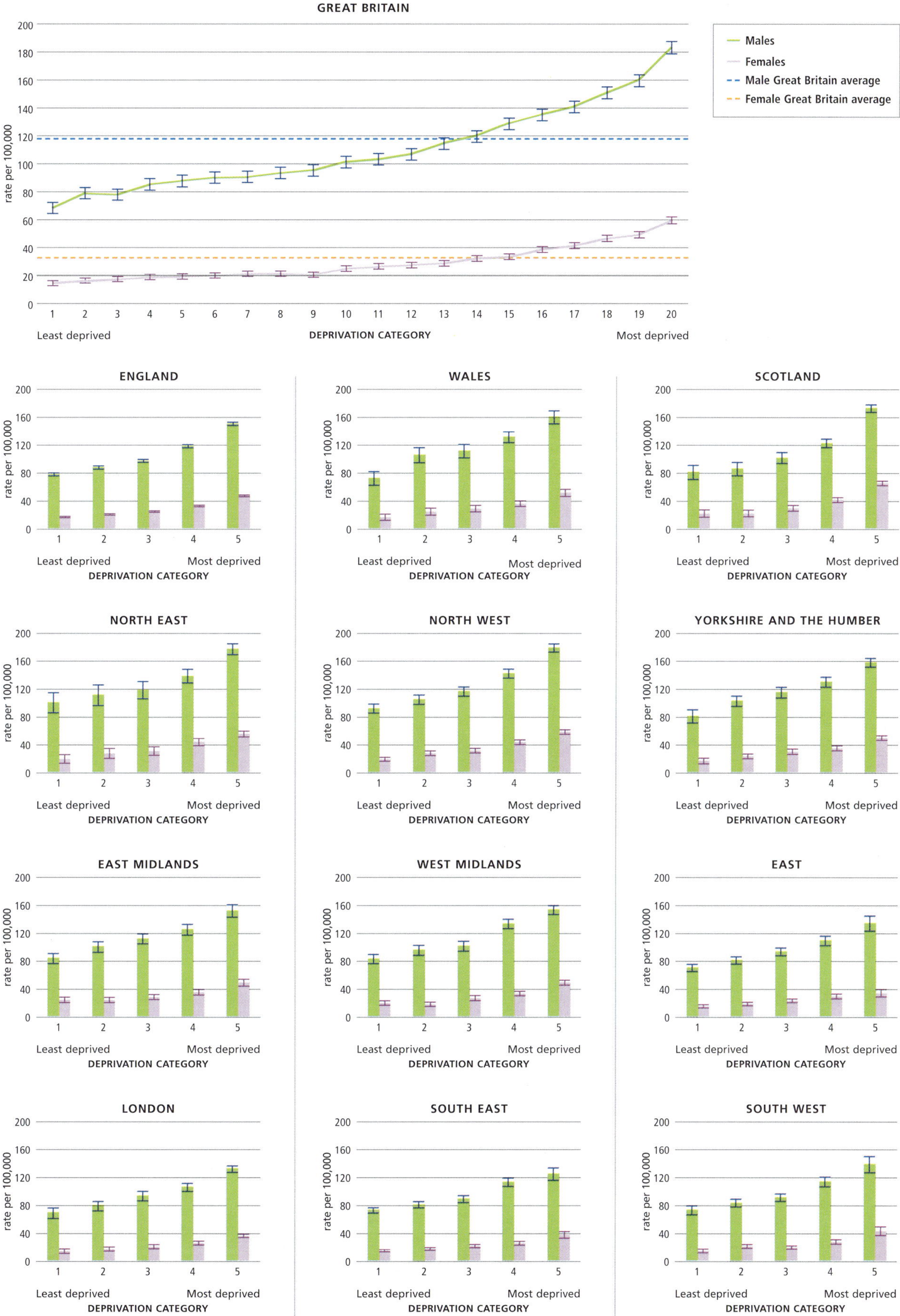

Figure 11.3

Age-standardised mortality rates for stroke by deprivation, country and region, ages 15-64
Great Britain 1991-1993

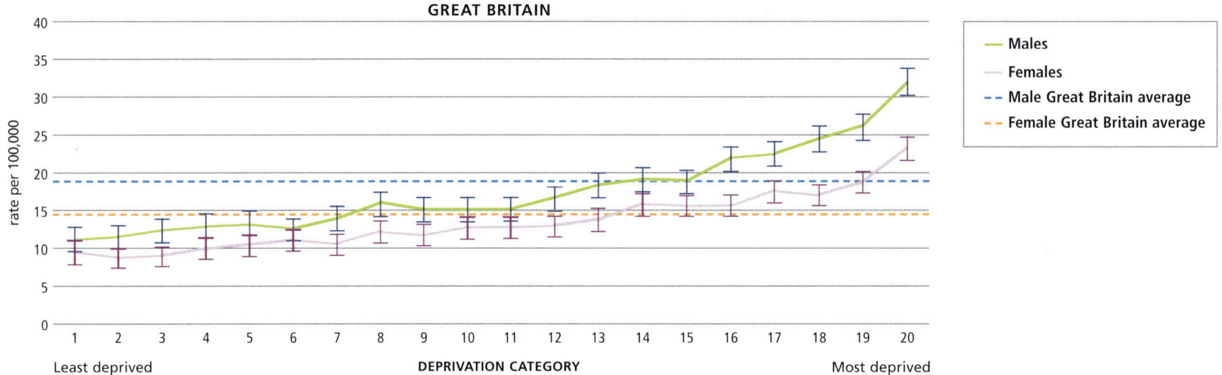

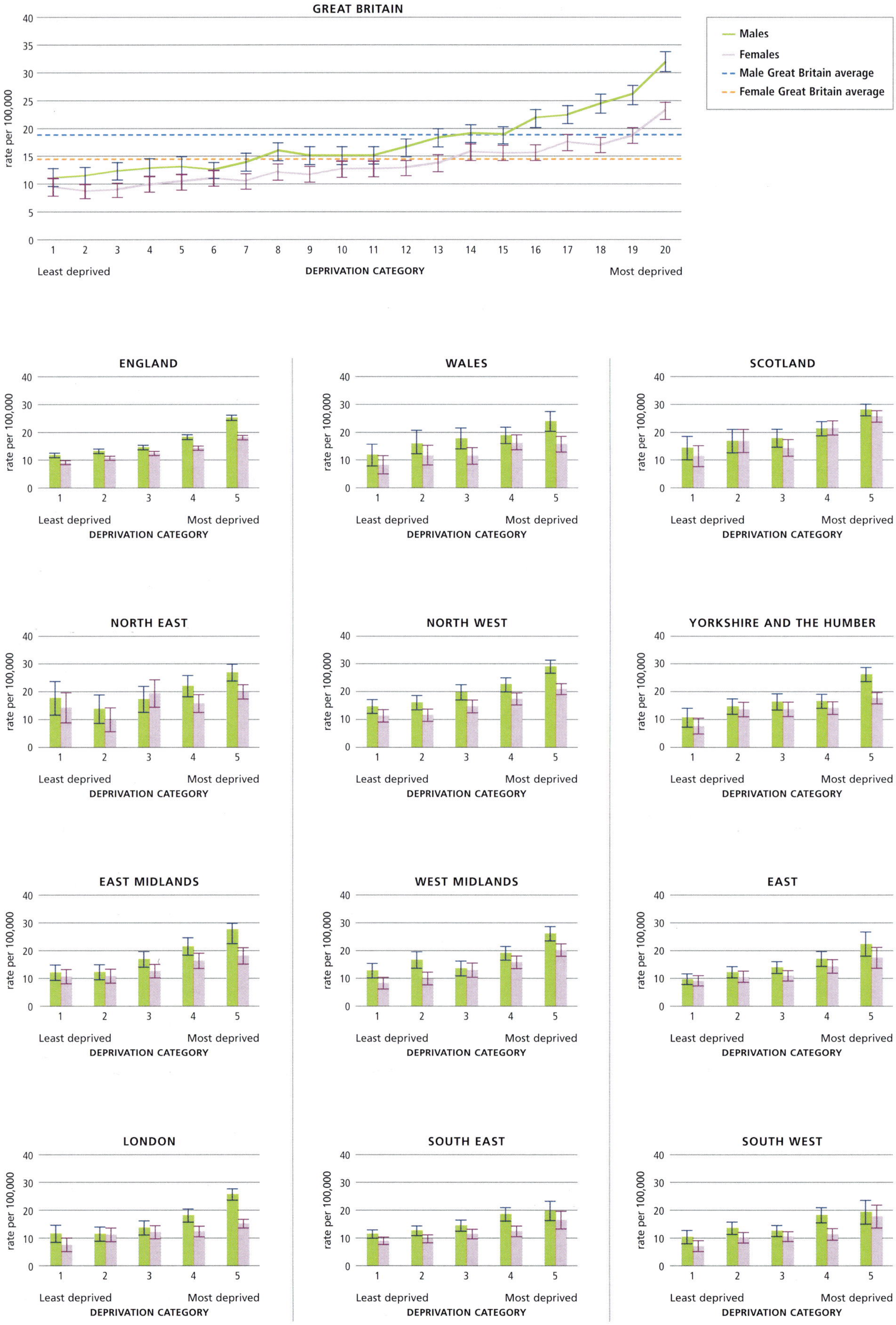

Figure 11.4

Age-standardised mortality rates for all cancers by deprivation, country and region, ages 15-64
Great Britain 1991-1993

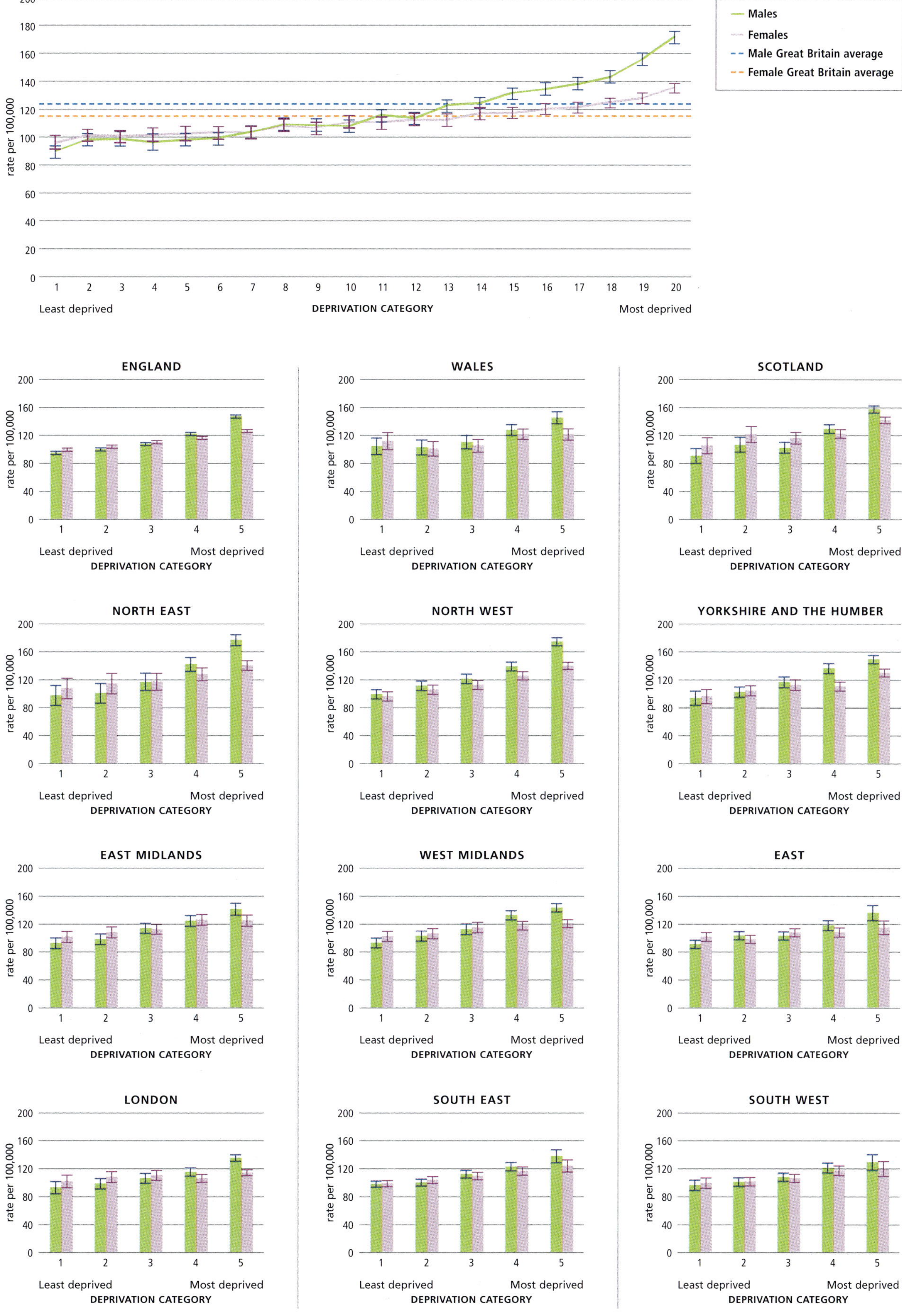

rates for males and females. Previous analysis has shown that mortality from lung cancer, the most common cancer in males, more closely follows the traditional relationship with deprivation than breast cancer, the most common cancer in females.[7] Lung cancer mortality makes up a greater proportion of all cancer mortality in males than females; approximately 29 per cent for males compared to 16 per cent for females. Chapter 10 of this volume, looking at the relationship between breast cancer mortality and ONS classification Group, showed that there was little variation between Groups.

Analysis of cancer mortality by deprivation quintile within countries of Great Britain and regions of England also shows a flatter gradient than was seen for all causes of death. Similarly this may be explained because mortality from certain cancers such as breast and prostate cancer have an inverse relationship with deprivation.[7] The results indicate that, for females, in some countries and regions the mortality level for those in quintile 2 was equivalent to, or in some cases was less than, mortality levels in deprivation quintile 1 (for example, Wales and the East of England). The greatest relative differences in mortality rates between deprivation quintiles were found in the North East, the North West and Scotland for males, and the North West, Yorkshire and the Humber and Scotland for females.

There was little difference between the mortality experiences of those in the least deprived quintile across Great Britain. However, there were considerable regional differences in cancer mortality for those in the most deprived quintile. The ratio of the male mortality rates in the North East and the South West, the regions with the highest and lowest mortality within this most deprived group, was 1.4.

11.7 Lung cancer

Mortality from lung cancer shows a much clearer gradient of an increase in mortality with increasing deprivation than that seen for all cancers (Figure 11.5). In addition, the distribution of mortality by deprivation twentieth reveals that the mortality rates of those in the highest deprivation category (twentieth 20) were significantly higher than for the next lower deprivation score (twentieth 19). For example those in twentieth 20 had 3.7 and 3.4 times higher mortality than those in twentieth 1 for males and females respectively and 1.2 times higher mortality than those in deprivation twentieth 19 for both males and females.

Examination of mortality by deprivation quintile for males indicates that this general pattern was evident within the different countries and regions of Great Britain. However, for females, in many countries and regions, the first three deprivation quintiles often had quite similar mortality levels. Those in the most deprived category experienced significantly higher lung cancer mortality than those in deprivation quintile 4 for the majority of areas for both sexes. The greatest relative differences between the highest and lowest deprivation quintiles for males were found in Scotland and the North East with smaller differences in the southern regions. This north-south distinction was not so clear for females.

Within deprivation categories the geographic variation was greatest for females. For example within the least deprived (quintile 1), the female mortality rates differed by two fold between the North East, the area with the highest mortality, and the West Midlands. In contrast the ratio was only 1.4 between the North West, the area with the highest mortality, and Scotland for males. However, the analysis of the geographic variation for the most deprived (quintile 5) reveals that the regional distribution of mortality was more pronounced. The difference between areas with high and low mortality in this deprivation group was 1.8 and 2.0 for males and females respectively. Mortality among the most deprived tended to be higher in the north of England compared to the south of England.

11.8 Accidents

The relationship between deprivation and accident mortality differed between the two sexes. For males there was a gradual increase in mortality as deprivation increased (Figure 11.6). The difference between the highest and lowest deprivation twentieths for males was 2.1. However for females there was no relationship between accident mortality and deprivation.

For male accident mortality, the difference between the most deprived and the least deprived was generally smaller than for other causes of death. For example, the region of England with the largest difference was London, where the most deprived had 1.4 times the mortality of the least deprived. In Scotland the differences in mortality by deprivation were high, but the least deprived had higher mortality than those that were more deprived (in deprivation quintile 2). In addition, for males in the North West, Yorkshire and the Humber and London mortality in deprivation quintile 1 was higher than for quintile 2.

11.9 Suicide and undetermined injury

The association between suicide mortality and deprivation in Great Britain also differed between the two sexes. The analysis of the relationship between mortality and deprivation twentieth revealed that for males a gradient between the two variables existed (Figure 11.7). Those considered the most deprived (deprivation twentieth 20) had significantly higher mortality from suicide than any other deprivation group. The male gradient was, however, relatively flat between deprivation twentieths one and fourteen, and then increased as deprivation increased in the most deprived twentieths. However for females there was no specific relationship between the two variables.

A similar unclear pattern is evident by deprivation quintile for the countries of Great Britain and regions of England. For male mortality, the country within Great Britain with the greatest difference between the least deprived and most deprived was Scotland. However, in Wales there was little difference in mortality by deprivation quintile. For the regions of England, the pattern of suicide mortality by deprivation was variable.

Figure 11.5

Age-standardised mortality rates for lung cancer by deprivation, country and region, ages 15-64
Great Britain 1991-1993

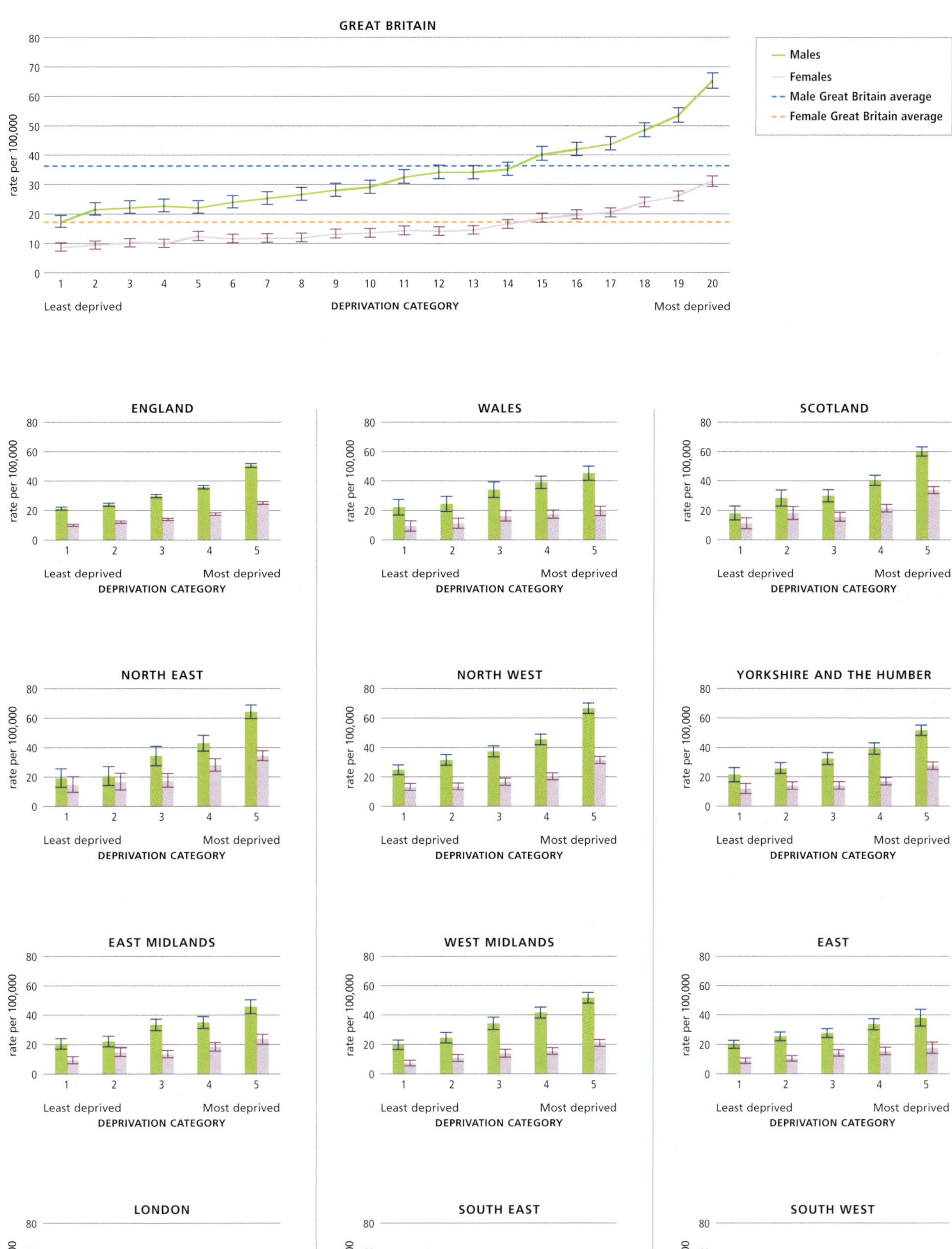

Figure 11.6

Age-standardised mortality rates for accidents by deprivation, country and region, ages 15-64
Great Britain 1991-1993

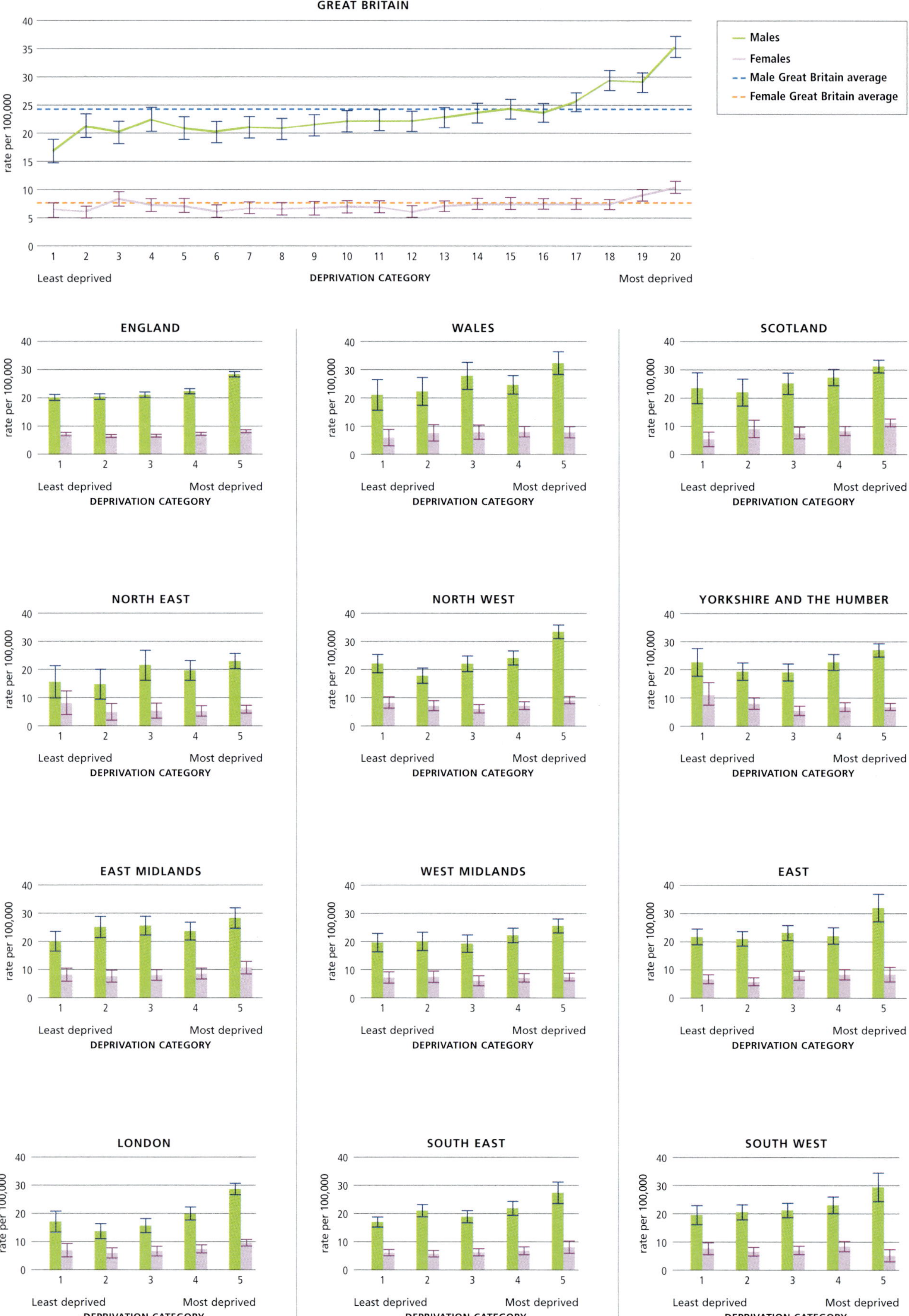

Figure 11.7

Age-standardised mortality rates for suicide and undetermined injury by deprivation, country and region, ages 15-64 Great Britain 1991-1993

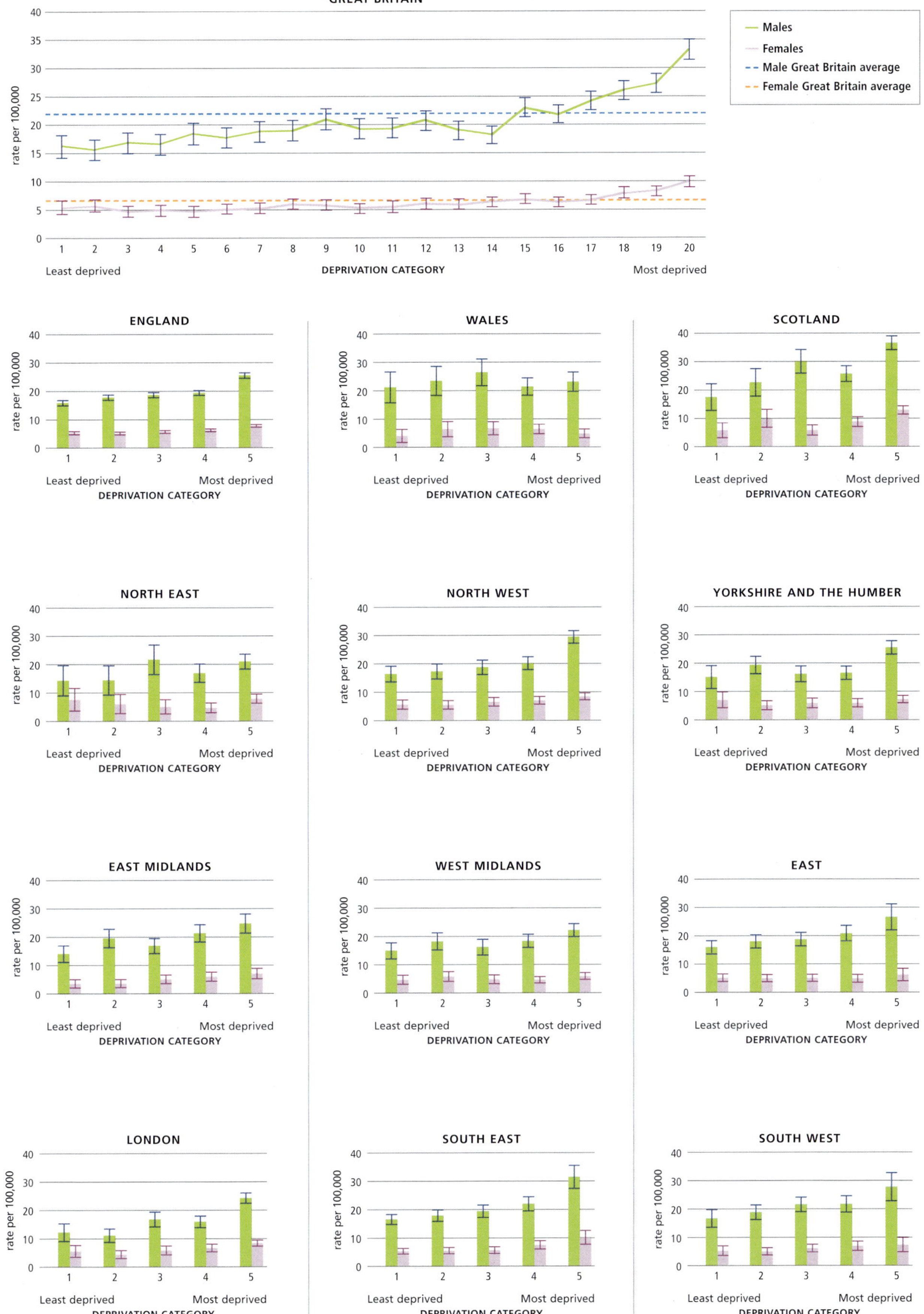

However, rates in the North West, Yorkshire and Humber, London and the South East were significantly higher for the most deprived (quintile 5) than elsewhere.

11.10 Discussion

This chapter demonstrates a clear gradient of increasing all-cause mortality with increasing deprivation for all countries of the United Kingdom and regions of England. However, the gradient and the ratio of mortality rates between the most and the least deprived was not consistent for all causes of death. Mortality from IHD and lung cancer showed large differences between the most and the least deprived. In contrast mortality from stroke, all cancers, accidents and suicide showed a weaker relationship with deprivation.

It is also clear from the data presented in this chapter that geographic differences in mortality rates existed between those living in areas with an equal level of deprivation as measured by the Carstairs and Morris index. For all cause mortality, for those living in areas with an equivalent level of deprivation, regions in the north had higher mortality than regions in the south. This was also true for mortality from IHD, stroke and lung cancer. Other causes did not show such a difference.

An analysis of variance was conducted to examine how much of the variation in mortality rates presented in this chapter was accounted for by the country and region of location (country/region) and how much was accounted for by deprivation. The results indicate that both country/region and deprivation contributed to the variation in mortality. For IHD, stroke, cancer and lung cancer approximately 80-90 per cent of the variation in rates was explained by these two factors. A smaller percentage of the variation was explained for other causes of death. The analysis also showed that deprivation is more strongly correlated with mortality than country/region for all causes of death examined.

The major problem with measuring the association between mortality and deprivation at the area level is that the relationship is subject to the ecological fallacy.[8] The existence of a positive relationship between area level deprivation and mortality does not mean that all individuals in the deprived areas are 'deprived' and, therefore, subject to this increased mortality risk. The extent of this effect is dependent on the proportion of people suffering material deprivation in the deprived area.[2] Regional differences in the proportion of 'deprived' people in areas classified as deprived may be effecting the results presented in this chapter. However, what is not yet fully understood about the relationship between deprivation and mortality at the area level is whether the differences observed are merely a result of the concentration of people of low socio-economic status within deprived areas, or whether there are other area effects in operation that have not been measured.

Chapter 12 of this volume demonstrates that the gradients in mortality observed when using individual social class

information from a death certificate or area level deprivation scores are very similar. What has not been demonstrated in this chapter, but has been concluded elsewhere, is that if social class is controlled for, a variation in mortality by area level deprivation still exists and vice versa.[9] This would suggest that there is some other effect of area or geography on mortality, other than that being measured in the deprivation index. In some cases the area effect may be related to factors that are not measured in the study or by the deprivation index such as crime, pollution and environmental factors.[10] For example, it has been reported that there is a decrease in coronary heart disease mortality with increasing water hardness.[11]

However, another study has found that the relationship between deprivation and mortality at the area level is largely eliminated if the socio-economic characteristics of individuals are controlled for.[2] Thus this would imply that non-deprived people living in deprived areas are not subject to an increased risk of death. In addition, deprived people living in non-deprived areas are not subject to a protective effect of living in these areas. Therefore it is individual factors that are most important in determining mortality risk. As discussed in chapter 10, analysis examining the association between suicide and area-based deprivation and social fragmentation showed that suicide mortality was more strongly associated with social fragmentation than deprivation, whereas deaths from other causes were more closely related to deprivation.[12] The relative importance of behavioural and material factors in determining inequalities in health has been debated extensively and is beyond the analysis of this volume.[13, 14]

References

1 Drever F and Whitehead M. Mortality in regions and local authority districts in the 1990s: exploring the relationship with deprivation. *Population Trends* 82 (1995), 19-26.

2 Sloggett A and Joshi H. Higher mortality in deprived areas: community or personal disadvantage? *British Medical Journal* 309 (1994), 1470-1474.

3 Eames M, Ben-Shlomo Y and Marmot M. Social deprivation and premature mortality: regional comparison across England. *British Medical Journal* 307 (1993), 1097-1102.

4 Jessop E. Deprivation and mortality in non-metropolitan areas of England and Wales. *Journal of Epidemiology and Community Health* 50 (1996), 524-526.

5 McLoone P and Boddy F. Deprivation and mortality in Scotland, 1981 and 1991 *British Medical Journal* 390 (1994), 1465-1469.

6 Carstairs V and Morris R. *Deprivation and health in Scotland*. Aberdeen University Press (Aberdeen: 1991).

7 Quinn MJ, Babb P, Brock A, Kirby L and Jones J. *Cancer Trends in England and Wales 1950-1999*. SMPS No. 66. The Stationery Office (London: 2001).

8 Robinson W. Ecological correlations and the behaviour of individuals. *American Sociological Review* 15 (1950), 351-357.

9 Carstairs V and Morris M. Deprivation and mortality: an alternative to social class? *Community Medicine* 11 (1989), 210-219.

10 Hann M, Kaplan G and Camacho T. Poverty and health: prospective evidence from the Alameda County study. *American Journal of Epidemiology* 125 (1987), 989-997.

11 Pocock S, Cook D and Shaper A. Analysing geographic variations in cardiovascular mortality: methods and results. *Journal of the Royal Statistical Society* 145 (1982), 313-341.

12 Whitley M, Gunnell D, Dorling D and Davey Smith G. Ecological study of social fragmentation, poverty and suicide. *British Medical Journal* 319 (1999), 1034-1037.

13 Townsend P, Whitehead M and Davidson H. (eds.) *Inequalities in health: The Black Report and the health divide*. Penguin (London: 1992).

14 Davey Smith G, Blane D and Bartley M. Explanations for socio-economic differentials in mortality: evidence from Britain and elsewhere. *European Journal of Public Health* 4 (1994), 131-144.

Geographic variation in mortality by Social Class and alternative social classifications

Zoe Uren, Justine Fitzpatrick, Alison Reid and Peter Goldblatt

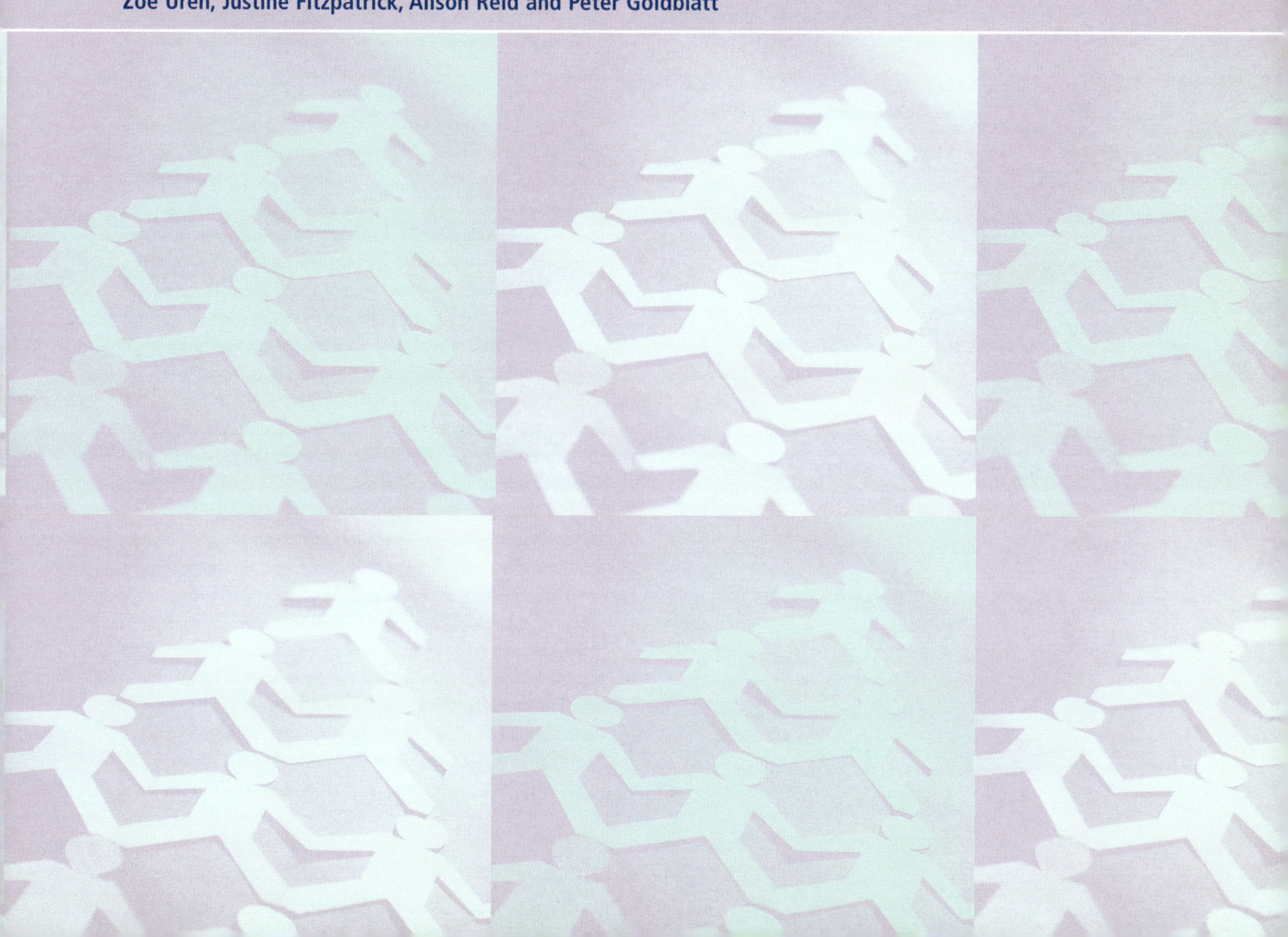

Chapter 12

Geographic variation in mortality by Social Class and alternative social classifications

Summary

- There was a clear socio-economic gradient in all-cause mortality for all countries of the United Kingdom and regions of England, with mortality increasing between Social Class I and V.

- The relative mortality difference between the Social Classes was greater in Wales, Scotland and Northern Ireland and the northern regions of England than in the southern regions of England.

- This pattern was similar for ischaemic heart disease, stroke and cancer mortality, but was less evident for accidents and suicide.

- There was little geographic variation in mortality rates among those in Social Class I.

- Geographic differences in Social Class V were considerably greater than in all other classes.

- Although both Social Class and country/region of residence contributed to mortality variation, the contribution made by Social Class was greater.

- There were clear gradients in mortality between car access and housing tenure categories in all regions of England and Wales.

- Within each car access and housing tenure category, those in the north of England had higher mortality than those in the south.

12.1 Introduction

There is a long history to measuring socio-economic differentials in mortality and relating these to geographic variations. The analyses developed by the General Register Office, following its foundation in 1837, focused on representing inequalities in health in both geographic and occupational terms. The links with socio-economic status of both these dimensions were fully appreciated.

"The state of health among the people differs in different times and in different places: and the principle purpose of the registration of disease is to determine the degree of their variation in each district, and in each class of the population, as well as the extent to which they are modified by circumstances"

Sixteenth annual report of the Registrar General[1]

Concern about health inequalities in modern Britain had previously appeared in the reports submitted by the Poor Law Commissioners, set up to review the workings of the New Poor Law Act 1834. They had presented evidence from inspectors[2] on the *"pestilential places the industrious poor are obliged to take their abode"* and given figures on *"the final results of that suffering."*

In 1864, the Registrar General published the first decennial supplement to his annual reports, providing greater detail on mortality in the period 1851-1860. The commentary, contributed by William Farr, drew attention to the relationship between mortality, geography and social conditions.[3]

In the second decennial supplement, published in 1875, Farr further developed his analysis of the contrast between the healthiest districts, the unhealthiest and the impact of the social conditions of their inhabitants on these differences:

"The thousands of families of the Liverpool district are of various grades, and live in very different sanitary conditions; some may be as healthy as groups of families anywhere else, and others may suffer to the extremest extent; but the general result is seen in the Table, which may for the moment represent the unhealthy classes [this table contrasted the high mortality rates in Liverpool with those in London, Manchester and 51 "healthy districts"]... *Every great city has in it a bit of Liverpool."*

Supplement to the thirty-fifth annual report of the Registrar General[4]

In later decennial supplement analyses, based on censuses between 1911 and 1991, ONS and its predecessors used Social Class (based on occupation) as the principal indicator of socio-economic status. The most recent in this series[5] focused on health inequalities. It confirmed earlier findings that although mortality rates in England and Wales are falling, Social Class differentials have been widening since the 1930s.[6] In 1991-3, all cause mortality in Social Class V was almost three times that of Social Class I[7] and, for some causes of death, these differentials were even greater.

The most recent previous decennial supplement on geographic differences in mortality, *Mortality and Geography*,[8] included an analysis that grouped local authorities according to the percentage of households with the head in Social Class I or II and examined mortality rates within these groups of local authorities. This showed that, within each region of England and within Wales, local authorities with a higher percentage of households with the head in Social Class I or II had lower mortality than those with a low percentage in these social groups.[9] Using the ONS Longitudinal Study (LS), the analysis also showed broad regional, Social Class and housing tenure differences in mortality in 1971-81 between those living in wards with similar socio-economic characteristics in 1971.

More recent analyses, using the LS, have related mortality data in 1988-94 to 1981 population characteristics. These analyses showed that in men aged 25 to 64 there were clear social gradients in mortality in the North, North West and the South East.[10] In Section 12.2, we build on these earlier results to examine the relationship between mortality and Social Class in men aged 20-64 in the countries of the United Kingdom and the regions of England from 1991 to 1993 for particular causes of death.

Using the LS, inequalities in health have been examined using household-based markers of socio-economic position, such as household access to cars and housing tenure.[11] These indicators have been argued to act as a proxy for disposable income and wealth respectively. These analyses have consistently shown that those living in owner-occupied accommodation experienced lower mortality rates than those living in rented accommodation and those living in households with access to cars had considerably lower mortality than those without access.

Recently Reid and Harding[12] extended earlier LS analyses to look at mortality among those who experienced multiple deprivation. They found that although mortality of those aged 20 to 64 in England and Wales was highest in the north and lowest in the south between 1991 and 1997, the death rate of the most deprived individuals (defined as having at least three of the following four characteristics – being in Social Class IV or V, living in rented accommodation, having no access to a car and being unemployed) was more than twice that of the least deprived individuals (defined as being in Social Class I, II or III, living in owner occupied housing, having car access and being employed) in both the north and in the south. They also found that the death rates of the most deprived individuals had not declined in the 1990s, whereas those of the least deprived individuals had declined substantially. In another paper,[13] they found that adjusting for differences in long-term disadvantage did not explain the north-south divide in mortality.

Section 12.3 in this chapter examines the variation in mortality rates between regions of England and for Wales by housing tenure and car access using the ONS Longitudinal Study.

12.2 Mortality by Social Class

Methods and data

In this analysis deaths among men aged 20-64 are examined for the three years 1991-1993. The analysis is focused on this period to ensure consistency with population denominator information from the 1991 Census (as the ten-yearly Census provides the only national breakdown of the whole population by occupation and Social Class). It was necessary to combine three years of death registration data to ensure that sufficient numbers of deaths were available to present data for each Social Class by age group and by cause. Only deaths allocated to a Social Class were included.

The last gainful occupation of the deceased is recorded at death registration and is routinely coded for all men over the age of 16 and under the age of 75, using the latest available occupational classification. For the deaths analysis here, the 1990 Standard Occupational Classification (SOC90) was used. For those who have a stated occupation at death registration, their employment status is also recorded. These two pieces of information together determined the Social Class of the deceased. For further details and a description of the Social Class classification see chapter 3, Box 3.1.

The analyses presented relate only to men. Social Class for mortality and for the population at risk was obtained from different sources (death registration and the 1991 Census). As very different percentages of women have an occupation recorded at death than at Census, and these differences are unlikely to be independent of Social Class, we have excluded women from this analysis.

Figure 12.1

Age-standardised all-cause mortality rates by Social Class, country and region, males aged 20-64
United Kingdom 1991-1993

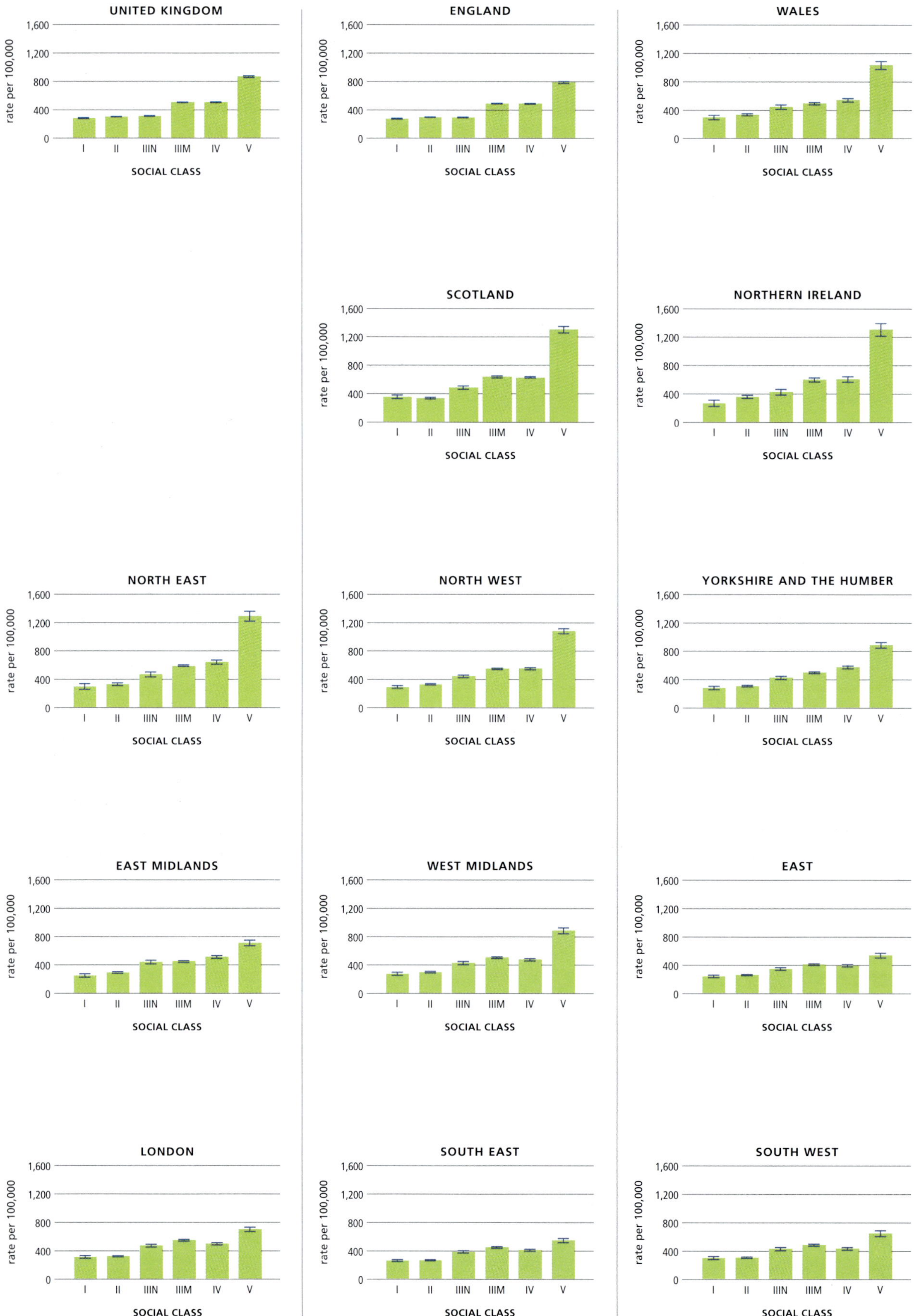

Figure 12.2

Age-standardised all-cause mortality rates for Social Classes I and V by country and region, males aged 20-64 United Kingdom 1991-1993

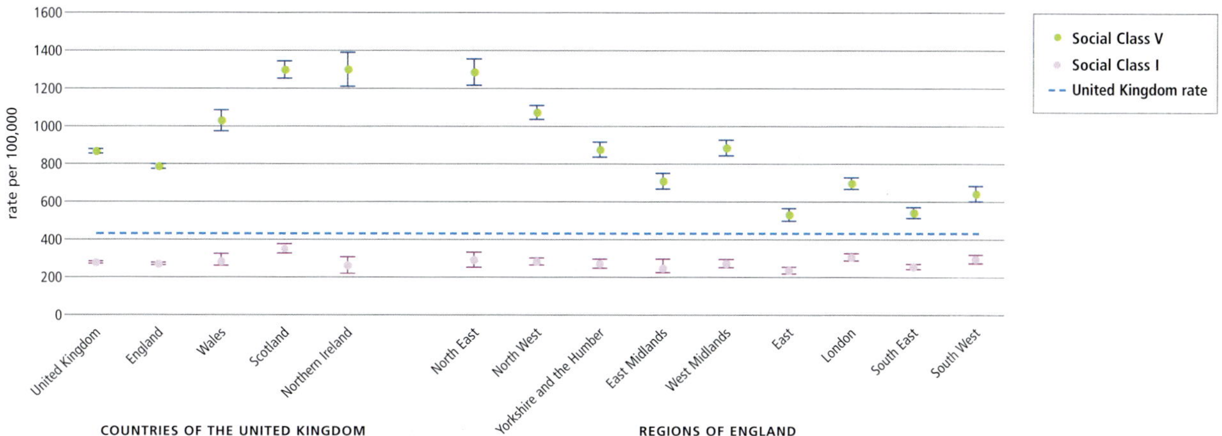

All cause mortality

Figure 12.1 shows that, consistent with other studies, mortality increased with decreasing Social Class. The graphs indicate that there was a clear social gradient in mortality. The highest mortality rates occurred in Social Class V, and in the United Kingdom as a whole these rates were three times higher than mortality in Social Class I. This general pattern existed in each country of the United Kingdom and region of England. However the relative difference between Social Classes did vary by region. Generally the largest relative difference between Social Classes was seen in the northern regions of England, Wales, Scotland and Northern Ireland. For example, in Northern Ireland mortality rates for Social Class V were five times those for Social Class I. In contrast, the southern regions of England had the most favourable mortality rates within the United Kingdom. Specifically the East of England had the best mortality experience for each Social Class and smaller differences between Social Classes. The smallest ratio between Social Class I and Social Class V was found in the South East, where the difference was two-fold.

Figure 12.2 shows age-standardised mortality rates for all causes of death, for Social Classes I and V for countries and regions of the United Kingdom. Comparison between the two graphs indicates that there was less geographic variation among men in Social Class I than in Social Class V. While mortality in Social Class I was largely uniform throughout the regions and countries of the United Kingdom, there were significant regional differences in Social Class V mortality. Scotland and the East of England experienced the highest and lowest rates respectively for both Social Classes I and V. However, while Social Class V mortality was 2.5 times greater in Scotland than in the East of England, the comparable ratio for Social Class I was just 1.5. For Social Class V, the southern areas of England and the East Midlands had significantly lower mortality rates than the United Kingdom as a whole while rates were significantly higher in the North East, Scotland and Northern Ireland. The regions in which Social Class V mortality was highest were not necessarily those with the highest mortality for Social Class I. For example, Social Class I mortality in London exceeded that of Northern Ireland while the reverse was true for Social Class V.

Figure 12.3

Age-standardised mortality rates for ischaemic heart disease by Social Class, country and region, males aged 20-64
United Kingdom 1991-1993

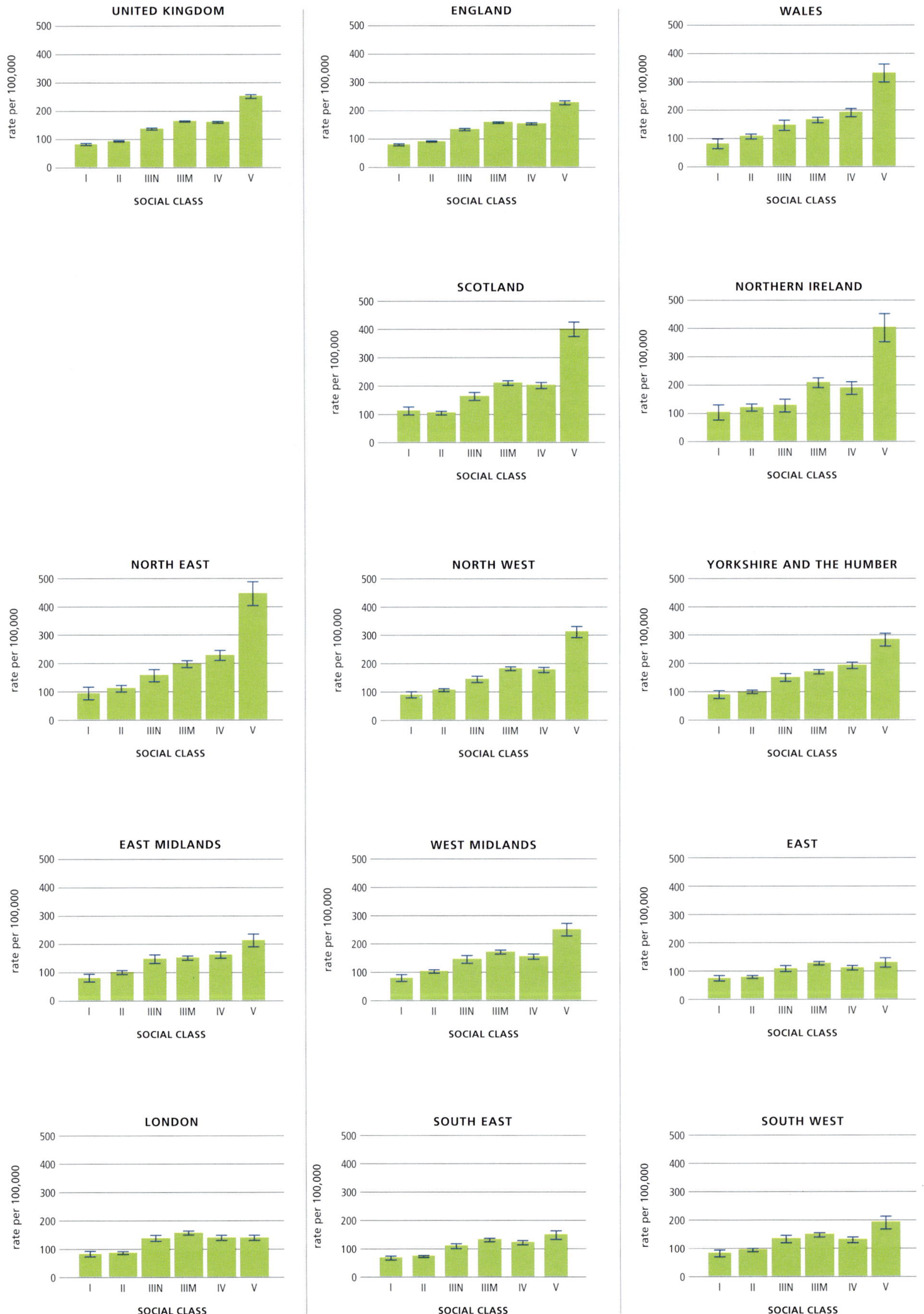

Figure 12.4

Age-standardised mortality rates for ischaemic heart disease for Social Classes I and V by country and region, males aged 20-64
United Kingdom 1991-1993

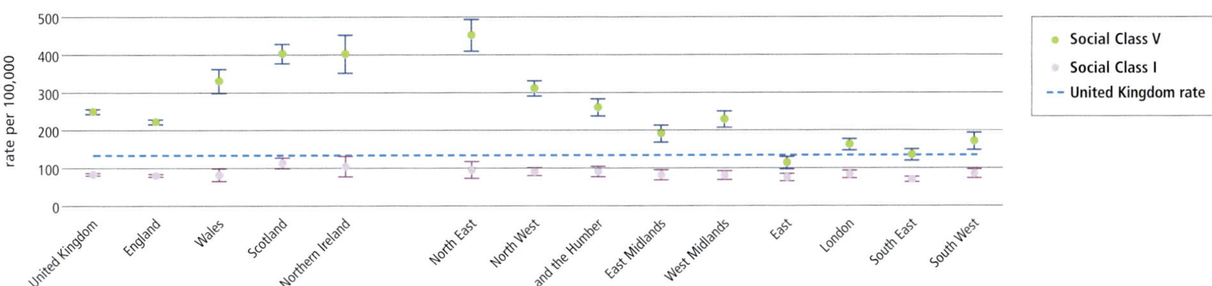

Ischaemic heart disease

Figure 12.3 shows that in the United Kingdom as a whole during the period 1991 to 1993, men in Social Class V were 3.1 times more likely to die from ischaemic heart disease than those in Social Class I. However there was a geographic difference in this social gradient. As for all-causes, the Social Class gradient was flatter in England than in Wales, Scotland and Northern Ireland. Within England, gradients in the southern regions were flatter than those in the north. Specifically, the greatest difference between classes was in Northern Ireland, where mortality in Social Class V was 4 times greater than in Social Class I. In contrast, the area with the smallest difference was the South West region, where the ratio of mortality rates between Social Classes I and V was 2.3.

The pattern of mortality rates for ischaemic heart disease by region within Social Classes I and V was very similar to that seen for all causes (Figure 12.4). For Social Class I mortality rates in each country and region were generally similar to those of the United Kingdom, with the exception of Scotland and Northern Ireland which had higher rates. In Social Class V the southern regions of England had more favourable mortality rates than the United Kingdom as a whole, while the North East region, Wales, Scotland and Northern Ireland had less favourable rates.

Figure 12.5

Age-standardised mortality rates for stroke by Social Class, country and region, males aged 20-64
United Kingdom 1991-1993

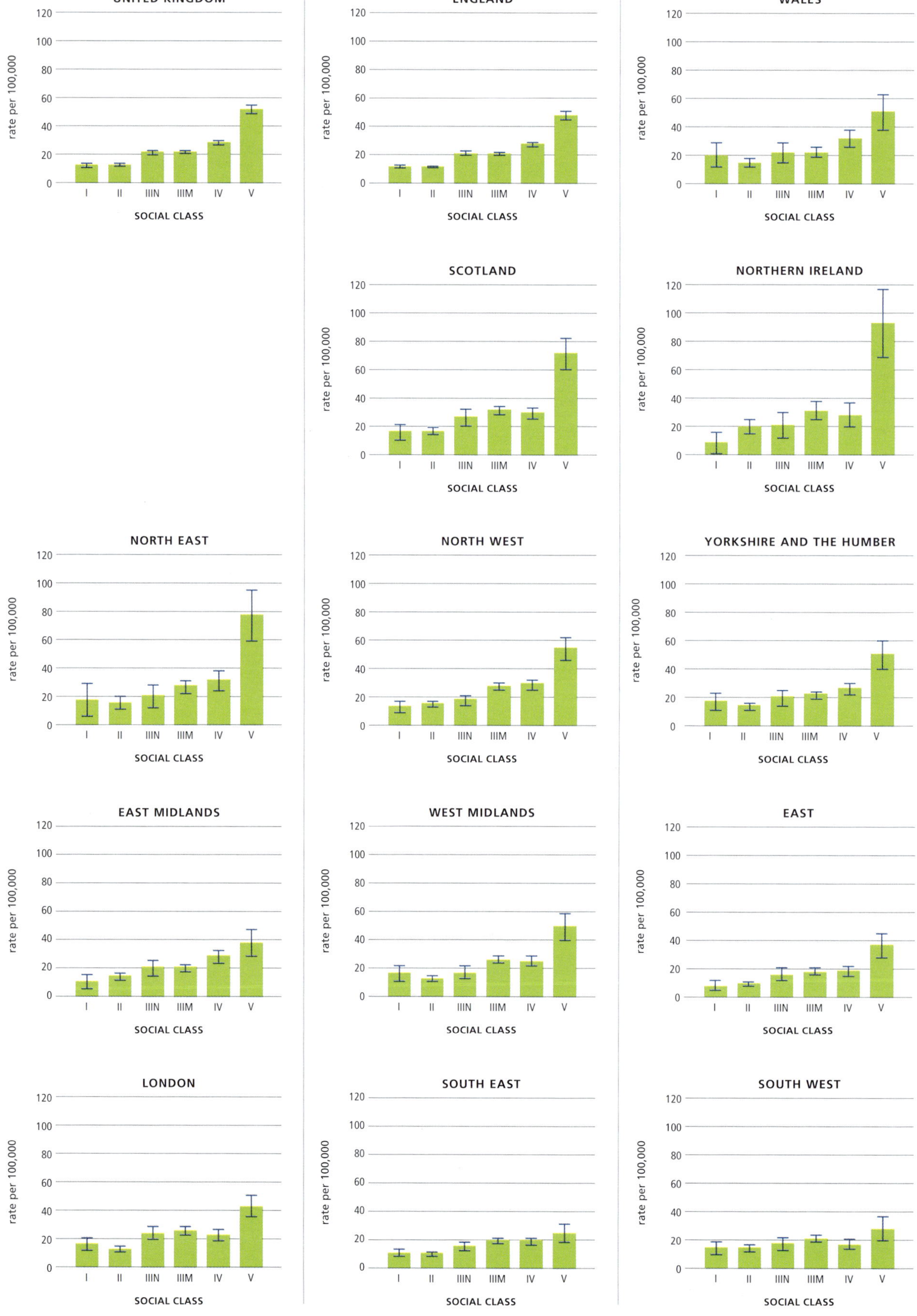

Figure 12.6

Age-standardised mortality rates for stroke for Social Classes I and V by country and region, males aged 20-64 United Kingdom 1991-1993

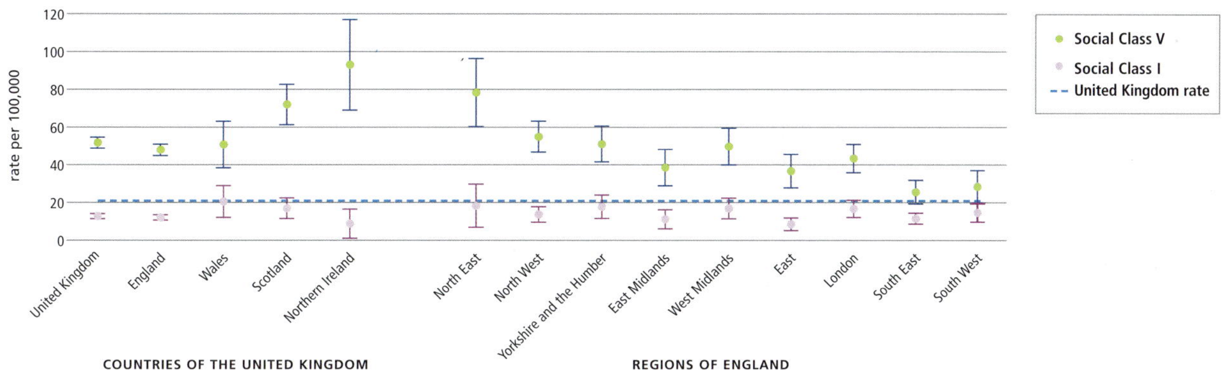

Stroke

Regional differences in Social Class mortality gradients were also evident in deaths from stroke, as Figure 12.5 shows. The difference between classes was greater in the northern regions of England, Scotland and Northern Ireland than in the southern regions of England. The Social Class gradient was steepest in Northern Ireland, where the difference between Social Class V and Social Class I was 10.6. This large difference was due to the combination of a particularly high rate for Social Class V and a slightly lower than average Social Class I rate. In the East of England, there were large disparities between Social Classes I and V (ratio of 4.3), despite mortality rates in every Social Class being lower than the national average. This was particularly interesting because a mortality gradient was not evident for all causes of death and for ischaemic heart disease in this region. The areas with the smallest class differences in stroke mortality were the South West and the South East.

Figure 12.6 summarises regional variation in class-specific stroke mortality. In Social Class I there was more geographic variation than for all causes of death. Although this variability was in part due to the smaller number of deaths available for analysis, mortality from stroke was significantly lower in the East of England than in the rest of the United Kingdom in Social Class I. The areas with the highest and lowest Social Class V mortality were Northern Ireland and the South East of England, respectively, with a ratio of 3.6 between the rates for the two areas.

Figure 12.7

Age-standardised mortality rates for all cancers by Social Class, country and region, males aged 20-64
United Kingdom 1991-1993

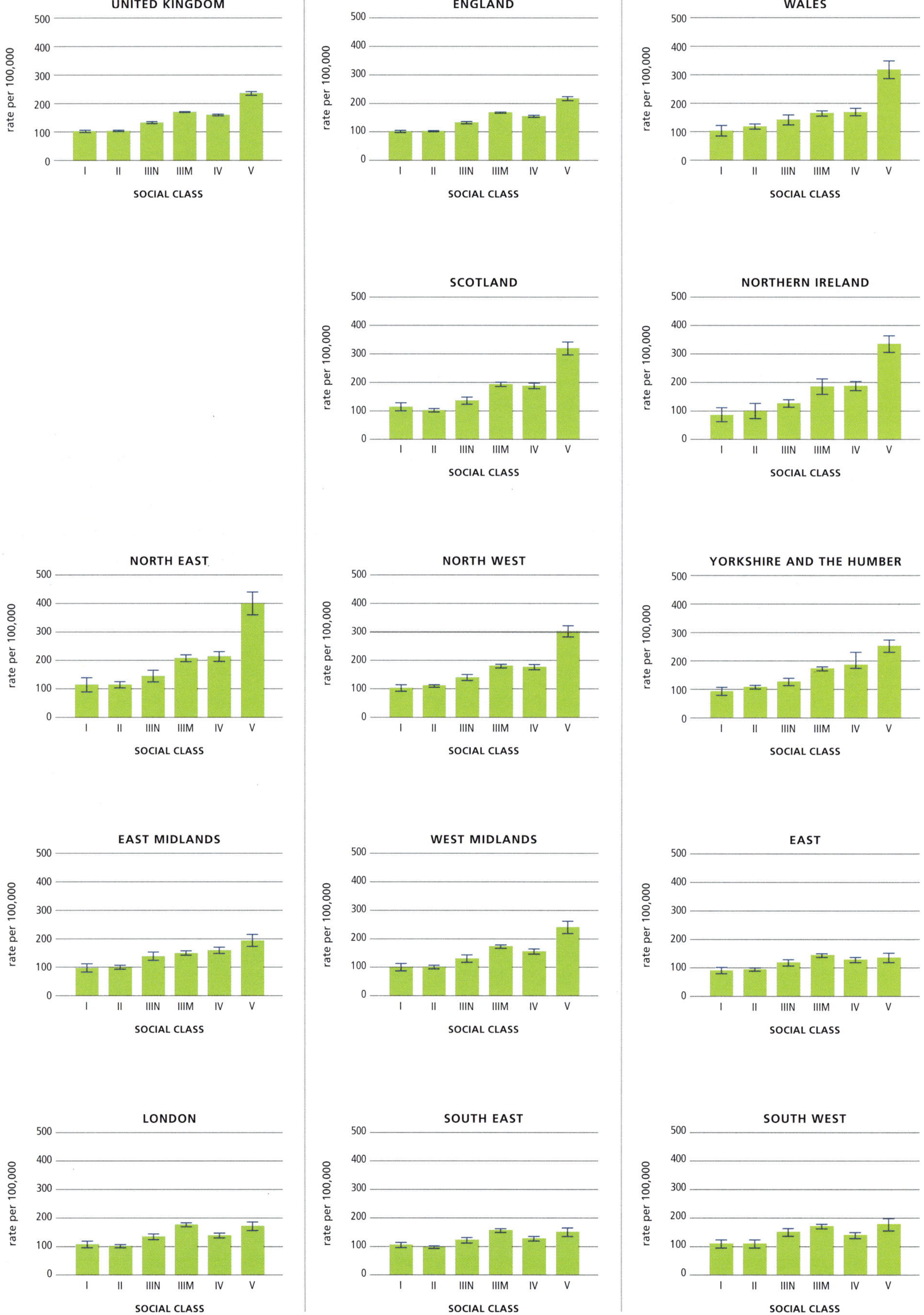

Figure 12.8

Age-standardised mortality rates for all cancers for Social Classes I and V by country and region, males aged 20-64 United Kingdom 1991-1993

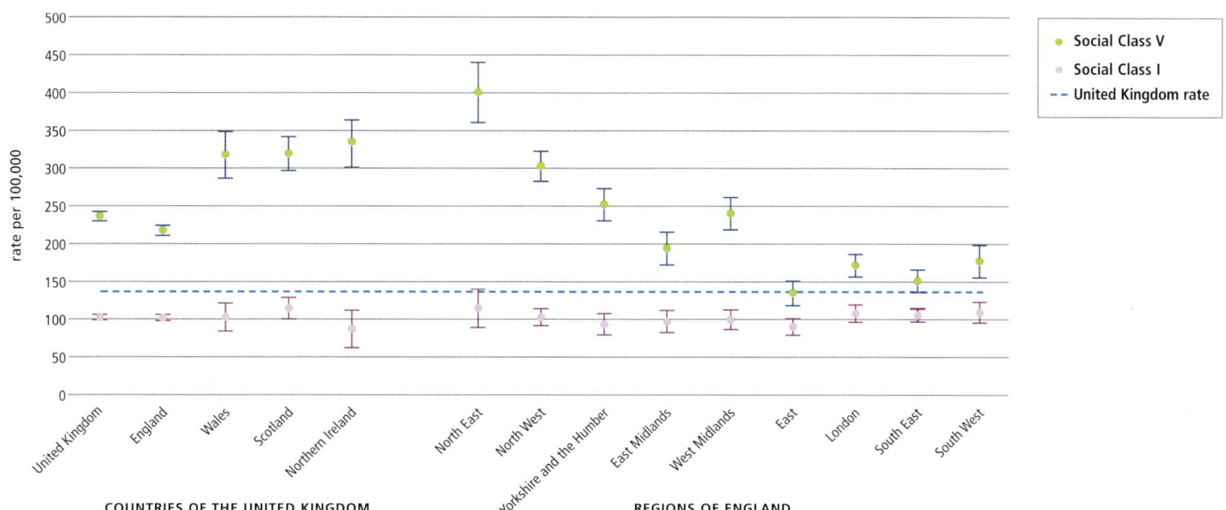

All cancers

In general there was a clear social gradient for cancers, with high mortality in Social Class V and low mortality in Social Classes I and II (Figure 12.7). For the United Kingdom as a whole, mortality in Social Class V was twice that in Social Class I. However, this ratio varied by country and region. A gradient was less apparent in the South East, South West, East of England and London where the ratio between Social Classes V and I was closer to 1.5. The North East showed the greatest relative mortality differences between Social Class V and other Social Classes (three and a half times greater than Social Class I and almost twice that of Social Class IV). A similar, but not as marked pattern, was present in the North West and Northern Ireland.

As for all cause mortality, regional differences were most apparent for Social Class V (Figure 12.8). Cancer mortality in Social Class V was greatest in the North East, Scotland, Northern Ireland and Wales. The rate in the North East was 1.7 times that for Social Class V in the United Kingdom as a whole. Within Social Class I there was very little difference in rates between countries and regions.

Figure 12.9

Age-standardised mortality rates for lung cancer by Social Class, country and region, males aged 20-64
United Kingdom 1991-1993

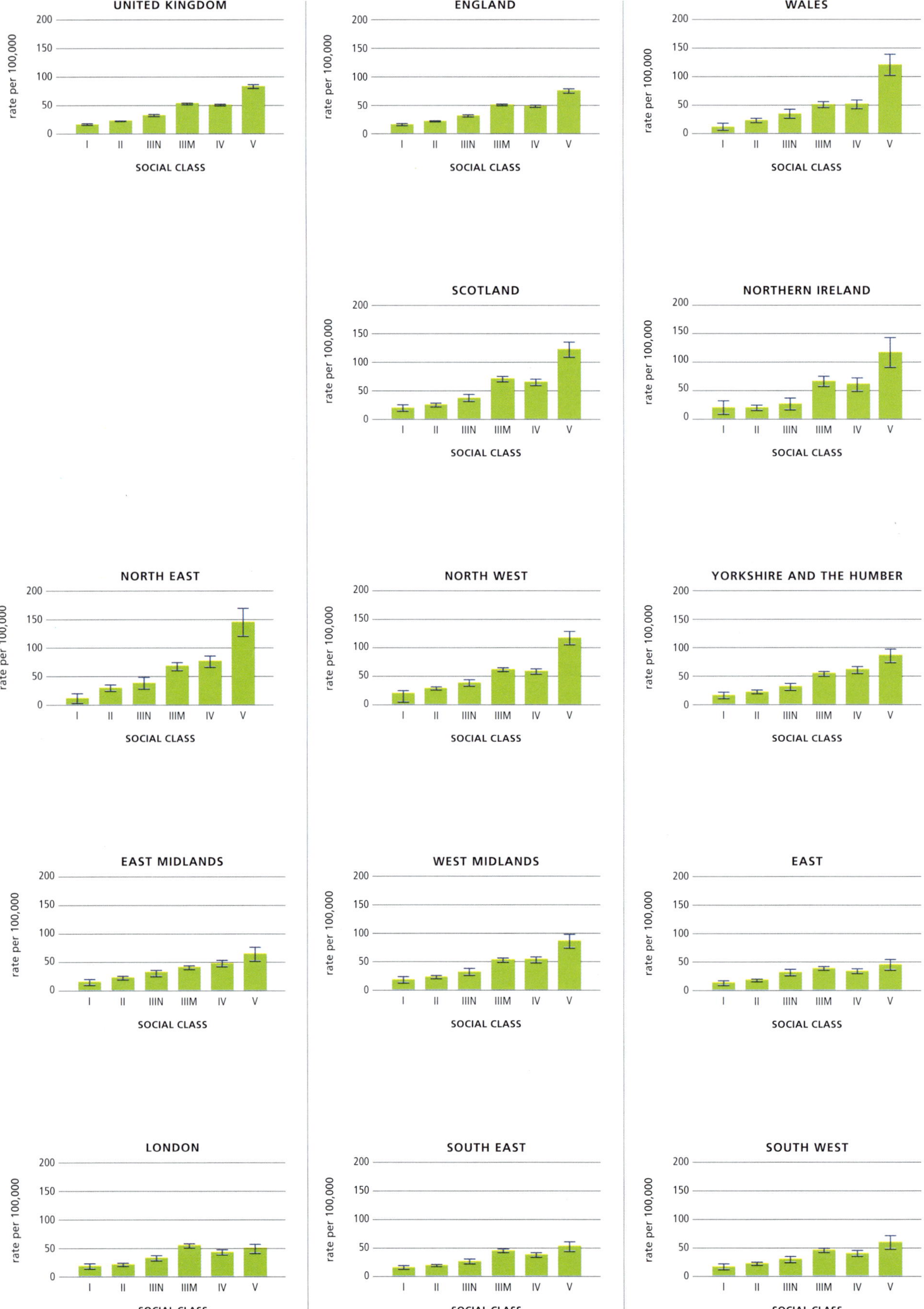

Figure 12.10

Age-standardised mortality rates for lung cancer for Social Classes I and V, lung cancer by country and region, males aged 20-64
United Kingdom 1991-1993

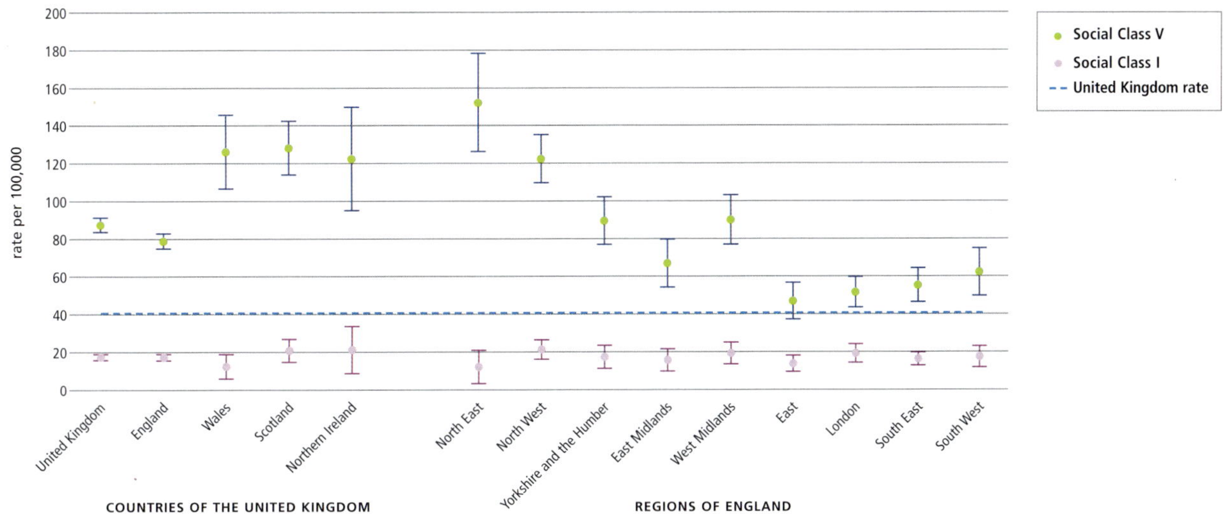

Lung cancer

The Social Class gradient in mortality from lung cancer was steeper than for all cancers combined (Figure 12.9). For the United Kingdom as a whole, mortality rates were five times greater for Social Class V than for Social Class I. The greatest geographic differences were once again within Social Class V. Mortality in this class was approximately twice as high as that in Social Class IV in the North East, North West, Wales, Scotland and Northern Ireland. In contrast the difference between this class and others was least in southern England.

Figure 12.10 summarises this sharp geographic gradient in Social Class V lung cancer mortality, with the lowest rate in the East of England and the highest in the North East. It also shows that for Social Class I there was little significant difference in rates between the regions and countries of the United Kingdom.

Figure 12.11

Age-standardised mortality rates for accidents by Social Class, country and region, males aged 20-64 United Kingdom 1991-1993

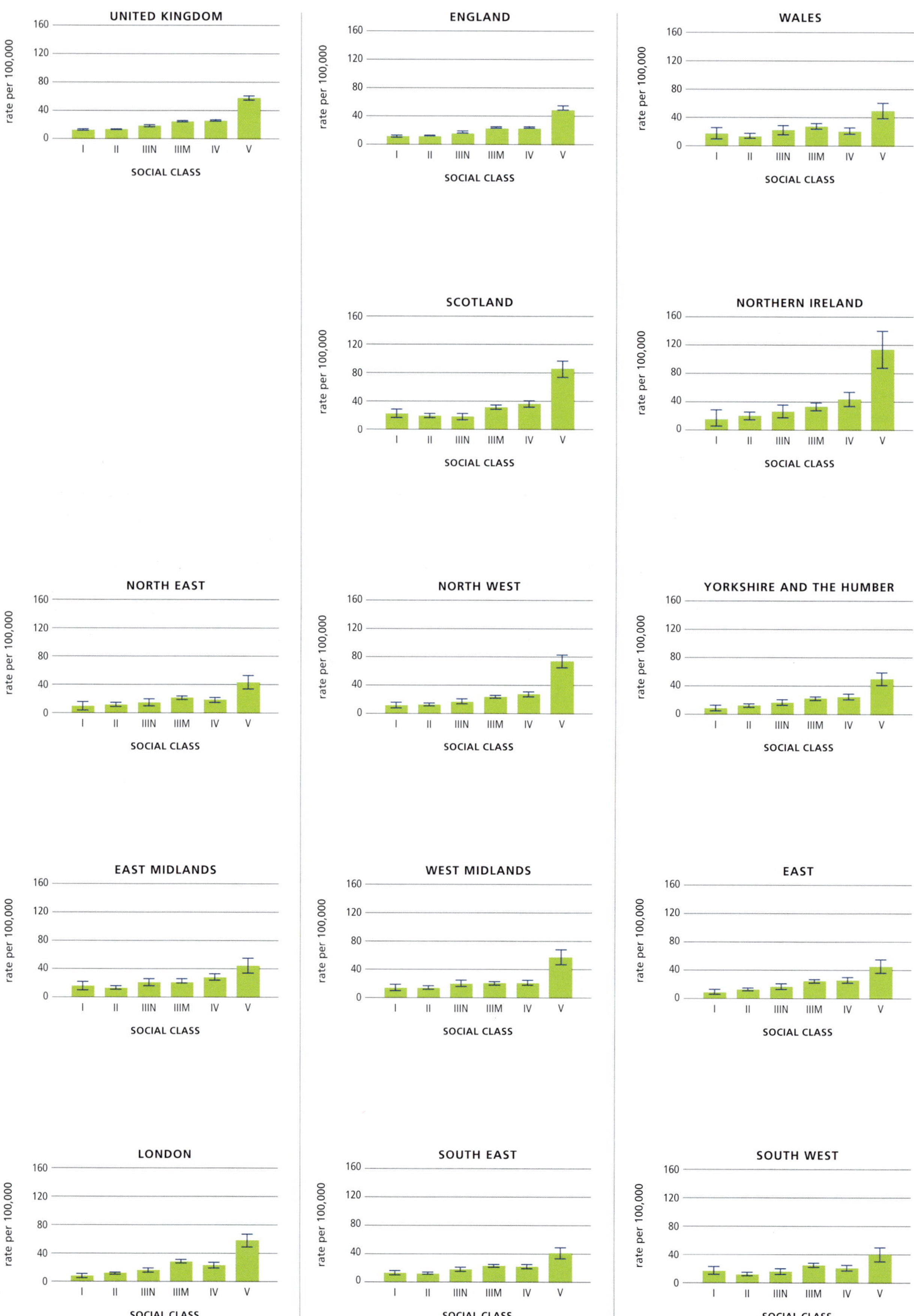

Figure 12.12

Age-standardised mortality rates for accidents for Social Classes I and V by country and region, males aged 20-64 United Kingdom 1991-1993

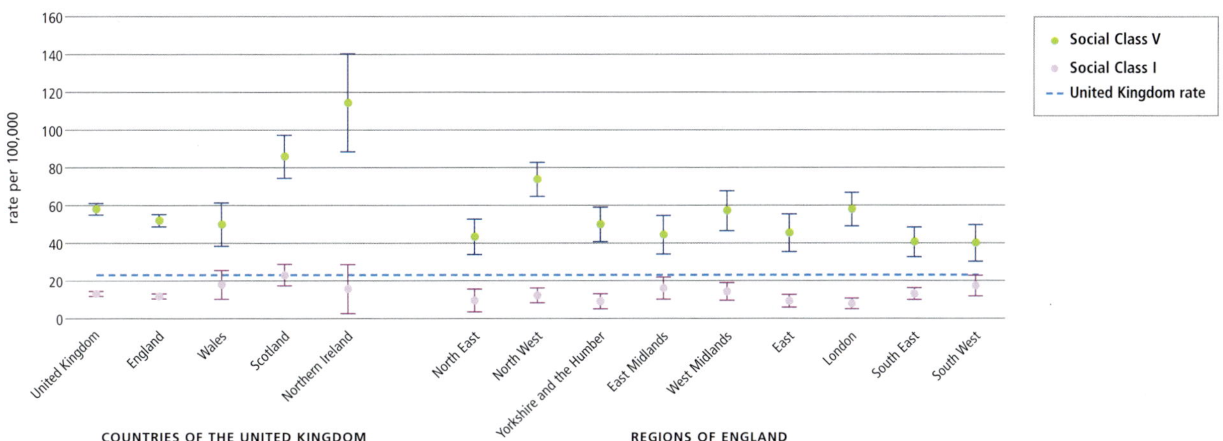

Accidents

There was a Social Class gradient in accident mortality for the United Kingdom as a whole, with Social Class V rates 4.4 times those in Social Class I (Figure 12.11). There were substantial differences between these classes in every region and country. The gradient between Social Classes I and IV was however noticeably less in every area. In Northern Ireland mortality from accidents was higher than the rest of the United Kingdom for all Social Classes and the seven-fold difference between Social Classes I and V in this area was greater than elsewhere.

Regional differences in accident mortality were evident in both Social Classes I and V (Figure 12.12). Mortality in Social Class I was highest in Scotland (1.8 times the United Kingdom rate for this class) and lowest in London. Rates for Social Class V were greatest in Northern Ireland (twice as great as the United Kingdom figure for this class) and least in the South West. Noticeably, accident mortality was low in both these Social Classes in the North East region, in contrast to findings for other causes.

Figure 12.13

Age-standardised mortality rates for suicide by Social Class, country and region, males aged 20-64
United Kingdom 1991-1993

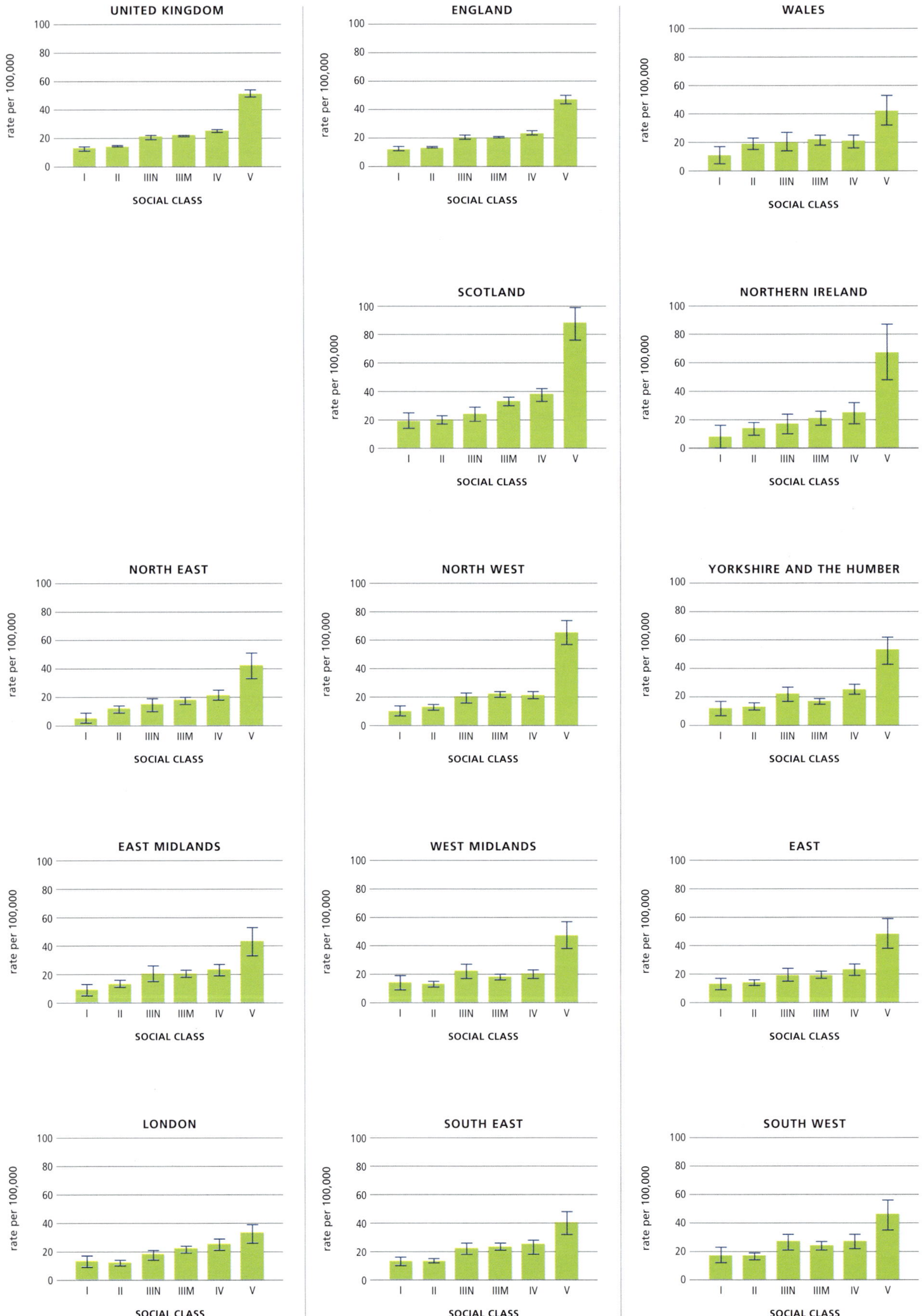

Figure 12.14

Age-standardised mortality rates for suicide for Social Classes I and V by country and region, males aged 20-64 United Kingdom 1991-1993

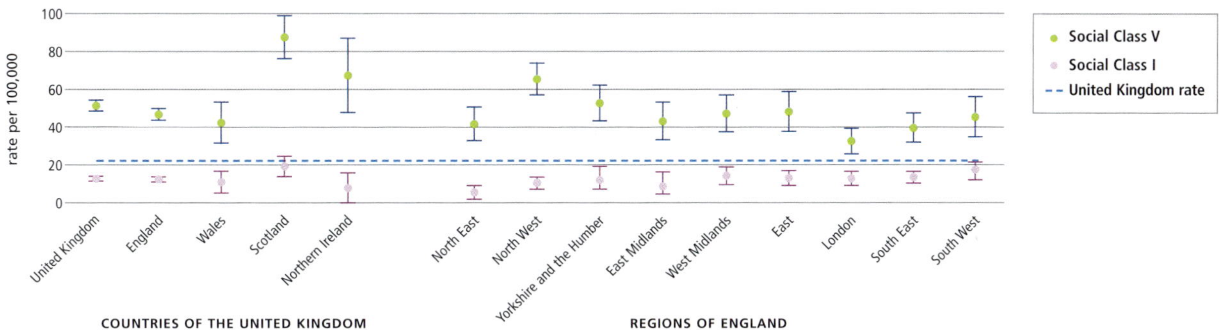

Suicide

There was a clear social gradient in suicide mortality between Social Classes (Figure 12.13), with a four-fold difference in mortality between Social Classes I and V for the United Kingdom as a whole. However, this was mainly associated with excess mortality in Social Class V, as the gradient was less apparent when the experiences of Social Class V were excluded. Scotland had the worst level of suicide mortality, with higher rates in each Social Class than all other countries and regions (with the sole exception of Social Class IIIN in the South West).

Figure 12.14 highlights considerable geographic variation in suicide mortality for both Social Classes I and V. For Social Class I, suicide mortality rates in Scotland were 3.5 times those in the North East (the region with the lowest mortality in this class). For Social Class V, rates in Scotland were 2.7 times higher than in London (where rates for this class were significantly below most other areas in the United Kingdom).

Figure 12.15

Age-standardised mortality rates for all causes of death by housing tenure, males all ages England and Wales 1991-1997

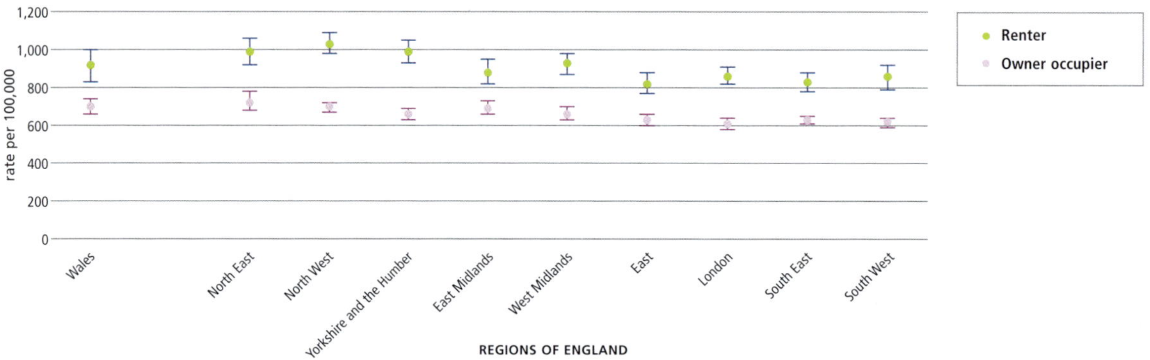

12.3 Mortality for the regions of England and for Wales by alternative social classifications

Methods and data

This analysis is based on data from the ONS Longitudinal Study, which is described in more detail in Appendix A. The study is based on a sample of approximately one per cent of the population of England and Wales. It includes records from each Census since 1971 and deaths in the inter-censal periods. This analysis is based on 1991 Census data and deaths between 1991 and 1997. Mortality rates are presented using directly standardised rates as in the rest of this chapter (see Section 12.2 for more details of methods and data). However, the method used in this section is slightly different to all the other sections. In previous sections the population used as the standard was the European Standard Population. In this section the Longitudinal Study population is used as the standard.

Housing tenure

Figures 12.15 and 12.16 show age-standardised mortality rates by housing tenure, for the regions of England and for Wales between 1991 and 1997. Both males and females living in owner-occupied housing experienced lower mortality in every region than those living in either local authority or privately rented housing. Within tenure categories there was evidence of a north-south divide in mortality rates. Mortality rates generally increased from the southern regions of England (East of England, London, South East and South West) to the Midlands and north. In particular, for both sexes and both tenure categories, mortality was significantly higher in the North East and North West than in each of the southern regions.

Car access

Figures 12.17 and 12.18 show age standardised mortality rates by car access for the regions of England and for Wales between 1991 and 1997. Both males and females with access to a car experienced lower mortality in every region than those without access to a car. Within car access categories there was evidence of a similar north-south divide in mortality rates to that for housing tenure, although not quite as consistent. While both sexes in the North East and North West had higher mortality than all southern regions for both car access categories, these differences were not statistically significant for males with no car access in the East of England and South West and for females with car access in London.

12.4 Discussion

In 1991 to 1993 there were clear socio-economic gradients in all-cause mortality for all countries of the United Kingdom and regions of England although the differences between Social Classes varied geographically. Generally differences in all cause mortality between Social Classes in the northern regions of England were larger than those in the southern regions. In addition larger differences were seen in Northern Ireland, Scotland and Wales than in England. This was true for mortality for each of the causes examined, but was less evident for accidents and suicide.

This chapter also demonstrates differences in the amount of geographic variation in mortality rates within Social Classes. Geographic variation was particularly great in Social Class V. For most causes of death, Social Class V mortality rates in the southern regions of England were considerably lower than in the northern regions of England, Northern Ireland, Scotland and Wales. In contrast there was little geographic variation in mortality rates for those in Social Class I.

An analysis of variance was conducted to examine how much of the variation in mortality rates by Social Class presented in this chapter was accounted for by the country and region of location (country/region) and how much was accounted for by Social Class. The results indicate that both country/region and Social Class contributed to the variation in mortality and in most cases approximately 80 per cent of the variation was explained by these two factors. The analysis also showed that Social Class was more highly correlated with mortality than country/region for all causes of death examined.

Figure 12.16

**Age-standardised mortality rates for all causes of death by housing tenure, females all ages
England and Wales 1991-1997**

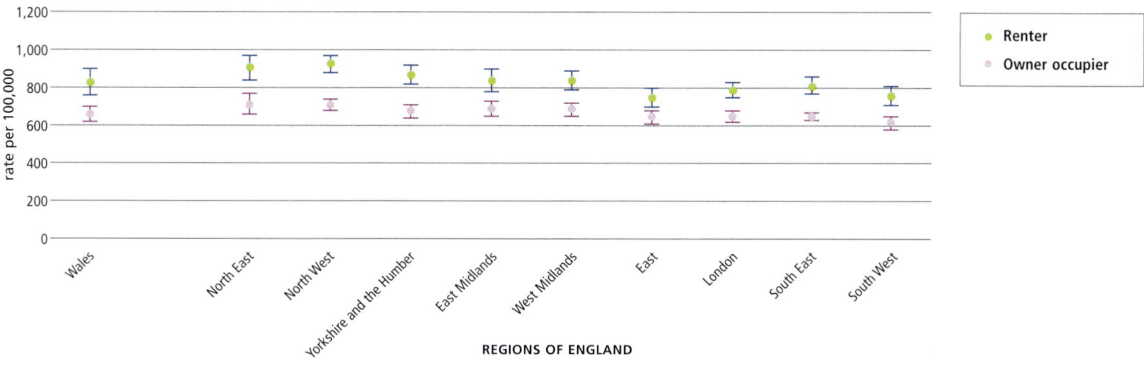

Figure 12.17

**Age-standardised mortality rates for all causes of death by car access, males all ages
England and Wales 1991-1997**

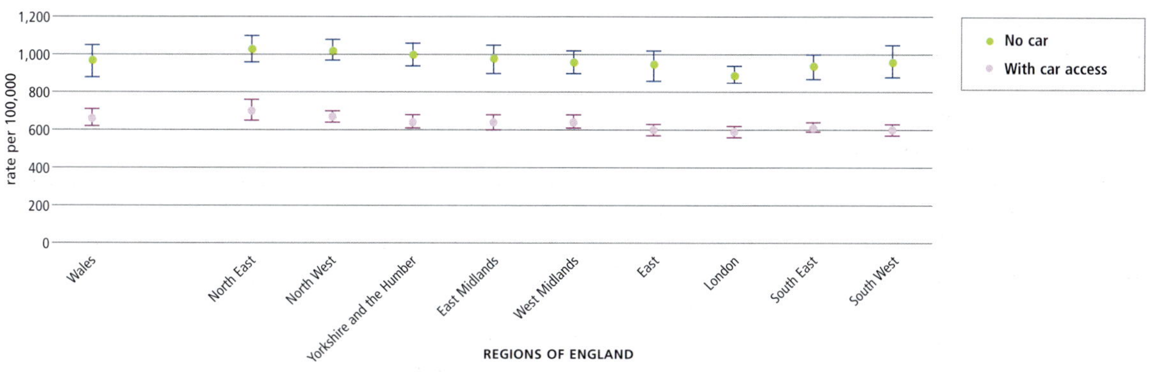

Figure 12.18

**Age-standardised mortality rates for all causes of death by car access, females all ages
England and Wales 1991-1997**

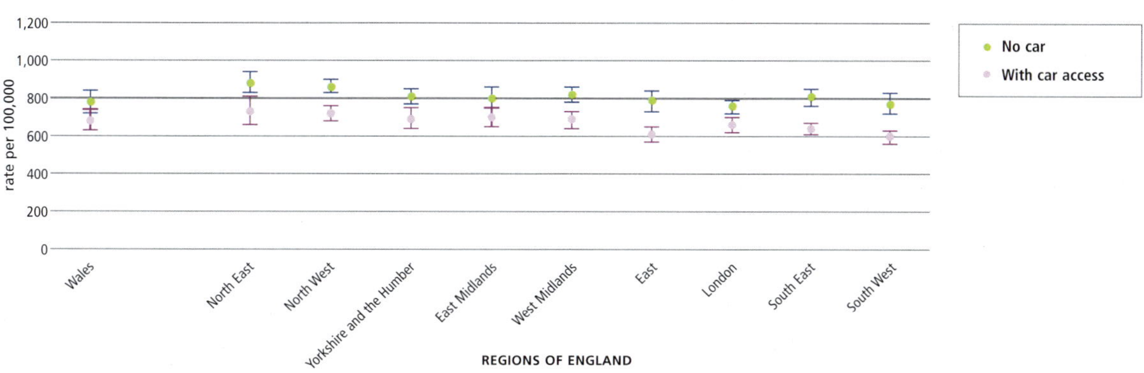

Analysis of mortality by housing tenure and car access confirms findings from other studies that those in owner occupied accommodation had lower mortality than those in rented accommodation and those with access to a car had lower mortality than those without. This was found to hold in each region of England and in Wales. Within car access and housing tenure categories, those living in the north of England had higher mortality than those living in the south.

What can we deduce from this strong and persistent relationship between geographic and socio-economic variation in mortality? In particular, the contrast between the very much higher mortality of the most deprived groups (such as Social Class V) in the northern regions of England, Wales, Scotland and Northern Ireland and the limited geographic variation among the most advantaged. Several generic models have been suggested which may help in explaining these patterns.

From their examination of the evidence, Shaw and colleagues[14] argue that *"social circumstances across the entire life-course – from birth through to late adulthood – influence people's health and well-being. The characteristics of the areas in which people live, as well as their individual characteristics, influence their health......Health inequalities are produced by the clustering of disadvantage – in opportunity, material circumstances and behaviours related to health – across people's lives. Health-related behaviours – such as smoking and diet – are strongly influenced by the social environment in which people live."*

On the other hand, Brunner and Marmot[15] hypothesise that the social determinants of health may be psychosocial, based on chronic stress associated with *"the organisation of work, degree of social isolation, and sense of control over life."* A key element of this are the gradients in health observed in the Whitehall Study, as well as in studies based on Social Class. These, they argue, indicate that *"position in the hierarchy (rather than absolute deprivation) is important. This suggests some concept of relative rather than absolute deprivation."*

Wilkinson[16] then argues that *"greater income inequality is one of the major influences on the proportion of the population who find themselves in situations that deny them a sense of dignity, situations that increase the insecurity they feel about their personal worth and competence, and that carry connotations of inferiority in which few can feel respected, valued and confident."*

In contrast to views which might emphasise the importance of area, in looking at the contribution of small areas and personal disadvantage in the LS, Sloggett and Joshi[17] concluded that *"higher death rates in areas identified as deprived by use of Census variables occur because a disproportionate number of socially disadvantaged people live there."*

Dahlgren and Whitehead[18] have proposed a generic model of health that represents the various determinants of health as layers of influence, one over another. This emphasises that individuals are endowed with age, sex and constitutional factors which influence their health potential, but which are fixed. Surrounding the individuals are layers of influence that, in theory, could be modified. These range from personal behaviour and way of life, to social and community influences in interactions with friends, family and neighbours, to wider influences on a person's ability to maintain health, such as living and working conditions and access to essential goods and services, and finally to the overall economic, cultural and environmental conditions prevailing in a society.

References

1 Registrar General. *Sixteenth annual report.* HMSO (London: 1856).

2 Smith S. Quoted in Simon J. *English sanitary institutions.* Cassell (London: 1890).

3 Registrar General. *Supplement to the twenty-fifth annual report.* HMSO (London: 1864).

4 Registrar General. *Supplement to the thirty-fifth annual report.* HMSO (London: 1875).

5 Drever F and Whitehead M. (eds.) *Health Inequalities.* Series DS No.15. The Stationery Office (London: 1997).

6 Pamuk ER. Social class inequality in mortality from 1921 to 1972 in England and Wales. *Population Studies* 39 (1985), 17-31.

7 Drever F and Bunting J. Patterns and trends in male mortality. In Drever F and Whitehead M. (eds.) *Health Inequalities.* Series DS No.15, The Stationery Office (London: 1997).

8 Britton M. (ed.) *Mortality and Geography.* Series DS No. 9. HMSO (London: 1990)

9 Britton M, Fox AJ, Goldblatt P, Jones DR and Rosato M. The influence of socio-economic and environmental factors on geographic variation in mortality. In Britton M (ed.) *Mortality and Geography.* Series DS No. 9. HMSO (London: 1990)

10 Rosato M, Harding S, McVey E and Brown J. Research implications of improvements in access to the ONS Longitudinal Study. *Population Trends* 91 (1998), 35-42.

11 Goldblatt PO. Mortality and alternative social classifications. In Goldblatt PO. (ed.) *Longitudinal Study: mortality and social organisation.* Series LS no. 6 HMSO (London: 1990), 164-192.

12 Reid A and Harding S. Trends in regional deprivation and mortality using the Longitudinal Study. *Health Statistics Quarterly* 5 (2000), 17-25.

13 Reid A and Harding S. An examination of persisting disadvantage and mortality in the regions using the Longitudinal Study. *Health Statistics Quarterly* 6 (2000), 17-25.

14 Shaw M, Dorling D, Gordon D and Davey Smith G. *The Widening Gap: health inequalities and policy in Britain* The Policy Press (Bristol: 1999).

15 Brunner E and Marmot M. Social organisation, stress and health. In Marmot M and Wilkinson RG (eds.). *Social Determinants of Health.* Oxford University Press (Oxford: 1999).

16 Wilkinson RG. Putting the picture together: prosperity, redistribution, health and welfare. In Marmot M and Wilkinson RG (eds.) *Social Determinants of Health.* Oxford University Press (Oxford: 1999).

17 Sloggett A and Joshi H. Higher mortality in deprived areas: community or personal disadvantage. *British Medical Journal* 309 (1994), 1470-1474.

18 Dahlgren G and Whitehead M. *Policies and strategies to promote social equity in health.* Institute for Future Studies (Stockholm: 1991).

Geographic variations in health: main findings and implications for the future

Clare Griffiths, Peter Goldblatt and Justine Fitzpatrick

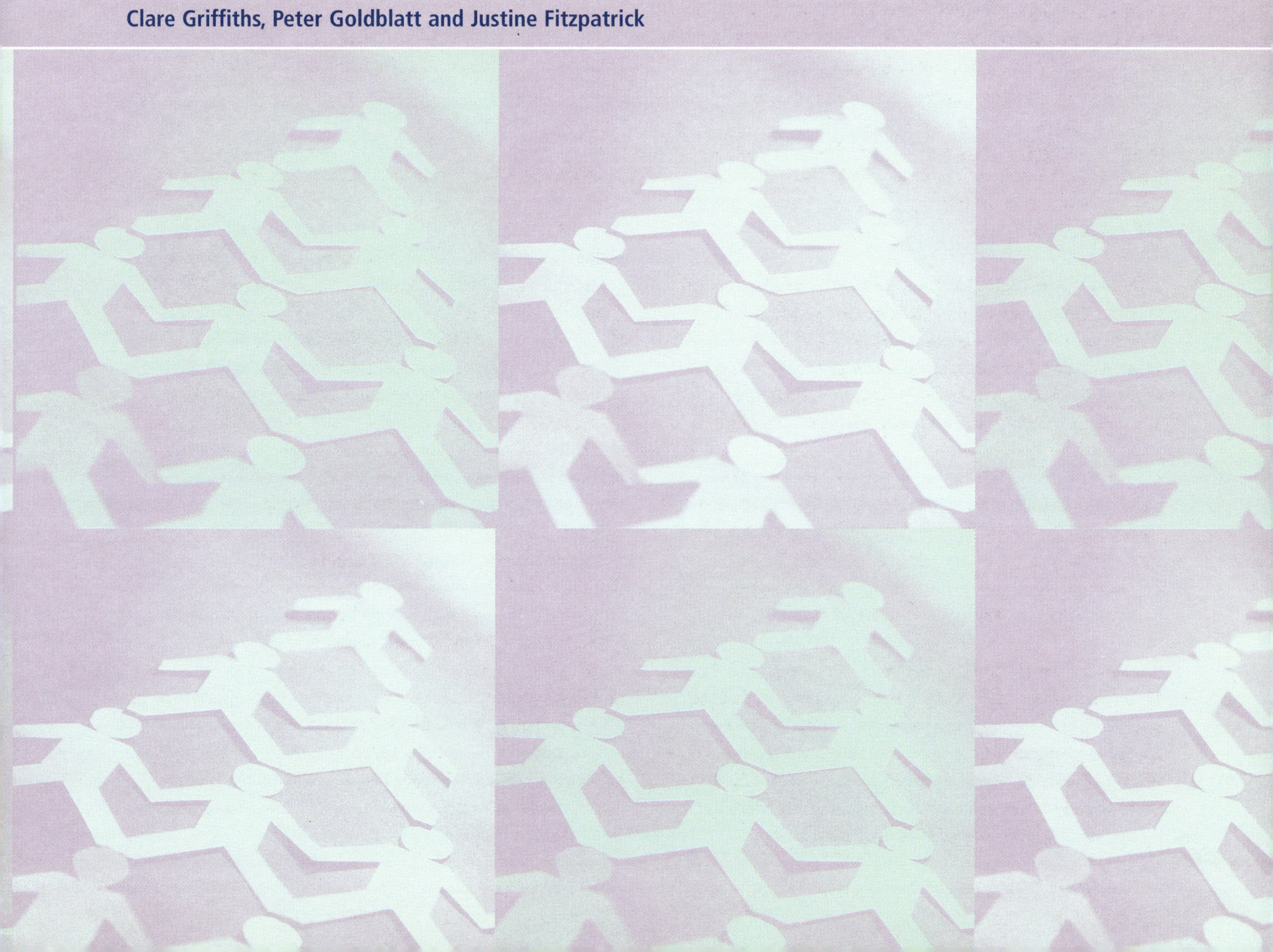

Chapter 13

Geographic variations in health: main findings and implications for the future

Summary of findings

- Age-standardised mortality rates for Scotland, Wales and Northern Ireland were higher than for England for both sexes. Within England, rates in the north were greater than those in the south.

- With some significant exceptions, this pattern was reflected in each age group for the major causes of death.

- Variations between local authorities within regions were greater than variations between regions throughout the United Kingdom.

- There were clear gradients with increasing levels of area deprivation throughout Great Britain in mortality from ischaemic heart disease, lung cancer and stroke and in infant mortality and stillbirth rates. For areas with similar levels of deprivation, mortality rates were higher in the north of England than in the south.

- Those living in more deprived areas had a higher incidence of lung cancer than those in less deprived areas. In contrast, the incidence of breast and prostate cancer shows an inverse association with deprivation; those living in less deprived areas were more likely to develop these cancers.

- Teenage fertility was seven times higher in the more deprived areas of Great Britain than in the least deprived areas. In contrast, higher fertility among older women was generally associated with areas in London, its surroundings and the more prosperous parts of Great Britain.

- Among men, there was a gradient of increasing mortality from ischaemic heart disease, lung cancer and stroke between Social Classes I and V in all countries and regions. The relative difference between these two classes was greatest in Wales, Scotland, Northern Ireland and the northern regions of England and least in the southern regions of England.

- Geographic variation in male mortality across the United Kingdom was minimal among those in Social Class I and increased across the Social Classes. Geographic variations among men in Social Class V were significantly greater than those in any other Social Class.

- Social Class made a larger contribution to male mortality variation than country or region of residence.

- Regional differences in stillbirth and infant mortality rates were reduced when factors such as Social Class were taken into account.

- Regional variations in notifications of congenital anomalies were affected by notification procedures. However, for those anomalies where the risk varies with mother's age, the geographic distribution was closely linked to variations in the mean age of mothers at the birth of their child.

13.1 Introduction

This chapter presents an overview of the main findings in this volume. It points to areas of concern where geographic inequalities have been increasing and comments on those areas where geographic inequalities are reducing. We draw together explanations for the patterns in health presented in the volume and highlight implications for future research.

13.2 Geographic differences in health described in this volume

From the analysis presented in this volume a number of patterns emerge. At country level, Scotland had the highest rates of lung cancer incidence and mortality; ischaemic heart disease (IHD), stroke and accident mortality; suicide; alcohol-related mortality and drug-related poisonings. Wales had the highest incidence of breast, prostate and colorectal cancer. Northern Ireland had the highest mortality from respiratory diseases. There was little variation between countries in stillbirths and infant mortality, although Scotland had a higher stillbirth rate than the other countries. England fared much better than the other countries, having the lowest rates for most of the outcomes discussed above.

However, at regional level within England, a north-south divide in health was evident for many outcomes discussed in this volume. Regions in the north had higher mortality from IHD, stroke, lung cancer and accidents, higher stillbirth and infant mortality rates and higher lung cancer incidence rates. Regions in the north also had higher pregnancy and birth rates for under 18s than those in the south.

A north-south divide in England was not evident in some of the other outcomes presented in this volume. London stood out as having the highest rates of mortality from infectious diseases and respiratory diseases. Suicide, drug-related poisonings and alcohol-related mortality did not show the north-south gradient that was evident for all-cause mortality. There was little geographic variation in breast, prostate and colorectal cancer mortality. There was, similarly, little variation in the incidence of colorectal cancer, while for breast and prostate cancer incidence rates in the south were higher than in the north. The geographic pattern in mean age at live birth showed that mothers in the south were more likely to be older at the birth of their child than those in the north. Abortion rates were highest in London for women in all age groups. There was not a clear north-south divide in congenital anomaly rates, but for those conditions known to be related to the age of the mother[1,2,3] rates were related to the average age at childbirth in the area.

Geographic patterns in mortality also differed by age as well as cause. At younger ages all-cause mortality rates in London were higher than average, whereas London had lower than average all-age rates. For IHD mortality, rates at ages 45-64 in London were lower than average, whereas stroke mortality rates at these ages in London were very high. No clear north-south divide in all-cause mortality was evident for those aged 15-44.

Differences in infant mortality rates by region were much reduced by accounting for factors such as birthweight, mother's age, Social Class, registration type and mother's country of birth. However, part of the differences between areas remained, indicating that these factors contribute to, but do not wholly account for, geographic differences in infant mortality. Regional differences were also seen in specific causes of infant death, particularly congenital anomalies and immaturity-related conditions.

A central finding in this volume is that differences between countries and regions masked wide differences within the regions themselves. In most cases 'within region' differences were much greater than 'between region' differences. We have used the ONS classification of local authorities[4] and the Carstairs and Morris index of deprivation[5] to describe these differences. Both of these measures group areas together on the basis of the characteristics of the individuals living there.

Urban and industrial areas, described using ONS classification Groups, had the highest stillbirth and infant mortality rates; all-cause mortality rates; mortality rates from major causes of death such as IHD, lung cancer and stroke; and teenage pregnancy rates. The characteristics of these areas include high unemployment, a high proportion of the population in Social Classes IV or V and a high proportion of terraced and social housing. In addition, using the Carstairs and Morris index of deprivation suggested that more deprived areas had higher rates of the outcomes described above than less deprived areas.

However, the pattern of cancer incidence by ONS classification Group varied by the site of the cancer. Urban and industrial areas and deprived areas had the highest rates of lung cancer incidence in both males and females. For colorectal cancer the pattern was unclear, while for prostate cancer and breast cancer the least deprived areas had the highest rates. In addition, fertility patterns by ONS classification Group varied with age; older mean ages at childbirth were found in prosperous areas, in areas immediately surrounding London and in London itself, whereas younger mean ages were found in the more urban and industrial areas, with high teenage pregnancy rates as described above.

From this discussion we can see that some of the differences highlighted between countries and regions can be explained by differences in the characteristics of the individual areas within these countries and regions. Countries and regions with a high percentage of the population living in authorities classified as urban and industrial or deprived had poorer health than those with low percentages living in these areas, although any potential health problems associated with older motherhood will be more prevalent in those areas classified as prosperous and least deprived.

13.3 Changes in geographic variation over time

It has been reported elsewhere that over recent decades, areas already experiencing the worst health have seen the smallest declines in mortality.[6,7] Generally in this volume, we have found that although mortality may be declining, differences between countries and regions have remained similar, or even widened - for example in the case of drug-related poisonings, the rate for London diverged from the rates in other regions during the 1990s.

Trends in fertility showed a slightly different pattern. Although rates have changed over the 1990s, the differences between countries and regions have remained relatively constant. For example, the effect of the 1995 pill scare appears to have been similar for all areas in Great Britain. One exception to this is the Total Fertility Rate, where the rate in Northern Ireland appeared to be converging with the rate in the other countries of the United Kingdom.

Although we have not analysed trends in health at the local level, it is possible at a broad level to compare patterns over time from earlier decennial supplements. It appears that although the names and precise boundaries of the authorities with highest and lowest mortality may have changed over time, they often cover similar geographic areas. For example, mortality in infants was noted by Farr in 1864[8] to be high in urban districts such as East London, Coventry, Whitechapel, Leeds, Wolverhampton, Manchester and Liverpool. Life expectancy at birth was also noted to be low in Manchester and Liverpool in 1911-1912,[9] and has recently been shown to be amongst the lowest in the United Kingdom in 1995-1997.[10] Reference to a north-south divide in mortality was made in 1921,[11] showing that standardised male mortality was highest in the north and lowest in the Midlands if London was included with the south. However, if London was excluded, the south had the lowest mortality. For females, mortality was lowest in the south whether London was included or not. These patterns have persisted into more recent times and were described in detail in the area mortality decennial supplements covering the 1970s[12] and 1980s,[13] as well as in this volume.

13.4 Interpretation of the results presented in this volume

In previous chapters we touched briefly on the interpretation of geographic inequalities in health and possible explanations for the findings in this volume. In this section we consider the following general issues in greater detail:

- Are the differences merely an artefact of the data presented here?
- Do migration patterns contribute to geographic variations in health across the United Kingdom?
- Are there geographic reasons for the differences presented, or are geographic inequalities merely a result of differences in the socio-economic structure of the areas?
- What contributions do health-related behaviour and the environment make to these differences?

Data issues

It is possible that issues such as differential completeness of data or levels of reporting, numerator-denominator biases and data quality may have contributed to some of the geographic differences reported in this volume.

The births and deaths data used in this volume are considered to be complete, as they are obtained from national registration data. However, data on congenital anomalies are not complete[14] and the level of completeness is known to vary by registry, as described in chapter 8 of this volume. Care must also be taken in interpreting variations in cancer incidence, as there are a number of factors that may affect variations between areas including geographic coverage of the cancer registries, methods of data collection and completeness of registration. These and other factors are described in more detail in the recent volume *Cancer Trends in England and Wales 1950-1999*.[15] There are potential biases in data on abortions by area, in particular abortion and conception rates calculated for local authorities may be inflated in areas where non-residents attend for abortion giving a temporary address as their address of usual residence.[16] Differences in the recording of abortions in Scotland compared to England and Wales were also described in detail in chapter 5.

Another issue to be considered is the stability of the geographic areas used in the analysis. The boundaries of areas change, due both to substantive administrative reorganisations and to a continual process of adjustment at small area level. Populations and events associated with individuals in that population may be assigned to one area one year and another the next. These boundary changes therefore pose problems of comparability when analysing data for geographic areas over time, as population exposure to risk is not held constant. One way to get round this problem is to allocate postcodes to boundaries at a fixed point in time and to match the data in other years with this geographic definition. This is the approach adopted in this volume for data for England, Wales and Scotland, using boundaries currently in use as the fixed spatial reference.

However, use of the postcode to allocate events such as births and deaths to geographic areas also poses problems. The post office administers postcodes, and can terminate and re-use them in a different area from the original postcode. This creates two problems for data analysis. First, it is difficult to allocate terminated postcodes to a current area. Second, it is difficult to avoid allocating an event to the wrong area if the postcode has been re-used elsewhere. While these problems can be overcome to some extent, this is far from straightforward. In addition, each postcode covers around 15 addresses. This may cross an area boundary, requiring arbitrary decisions to be taken as to which area to allocate an event with a postcode of this sort. Some events will necessarily be wrongly allocated.

Grid referencing of data - linking addresses to a fixed point on a map - reduces many of the above problems. Data can easily be recast using different boundaries to provide statistics for different areas, independently of the time period during which the boundaries were in use. By choosing a grid referencing system with a suitable degree of spatial definition, the chances of misallocating an address across a boundary are substantially reduced. ONS strategy is to progressively adopt grid referencing. This will enable the Office to respond more easily to boundary change and be more flexible in the outputs it produces.

Artefact explanations

The main problem in inferring causality from geographic patterns is the so-called 'ecological fallacy.' Statistics for areas show the average health experience for people living in that area during a particular time period, as well as the average values for possible causal factors. However, the fact that there is a statistical relationship between health outcomes and other factors at an area level does not imply causality. Robinson was among the first to point out that the behaviour of individuals cannot be inferred from analysis based on aggregate units.[17] Within an area, the individuals with the worst health may not be those with the highest levels of the suspected causal factor. Indeed, those currently experiencing adverse health outcomes in an area may not have been exposed to the risk at all, for sufficient duration or at a point in time that would make the relationship plausible.

A significant issue in looking at area correlations in general, and deprivation in particular, is the effect of collinearity, i.e. that risk factors cluster together. In geographic analyses, this means that if clustering occurs at the area level being analysed, it may be impossible to tell which of the factors is having a causal effect on outcomes. Any inferences may therefore be subject to the ecological fallacy.

Selective migration

The effect of migration on geographic variations in health is always of concern when looking at differences at one point in time. Welton[18] noted this problem in looking at migration into and out of London between 1851 and 1860. He hypothesised a dual effect. Migrants were generally stronger than those who remained, resulting in a relatively unhealthy rural population at ages affected by migration to towns. Also, migrants who then lost their health in the towns returned home to die, or long-standing town-dwellers may have moved to the countryside after becoming ill. Stevenson,[19] in 1913, also noted the problem of town-dwellers returning to the countryside to die and pointed out that this was difficult to resolve as previous residence in a town would not have been noted anywhere in the death registration. Hill,[20] in 1925, reported on a study carried out to look in more detail at this effect. He concluded that migration of healthy people to the towns was very important, but that the returning home of migrants to die seemed to be less important in affecting death rates. Fox and Goldblatt[21] reviewed this hypothesis using data from the ONS Longitudinal Study and put forward the view that migration selects out two principal groups - those with existing serious health problems, who are more likely to move locally and have high mortality in the short term, and those with very good health over the long term - who tend to predominate among those moving greater distances.

Analysis by Davey Smith and colleagues showed that those areas experiencing the greatest population decline in the 1980s also experienced increases in their mortality rates throughout this period.[22] They suggest that the 'healthy migrant effect' described by Hill was probably responsible for this. Analysis in the previous Decennial Supplement on geography found that movers into more affluent areas tended to have similar or lower mortality than the area they moved into and that the pattern of mortality for migrants across England and the net effect of migration on mortality rates in the area of origin and destination were variable.[23] Another study by Strachan *et al* examined migration into London and showed that movers into London acquired the low mortality rates from IHD seen in London as a whole.[24]

Brimblecombe *et al*, using the mortality data so far available from the British Household Panel Survey, found that migration appeared to make little difference to regional mortality rates,[25] but that it could account for most of the difference in male mortality rates between districts[26] and between deprived and non-deprived areas.[27] However, selective attrition, the method used in collecting the mortality data and small numbers of events may have had an impact on these findings.

Analysis by Reid and Harding[28] attempted to overcome some of the effects of migration on mortality patterns by looking at the mortality of those who remained within the same region between 1981 and 1991, by disadvantage in 1981 and 1991. They found that both region of residence and long-term disadvantage appeared to have independent effects on mortality.

Migration may also have an impact on the fertility patterns seen in chapter 5 as migration occurs more in the childbearing years.[29] Migration appears to be associated with childbearing itself, with the desire to move to more spacious accommodation around the birth of a child. The ability to move depends on housing tenure, income and resources, with those living in shared accommodation before the birth of a child being more likely to move. Fertility rates in under 18s and 18-19s may also be altered by the movements of students to university towns and cities. However, it is difficult to quantify what effect this has on rates.

Differences in the socio-economic structure of the population within areas

One explanation put forward for geographic differences in health is that they simply reflect a concentration of people of lower socio-economic status, with their concordant health problems. This can only be a partial explanation, as the results in this volume demonstrate. Other factors also appear to influence geographic patterns of health in the United Kingdom.

Within the countries of the United Kingdom and the regions of England there are differences in the health of the population by socio-economic status. Within all regions of England babies born to fathers in Social Class V had higher infant mortality rates than those born to fathers in Social Class I, although regional differences persisted across all Social Classes. Both area and individual effects were important in determining geographic differences in adult mortality, with individual Social Class and local area deprivation making a larger contribution to male mortality than country or region of residence. Men aged 20-64 in Social Class V had higher mortality than those in Social Class I living in the same region. Men in Social Class V living in the northern regions of England had higher mortality than men aged 20-64 in Social Class V living in the southern regions of England, while there was little geographic variation within Social Class I.

The extent and causes of socio-economic differences in health, such as these, have been analysed in this country for over 150 years, based on both geographic and occupational differences in mortality. In the mid-1970s, concern at *"Britain's failure to match the improvement in health in some other countries"*[30] focused attention on the contribution made by persistent inequalities in health. The Black report[30] brought together evidence available at that time on inequalities in mortality, longstanding illnesses and utilisation of health services (particularly preventative services). It concluded that, while genetic and cultural or behavioural explanations played their part at different stages of the life course - including smoking patterns and access to and uptake of health care (in particular preventative services such as antenatal care) - the predominant or governing explanation for inequalities in health lay in material deprivation and specific features of the socio-economic environment such as working and housing conditions. Since that report, several generic models, described in more detail in chapter 12, have been suggested which may help in explaining geographic and social patterns of health.

From their examination of the evidence on geographic differences, Shaw and colleagues[7] argue that social circumstances across the entire life course influence health, as do characteristics of the areas in which people live. Thus health inequalities are produced by clusters of disadvantage, and health-related behaviours are strongly related to people's social environment. Brunner and Marmot[31] hypothesise that the social determinants of health may be psychosocial, based on chronic stress associated with organisation of work, degree of social isolation and sense of control over life. They argue that position in the hierarchy is important, suggesting some concept of relative rather than absolute deprivation.

Wilkinson[32] has hypothesised that greater income inequality is one of the major influences on the proportion of the population who find themselves relatively deprived. In contrast to views emphasising the influence of area on individual health, in looking at the contribution of small areas and personal disadvantage in the ONS Longitudinal Study, Sloggett and Joshi[33] concluded that higher death rates in deprived areas occur because a disproportionate number of socially disadvantaged people live there.

Dahlgren and Whitehead[34] proposed a generic model of health that represents the various determinants of health as layers of influence, one over another. This emphasises that individuals are endowed with fixed characteristics such as age and sex, which influence their health potential. Surrounding the individuals are layers of influence that, in theory, could be modified. These range from personal behaviour, to social and community influences, to wider influences on a person's ability to maintain health and finally to the overall economic, cultural and environmental conditions prevailing in a society.

Health-related behaviour

Geographic variation in behaviours affecting health may have a role in determining the geographic patterns of some of the outcomes described in this volume, most obviously mortality and the incidence of cancer.

Levels of smoking vary quite markedly across the United Kingdom. It is also clear from the analysis in chapters 9 and 10 that the regional pattern of lung cancer incidence and mortality closely follows the regional pattern of smoking described in chapter 3. The effect of deprivation on both lung cancer incidence and mortality also follows the pattern of smoking by deprivation. It is well known that those of lower social status are more likely to be heavy smokers than those of higher status[35] and it is this fact that drives the pattern of lung cancer by deprivation.

Studies have suggested that diet has little influence on regional differences in mortality and alcohol some influence, whereas smoking has a substantial degree of influence.[36] Data presented in chapter 3 of this volume show that alcohol consumption and diet seem to vary only a little between regions and are therefore likely to have limited influence on the regional geographic patterns of health described.

The effect of behaviours where the influence on health is not as clear-cut is difficult to interpret. It is likely that differences in attitude to health and disease across regions and across Social Classes also have an impact on the geographic variation described in this volume but it is far from straightforward to quantify the effects. For example, while physical activity varies across groups with differing social status and shows a north-south divide within England,[37] the contribution this makes to the patterns of health described is unclear.

Genetics

Genetic factors and their differential distribution within the United Kingdom may also have a role to play. Some of the outcomes we have examined in this volume are known to have a genetic cause, for example Down syndrome. Genetics may also influence health and disease in a less direct way. It is possible that the distribution of ancestral populations based on different origins and modes of settlement still influences spatial patterns of health and disease today, despite blurring by centuries of migration and intermarriage. Migration of modern immigrant groups may also play a part in localised clustering of conditions such as sickle-cell anaemia, thalassaemia and polydactyly. Immigrant groups may also carry with them diseases that are more prevalent in their countries of origin. This may, for example, partly explain the higher rates of infectious disease mortality in London, although the role of HIV should not be underestimated.[38]

There is strong evidence of a relationship between blood group and disease.[39] The distribution of blood groups differs across the country and does seem to show a very broad relationship with regional mortality, with those areas having a higher percentage of blood group A genes being lower mortality areas, and those with a higher percentage of O genes being higher mortality areas.[40]

There is also evidence of a relationship between genetics and some diseases. For example, some forms of breast cancer have been shown to be genetically determined.[41,42] Some patients with severe heart problems have a gene that prevents cholesterol being removed from the blood.[43] In addition, the inherited form of Alzheimer's is probably the commonest severe mental illness with an unequivocally genetic basis.[43] However, the effect of these relationships on regional and local mortality variations is difficult to assess.

The environment

Much work has been carried out into the associations between environment and health. In this section we examine some of the aspects briefly and speculate as to whether these associations could have an effect on the geographic patterns of health described in earlier chapters. For example, the environment might have a much stronger role in congenital anomalies than other health measures studied in this volume.[44] The relationship between weather and various aspects of health has been much studied, for example relationships have been found between temperature and IHD,[45] stillbirths and infant mortality,[46] stroke and pneumonia, but not cancer.[47] IHD mortality has also been found to be correlated with rainfall, and it is possible that this has an impact on regional differences in IHD mortality.[45] However, it is thought that the association between IHD and temperature is likely to explain relatively little inter-regional variation, explaining more seasonal variation.[48] Analysis of infant mortality and stillbirths also suggests that it is seasonal variation in temperature that has an effect.[49] Seasonality in mortality has declined since the 1960s, possibly due to increased usage of central heating, but also a decline in air pollution.[50]

The impact of background radiation may be a factor in some diseases. The sedimentary rocks of the south and east (lowland) have a lower content of radioactive elements, and therefore gamma radiation, than the north and west (highland).[40] In addition, doses of radiation that are not permitted in the nuclear industry are not uncommon from natural sources in the high radon areas of Devon and Cornwall.[51] This raises concern as studies of miners occupationally exposed to radon have consistently shown them to be at increased risk of lung cancer.[52] Evidence suggests that residential radon exposure increases the risk of lung cancer by about the same level as this occupational exposure, implying that residential radon may be responsible for about one in 20 lung cancers in the United Kingdom.[53]

Issues of water quality, particularly water hardness, have been much reviewed. Hard water is found in the south and east, soft water in the north and west. A consistent relationship has also been shown between soft water and high levels of heart disease. The most detailed study is the British Regional Heart Study, which studied 253 towns. Water hardness was found to be one of several factors involved in geographic variations in heart disease. Other independent variables were temperature, rainfall, manual employment and car ownership.[54]

Both deficiencies and excesses of certain trace elements, in water and elsewhere, are known to be harmful to health.[55,56] Excesses of nickel, cadmium, mercury and lead are considered hazardous. However, the effect that high levels of cadmium from a disused zinc mine near the village of Shipham has had on the mortality of residents of the village is unclear. The latest study of this village shows all-cause mortality lower than expected, but with a significant excess of cancer incidence and a borderline significant excess of stroke mortality.[57] The potential hazards of lead poisoning from drinking soft water after exposure to lead pipes has also been highlighted,[58] although this is less of a problem today. High concentrations of aluminium in water have been put forward as an explanation of geographic variation in the distribution of Alzheimer's disease,[59] although the strength of the association has since been debated.[60]

Atmospheric pollution is certainly associated with excess mortality from respiratory diseases, a classic example being the great smog of 1952 in London,[61] which caused 4,000 deaths in the period between the 6th and 10th December, and air pollution may be partly responsible for the raised levels of respiratory disease mortality in London. In addition, problems with pollution from petrochemical and chemical complexes may be associated with mortality. This has been demonstrated for cancer in the city of Houston in the United States.[62] A heavy concentration of lung cancer in industrial areas may be indicative of a link with pollution as hypothesised by Haynes,[63] although this is confounded by differential levels of smoking. Doll and Peto have hypothesised that smoking is more responsible for urban excesses of lung cancer than is atmospheric pollution.[64] Particular local problems also exist, for example lead poisoning near roads, and associations with particular industries, for example asbestos, coal, slate, tin and china clay.[65]

Access to services

Before the establishment of the NHS in 1946, the regional distribution of healthcare facilities favoured the south and east of the country, because of the attraction of services to client wealth. These regional differences in England and Wales continued well into the 1970s, because of the maintenance of inherited stock.[40] In 1971, Tudor Hart hypothesised the 'inverse care law', whereby those most in need of health services and health care were the least likely to receive the services and care they required.[66] Since 1976 regional resources have been allocated based on formulae intended to meet health needs, rather than reflecting demand, existing utilisation or supply.[67,68] However, expansion of private services has been concentrated in the south[69] and it is acknowledged that the inverse care law continues to operate in many parts of the NHS.[70] Poverty itself may pose problems in accessing health care services,[71] and an inequitable system may reinforce poverty.[72]

13.5 Discussion

This volume set out to provide a broader view of geographic variations in health than its predecessors. In terms of topics covered, this was achieved by examining mortality (including infant mortality and stillbirths), fertility-related topics (including conceptions, abortions, live births and congenital anomalies) and cancer incidence. In geographic terms, the analyses were extended to cover the whole of the United Kingdom wherever possible. The previous decennial supplement, *Health Inequalities,*[73] had confirmed a widening of socio-economic differences in health. There is also growing concern that the quality of life in many poor neighbourhoods has become increasingly detached from the rest of society.[74] This prompted us to place particular attention on the characteristics of areas and the interplay between place and person in the analyses presented.

This report has confirmed that in the 1990s, mortality from the major causes was higher in Scotland, Wales and Northern Ireland than in England for both sexes and that, within England, the north-south divide persisted. However, variations between local areas within each region were greater than the variations between regions and there were clear gradients with increasing levels of area deprivation across the United Kingdom in mortality from ischaemic heart disease, lung cancer and stroke, and in infant mortality and stillbirth rates. For areas with similar levels of deprivation, mortality rates were higher in the north of England than in the south.

At an individual level, Social Class made a larger contribution to adult male mortality variation than country or region of residence and regional differences in stillbirth and infant mortality rates were partially explained by factors such as Social Class. Among men there was a gradient of increasing mortality from ischaemic heart disease, lung cancer and stroke between Social Classes I and V in all countries and regions. The relative difference between these two classes was greatest in Wales, Scotland, Northern Ireland and the northern regions of England and least in the southern regions of England. There was little geographic difference in mortality among those in Social Class I. Regional and country differences increased substantially across the Social Classes and were significantly greater in Social Class V than in any other Social Class.

Patterns of cancer incidence varied by site. Those living in more deprived areas had a higher incidence of lung cancer than those in less deprived areas, while the reverse was true for breast and prostate cancers. Teenage fertility was seven times higher in the more deprived areas of the United Kingdom than in the least deprived areas. In contrast, higher fertility among older women was generally associated with areas in London, its surroundings and the more prosperous parts of the United Kingdom. Although regional variations in notifications of congenital anomalies were affected by notification procedures, for those anomalies where the risk varies with mother's age, the geographic distribution was closely linked to variations in the mean age of mothers at the birth of their child.

Each of the administrations in the United Kingdom has developed strategies for health in which the reduction of inequalities is an integral part. The *NHS Plan*[75] for England aims to bring improvements in health across the board and to reduce health inequalities. The White Paper *Towards a Healthier Scotland*[76] calls for a *"coherent attack on health inequalities with a special focus on improving the health of children and young people."* The recent consultation paper produced by the Department of Health, Social Security and Public Safety in Northern Ireland *Investing for Health*[77] and the Health Strategy for Wales *Better Health Better Wales*[78] both have a commitment to targeting health inequalities.

The information provided in this volume on health status in different areas, its spatial patterning and its relationship to disadvantage will provide the background against which decisions can be made to target action and ensure that appropriate baselines are set to monitor the impact of policies and initiatives on outcomes. In the future, the opportunities provided by the ONS geographic referencing strategy and the greater availability of data on health at local level will improve the quality of local area monitoring and hence bring greater accuracy in assessing the role of neighbourhood characteristics on individuals' health.

References

1 Botting B, Rosato M and Wood R. Teenage mothers and the health of their children. *Population Trends* 93 (1998), 19-28.

2 Makinson C. The health consequences of teenage fertility. *Family Planning Perspectives* 17 (1985), 132-139.

3 Mutton D, Alberman E and Hook EB. Cytogenetic and epidemiological findings in Down syndrome, England and Wales 1989 to 1993. *Journal of Medical Genetics* 33 (1996), 387-394.

4 Office for National Statistics. *The ONS classification of local and health authorities: revised for authorities in 1999.* The Stationery Office (London: 1999).

5 Carstairs V and Morris R. *Deprivation and health in Scotland.* Aberdeen University Press (Aberdeen: 1991).

6 Dorling D. *Death in Britain: How local mortality rates have changed 1950s-1990s.* Joseph Rowntree Foundation (York: 1997).

7 Shaw M, Gordon D, Dorling D and Davey Smith G. *The Widening Gap. Health inequalities and policy in Britain.* The Policy Press (Bristol: 1999).

8 General Register Office. *Supplement to the twenty-fifth annual report of the Registrar General.* HMSO (London: 1864).

9 General Register Office. *Supplement to the seventy-fifth annual report of the Registrar General.* HMSO (London: 1914).

10 Griffiths C and Fitzpatrick J. Geographic inequalities in life expectancy in the United Kingdom, 1995-97. *Health Statistics Quarterly* 9 (2001), 16-28.

11 General Register Office. *Registrar General's decennial supplement. England and Wales 1921.* HMSO (London: 1933).

12 Office of Population Censuses and Surveys. *Area mortality decennial supplement. England and Wales 1969-1973.* Series DS No. 4. HMSO (London: 1981).

13 Britton M. (ed.) Mortality and Geography. *A review in the mid 1980s. England and Wales.* Series DS No. 9. HMSO (London: 1990).

14 Office of Population Censuses and Surveys. *The OPCS monitoring scheme for congenital malformations. A review by a Working Group of the Registrar General's Medical Advisory Committee.* Occasional Paper 43. OPCS (London: 1995).

15 Quinn M, Babb P, Brock A, Kirby L and Jones J. *Cancer Trends in England and Wales 1950-1999.* Series SMPS No. 66. The Stationery Office (London: 2001).

16 Office for National Statistics. Series AB. *Abortion Statistics, England and Wales.* The Stationery Office (London: 1997).

17 Robinson WS. Ecological correlations and the behaviour of individuals. *American Sociological Review* 15 (1950), 351-357.

18 Welton TA. The effects of migration in disturbing local rates of mortality as exemplified in the statistics of London and the surrounding country for the years 1851-60. *Journal of the Institute of Actuaries* 16 (1872), 153-186.

19 General Register Office. *Seventy-fourth annual report of the Registrar General for the year 1911.* HMSO (London: 1913).

20 Hill AB. *Internal migration and its effect upon the death rates: with special reference to the county of Essex*. MRC Special Report Series No. 95. HMSO (London: 1925).

21 Fox AJ and Goldblatt PO. *Longitudinal Study: socio-demographic mortality differentials 1971-1975*. Series LS No. 1. HMSO (London: 1982).

22 Davey Smith G, Shaw M and Dorling D. Shrinking areas and mortality. *Lancet* 352 (1998), 1139-1140.

23 Britton M, Goldblatt PO, Jones DR and Rosato M. The influence of migration on geographic variation in mortality. In Britton M. (ed.) *Mortality and Geography. A review in the mid 1980s. England and Wales*. Series DS No. 9. HMSO (London: 1990), 79-94.

24 Strachan DP, Leon DA and Dodgeon B. Mortality from cardiovascular disease among interregional migrants in England and Wales. *British Medical Journal* 310 (1995), 423-427.

25 Brimblecombe N, Dorling D and Shaw M. Mortality and migration in Britain - first results from the British Household Panel Survey. *Social Science and Medicine* 49 (1999), 981-988.

26 Brimblecombe N, Dorling D and Shaw M. Migration and geographical inequalities in health in Britain. *Social Science and Medicine* 50 (2000), 861-878.

27 Dorling D, Shaw M and Brimblecombe N. Housing wealth and community health: exploring the role of migration. In Graham H. (ed.) *Understanding health inequalities*. Open University Press (Buckingham: 2000), 186-199.

28 Reid A and Harding S. An examination of persisting disadvantage and mortality in the regions using the Longitudinal Study. *Health Statistics Quarterly* 6 (2000), 7-13.

29 Grundy E. Migration and fertility behaviour in England and Wales: a record linkage study. *Journal of Biosocial Science* 18 (1986), 403-423.

30 Townsend P and Davidson N. (eds.) *Inequalities in Health. The Black Report*. Penguin (London: 1992).

31 Brunner E and Marmot M. Social organisation, stress and health. In Marmot M and Wilkinson RG. (eds.) *Social Determinants of Health*. Oxford University Press (Oxford: 1999).

32 Wilkinson RG. Putting the picture together: prosperity, redistribution, health and welfare. In Marmot M and Wilkinson RG. (eds.) *Social Determinants of Health*. Oxford University Press (Oxford: 1999).

33 Sloggett A and Joshi H. Higher mortality in deprived areas: community or personal disadvantage. *British Medical Journal* 309 (1994), 1470-1474.

34 Dahlgren G and Whitehead M. *Policies and strategies to promote social equity in health*. Institute for Future Studies (Stockholm: 1991).

35 Drever F, Fisher K, Brown J and Clark J. *Social Inequalities 2000*. The Stationery Office (London: 2000).

36 Law MR and Morris JK. Why is mortality higher in poorer areas and more northern areas of England and Wales? *Journal of Epidemiology and Community Health* 52 (1998), 344-352.

37 Office for National Statistics. *Living in Britain. Results from the 1996 General Household Survey*. The Stationery Office (London: 1998).

38 Hickman M, Bardsley M, De Angelis D and Ward H. Impact of HIV on adult (15-54) mortality in London: 1979-96. *Sexually Transmitted Infections* 75 (1999), 385-388.

39 Mourant A. *Blood Groups and Diseases*. Oxford University Press (Oxford: 1978).

40 Jones HR. *Population Geography. Second Edition*. Paul Chapman (London: 1990).

41 Ford D, Easton DF and Peto J. Estimates of the gene frequency of BRCA1 and its contribution to breast and ovarian cancer incidence. *American Journal of Human Genetics* 57 (1995), 1457-1462.

42 Wooster R, Bignell G, Lancaster J, Swift S, Seal S, Mangion J, Collins N, Gregory S, Gumbs C and Micklem G. Identification of the breast cancer susceptibility gene BRCA2. *Nature* 378 (1995), 789-792.

43 Jones S. *In the blood. God, genes and destiny*. Harper Collins (London: 1996).

44 Brent RL and Beckman DA. The contribution of environmental teratogens to embryonic and fetal loss. *Clinical Obstetrics and Gynecology* 37 (1994), 646-670.

45 West RR and Lowe CR. Mortality from ischaemic heart disease – inter-town variation and its association with climate in England and Wales. *International Journal of Epidemiology* 5 (1976), 195-201.

46 Hare EH, Moran PA and Macfarlane A. The changing seasonality of infant deaths in England and Wales 1912-78 and its relation to seasonal temperature. *Journal of Epidemiology and Community Health* 35 (1981), 77-82.

47 Bull GM and Morton J. Environment, temperature and death rates. *Age and Ageing* 7 (1978), 210-224.

48 Eldwood PC, Beswick A, O'Brien JR, Renaud S, Fifield R, Limb ES and Bainton D. Temperature and risk factors for ischaemic heart disease in the Caerphilly prospective study. *British Heart Journal* 70 (1993), 520-523.

49 Hawe E, Macfarlane A and Bithell J. Daily and seasonal variation in live births, stillbirths and infant mortality in England and Wales, 1979-96. *Health Statistics Quarterly* 9 (2001), 5-15.

50 McDowall M. Long-term trends in seasonal mortality. *Population Trends* 26 (1981), 16-19.

51 Darby S. Editorial: Radiation risks. *British Medical Journal* 319 (1999), 1019.

52 National Research Council. *Committee on health risks of exposure to radon: Beir VI, health effects of exposure to radon*. National Academic Press (Washington DC: 1999).

53 Darby S, Whitley E, Silcocks P, Thakrar B, Green M, Lomas P, Miles J, Reeves G, Fearn T and Doll R. Risk of lung cancer associated with residential radon exposure in south-west England: a case-control study. *British Journal of Cancer* 78 (1998), 394-408.

54 Shaper A. Geographic variations in cardiovascular mortality in Great Britain. *British Medical Bulletin* 40 (1984), 366-373.

55 Cannon H and Hopps H. *Geochemical environment in relation to health and disease*. Geological Society of America Special Paper 140. Boulder (Colorado: 1972).

56 Warren H. Geology, trace elements and health. *Social Science and Medicine* 29 (1989), 923-926.

57 Elliott P, Arnold R, Cockings S, Eaton N, Jarup L, Jones J, Quinn M, Rosato M, Thornton I, Toledano M, Tristan E and Wakefield J. Risk of mortality, cancer incidence and stroke in a population potentially exposed to cadmium. *Occupational and Environmental Medicine* 57 (2000), 94-97.

58 Bacon AP, Froome K, Gent AE, Cooke TK and Sowerby P. Lead poisoning from drinking soft water. *Lancet* 1 (1967), 264-266.

59 Martyn CN, Barker DJ, Osmond C, Harris EC, Edwardson JA and Lacey RF. Geographical relation between Alzheimer's disease and aluminium in drinking water. *Lancet* 1 (1989), 59-62.

60 Martyn CN, Coggon DN, Inskip H, Lacey RF and Young WF. Aluminium concentrations in drinking water and risk of Alzheimer's disease. *Epidemiology* 8 (1997), 281-286.

61 Logan WPD. Mortality in the London fog incident, 1952. *Lancet* 1 (1953), 336.

62 Mason T. *Atlas of cancer mortality of US Counties 1950-1969.* Government Printing Office (Washington DC: 1975).

63 Haynes R. The urban distribution of lung cancer mortality in England and Wales 1980-83. *Urban Studies* 25 (1988), 497-506.

64 Doll R and Peto R. The causes of cancer: quantitative estimates of avoidable risks of cancer in the United States today. *Journal of the National Cancer Institute* 66 (1981), 1191-1308.

65 Greenberg M and Coleman MP. *Medical Research at the Office for National Statistics: a review.* Series SMPS No. 65. The Stationery Office (London: 2000).

66 Tudor Hart J. The inverse care law. *Lancet* 1 (1971), 405-412.

67 Department of Health and Social Security. *Sharing resources for health in England: report of the Resource Allocation Working Party.* HMSO (London: 1976).

68 NHS Executive. *HCHS revenue resource allocation to health authorities: weighted capitation formulas.* NHS Executive (Leeds: 1997).

69 Mohan J. Restructuring, privatisation and the geography of health care provision in England 1983-87. *Transactions of the Institute of British Geographers* 13 (1988), 449-465.

70 Acheson D. *Independent inquiry into inequalities in health.* The Stationery Office (London: 1998).

71 Mackintosh M. Do health care systems contribute to inequalities? In Leon DA and Walt G. (eds.) *Poverty, inequality and health. An international perspective.* Oxford University Press (Oxford: 2001), 175-193.

72 Barnes M. Users as citizens: collective action and the local governance of welfare. *Social Policy and Administration* 33 (1999), 73-90.

73 Drever F and Whitehead M. (eds.) *Health inequalities.* The Stationery Office (London: 1997).

74 Social Exclusion Unit. *Bringing Britain together, a national strategy for neighbourhood renewal.* Cabinet Office (London: 1998).

75 Department of Health. White Paper. *The NHS Plan.* The Stationery Office (London: 2000).

76 Scottish Executive. White Paper. *Towards a Healthier Scotland.* The Stationery Office (Edinburgh: 1999).

77 Department of Health. Social Security and Personal Services. *Investing for Health.* Department of Health, Social Security and Personal Services (Belfast: 2000).

78 Welsh Office. *Better Health Better Wales.* The Stationery Office (Cardiff: 1998).

Appendices

Appendix A
Sources and methods

This appendix briefly discusses the data sources and methods used by the authors of this volume. A guide to the maps and details on the geography used are also included. Generally this appendix only discusses issues that are relevant to more than one chapter to avoid duplication between individual chapters.

Data sources

A wide variety of sources have been used in this volume, including birth and death registration data, cancer registration data, abortion notifications and congenital anomaly notifications. More details on these data sources can be found within the relevant chapters. These sources have been supplemented, where possible, using data from the ONS Longitudinal Study, and the introductory chapters make use of both Census and survey data.

The ONS Longitudinal Study
The ONS Longitudinal Study (LS) is a representative one per cent sample of the population of England and Wales containing linked Census and vital events data for approximately 500,000 people. The LS was begun in the early 1970s by selecting everyone born on one of four particular dates who was enumerated at the 1971 Census. Subsequent samples have been drawn and linked from the 1981 and 1991 Censuses using the LS dates of birth and data from the 2001 Census will also be linked. Population change is reflected by the addition of new sample members born on the LS dates together with the recording of exits via death or emigration. Routinely collected data on mortality, fertility and cancer registration for sample members are linked using the National Health Service Central Register (NHSCR) to perform the link. More details on the LS can be found in the LS Technical Volume.[1]

Methods

Method of age-standardisation
All rates in chapters 9-12 of this volume are age-standardised. Mortality and cancer incidence increase with age and therefore areas with older populations would generally experience higher crude rates than those with young populations. Age-standardisation enables comparisons of mortality and cancer incidence rates between different areas while allowing for differences in the age structure of the population.

All mortality and cancer rates in this volume are directly standardised using the European Standard Population (Table A1). This is used because it is closest to the demographic profile of the United Kingdom, having a high proportion of the population in the older age groups. The same population is used for both males and females.

Directly standardised rates measure the number of events per 100,000 population that would occur in the standard population if it had the same age-specific rates as the population being studied. Further details of direct standardisation can be found in numerous demography and statistical textbooks.[2,3]

Table A1
The European Standard Population

Age group	European Standard Population
0	1,600
1-4	6,400
5-9	7,000
10-14	7,000
15-19	7,000
20-24	7,000
25-29	7,000
30-34	7,000
35-39	7,000
40-44	7,000
45-49	7,000
50-54	7,000
55-59	6,000
60-64	5,000
65-69	4,000
70-74	3,000
75-79	2,000
80-84	1,000
85+	1,000
Total	100,000

Calculation of confidence intervals
Standard methods for the calculation of the confidence interval for a directly standardised rate are used.[2,3] All confidence intervals for data for countries and regions have been calculated at the 95% level, using the appropriate methods for the rate or percentage under discussion. Where necessary, further details have been discussed within individual chapters. All confidence intervals for local authorities used in the presentation of maps have been calculated at the 90% level.

Guide to maps

Two main types of map are presented in this volume:

The first are those which divide authorities up into categories based on their value for a particular measure. These categories may be quintiles, in the case of cancer data, or predetermined categories, such as in the data for country of birth, Social Class and so on. These maps are single colour maps, with shading graded from blue to white, where blue denotes high values and white low values.

The second type of map, used in the majority of the chapters that include analysis at local authority level, compares the values for a particular measure with the national value. For different chapters this may be United Kingdom, Great Britain or England and Wales. For this type of map, we have allocated local authorities to categories on the basis of statistical significance, since there may only be a small number of events in any given local authority in a particular age group. We have attached 90% confidence intervals to all rates and percentages. The maps are constructed using the values for these confidence intervals in order to highlight true geographic variation. An authority is:

- Shaded purple if the 90% confidence interval around the rate or percentage excludes and is higher than the 90% confidence interval around the national value. Therefore, all authorities shaded purple had higher rates or percentages than the national value. Those shaded purple are divided into two groups with an equal number of authorities in each. Those shaded dark purple had the highest rates or percentages.

- Shaded green if the 90% confidence interval around the rate or percentage excludes and is lower than the 90% confidence interval around the national value. Therefore, all authorities shaded green had lower rates or percentages than the national value. Those shaded green are divided into two groups with an equal number of authorities in each. Those shaded dark green had the lowest rates or percentages.

- Unshaded if the 90% confidence interval around the rate includes the national 90% confidence interval. These authorities either had similar rates or percentages to the national value, or had large confidence intervals attached to their rates as the number of events in the authority was small.

Geography

England and Wales

Data for England and Wales are presented for authorities as they existed in April 1999. Data for abortions, conceptions, births, mortality, cancer and congenital anomalies have been recast to the latest administrative boundaries using the postcode of usual residence. Postcodes recorded at the time of event were matched to the Central Postcode Directory (CPD) for 1999 to obtain the corresponding administrative area for 1999. Generally, the Isles of Scilly and City of London have been excluded from the analysis due to small numbers in their populations.

Census data was produced for 1999 authorities by re-aggregating original Census data. ONS Census Division supplied us with a listing of the constituent of each new local authority in terms of its census authorities, wards and enumeration districts.

Scotland

Data for Scotland are presented for authorities as they existed in April 1999. This data was supplied directly to us by the General Register Office for Scotland (GROS) and the Information and Statistics Division of the NHS in Scotland (ISD).

Northern Ireland

Data for Northern Ireland are presented for local authorities as they existed at the time the data was collected. There was one boundary change in Northern Ireland during the period of analysis (Rathfriland ward was reallocated to Banbridge from Newry and Mourne in 1993). This data was supplied directly to us by the General Register Office for Northern Ireland (GRONI) and the Northern Ireland Statistics and Research Agency (NISRA).

Confidentiality

In each chapter, for all countries, rates and percentages are not included for any local authority where there are less than ten cases in any one category.

Data for non-residents

Generally data for non-residents are excluded from the analyses in this volume. There are two exceptions to this. In chapter 5, births data for England, Wales, Scotland and Northern Ireland at local authority level refer to residents of these countries only. However, data at country level for Scotland and Northern Ireland include approximately 280 and 190 births to non-residents respectively.

In chapter 10, data for England, Wales and Scotland at local authority level refer to residents of these countries only. However, data for Northern Ireland at both country and local authority level include approximately 90 deaths per year to non-residents. These deaths to non-residents are allocated to the local authority of occurrence. In addition, data for Scotland at country level include approximately 330 deaths per year to non-residents.

Data on conceptions, abortions, congenital anomalies and cancer refer to residents only, as do all data in chapters 2-4.

References

1 Hattersley L and Creeser R. *Longitudinal Study 1971-1991. History, organisation and quality of data.* Series LS 7. HMSO (London: 1995).

2 Breslow N and Day N. *Statistical Methods in Cancer Research, Volume II: The Design and Analysis of Cohort Studies.* International Agency for Research on Cancer, WHO (Lyon: 1987).

3 Armitage P and Berry G. *Statistical Methods in Medical Research,* 2nd edition. Blackwell Scientific Publications (Oxford: 1987).

Appendix B
Reference maps

Map A

Countries of the United Kingdom and Government Office Regions of England 1999

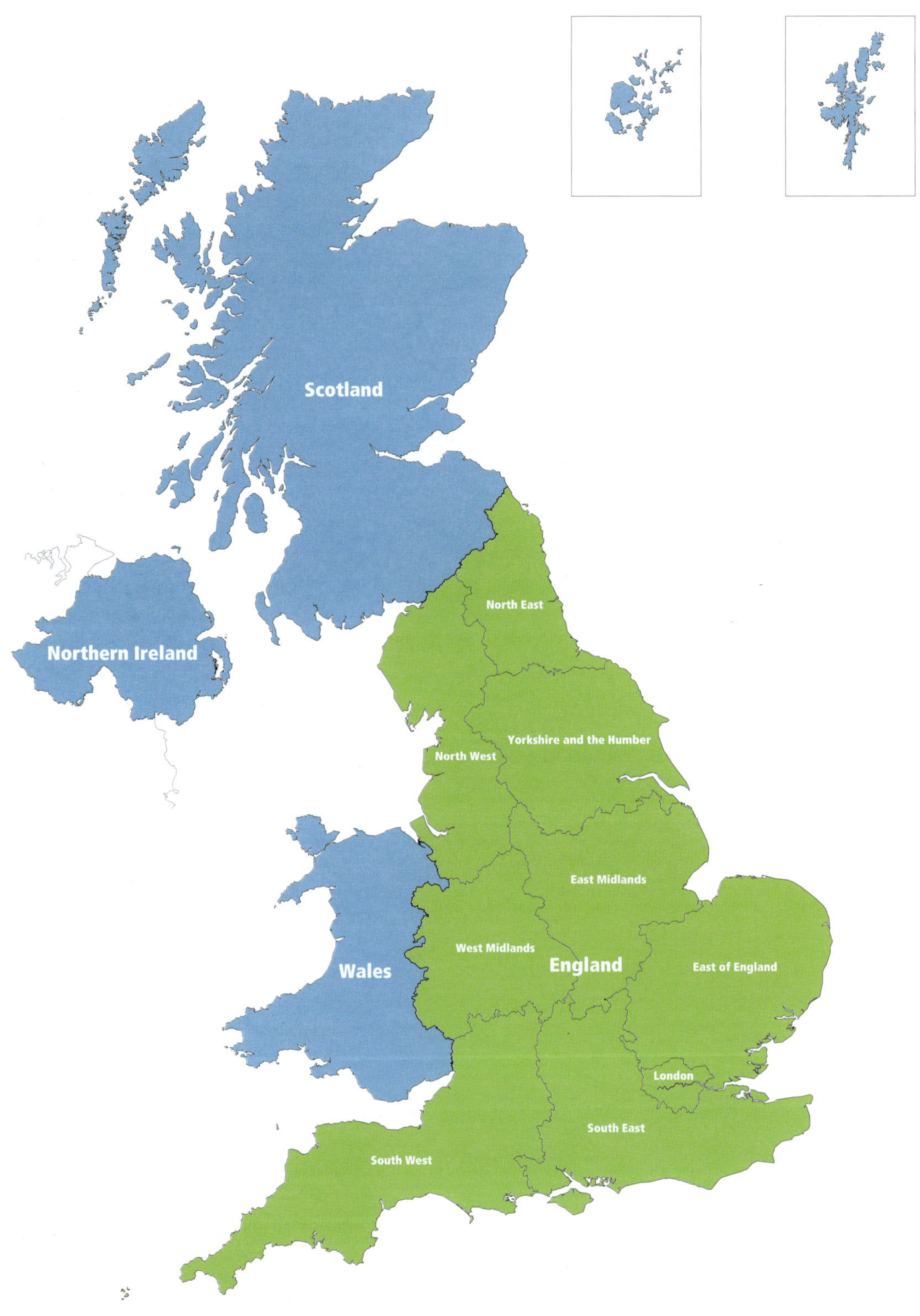

Map B

Local and Unitary Authorities, England 1999

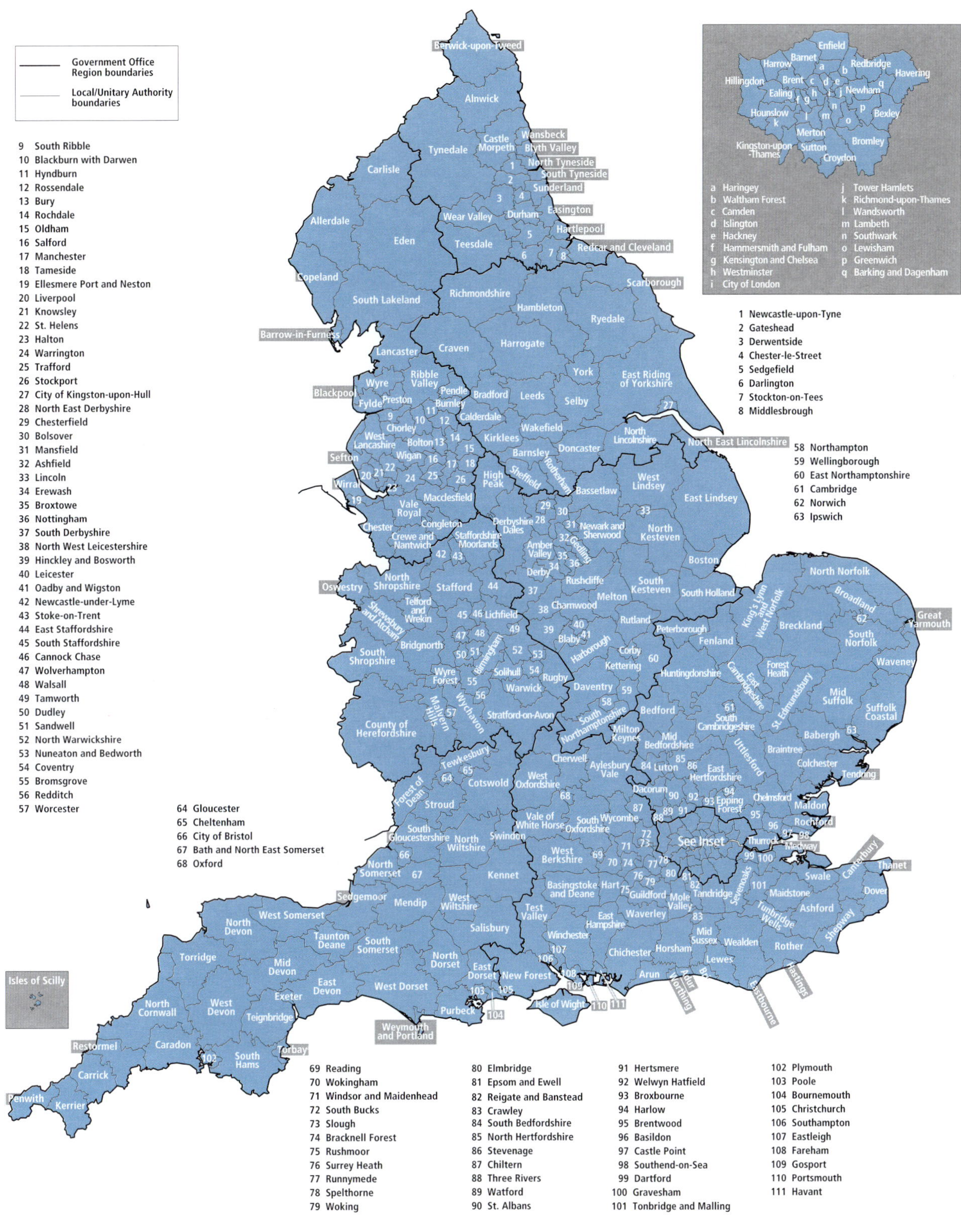

Map C

Unitary Authorities, Wales 1999

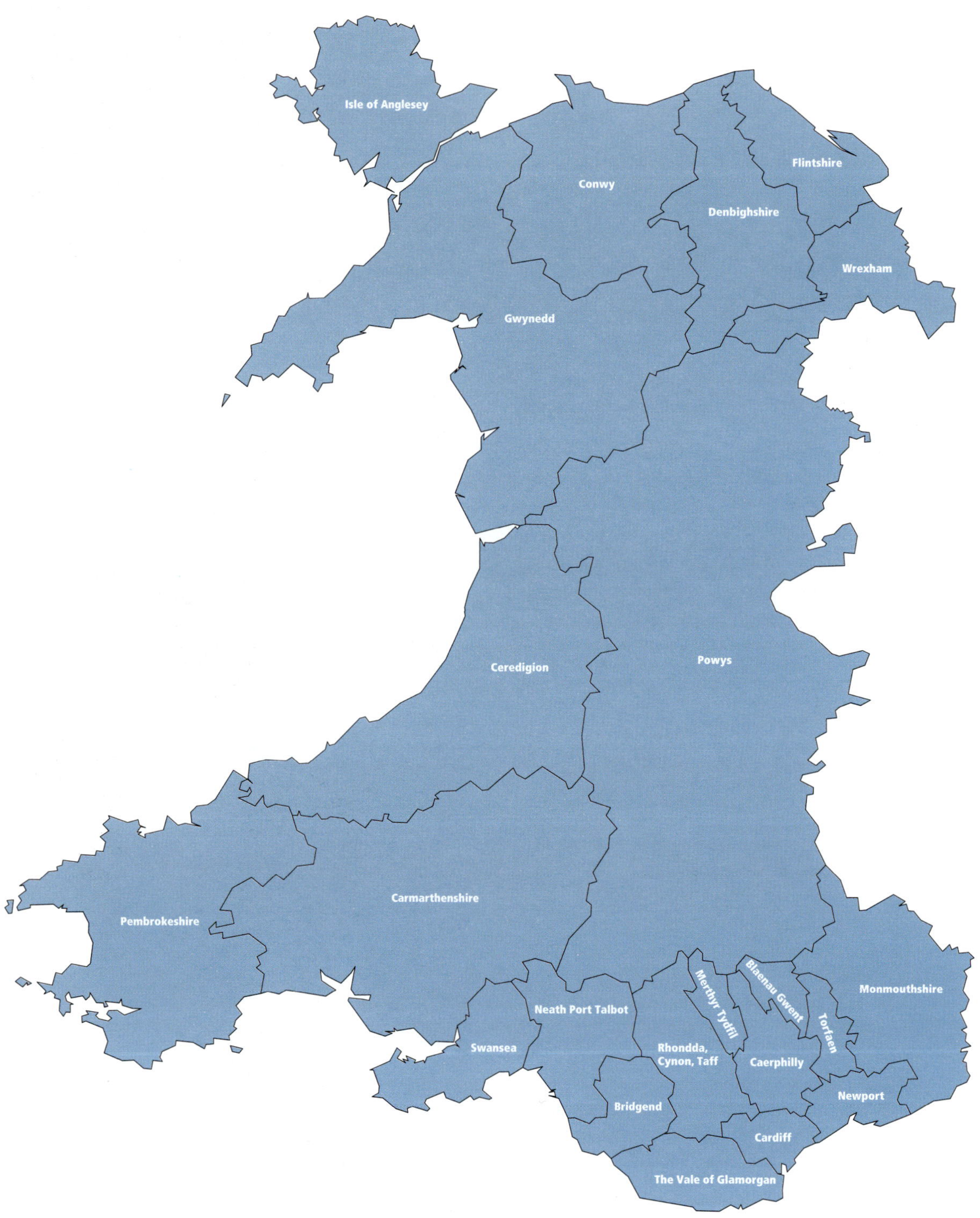

Map D

Local Councils, Scotland 1999

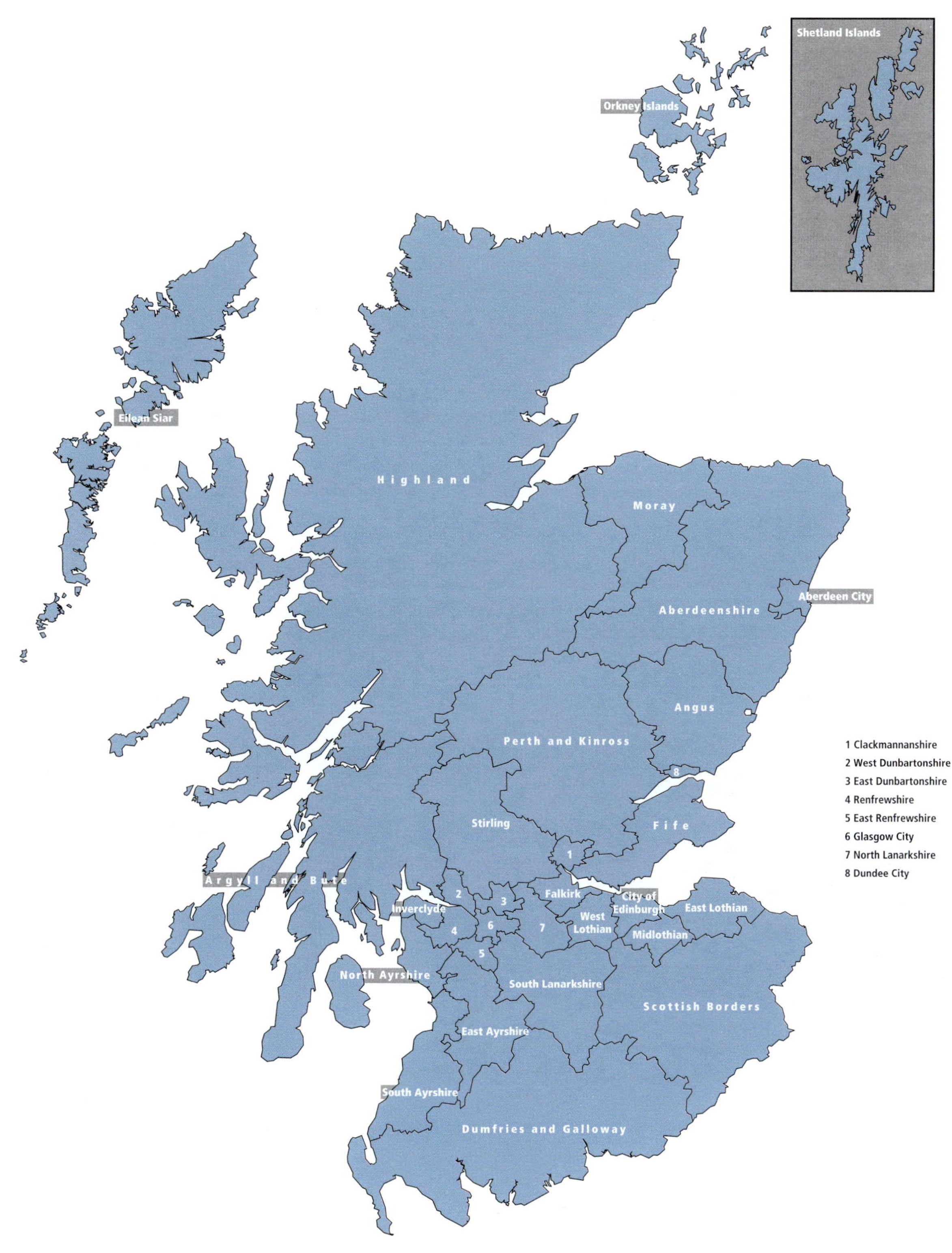

Map E

District Councils, Northern Ireland 1999

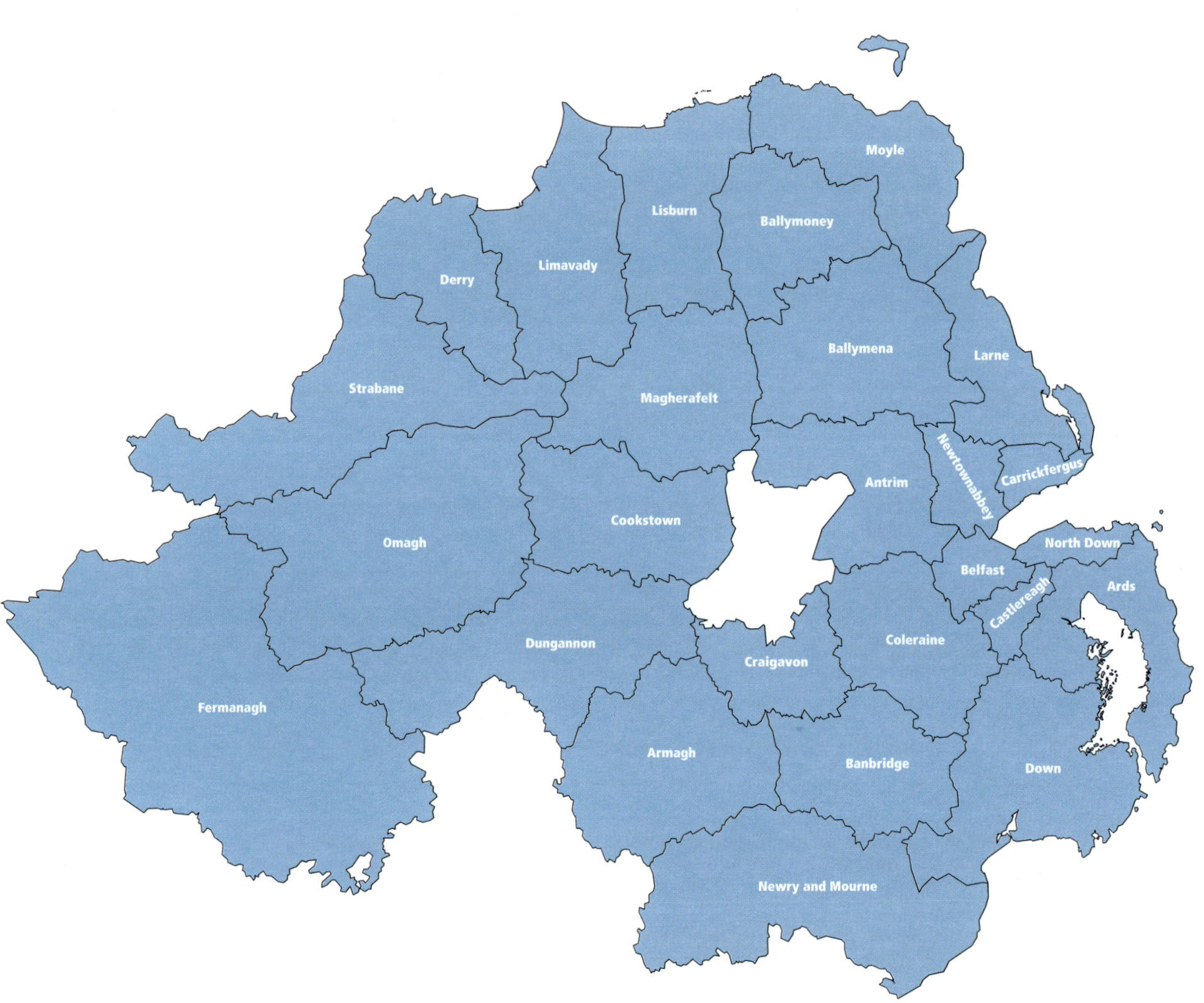

Appendix C
External referees

The help received from independent referees is greatly appreciated. They made very valuable comments about the chapters at draft stage and helped to clarify content and consistency of approach across chapters. The overall responsibility for each chapter rests with the chapter authors. No responsibility for the contents or comments within a chapter rests with the referees. The following provided comments on one or more of the chapters:

Professor Danny Dorling
School of Geography
University of Leeds
Woodhouse Lane
Leeds
LS2 9JT

Professor Phil Rees
School of Geography
University of Leeds
Woodhouse Lane
Leeds
LS2 9JT

Ms Alison Macfarlane
National Perinatal Epidemiology Unit
Institute of Health Sciences
Old Road
Headington
Oxford
OX3 7LF

Professor David Stone
Paediatric Epidemiology and Community Health (PEACH) Unit
Department of Child Health
Royal Hospital for Sick Children
Yorkhill
Glasgow
G3 8SJ

Professor Helen Dolk
School of Health Sciences
University of Ulster at Jordanstown
Shore Road
Newtownabbey
County Antrim
BT37 0QB

Professor George Davey Smith
Department of Social Medicine
University of Bristol
Canynge Hall
Whiteladies Road
Bristol
BS8 2PR

Dr David Brewster
Scottish Cancer Intelligence Unit
Information and Statistics Division (NHS in Scotland)
Trinity Park House
South Trinity Road
Edinburgh
EH5 3SQ

Printed in the United Kingdom for The Stationery Office.
TJ004379 c12 05/01 5673.